Dimensional Analysis Style Examples

Ordered: Medication Y, 1 g PO daily
Available: 500 mg per tablet
How many tablets will you give?
Conversion factor needed: 1000 mg = 1 g
Estimate: Will give 2 tablets (500 mg × 2 = 1000 mg = 1 g)

$$\frac{\text{tablet}}{\text{dose}} = \frac{1 \text{ tablet}}{\cancel{500 \text{ mg}}} \times \frac{\overset{2}{\cancel{1000 \text{ mg}}}}{1 \cancel{\text{ g}}} \times \frac{1 \cancel{\text{ g}}}{\text{dose}} = 2 \text{ tablets per dose}$$

Evaluation: The equation is balanced. Only tablets remain.

Ordered: Medication Y, 30 mg PO daily
Available: 20 mg per 5 mL
How many mL will you give?
Estimate: Will give more than 5 mL but less than 10 mL

$$\frac{\text{mL}}{\text{dose}} = \frac{5 \text{ mL}}{\underset{2}{\cancel{20 \text{ mg}}}} \times \frac{\overset{3}{\cancel{30 \text{ mg}}}}{\text{dose}} = 7.5 \text{ mL per dose}$$

Evaluation: The equation is balanced. Only mL remain.

Ordered: 1000 mL q8h
Available: IV administration set: Drop factor (DF) = 10 drops per mL
At how many drops per minute will the flow rate be set?

$$\frac{\text{drops}}{\text{minute}} = \frac{\overset{1}{\cancel{10} \text{ drops}}}{1 \cancel{\text{ mL}}} \times \frac{\overset{125}{\cancel{1000 \text{ mL}}}}{\underset{1}{\cancel{8 \text{ hr}}}} \times \frac{1 \cancel{\text{ hr}}}{\underset{6}{\cancel{60} \text{ minutes}}}$$

$$= 21.83, \text{ rounded to } 21 \text{ drops per minute}$$

Evaluation: The equation is balanced. Only drops per minute remain.

Ordered: IV antibiotic to infuse in 30 minutes 4 times daily
Available: 50 mL of IV antibiotic
At how many mL per hour will the flow rate be set?
Conversion factor needed: 60 minutes = 1 hour
Estimate: 100 mL rate in 60 minutes will deliver 50 mL in 30 minutes

$$\frac{\text{mL}}{\text{hr}} = \frac{50 \text{ mL}}{\underset{1}{\cancel{30 \text{ minutes}}}} \times \frac{\overset{2}{\cancel{60 \text{ minutes}}}}{1 \text{ hr}} = 100 \text{ mL per hour}$$

Evaluation: The equation is balanced. Only mL per hour remain.

Standard Abbreviations for Medications

Abbreviation	Meaning	Abbreviation	Meaning
a or ā	before	ml or mL	milliliter
aa or āā	of each	NKA	no known allergies
āc	before meals	NKDA	no known drug allergies
ad lib	as desired, freely	NPO	nothing by mouth
ADE	adverse drug event	NS	normal saline
A.M., a.m., AM, ᴀᴍ	in the morning, before noon	oz	ounce
amp	ampule	OTC	over the counter
aq	water	p̄	after
bid	twice a day	p̄c	after meals
BSA	body surface area	PCA	patient-controlled analgesia
C	Celsius	per	through, by (route)
c̄	with	per	each (math term)
cap or caps	capsule	PO, po, per os	by mouth
CD*	controlled dose	P.M., p.m., PM, ᴘᴍ	afternoon, evening
comp	compound	prn	as needed, when necessary
CR*	controlled release	q	each, every
dil.	dilute	qh or q1h	every hour
DR*	delayed release	qid	four times daily
DS*	double strength	q2h, q4h, etc.	every 2 hours, every 4 hours, etc.
elix	elixir	qs	as much as needed; quantity sufficient
E-R*	extended release		
ext	external, extract	rep.	repeat
F	Fahrenheit	Rx	give, treatment, prescription
fl. or fld	fluid	s̄	without
g	gram	SL, subl	sublingual (under the tongue)
gtt	drop	sol. or soln.	solution
h or hr	hour	SR*	slow, sustained release
ID	intradermal(ly)	stat.	immediately, at once
IM	intramuscular(ly)	subcut	subcutaneous(ly)
Inj	injection	supp	suppository
IV	intravenous(ly)	susp.	suspension
IVPB	intravenous piggyback	Syr	syrup
kg	kilogram	tab	tablet
KVO	keep vein open	tbs., Tbsp, or T	tablespoon
L	liter	tid	three times a day
LA*	long acting	tinct	tincture
lb	pound	TKO	to keep open
liq.	liquid	tsp	teaspoon
m	meter	ung	ointment
m²	square meter	vag	vaginal
mcg	microgram	XL*	long acting
mEq	milliequivalent	XR*	extended release
mg	milligram		

➤ Clinical Alert: *The manufacturer acronyms that follow medication names have caused confusion and errors. CD, CR, DR, E-R, LA, SA, SR, TR, XL, XR, XT all refer to various timed-release forms of the drug. They cannot be used interchangeably. Some need to be taken more than once a day, some tablets can be cut, others cannot. Double check the order and the acronym with a current drug reference and the patient medication history to protect the patient from a medication type or dose error.

5TH EDITION

MULHOLLAND'S

THE NURSE,

THE MATH,

THE MEDS

DRUG CALCULATIONS USING DIMENSIONAL ANALYSIS

SUSAN J. TURNER,

RN, MSN, FNP-BC

Professor of Nursing

Gavilan Community College, Gilroy, California

Family Nurse Practitioner

Rota-Care Free Clinic, Gilroy, California

Indian Acres & Forest Acres Summer Camps, Fryeburg, Maine

FNP, State University of New York (SUNY) at Stony Brook

MSN, San Jose State University, San Jose, California

BSN, California State University, Bakersfield, California

ELSEVIER

ELSEVIER

3251 Riverport Lane
St. Louis, Missouri 63043

MULHOLLAND'S THE NURSE, THE MATH, THE MEDS: DRUG
CALCULATIONS USING DIMENSIONAL ANALYSIS, FIFTH EDITION

ISBN: 978-0-323-79201-1

Senior Content Strategist: Yvonne Alexopoulos
Senior Content Development Manager: Lisa Newton
Senior Content Development Specialist: Danielle M. Frazier
Publishing Services Manager: Deepthi Unni
Book Production Specialist: Aparna Venkatachalam
Design Direction: Brian Salisbury

Printed in the United States of America.

Last digit is the print number: 9 8 7 6 5 4 3 2 1

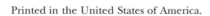

Working together
to grow libraries in
developing countries

www.elsevier.com • www.bookaid.org

To my smart and beautiful daughters,

Sara and *Amy,*

you have brought joy to me every day of my life.

And to my husband,

Warren,

thank you for supporting

everything I do, always.

Susan Turner

Content and Math Reviewers

Bethany C. Callaway, MSN, RN
Director of Nursing
Frank Phillips College
Borger, Texas

Paula Denise Silver, PharmD, MEd, BS
Medical Instructor
ECPI University
School of Health Science
Newport News, Virginia

Bobbi Steelman, CPhT, MAEd
Pharmacy Technician Educator
American National University
Bowling Green, Kentucky

Rosalynn Thyssen, PhD, MSN, MHA, RN
Assistant Professor
School of Nursing
Southern University and A&M College
Baton Rouge, Louisiana

To the Student

Mulholland's The Nurse, The Math, The Meds: Drug Calculations Using Dimensional Analysis, 5th edition has been designed not only to teach you what you need to know but also to save your valuable time. Here are a few time-tested tips:

1. First, take an hour or so to review and master Chapters 1 and 2. They contain all the math and concepts of dimensional analysis you will need.

2. Set aside multiple study periods for each chapter—the first shortly after the initial presentation and the last shortly before the next class session or quiz. Working with a study buddy can help a lot.

3. Take the time to review the Vocabulary provided at the beginning of each chapter. This is a very useful reference as you proceed through each chapter.

4. Try to complete a topic and quiz in one sitting. The quizzes are brief.

5. Fifteen minutes spent studying medication labels in the over-the-counter drug section of a pharmacy will be of great help to clarify information needed about medication labels and drug measurements.

6. Be sure to estimate reasonable answers. This gives you the ability to perform an independent verification of the math answers.

7. Ask yourself "Does my answer make sense?" Many errors would be caught if only this question were asked.

8. As you proceed through the text, some useful math operation shortcuts may occur to you. They have their place, but only after you are sure you understand what you are doing.

9. Write numbers as neatly as you can. Sloppy writing of numbers, decimals, and commas contributes to major errors.

10. Be sure to label the units of measurement at each step; failing to do this makes errors much easier to make.

11. Be sure to review and refresh your memory after holidays and long breaks as well as before entering new clinical areas. And remember, think metric!

This text also offers key features to enhance your learning experience. Take a look at the following features so that you may familiarize yourself with this text and maximize its value.

Vocabulary boxes are provided for convenient reference at the beginning of each chapter.

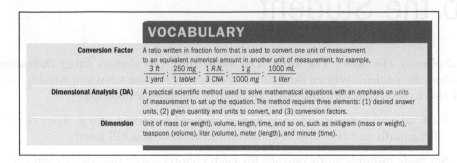

Quizzes consisting of five questions are placed throughout each chapter. They can be finished in one sitting and provide quick content review. Answers are worked out and provided at the end of each chapter so that you can self-correct and have immediate feedback.

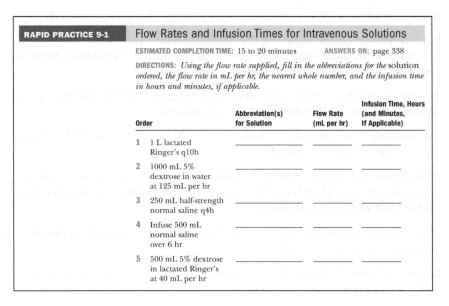

High-risk drug icon ▶ serves as a visual reminder of the high-risk drugs in the text. High risk drugs have the potential to do great harm if given at the wrong dosage or route.

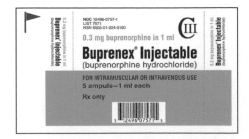

Mnemonics are supplied so that you can conserve learning time to retain important concepts.

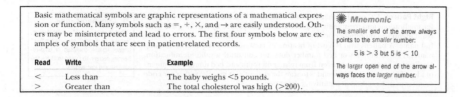

Basic mathematical symbols are graphic representations of a mathematical expression or function. Many symbols such as =, ÷, ×, and → are easily understood. Others may be misinterpreted and lead to errors. The first four symbols below are examples of symbols that are seen in patient-related records.

Read	Write	Example
<	Less than	The baby weighs <5 pounds.
>	Greater than	The total cholesterol was high (>200).

✳ *Mnemonic*
The smaller end of the arrow *always* points to the *smaller* number:

5 is > 3 but 5 is < 10

The larger open end of the arrow always faces the *larger* number.

Cultural Notes describe selected math and medication-related cultural practices.

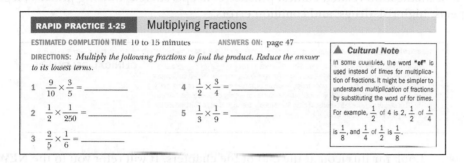

RAPID PRACTICE 1-25   Multiplying Fractions

ESTIMATED COMPLETION TIME 10 to 15 minutes   ANSWERS ON: page 47

DIRECTIONS: *Multiply the following fractions to find the product. Reduce the answer to its lowest terms.*

1 $\dfrac{9}{10} \times \dfrac{3}{5} =$ _____

2 $\dfrac{1}{2} \times \dfrac{1}{250} =$ _____

3 $\dfrac{2}{5} \times \dfrac{1}{6} =$ _____

4 $\dfrac{1}{2} \times \dfrac{3}{4} =$ _____

5 $\dfrac{1}{3} \times \dfrac{1}{9} =$ _____

▲ *Cultural Note*
In some countries, the word **"of"** is used instead of *times* for multiplication of fractions. It might be simpler to understand *multiplication* of fractions by substituting the word of for *times*.
For example, $\dfrac{1}{2}$ of 4 is 2, $\dfrac{1}{2}$ of $\dfrac{1}{4}$ is $\dfrac{1}{8}$, and $\dfrac{1}{4}$ of $\dfrac{1}{2}$ is $\dfrac{1}{8}$.

Red Arrow Alerts are included throughout to call attention to critical math and patient safety theory as well as issues related to practice.

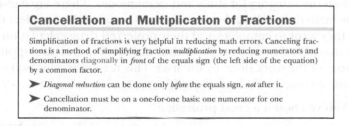

Cancellation and Multiplication of Fractions

Simplification of fractions is very helpful in reducing math errors. Canceling fractions is a method of simplifying fraction *multiplication* by reducing numerators and denominators diagonally in *front* of the equals sign (the left side of the equation) by a common factor.

➤ *Diagonal reduction* can be done only *before* the equals sign, *not* after it.

➤ Cancellation must be on a one-for-one basis: one numerator for one denominator.

FAQ and Answers included in each chapter are derived from years of medication and math-related classroom questions compiled by the author. They break up text, add to comprehension, and provide needed additional knowledge.

FAQ   *When are squares used in medication administration?*

ANSWER   Squares are used to denote square meters of body surface area (BSA). The most appropriate dosage for powerful drugs for pediatric patients and patients with cancer may be determined by milligrams per square meter (m²) of BSA rather than by weight. This type of notation is often found when consulting a pharmacology reference for safe dosage ranges.

Ask Yourself questions within each chapter are based on content previously covered in the chapter to help you synthesize and reinforce comprehension of content.

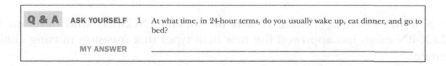

Q & A   ASK YOURSELF   1   At what time, in 24-hour terms, do you usually wake up, eat dinner, and go to bed?

MY ANSWER   _____

Communication boxes display sample nurse-patient and nurse-prescriber dialogues that can help reduce medication errors.

> **Right Patient** TJC requires that at least two methods be used to identify the patient for medications and treatments. You may identify the patient by checking the wristband identification number or birth date and asking the patient to state his or her full name. A patient who is hard of hearing or confused may respond to a wrong name. A room number or bed number does not constitute a valid identification. Medication errors have occurred from relying on room and bed numbers as means of identifying patients. The trend is to scan the patient's ID bracelet with a bar code scanner as one method of identifying the patient.
>
> ✷ **Communication**
> "What is your name?" is best. Asking, "Are you Mr. Smith?" may yield a "Yes" answer from a confused or hard-of-hearing patient. You need to check the full first and last names.

Clinical Relevance boxes in each chapter offer additional information for integration of medication-related clinical practice concepts such as nursing practice, legal aspects, high-risk drugs, and common errors.

> **CLINICAL RELEVANCE**
> Epinepherine is frequently given in emergency situations to treat anaphylaxis (severe allergic reactions). When the medication was expressed in terms of a ratio, providers needed to calculate the dosage differently than most other drugs, which are expressed in mg/mL. In an emergency situation, calculating the dosage of a medication expressed in entirely different terms (such as 1 : 10,000) can increase the chances of error. Standardizing the units to mg/mL will reduce the chances for an error being made.

ⓔvolve   Look for this icon at the end of the chapters. It will refer you to the **NEW! Elsevier's Interactive Drug Calculation Application, Version 1.** This interactive drug calculations application provides hands on, interactive practice for the user to master drug calculations. Users can select the mode (Study, Exam, or Comprehensive Exam) and then the category for study and exam modes. There are eight categories that cover the main drug calculation topics. Users are also able to select the number of problems they want to complete and their preferred drug calculation method. A calculator is available for easy access within any mode, and the application also provides history of the work done by the user. This resource is located on Evolve at *http://evolve.elsevier.com/Mulholland/themath/*.

Best wishes. You've chosen a great profession!

Susan Turner

Next-Generation NCLEX™ (NGN) Item Types - Beginning in 2023 the NCLEX-RN exam will have Next-Generation NCLEX™ (NGN) Case Studies. These will include extended multiple response, extended drag and drop items, Cloze (drop-down) items, enhanced hot spot (highlighting), and matrix grid items.

The NGN exam asks better questions to help nurses think critically when providing care and make the right decisions. It uses case studies like you would see in the real world. It focuses on interactions between nurse and client, the clients needs and expected outcomes.

The National Council of State Boards of Nursing (NCSBN) who develops the NCLEX-RN exam has approved five new item types that measure nursing clinical judgment.

1. Extended Multiple Response:
Extended Multiple Response items allow candidates to select one or more answer options at a time. This item type is similar to the current NCLEX multiple response items but with more options and using partial credit scoring.

2. Extended Drag and Drop:

Extended Drag and Drop items allow candidates to move or place response options into answer spaces. This item type is like the current NCLEX ordered response items but not all of the response options may be required to answer the item. In some items, there may be more response options than answers spaces.

3. Cloze (Drop – Down):

Cloze (Drop-Down) Items allow candidates select one option from a drop-down list. There can be more than one drop-down list in a cloze item. These drop-down lists can be used as words or phrases within a sentence, within tables and charts.

4. Enhanced Hot Spot (Highlighting):

Enhanced Hot Spot items allow candidates to select their answer by highlighting predefined words or phrases. Candidates can select and deselect the highlighted parts by clicking on the words or phrases. These types of items allow an individual to read a portion of a client medical record, (e.g., a nursing note, medical history, lab values, medication record, etc.) and then select the words or phrases that answer the item.

5. Matrix/Grid:

Matrix/Grid items allow the candidate to select one or more answer options for each row and/or column. This item type can be useful in measuring multiple aspects of the clinical scenario with a single item.

To the Instructor

Welcome to the fifth edition of *Mulholland's The Nurse, The Math, The Meds*. It is designed for students in nursing, physician assistant programs, and those refreshing their math skills in their profession. This text presents thorough coverage of dimensional analysis. The use of dimensional analysis offers a systematic easy method for setting up each math problem correctly. Additionally, all the equations can be set up in one step. These two features prevent many common math mistakes that can result in medication dose errors.

The text has been updated with the latest medications, drug labels, and illustrations including IV equipment, recommendations from the Joint Commission (TJC), Institute for Safe Medication Practices (ISMP), and Quality and Safety Education for Nurses (QSEN) organizations. A new Medication Error Chart with Clinical Implications has been added to the Appendix. Answer keys with worked-out answers for all quizzes and tests are at the end of each chapter to facilitate access. The two test banks have been revised with additional questions added. A large drug label glossary is available online from which you can copy, cut, and paste to create your own questions. PowerPoint slides have been created for each chapter for instructor use.

Continuing features of earlier editions include emphasis on clinical relevance of the math to its application in the clinical setting. This makes the math meaningful, increases retention, and highlights patient safety issues and the role of the nurse. Each chapter provides ample brief sequential quizzes that can be completed in one sitting and a longer chapter final practice test that covers all the chapter concepts. Multiple-choice quizzes provide an alternate way of understanding the material. The instructor always has the option to require that student show all work for the selected answer. A high-risk drug icon ▶ serves as a visual reminder of ISMP-identified high-alert medications mentioned throughout the text. A Math Self-Assessment, Math Review, and ample practice problems with w0orked-out answers are provided at the beginning of the text so that students can assess, review, and correct their math before proceeding to subsequent chapters. Mastery of these essential math skills will ensure that students have the ability to complete the dosage calculations throughout the other chapters. This is followed by the introduction of Dimensional Analysis in Chapter 2 with simple equations to permit maximum reinforcement of DA throughout the text, and to ease the transition from simple to more complex equations in later chapters.

Two high-risk drug categories, Insulin and Anticoagulants, are singled out for emphasis in separate later chapters because of their prescribed frequency, frequent dose changes, and to illustrate integration of broader knowledge needed for the nurse role in safe medication administration including teaching needs for discharge. Additional oral anticoagulants have been added to reflect current patient use. Pediatric safety issues are covered in a separate chapter.

QSEN competencies are also emphasized in Communications and Clinical Relevance text boxes including illustrations of medication resolution at time of transfer.* The appendices further address safe practice with a Sample Verbal Hand-off Report that highlights medication transfer information.**

NGN test questions are included in multiple chapters to help give you exposure to the new testing format that has been added to the NCLEX-RN exam.

---

*Refer to Chapter 12, p. 447 text boxes.
**Appendix C

Ancillaries

Instructor Resources for Mulholland's The Nurse, The Math, The Meds: Drug Calculations Using Dimensional Analysis, fifth edition are available to enhance student instruction. These resources correspond with the main book and include:

- TEACH for Nurses
- Test bank
- PowerPoint slides
- Drug Label Glossary

These resources are available online on the **Evolve** site at *http://evolve.elsevier.com/ Mulholland/themath/*.

Acknowledgments

I would like to thank the readers who selected this fifth edition of *Mulholland's The Nurse, The Math, The Meds*—the **students** on their journey to becoming nurses, the **instructors** who guide students to adopt safe nursing practices, and the **practitioners** who role model best practice patient care. We hope that this book will provide the foundation to ensure safe medication administration in your practice.

Thank you to those reviewers who contributed detailed recommendations for this text. This edition includes as many of those ideas as practicable. We are also very appreciative of the pharmacists who provided information about current medications, labels, and prescribing practices at their respective agencies. Last but not least, my gratitude to the editors at Elsevier, Yvonne Alexopoulos, Sr. Content Strategist; Danielle Frazier, Sr. Content Development Specialist; and Aparna Venkatachalam, Book Production Specialist, and the rest of the staff who made the text happen.

Susan Turner

Contents

CHAPTER 2   **Dimensional Analysis Method,** 50

PART II   **Metric System and Medication Calculations**

CHAPTER 3   **Metric Units and Conversions,** 72

PART V   Common High-Alert Medications

Math Review

Math Self-Assessment

ESTIMATED COMPLETION TIME: 30 minutes   ANSWERS ON: page 5

The basic mathematic skills required in this self-assessment are essential for success with medication calculations. Review Chapter 1 if material is unfamiliar or if Self-Assessment calculation results are incorrect. It is important to be able to do all of the operations in Chapter 1 with ease before proceeding to Chapter 2 or other chapters.

The material is organized in a specific sequence, increasing in complexity, and builds on math skills learned within the chapter.

Many medication calculations require only simple math. A calculator may be helpful for more complex problems encountered later.

DIRECTIONS: *Answer all of the questions. Circle the problems that may need review. After you are finished, check your answers on p. 5. Review Chapter 1 for the areas needing further study.*

Whole Numbers (explanation on p. 8)

1 Write the whole number as a fraction without changing the value: 75 _____

2 Write the whole number 333 with a decimal point in the implied decimal place for whole numbers. _____

3 Edit the whole number to avoid misinterpretation: 275.00 _____

4 Use the whole number 352 to write a fraction that equals the number one (1). _____

Symbols (explanation on p. 7)

Write out the meaning of the following symbols:

5 ≥ _____

6 ≤ _____

7 Fill in the appropriate symbol: Take two Tylenol if your fever is _____ (greater than or equal to) 100.4° F.

8 > _____

9 < _____

Squares, Square Roots, and Powers of 10 (explanation on pp. 13–15)

10 Which number is the *base?* 10^2 _____

11 Which number is the *exponent?* 10^6 _____

12 Write the *square* of 5. _____

13 Write the *square root* of 16. _____

14 Write 10^3 out in the sequence, illustrating the process you would use to calculate it. _____

Products, Factors, Common Factors, and Multiples (explanation on pp. 11–12)

15 Write the *product* of 7 and 8. _____

16 Write the *common factors* of the numbers 10 and 20. _____

17 Write the first 3 *multiples* of the number 15. _____

18 Write 5 *factors* of the number 16. _____

Decimals (explanation on pp. 17–24)

19 Change the following fractions to a decimal and round to the nearest hundredth:

a. $\frac{3}{4}$ _____

b. $\frac{1}{8}$ _____

20 Write the following decimals in fraction form:

a. 0.15 _____

b. 0.045 _____

(Do not reduce the result.)

21 Divide 0.5 by 0.125. _____

22 Which is greater? 0.23 or 0.023 _____

23 Round the following decimals to the nearest tenth:

a. 0.54 _____

b. 0.08 _____

24 Change the following decimals to a fraction and reduce to lowest terms:

a. 0.3 _____

b. 0.5 _____

c. 0.125 _____

25 Multiply 0.4 by 1.2 and round to the nearest tenth. _____

26 Round the decimals to the nearest thousandth: 0.23456 _____

27 Which is smaller? 0.15 or 0.1 _____

28 Round the decimals to the nearest hundredth: 1.344 _____

Fractions (explanation on pp. 24–35)

29 Write 4 divided by 5 as a fraction and label the numerator and denominator.

30 Which is greater:

a. $\frac{1}{8}$ or $\frac{1}{800}$? _____

b. $\frac{1}{2}$ or $\frac{1}{8}$? _____

31 Change the mixed fraction $7\frac{1}{5}$ to an improper fraction. _____

32 Find the lowest common denominator (LCD) in the pairs of fractions:

a. $\frac{1}{2}$ and $\frac{5}{8}$ _____

b. $\frac{2}{3}$ and $\frac{9}{10}$ _____

33 Change the improper fraction $\frac{31}{6}$ to a whole number and a fraction. _____

34 Find a common factor (if available) other than 1 for the numerator and denominator: $\frac{9}{12}$ _____

35 Write each of the following expressions in fraction form:

    a. 5 diapers *per* package _____
    c. $15 *an* hour _____

    b. $2.00 *each* gallon _____

36 Divide the fractions and use cancellation to simplify. Reduce to lowest terms.

    a. $\frac{1}{2} \div \frac{1}{8}$ _____
    b. $2\frac{2}{3} \div \frac{1}{6}$ _____

37 Find the product and use cancellation to simplify. Reduce to lowest terms.

    a. $\frac{2}{3} \times \frac{6}{8}$ _____
    b. $\frac{4}{5} \times \frac{3}{4}$ _____

38 Subtract the fractions: $\frac{5}{8} - \frac{1}{4}$ _____

39 Add the fractions: $\frac{3}{4} + \frac{2}{3}$ _____

40 Reduce the fractions to lowest terms:

    a. $\frac{8}{10}$ _____
    b. $\frac{4}{100}$ _____

Percent   (explanation on pp. 35–38)

41 What is the numerical value of the *constant* used to convert hours to minutes?

_____

42 Change the following decimals to a percent:

    a. 0.1 _____
    b. 0.75 _____
    c. 0.075 _____

43 What is the written spatial placement for a decimal point in this text: baseline or midline (e.g., 2.4 or 2 · 4)?

_____

44 How would you interpret a period inserted midway between numbers as illustrated below: *add* or *multiply*?

    $5 \cdot 6 \cdot 3$ _____

45 What is 25% of 200?

MATH SELF-ASSESSMENT (p. 2)

1 $\dfrac{75}{1}$

2 333.

3 275

4 $\dfrac{352}{352}$

5 greater than or equal to

6 less than or equal to

7 >

8 greater than

9 less than

10 10

11 6

12 $5^2 = 25$

13 $\sqrt{16} = 4$

14 $10 \times 10 \times 10 = 1000$

15 56

16 1, 2, 5, 10

17 15, 30, 45

18 1, 2, 4, 8, 16

19 **a.** 0.75; **b.** 0.13

20 **a.** $\dfrac{45}{100}$; **b.** $\dfrac{45}{1000}$

21 4

22 0.23

23 **a.** 0.5; **b.** 0.1

24 **a.** $\dfrac{3}{10}$; **b.** $\dfrac{5}{10} = \dfrac{1}{2}$; **c.** $\dfrac{125}{1000} = \dfrac{1}{8}$

25 0.5

26 0.235

27 0.1

28 1.34

29 $\dfrac{4}{5}$ $\quad\dfrac{\text{numerator}}{\text{denominator}}$

30 **a.** $\dfrac{1}{8}$; **b.** $\dfrac{1}{2}$

31 $\dfrac{36}{5}$

32 **a.** 8; **b.** 30

33 $5\dfrac{1}{6}$

34 3

35 **a.** $\dfrac{5 \text{ diapers}}{1 \text{ pkg}}$; **b.** $\dfrac{\$2}{1 \text{ gallon}}$; **c.** $\dfrac{\$15}{1 \text{ hour}}$

36 **a.** 4; **b.** 16

37 **a.** $\dfrac{4}{8} = \dfrac{1}{2}$; **b.** $\dfrac{3}{5}$

38 $\dfrac{3}{8}$

39 $\dfrac{9}{12} + \dfrac{8}{12} = \dfrac{17}{12}$ or $1\dfrac{5}{12}$ reduced

40 **a.** $\dfrac{4}{5}$; **b.** $\dfrac{1}{25}$

41 60

42 **a.** 10%; **b.** 75%; **c.** 7.5%

43 baseline (as in 2.4)

44 "times"—a multiplication sign $(5 \times 6 \times 3)$

45 50

1 Math Review

- Define and interpret the symbols and vocabulary of basic mathematics.
- Insert leading zeros and eliminate trailing zeros.
- Calculate sums, products, and multiples of numbers.
- Identify factors and multipliers.
- Calculate squares and square roots.
- Calculate powers of base 10.
- Read, write, multiply, divide, and round decimal numbers.
- Add, subtract, multiply, cancel, divide, and reduce simple, mixed, and improper fractions.
- Compare fraction size by creating equivalent fractions.
- Convert fractions, decimal numbers, and percents.
- Solve basic equations.
- Estimate and evaluate answers.
- Calculate unit values.

ESTIMATED TIME TO COMPLETE CHAPTER: 1 to 2 hours

➤ Please do not skip this chapter if you missed questions on the Math Self-Assessment.

This chapter contains all of the mathematics needed for calculating medication dosages. Being confident in your own ability to understand and interpret basic arithmetic and do the basic math reduces chances of error.

Time is precious for both students and staff nurses. Being skilled with medication dosage calculation frees up time needed for other aspects of nursing care. No one wants to wait a half-hour for a medication while you laboriously attempt to calculate the dosage.

Directions

Set aside the time to complete this chapter in one sitting if you have mastered the basic math, or complete the chapter in two or three sittings if you need a refresher.
- Skim the chapter objectives.
- Skim each topic in the chapter.
- When more review of a topic is needed, take the designated Rapid Practice quiz for that topic.
- The depth of your review depends on your understanding of the math concepts.
- A review *before* taking a test helps boost your score.
- Be sure you can answer all of the questions provided.
- Revisit any content areas where questions are missed.
- When your review is completed, take the Multiple-Choice Review and the Chapter 1 Final Practice.

- Refer to a basic mathematics text or online resources if further explanation is needed.
- See website recommendations at the end of the chapter.

➤ Remember: An investment of an hour or two in the math basics will greatly accelerate your mastery of the rest of the text.

Essential Math Vocabulary and Concepts

Basic mathematical symbols are graphic representations of a mathematical expression or function. Many symbols such as $=$, $\div$, $\times$, and $\rightarrow$ are easily understood. Others may be misinterpreted and lead to errors. The first four symbols below are examples of symbols that are seen in patient-related records.

Read	Write	Example
$<$	Less than	The baby weighs <8 pounds.
$>$	Greater than	The total cholesterol was high (>200).
$\geq$	Greater than or equal to	Give the medications if the systolic blood pressure ≥180.
$\leq$	Less than or equal to	Hold the medication if his temperature is $\leq100°F$.
$\sqrt{}$	Square root	$\sqrt{25}$ means the square root of 25.

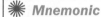 *Mnemonic*

The smaller end of the arrow *always* points to the *smaller* number:

5 is $>$ 3 but 5 is $<$ 10

The larger open end of the arrow always faces the *larger* number.

CLINICAL RELEVANCE

Keep in mind the potential effect on a patient receiving a medication that was supposed to be withheld if the pulse is <50 because the nurse misinterpreted the symbol as "greater than." If this results in a patient medication error, remember that ignorance is not a defense.

FAQ *Are these symbols really seen very frequently in medicine and nursing?*

ANSWER Yes. These symbols are frequently seen in printed materials, such as drug and laboratory literature, medication references, and medication orders. Misinterpretation has led to medication errors.

➤ Be able to read and interpret them. Do <u>not</u> write them. Write out the meaning. Refer to pp. 111–114 for The Joint Commission and Institute for Safe Medication Practices recommendations for writing out certain abbreviations that are frequently misinterpreted.

RAPID PRACTICE 1-1 | Interpreting Symbols

ESTIMATED COMPLETION TIME: 5 minutes   **ANSWERS ON:** page 45

DIRECTIONS: *Circle the correct definition for the symbols.*

TEST TIP Keep the initial statement (stem) of the multiple-choice test questions in mind, and as you read each choice, say to yourself, "true or false."

Put a mark to the right of the incorrect responses as you go through them. Marks on the right are suggested because if the answers are entered on a computer response sheet, any stray marks on the left or within the choices may cause the scanner to read them as a desired response.

1   A blood pressure goal for healthy adults is ≤120/80.

   a.   less than
   b.   greater than
   c.   less than or equal to
   d.   greater than or equal to

2   When a blood pressure is ≥120/80 in an otherwise healthy adult, lifestyle changes need to be instituted.

   a.   less than
   b.   greater than
   c.   less than or equal to
   d.   greater than or equal to

3   According to the Centers for Disease Control and Prevention (CDC), one of the characteristics of severe acute respiratory distress syndrome (SARS) disease is a temperature >100.4°F (38°C).

   a.   less than
   b.   greater than
   c.   less than or equal to
   d.   greater than or equal to

4   Identify the symbol used for square root.

   a.   £
   b.   ®
   c. $\sqrt{\ }$
   d.   ≥

5   If the pulse is <50, notify the physician.

   a.   less than
   b.   greater than
   c.   less than or equal to
   d.   greater than or equal to

RAPID PRACTICE 1-2   **Writing Math Symbols**

ESTIMATED COMPLETION TIME: 5 minutes   **ANSWERS ON:** page 45

DIRECTIONS: *Write in the appropriate symbol in the space provided.*

TEST TIP   It is important to correctly identify math symbols. Unfortunately, they are frequently misinterpreted. Write out the definition for the symbols in their notations on the medical record to avoid misinterpretation.

1   If the systolic blood pressure is _____ 180, notify the physician. (greater than)

2   Inject the medicine in the baby's thigh if he has walked _____ a year. (less than)

3   The _____ symbol is used in medication math to determine body surface area for safe dosages for very powerful medicines. (square root)

4   The risk of getting cancer from smoking is greatly accelerated when the patient has a history of smoking _____ 20 years. (greater than or equal to)

5   Give the patient 1 teaspoonful of medicine if his age is _____ 5 years. (less than or equal to)

Whole Numbers

A whole number is a number that is evenly divisible by the number 1.

Multiplying and dividing whole numbers by the number 1

Working with whole numbers is easier than working with fractions and decimals.

➤ A number divided by or multiplied by 1 will not change in value.

To write a whole number as a fraction, write the whole number as a numerator with the number 1 as the denominator.

The *numerator (N)*, the number above the dividing line, indicates the number of parts out of a total number of equal parts; the *denominator (D)* is designated below the dividing line.

Division by 1:

$$\frac{500}{1} \begin{matrix} \text{Numerator} \\ \text{Denominator} \end{matrix} = 500 \qquad 30 = \frac{30}{1} \begin{matrix} \text{N} \\ \text{D} \end{matrix} = 30 \qquad \frac{10}{1} \begin{matrix} \text{N} \\ \text{D} \end{matrix} = 10$$

Implied Decimal Points and Trailing Zeros

A *whole* number has an *implied* decimal point immediately *following* the whole number (e.g., 1. and 20.).

➤ Do write 1 and 20; do *not* write 1. and 20.

Implied decimal points, if handwritten, can be misread as commas, zeros, or the number one.

Zeros that follow the last number after a decimal point are called *trailing zeros*. Do write 1.3, do *not* write 1.30.

➤ **Never write implied decimal points and trailing zeros.**

Decimal points can be mistaken for commas. Trailing zeros contribute to reading errors.

20.0   403.00   8.000   50.90   400.000   2.400

➤ Do *not* remove zeros that occur *within* a number. The number 3.08 would be read as 3.8 if this error was made. This would result in a tenfold error.

➤ Do not remove zeros that occur before a decimal point. They *alert* the reader to a decimal that follows the zero immediately:

0.04   0.4   0.004

➤ **Always place a zero in front of a decimal point that is not preceded by a whole number. This is called a *leading zero*.**

➤ Always eliminate implied decimal points and trailing zeros that follow a whole number. Implied decimal points and trailing zeros do not change the value, but they do lead to reading errors and medication dosage errors.

Dividing a number or fraction by itself

A number or fraction divided by itself equals 1.
A number or fraction divided by 1 equals itself.

Equals the number 1: $\quad \frac{500}{500} = 1 \qquad \frac{3}{3} = 1 \qquad \frac{10}{10} = 1$

Equals itself: $\qquad \frac{500}{1} = 500 \qquad \frac{3}{1} = 3 \qquad \frac{10}{1} = 10$

RAPID PRACTICE 1-3 | Whole Numbers

ESTIMATED COMPLETION TIME: 5 minutes   ANSWERS ON: page 45

DIRECTIONS: *Circle the correct equivalent for the whole number supplied.*

1 When a whole number such as 30 is divided by itself, the numerical result is:
  a. 1
  b. 3
  c. 30
  d. 900

2 Identify the correct editing of decimals and trailing zeros for the number 350000:
  a. 350,000
  b. 350000:
  c. 350,000.0
  d. 35,000

3 Which fraction retains the value of the whole number 30?
  a. $\dfrac{30}{1}$
  b. $\dfrac{30}{10}$
  c. $\dfrac{30}{30}$
  d. $\dfrac{30}{1000}$

4 What is the numerical value of 50 multiplied or divided by 1?
  a. 1
  b. 5
  c. 10
  d. 50

RAPID PRACTICE 1-4 | Whole Numbers

ESTIMATED COMPLETION TIME: 5 minutes   ANSWERS ON: page 45

DIRECTIONS: *Fill in the answers pertaining to whole numbers in the space provided.*

1 Why is it necessary to remove decimals and trailing zeros after whole numbers? _____

2 Edit the number 125.50 to eliminate any trailing zeros. _____

3 Write the whole number 300 as a fraction without changing the value of the whole number. _____

4 Write the whole number 80 as a fraction without changing the value of the whole number. _____

5 Write a fraction that equals 1 with 300 in the numerator. _____

Sum

A sum is the result of *addition.*

EXAMPLES   The sum of 3 and 6 is 9.   The sum of 2 and 2 is 4.

Product

A product is the result of *multiplication* of numbers, decimals, fractions, and other numerical values.

The product of 3 and 6 is 18.　　　The product of $\frac{1}{3}$ and $\frac{1}{8}$ is $\frac{1}{24}$.

EXAMPLES

Factor

A factor is any whole number that can *divide another number evenly without a remainder*. For example, in addition to 1 and 18, the numbers 2, 3, 6, and 9 are factors of 18. Seventeen only has factors of 1 and 17. No other whole numbers divide 17.

3 has factors of 1 and 3.

25 has factors of 1, 5, and 25.

60 has factors of 1, 2, 3, 4, 5, 6, 10, 12, 15, 20, 30, and 60.

EXAMPLES

➤ A factor can only be less than or equal to a given whole number. One and the number itself are always factors. "Factoring" the number 9 gives you 1, 3, and 9.

➤ *Factor* also has other meanings. It also can be used as a general term to describe relevant data, such as, "He examined all the factors in the case" or "A dimensional analysis equation permits all the factors to be entered in one equation."

Common Factors

A common factor is a whole number that divides every number in a pair or group of numbers evenly. The number 1 is always a common factor of whole numbers.

Common factors other than 1

5 and 10 have the common factor: 5. (It helps to see first whether the smaller or smallest number divides the other number or numbers evenly.)

4 and 16 have common factors of 4 and 2. 8 is not a common factor because the result of dividing 8 into 4 is not a whole number.

12 and 8 have common factors of 2 and 4.

EXAMPLES

➤ A common factor can never be greater than the smallest number in the group. First, try to divide the numbers in the group by the smallest number. If that does not work, try to divide them by 2, 3, and so on.

Multiple

A multiple is the product of a *whole* number multiplied by two or more factors (*whole* numbers).

EXAMPLES	Five *multiples* of the number 5 are 5 (5 × 1), 10 (5 × 2), 15 (5 × 3), 20 (5 × 4), and 25 (5 × 5). 50 is a multiple of factors 10 and 5, 25 and 2, and 50 and 1.

Factors Versus Multiples

EXAMPLES	5 has factors of 1 and 5. 5 has multiples of 5, 10, 15, . . . 8 has factors of 1, 2, 4, and 8. 8 has multiples of 8, 16, 24, . . .

Multiplier

A multiplier is the number used to multiply; it immediately follows the times sign.

EXAMPLES	Right: The *multiplier* of 9 × 4 is 4. Right: The *multiplier* of $10 \times \frac{1}{2}$ is $\frac{1}{2}$.

A multiplier does *not* need to be a whole number.

RAPID PRACTICE 1-5 | ## Multiplication Terms

ESTIMATED COMPLETION TIME: 10 minutes   **ANSWERS ON:** page 45

DIRECTIONS: *Multiply or factor the numbers as requested.*

1   Write the two common factors of 8 and 12 (excluding 1). _____

2   Write the first three multiples of the number 3. _____

3   Write the product of 5 and 6. _____

4   Write the product of 8 and 3. _____

5   Write four factors of the number 12 (excluding 1 and 12). _____

Divisor, Dividend, Quotient, and Remainder

A *divisor* is the opposite of a multiplier. It is the number used to *divide* another number into smaller parts.

A *dividend* is the number being divided up, or the number the divisor is dividing.

A *quotient* is the result of division, or the answer.

The *remainder* is the amount left over in the answer when a divisor does not divide a dividend *evenly*.

EXAMPLES

Dividend	Divisor	$\dfrac{\text{Dividend}}{\text{Divisor}}$	$20\dfrac{2}{5}$ (Quotient and Remainder)

$$100 \div 5 \qquad \dfrac{100}{5} \qquad 5 \text{ (Divisor) } \overline{)102} \text{ (Dividend)}$$

RAPID PRACTICE 1-6   Division Terms

ESTIMATED COMPLETION TIME: 5 minutes   **ANSWERS ON:** page 45

DIRECTIONS: *Identify the division terms requested.*

1 Circle the *divisor:* $\dfrac{500}{50} = 10$.

2 Circle the *divisor:* $20 \div 5 = 4$.

3 Circle the *remainder:* $\dfrac{45}{6} = 7\dfrac{1}{2}$.

4 Circle the *dividend:* $50\overline{)2000}$.

5 Circle the *quotient:* $\dfrac{100}{40} = 2.5$.

Square

The square is the product of a number multiplied by itself one time.

EXAMPLES

$$2 \times 2 = 2^2 = 4$$

$$4 \times 4 = 4^2 = 16$$

$$10 \times 10 = 10^2 = 100$$

Squares can also be written as follows:

4 squared (4^2) = 16; 16 is the square of 4.

10 squared (10^2) = 100; 100 is the square of 10.

Think of the dimensions of a square box. To be a square, the sides must all be of equal size.

FAQ   *When are squares used in medication administration?*

ANSWER   Squares are used to denote square meters of body surface area (BSA). The most appropriate dosage for powerful drugs for pediatric patients and patients with cancer may be determined by milligrams per square meter (m^2) of BSA rather than by weight. This type of notation is often found when consulting a pharmacology reference for safe dosage ranges.

➤ Large medication errors may occur if you do not understand the difference between m^2 and milligram (mg).

Square Root

The square root is the (root) number used to arrive at a square when multiplied *by itself*. It is the inverse of a square.

EXAMPLES   2 is the square *root* of 4.   10 is the square *root* of 100.

The square root symbol ($\sqrt{}$) is used as an abbreviation and to increase comprehension:

$$\sqrt{4} = 2 \qquad \sqrt{9} = 3 \qquad \sqrt{100} = 10$$

On most calculators a square root can be obtained by entering the number followed by the square root symbol.

RAPID PRACTICE 1-7   More Multiplication Terms

ESTIMATED COMPLETION TIME: 5 minutes   **ANSWERS ON:** page 45

DIRECTIONS: *Circle the correct answer.*

TEST TIP
- Narrow your choices by eliminating the obviously wrong answers with a lightly penciled mark on the right of the paper.
- Create a different type of penciled reminder if you wish a reminder to revisit a question or response.

1 Which is a multiple of 36?
   a. 6   c. 18
   b. 12   d. 72

2 What is the square of 4?
   a. 2   c. 8
   b. 4   d. 16

3 What is the square root of 25?
   a. 2   c. 5
   b. 4   d. 625

4 Which is a common factor of the numbers 8 and 10?
   a. $\frac{4}{5}$ c. 5
   b. 2   d. 80

5 Which is the multiplier of $8 \times \frac{1}{4}$?
   a. $\frac{1}{4}$ c. 8
   b. 2   d. 32

RAPID PRACTICE 1-8   Multiplication, Squares, and Division

ESTIMATED COMPLETION TIME: 5 minutes   **ANSWERS ON:** page 45

DIRECTIONS: *Fill in the answers to the multiplication and division problems.*

1 Write the *square* of 7 or 7^2. _____

2 Write the *divisor* of $10 \div \frac{1}{2}$. _____

3 Identify the *dividend* in 100 divided by 10. _____

4 Write the *product* of 3×4. _____

5 Write the *product* of 3 and 5. _____

Bases and Exponents

Bases and exponents are numbers written with two parts: $2^{3\leftarrow\text{exponent}}_{\uparrow\text{base}}$

The *base* is the number that must be multiplied by *itself*. The *exponent*, also known as *power*, is the small superscript number that indicates *how many times* the base must be multiplied *by itself*. Some examples were given in the section on squares. The expression 2^3 is a type of shorthand for $2 \times 2 \times 2$.

EXAMPLES

Examine the difference in the values for 3^2 and 2^3.

$3^2 = 3 \times 3 = 9$

$2^3 = 2 \times 2 \times 2 = 8$

$4^5 = 4 \times 4 \times 4 \times 4 \times 4 = 1024$

Multiply the base the *specified number of times* by *itself*.

Read or say

You would *say* or *read* 2^3 as "2 to the third power" *or* "the third power of 2." The exponent is read as "power."

Powers of 10 Calculations

When working with powers of 10, such as 10^2, 10^3, 10^4, and so on, note the number of zeros in the answers.

EXAMPLES

$10^2 = 10 \times 10 = 100$

$10^3 = 10 \times 10 \times 10 = 1000$

$10^4 = 10 \times 10 \times 10 \times 10 = 10,000$

The number of zeros in the result is equal to the number in the exponent.

FAQ   *How are powers and exponents used in medication administration?*

ANSWER   Using powers of 10 and exponents makes it much easier to understand decimals and metric system conversions. The metric system is a decimal system based on powers of 10. Most medications are delivered in milligrams and grams, which are converted using powers of 10. Understanding these conversions will help you avoid medication errors. It only takes a few minutes to comprehend powers and exponents of 10.

Powers

ESTIMATED COMPLETION TIME: 5 to 10 minutes   **ANSWERS ON:** page 46

DIRECTIONS: *Use your understanding of powers and exponents to answer the following questions.*

1 Write in numerical shorthand: 10 to the eighth power. _____

2 Which number is the exponent in 10^4? _____

3 Write 2^5 out in the sequence to illustrate the process you would use to arrive at the answer. _____

4 Write 10^2 out in the sequence to illustrate the process you would use to arrive at the answer. _____

5 Which number is the base in 10^4? _____

Multiplying and Dividing by 10, 100, and 1000

Dividing and multiplying by a multiple of 10—such as 10, 100, and 1000—involves moving the decimal place to the left or right by the number of places *equal to the number of zeros* in the *divisor* or *multiplier.* 10, 100 or 1000, and so on. These three numbers are the most frequently used numbers in metric medication calculations. They are powers of 10: 10^1, 10^2, and 10^3.

- To divide, examine the *divisor*—10, 100, or 1000—for the number of zeros. In the dividend, move the decimal point (real or implied) to the left by the number of places equal to the number of zeros:

$$1000 \div 10 = 100$$

- To multiply, examine the *multiplier*—10, 100, or 1000—for the number of zeros. In the number being multiplied, move the decimal point to the right by the number of places equal to the number of zeros:

$$10 \times 1\underset{1\,2\,3}{000} = 10,000$$

Verify your answer.

EXAMPLES

Whole Number × Multiplier	= Answer	Whole Number ÷ Divisor	= Answer
50 × 10	= 500	500 ÷ 10	= 50.0̶ = 50
400 × 100	= 40,000	40 ÷ 100	= .4̶0̶ = 0.4
10 × 1000	= 10,000	4 ÷ 1000	= .004 = 0.004

➤ Whenever there are more than four numbers in a group, insert a comma in front of every three digits from right to left to ease the reading: e.g., 1000000 becomes 1,000,000 (1 million), and 20000 becomes 20,000 (20 thousand).

Insert zeros in front of decimals, and remove trailing zeros after whole numbers.

RAPID PRACTICE 1-10	Multiplying and Dividing by 10, 100, and 1000

ESTIMATED COMPLETION TIME: 10 minutes   **ANSWERS ON:** page 46

DIRECTIONS: *Fill in the answer in the table by moving decimal points to the left for division and to the right for multiplication.*

> **TEST TIP**   Only the multiplier or divisor determines the number of places to move the decimal point. First identify the multiplier or divisor and the number of zeros in it. Then move the decimal point to the left or the right.

	Number	÷ 10	÷ 100	÷ 1000		Number	× 10	× 100	× 1000
1	125	_____	_____	_____	4	0.25	_____	_____	_____
2	10	_____	_____	_____	5	0.5	_____	_____	_____
3	50	_____	_____	_____					

Decimal Fractions

A decimal fraction is any fraction with a denominator that is a *power of 10*. It is easier to read and write decimal *fractions* in *abbreviated* form with a decimal point to replace the denominator, for example, 0.1 for $\frac{1}{10}$ and 0.06 for $\frac{6}{100}$. In this abbreviated form, these decimal fractions are called *decimals*. Our money system is based on decimals.

EXAMPLES

Decimal = Fraction	Decimal = Fraction
$0.1 = \frac{1}{10}$	$0.4 = \frac{4}{10}$
$0.05 = \frac{5}{100}$	$0.35 = \frac{35}{100}$
$0.005 = \frac{5}{1000}$	$0.025 = \frac{25}{1000}$
$0.0009 = \frac{9}{10,000}$	$0.0005 = \frac{5}{10,000}$

> ➤ Decimals replace the division bar and the denominator of a fraction with a decimal point in the specified place that identifies power of 10 in the denominator. Zeros are used to hold the place values.

FAQ   *How does the denominator of a decimal fraction differ from the denominators of other fractions?*

ANSWER   The decimal fraction has a denominator that is a power of 10. Other fractions, such as $\frac{2}{3}$, $\frac{5}{6}$, and $\frac{1}{5}$, do not have a power of 10 in the denominator.

Fractions with denominators other than powers of 10 are covered in more detail on p. 24.

Like other fractions, decimal fractions—or decimals—are numbers that indicate less than a whole unit.

Observe the number line below, which represents numbers as points on a line. The numbers to the **left** of the decimal point are whole numbers. The numbers to the **right** of the decimal point are decimal fractions.

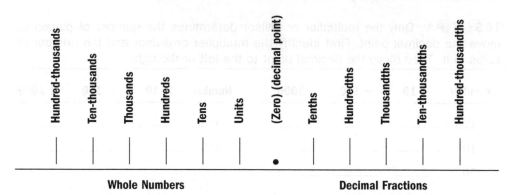

The number of places to the right of the decimal point determines the power of 10 in the denominator. One place denotes tenths, two places denote hundredths, three places denote thousandths, and so on.

EXAMPLES

1 Decimal Place	2 Decimal Places	3 Decimal Places	4 Decimal Places
0.5	0.12	0.375	0.0005
5 tenths	12 hundredths	375 thousandths	5 ten-thousandths

➤ A leading zero should always precede a decimal expression of less than 1 to alert the reader to the decimal.

Reading Numbers and Decimals

- Read the number or numbers that appear to the left of the decimal point out loud.
- Read the decimal *point* as "and" or "point."
- Read the number to the right of the decimal point as the denominator.
- Read the decimal in *fraction* form.

EXAMPLES

Written	Read and Spoken as a Fraction
0.5	"five tenths"
1.5	"one and 5 tenths" or "one point 5"
1.06	"one and 6 hundredths" or "one point zero 6"
42.005	"42 and 5 thousandths"
2.0008	"2 and 8 ten-thousandths" or "2 point zero, zero, zero, 8"

Reading Decimals

ESTIMATED COMPLETION TIME: 5 minutes   **ANSWERS ON:** page 46

DIRECTIONS: *Write the decimals in fraction form. Do not reduce to lowest terms.*

1   0.5   _____   4   0.25   _____

2   7.0628 _____   5   0.008 _____

3   2.76   _____

Decimal Point Spatial Placement

1.4 is 1 and four *tenths*.   1 · 4 is 1 times 4.

A change in the spatial placement of the decimal point can change its meaning.

EXAMPLES

Writing Decimals as Fractions

- Write the number or numbers that appear to the right of the decimal point as the *numerator.*
- Write the power of 10 (e.g., 10, 100, or 1000) according the decimal places in the *denominator.*
- The number of zeros in the denominator is equal to the number of decimal places.
- Eliminate the decimal point.

EXAMPLES

Decimal		Fraction Form	
0.5	5 "tenths"	$\dfrac{5}{10}$	One zero in the denominator because there is one place after the decimal point
0.05	5 "hundredths"	$\dfrac{5}{100}$	Two zeros in the denominator because there are two places after the decimal point
0.005	5 "thousandths"	$\dfrac{5}{1000}$	Three zeros in the denominator because there are three places after the decimal point

Be sure to include a zero for *each* decimal place, the *place value* of the decimal number (tenths, hundredths, thousandths, etc.), in the *denominator.*

➤ Insert leading zeros before decimal points and remove trailing zeros. Commas, decimal points, and the number 1 must be distinguished to avoid errors.

➤ To avoid 10-, 100-, and 1000-fold errors, the decimal point must be clearly identified and in the correct place:

0.5, *not* .5   0.025, *not* .025   625, *not* 625.00

EXAMPLES

Decimal	Fraction	Decimal	Fraction	Decimal	Fraction
0.5	$\dfrac{5}{10}$	0.01	$\dfrac{1}{100}$	0.025	$\dfrac{25}{1000}$

The decimal point replaces the division bar and the denominator of the decimal fraction.

RAPID PRACTICE 1-12 | ## Decimal Fractions in Decimal Form

ESTIMATED COMPLETION TIME: 5 to 10 minutes   **ANSWERS ON:** page 46

DIRECTIONS: *Write the decimal fractions in decimal form.*

1 $\dfrac{7}{100}$ _____

2 $\dfrac{6}{10}$ _____

3 $\dfrac{78}{1000}$ _____

4 $\dfrac{8}{10}$ _____

5 $\dfrac{48}{100}$ _____

RAPID PRACTICE 1-13 | ## Decimals in Fraction Form

ESTIMATED COMPLETION TIME: 5 minutes   **ANSWERS ON:** page 46

DIRECTIONS: *Write the decimal in fraction notation. Do not reduce to lowest terms.*

1 1.25 _____

2 0.015 _____

3 0.8 _____

4 0.25 _____

5 0.005 _____

➤ Tenths are the *largest* decimal fraction denominator. A tenth is 10 times larger than a hundredth.

Decimals: Which is Larger?

- Evaluate the **whole** number first. The higher number has the higher value (e.g., 1.21 < 2.21; 1.04 > 0.083).
- If the whole numbers are equal or there are no whole numbers, examine the *tenths* column for the higher number (e.g., 0.82 > 0.593; 0.632 < 0.71; 1.74 > 1.64).
- If the tenths columns are equal, examine the hundredths column (e.g., 0.883 > 0.87).

Decimals: Which is Larger?

ESTIMATED COMPLETION TIME: 5 to 10 minutes   **ANSWERS ON:** page 46

DIRECTIONS: *Circle the* **larger-value** *decimal in each pair.*

TEST TIP   Examine the place value of the denominators (e.g., tenths, hundredths, thousandths), and read them as decimal fractions. Do not reduce to lowest terms.

1 0.5 and 0.25	**5** 0.05 and 0.5	**8** 0.0006 and 0.006
2 1.24 and 1.32	**6** 1.06 and 1.009	**9** 0.1 and 0.5
3 0.01 and 0.05	**7** 0.6 and 0.16	**10** 0.01 and 0.005
4 0.3 and 0.03		

Rounding Decimals

1   Locate the *specified* place value (e.g., round to the nearest *tenth, hundredth, whole number,* etc.) in the quantity given.

2   If the number that immediately follows the *specified* unit is 0 to 4, leave the *specified* column *unchanged, e.g.,* a quantity of 0.34 *rounded to nearest tenth is 0.3, unchanged.*

3   If the number that immediately follows the *specified* unit is 5 or greater, round the *specified* column number up by one (1).

EXAMPLES

Quantity	Nearest Tenth	Nearest Hundredth	Quantity	Nearest Whole Number
0.25	0.3	0.25	1.2	1
0.0539	0.1	0.05	15.5	16
2.687	2.7	2.69	2.687	3

FAQ   *Why do nurses need to learn how to round numbers?*

ANSWER   Rounding doses of medicine will depend on the equipment available. This will become more apparent as you view the medication cups, various size syringes, and IV equipment in later chapters. Volumes less than 1 mL (milliliter) usually are rounded to the *nearest hundredth of a mL*, and volumes greater than 1 mL are usually rounded to the *nearest tenth of a mL*. Some intravenous solutions are delivered in drops per minute. Drops cannot be split. They must be rounded to nearest whole number.

Rounding Decimals

ESTIMATED COMPLETION TIME: 5 minutes   **ANSWERS ON:** page 46

DIRECTIONS: *Round to the desired approximate value in the space provided.*

1 Round to the nearest *tenth.*	**2** Round to the nearest *hundredth.*	**3** Round to the nearest *whole* number.
a. 1.27 _____	**a.** 0.051 _____	**a.** 0.9 _____
b. 0.34 _____	**b.** 3.752 _____	**b.** 3.47 _____
c. 0.06 _____	**c.** 2.376 _____	**c.** 1.52 _____
d. 1.92 _____	**d.** 0.888 _____	**d.** 2.38 _____
e. 0.788 _____	**e.** 0.6892 _____	**e.** 10.643 _____

Adding and Subtracting Decimals

- To add and subtract decimal numbers, line them up in a column with the decimal points directly under each other. Add or subtract the columns, proceeding from right to left, as with whole numbers. Insert the decimal point in the answer directly under the decimal points in the problem.

EXAMPLES

Addition		Subtraction	
0.26	1.36	4.38	12.4
+1.44	+2.19	−1.99	−0.6
1.70	3.55	2.39	11.8

It is important to keep the decimal points aligned in addition, subtraction, and division.

Multiplying Decimals

- To multiply decimals, multiply the numbers as for any multiplication of whole numbers.
- Counting from *right* to *left*, insert the decimal point in the answer in the place equal to the *total number of decimal places* in the two numbers that are multiplied.

EXAMPLES

1.2 1 Decimal Place		2.5 1 Decimal Place		3.4 1 Decimal Place	
×0.4 1 Decimal Place		×0.01 2 Decimal Places		×0.0001 4 Decimal Places	
0.48 2 Total Decimal Places		0.025 3 Total Decimal Places		0.00034 5 Total Decimal Places	

- **Insert a zero in front of the decimal point in the answer** if the answer does not contain a value to the left of the decimal point. The decimal points in multiplication are *not* aligned with other decimal points in the problem, as in addition, subtraction, and division.
- Insert zeros in the answer to hold the place for the decimal point if there are insufficient digits in the answer.

RAPID PRACTICE 1-16 ## Multiplying Decimals

ESTIMATED COMPLETION TIME: 10 minutes   **ANSWERS ON:** page 46

DIRECTIONS: *Multiply the numbers. Count the total decimal places and insert the decimal point in the answer as needed.*

1	1.5	**3**	2	**5**	0.25
	×6		×0.4		× 2

2	1	**4**	0.125
	×0.1		× 2

Dividing Decimals

Division of decimals is the same as division of whole numbers, with one exception: decimal point placement is emphasized.

Division of decimals when the divisor is a whole number

Examine the divisor. If it is a *whole* number, place the decimal point in the answer *directly above* the decimal point in the dividend, as shown in the examples that follow.

Proceed as with division for whole numbers.

```
        A                    B                    C
    2.6 Quotient         0.43 Answer          0.05 Answer
4 Divisor )10.4 Dividend  5)2.15              8)0.40
```

The alignment of decimal points must be exactly as shown in examples A, B, and C.

Insert a leading zero in front of a decimal that does not have an accompanying whole number, as shown in red in example B.

Add zeros if necessary to the dividend in order to arrive at a numerical answer, as shown in red in example C.

Division of decimals when divisor contains decimals

- If the divisor contains decimals, first change the divisor to a *whole* number by *moving* the real or implied decimal place in the dividend to the right by the number of decimal places *equal* to the decimal places in the *divisor.*
- *Place the decimal point in the answer directly* above the new decimal place in the dividend. Proceed with the division as for whole numbers.

```
        A                    B                    C
       45                    5                    2
0.4)18.0              0.5)2.5              1.25)2.50
```

- Add zeros if necessary as placeholders, as shown in example C.

  Moving the decimal place an equal number of places in both the divisor and the dividend to make a whole number in the divisor is the equivalent of multiplying both figures by 10, 100, or 1000. The value of the answer will be *unchanged,* as seen in the following example.

Dividend/Divisor = Quotient	Multiplying Divisor and Dividend × 10	Multiplying Divisor and Dividend × 100
$\frac{18}{0.4} = 45$	$\frac{180}{4} = 45$	$\frac{1800}{40} = 45$

FAQ	*Why do nurses need to understand division of decimals?*
ANSWER	Because medications may be ordered or supplied in decimal doses.

Dividing Decimals

ESTIMATED COMPLETION TIME: 10 to 15 minutes   **ANSWERS ON:** page 46

DIRECTIONS: *Perform the division. Do not use a calculator.*

> **TEST TIP**   Move the decimal points and place the decimal point prominently in the answer *before* proceeding with the division.

1   $250 \overline{)200}$ 3 $4 \overline{)1}$ 5 $0.25 \overline{)1}$

2   $0.025 \overline{)0.1}$ 4 $0.5 \overline{)2}$

Fractions

> ✳ *Mnemonic*
>
> DDD: Denominator, divisor, down under or down below the *divide by* line

A fraction is a number that describes the *parts* of a whole number. It is a form of division. A fraction has a numerator and a denominator. The numerator is the top number in the fraction and tells the number of parts in the fraction. The denominator is the bottom number in the fraction and tells the number of equal parts in which the whole number is divided. For math calculations or data entry on a calculator, the numerator is to be *divided by the denominator.*

➤ A denominator is the same as a divisor.

The fraction example below denotes two parts of a whole that is divided into three equal parts. The division line that divides the numerator and denominator, reading *top to bottom*, indicates "2 divided by 3."

EXAMPLES

$$\frac{2}{3} \begin{array}{l} \text{(numerator)} \\ \text{(denominator, divisor)} \end{array} = 2 \div 3$$

The whole pizza below is divided into six equal pieces (the denominator).

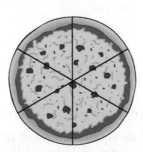

If you eat one piece of pizza, you have consumed $\frac{1}{6}$ of the pizza.

EXAMPLES

$\frac{1}{6}$ **Numerator**
   Division Bar, Dividing Line
   Denominator

$\frac{1}{6}$ part
   total number of equal parts

The denominator is a *divisor*.

Alternative Fraction Forms

The fraction $\frac{1}{2}$ can be expressed in the following forms:

1 decimal with a decimal point: 0.5 (numerator ÷ denominator, or 1 divided by 2)

2 percent with a percent sign: 50% (fraction × 100 with a percent sign added)

The forms above express one part of two equal parts.

Mixed Fractions

A fraction that consists of a *mixture* of a whole number and a fraction is called a *mixed fraction*.

	EXAMPLES
$1\frac{2}{3}$, $41\frac{5}{6}$, $8\frac{1}{8}$	

Be sure to leave a space between the whole number and the fraction to avoid misinterpretation as a larger number.

Improper Fractions

A fraction that consists of a numerator that is *equal to* or *larger than* the denominator is called an *improper fraction*.

	EXAMPLES
$\frac{10}{8}$, $\frac{12}{7}$, $\frac{4}{4}$	

Converting Mixed and Improper Fractions

- To convert a mixed fraction to an improper fraction, *multiply* the denominator by the whole number and *add* it to the numerator.
- Place the new numerator over the original denominator of the fraction.

	EXAMPLES
$3\frac{1}{2} = \frac{7}{2} (2 \times 3 + 1)$, $4\frac{1}{3} = \frac{13}{3} (3 \times 4 + 1)$, $1\frac{1}{5} = \frac{6}{5} (5 \times 1 + 1)$	

Converting an Improper Fraction to a Mixed Fraction

- To convert an improper fraction to a mixed fraction, *divide* the numerator by the denominator to obtain a whole number and a remainder.
- Write the remainder as a fraction.

EXAMPLES

$$\frac{20}{6} = 3\frac{2}{6} \quad \text{or} \quad 3\frac{1}{3} \qquad \frac{10}{8} = 1\frac{2}{8} \quad \text{or} \quad 1\frac{1}{4} \qquad \frac{27}{23} = 1\frac{4}{23}$$

➤ Be careful when writing mixed fractions. Leave space between the whole number and the fraction. The mixed number $3\frac{1}{2}$ without adequate space could be misread as $\frac{31}{2}$ (thirty-one over two, or $15\frac{1}{2}$).

RAPID PRACTICE 1-18 | Fraction Vocabulary

ESTIMATED COMPLETION TIME: 5 minutes   **ANSWERS ON:** page 46

DIRECTIONS: *Circle the appropriate terms and forms for the fractions.*

1 Identify the improper fraction.

   a. $\frac{1}{2}$

   b. $1\frac{1}{3}$

   c. $10\frac{1}{2}$

   d. $\frac{11}{2}$

2 Identify the correct conversion of an improper fraction to a mixed fraction.

   a. $\frac{1}{4} = \frac{4}{16}$

   b. $\frac{4}{3} = 1\frac{1}{3}$

   c. $\frac{21}{2} = 10\frac{1}{21}$

   d. $\frac{11}{3} = 33\frac{1}{3}$

3 Identify the correct conversion of a mixed fraction to an improper fraction.

   a. $\frac{1}{2} = \frac{4}{8}$

   b. $5\frac{1}{2} = \frac{11}{2}$

   c. $2\frac{1}{4} = 2\frac{2}{8}$

   d. $\frac{1}{3} = 1:3$

4 Identify the numerator of $\frac{5}{8}$.

   a. 1

   b. 5

   c. 8

   d. 40

5 Identify the denominator of $\frac{2}{6}$.

   a. 1

   b. 2

   c. 3

   d. 6

Reducing Fractions

Reducing fractions to the lowest (simplest) terms simplifies the math. Reducing a fraction is usually requested for the final answer to a fraction problem, but this step can be performed at any point in calculations to make it easier.

- To reduce a fraction, divide the numerator and the denominator by the same (common) factor until it *cannot be divided* further into whole numbers.
- Try using the numerator as the common factor. Divide it directly into the denominator, as shown in the first example that follows.
- If that does not work, try dividing the numerator and denominator by 2.
- If the numerator and denominator are not divisible by 2, find all factors of the numerator and denominator. The common factors will divide both the numerator and the denominator evenly.

➤ A fraction *cannot* be further reduced if the numerator is 1 $\left(\dfrac{1}{2}; \dfrac{1}{280}\right)$.

EXAMPLES

The numerator is the largest common factor.

Dividing the numerator and denominator by 100 reduces this fraction to its simplest terms.

$$\dfrac{\overset{1}{\cancel{100}}}{\underset{2}{\cancel{200}}} = \dfrac{1}{2}$$

Dividing the numerator and denominator by the common factor, 2, reduces this fraction to its lowest terms.

$$\dfrac{\overset{3}{\cancel{6}}}{\underset{4}{\cancel{8}}} = \dfrac{3}{4}$$

Note that the value of the fraction is unchanged by reduction.

$\dfrac{1}{8}, \dfrac{1}{200},$ and $\dfrac{1}{9}$ cannot be reduced because a numerator of 1 is not divisible by a whole number. $\dfrac{3}{7}$ cannot be reduced because there are no common factors.

RAPID PRACTICE 1-19	Reducing Fractions

ESTIMATED COMPLETION TIME: 5 minutes   **ANSWERS ON:** page 46

DIRECTIONS: *Identify the correctly reduced fraction.*

TEST TIP   Put a light "X" to the right of the obviously incorrect answers.

1 $\dfrac{100}{500}$ can be reduced to _____.

    a. $\dfrac{100}{250}$ **b.** $\dfrac{10}{25}$ **c.** $\dfrac{2}{5}$ **d.** $\dfrac{1}{5}$

2 $\dfrac{25}{75}$ can be reduced to which lowest terms? _____

    a. $\dfrac{1}{4}$ **b.** $\dfrac{1}{3}$ **c.** $\dfrac{2}{3}$ **d.** $\dfrac{5}{25}$

3 $\frac{4}{8}$ can be reduced to _____.

    a. $\frac{8}{4}$ **b.** $\frac{2}{3}$ **c.** $\frac{1}{2}$ **d.** $\frac{8}{16}$

4 The lowest terms for the fraction $\frac{1}{12}$ are _____.

    a. $\frac{1}{12}$ **b.** $\frac{2}{6}$ **c.** $\frac{2}{24}$ **d.** $\frac{3}{36}$

5 The lowest terms for the fraction $\frac{15}{26}$ are _____.

    a. $\frac{3}{13}$ **b.** $\frac{5}{26}$ **c.** $\frac{15}{26}$ **d.** $\frac{30}{52}$

Common (Same) Denominator

Fractions are easier to compare and interpret if they have the **same** denominator.

EXAMPLES

Comparing the size of $\frac{8}{24}$ and $\frac{9}{24}$ is easier than comparing the size of $\frac{1}{3}$ and $\frac{3}{8}$ because you only have to compare the numerators when the denominators are equal.

Lowest Common Denominator

Fractions can be added and subtracted if they share a common denominator. Finding the lowest common denominator simplifies the calculation.

Finding the lowest common denominator

- To find the lowest common denominator, reduce fractions first where applicable.
- If the larger denominator can be divided by the other denominator or denominators with a whole-number result, the larger denominator will be the lowest common denominator.
- *Or,* if the denominators are low numbers, multiply the denominators by each other.
- *Or* test each multiple of the largest denominator, starting with $\times 1$, $\times 2$, and so on, until a common multiple is located.
- Reduce the answer to lowest terms.

EXAMPLES

$\frac{1}{4}$ and $\frac{1}{8}$: 8 is the larger denominator. 4 will divide evenly into 8. $\frac{1}{4} = \frac{2}{8}$. 8 is the LCD.

$\frac{1}{2}$ and $\frac{1}{3}$: 3 is the larger denominator. 2 will not divide evenly into 3. Multiply the denominators by each other. $3 \times 2 = 6$. 6 is the lowest common denominator.

$\frac{1}{4}$ and $\frac{5}{6}$: 6 is the larger denominator. 4 will not divide evenly into 6. Try using multiples of 6. $6 \times 1 = 6$; $6 \times 2 = 12$. 12 is a multiple for both 4 and 6. 12 is the LCD.

RAPID PRACTICE 1-20   Lowest Common Denominator

ESTIMATED COMPLETION TIME: 15 minutes   **ANSWERS ON:** page 46

DIRECTIONS: *Calculate the lowest common denominator for the fractions supplied.*

TEST TIP   Since the lowest common denominator cannot be smaller than the largest denominator, start by examining the largest denominator to see if the smaller denominator or denominators divide the largest denominator evenly.

1   $\frac{1}{3}, \frac{1}{9},$ and $\frac{1}{18}$ _____   4 $\frac{1}{10}$ and $\frac{1}{25}$ _____

2   $\frac{1}{5}$ and $\frac{2}{6}$ _____   5 $\frac{1}{100}, \frac{1}{50},$ and $\frac{1}{200}$ _____

3   $\frac{1}{2}, \frac{1}{3},$ and $\frac{1}{4}$ _____

Equivalent Fractions

Equivalent fractions are fractions that have the same value.

- To create an equivalent fraction, multiply the denominator (D) and then the numerator (N) in that fraction by the **same factor**. The value will be *unchanged* because you are really multiplying by a fraction that equals 1 (e.g., $\frac{2}{2} = 1$).

- You can also divide the numerator and denominator by the same factor to arrive at smaller equivalent fractions.

EXAMPLES

Original Fraction	Factor 2	Equivalent Fraction	Original Fraction	Factor 3	Equivalent Fraction	Original Fraction	Factor 4	Equivalent Fraction
$\frac{5}{6}$	$\times \frac{2}{2}$	$= \frac{10}{12}$	$\frac{5}{6}$	$\times \frac{3}{3}$	$= \frac{15}{18}$	$\frac{5}{6}$	$\times \frac{4}{4}$	$= \frac{20}{24}$
$\frac{24}{36}$	$\div \frac{2}{2}$	$= \frac{12}{18}$	$\frac{24}{36}$	$\div \frac{3}{3}$	$= \frac{8}{12}$	$\frac{24}{36}$	$\div \frac{4}{4}$	$= \frac{6}{9}$

RAPID PRACTICE 1-21   Equivalent Fractions

ESTIMATED COMPLETION TIME: 5 to 10 minutes   **ANSWERS ON:** page 46

DIRECTIONS: *Using the common factor supplied, create an equivalent fraction.*

Fraction	Common Factor	Equivalent Fraction
1 $\frac{1}{3}$	2	_____
2 $\frac{1}{2}$	4	_____
3 $\frac{3}{4}$	2	_____
4 $\frac{3}{8}$	3	_____
5 $\frac{4}{5}$	3	_____

Comparing Fractions

- To compare fractions with the *same denominator*, compare the numerators. Comparing $\frac{1}{8}$, $\frac{3}{8}$, and $\frac{7}{8}$, the largest is $\frac{7}{8}$ and the smallest is $\frac{1}{8}$.

  There are two ways to compare fractions when the denominators are *different*.
  - The first way is to find the lowest common denominator and create equivalent fractions.
  - The faster way to compare sizes of fractions is to multiply diagonally from the numerator of one fraction to the denominator of the next fraction. This is called *cross-multiplication*.
- The *numerator* of the fraction with the higher product indicates which is the larger fraction. Examine the example of cross-multiplication that follows.

EXAMPLES

Cross-multiply the *numerator* of each fraction by the *denominator* of the other.

If the products are equal, the fractions are equivalent.

Equivalent	Larger	Larger
40 40	12 15	200 100
$\frac{5}{10} \times \frac{4}{8}$	$\frac{2}{3} \times \frac{5}{6}$	$\frac{1}{100} \times \frac{1}{200}$
40 = 40	15 is the larger product.	200 is the larger product.
$\frac{5}{10} = \frac{4}{8}$	$\frac{5}{6}$ is the larger fraction.	$\frac{1}{100}$ is the larger fraction.

RAPID PRACTICE 1-22

Comparing Fractions

ESTIMATED COMPLETION TIME: 5 to 10 minutes   **ANSWERS ON:** page 46

DIRECTIONS: *Circle the greater fraction in the pairs by calculating the lowest common denominator and creating equivalent fractions with common denominators.*

Fractions	Lowest Common Denominator	Equivalent Fractions	Greater Fraction
$\frac{3}{7}$ and $\frac{1}{2}$	14	$\frac{6}{14}$ and $\frac{7}{14}$	$\frac{1}{2}$ is larger
1. $\frac{1}{250}$ and $\frac{4}{50}$	_____	_____	_____
2. $\frac{4}{5}$ and $\frac{5}{6}$	_____	_____	_____
3. $\frac{1}{100}$ and $\frac{1}{200}$	_____	_____	_____
4. $\frac{1}{8}$ and $\frac{2}{24}$	_____	_____	_____

Adding and Subtracting Fractions

- To add or subtract fractions that have the *same denominator*, just add or subtract the numerators.
- Place the result over the denominator. Reduce the answer to simplest terms.
- If the denominators are *not* the same, identify the lowest common denominator, create an equivalent fraction, and then use the numerators to add and subtract while retaining the new common denominator.

Denominators the same

EXAMPLES

$$\frac{2}{4} - \frac{1}{4} = \frac{1}{4} \qquad \frac{1}{8} + \frac{3}{8} + \frac{5}{8} = \frac{9}{8} = 1\frac{1}{8}$$

EXAMPLES

Denominators not the same

EXAMPLES

Fractions (Lowest Common Denominator)	Equivalent Fractions with Lowest Common Denominator	Solution
$\frac{2}{3}$ $+\frac{1}{4}$ (12)	$\longrightarrow$ $\frac{8}{12}$ $+\frac{3}{12}$	$\longrightarrow$ $\frac{8}{12}$ $+\frac{3}{12}$ $\frac{11}{12}$
$1\frac{1}{4}$ $-\frac{1}{8}$ (8)	$\longrightarrow$ $1\frac{2}{8}$ $-\frac{1}{8}$	$\longrightarrow$ $1\frac{2}{8}$ $-\frac{1}{8}$ $1\frac{1}{8}$

RAPID PRACTICE 1-23 Adding Fractions

ESTIMATED COMPLETION TIME: 10 minutes   **ANSWERS ON:** page 46

DIRECTIONS: *Find the lowest common denominator, and create equivalent fractions if necessary. Add the fractions, as indicated. Reduce the answer to its lowest terms.*

1   $\frac{1}{100}$
    $+\frac{1}{200}$

3   $\frac{1}{2}$
    $+\frac{1}{2}$

5   $\frac{1}{2}$
    $+\frac{1}{4}$

2   $\frac{2}{3}$
    $+\frac{1}{4}$

4   $\frac{4}{8}$
    $+\frac{1}{3}$

Mixed fraction subtraction and borrowing

A mixed fraction consists of a whole number and a fraction (e.g., $1\frac{2}{3}$).

If the fractions have common denominators, subtract the numerator of the lower fraction from the numerator of the upper fraction and then subtract the whole numbers, if applicable (see Example A below).

If the lower fraction is larger than the upper one, *borrow* one whole number from the whole number accompanying the *upper* fraction and *add* it in *fraction form* to the upper fraction (see Example B below).

Subtract the numerators of the fractions. Reduce the answer (see Example B below).

Be sure the fractions have common denominators and that the upper fraction is larger than the lower fraction (see Examples A and B below).

EXAMPLES

A. $2\dfrac{3}{4}$
$-1\dfrac{1}{4}$
$\overline{1\dfrac{2}{4}=1\dfrac{1}{2}}$

The fractions have common denominators.

The upper fraction, $\dfrac{3}{4}$, is larger than the lower fraction, $\dfrac{1}{4}$.

Subtract the fraction numerators first. Then subtract the whole numbers.

B. $\overset{1}{\cancel{2}}\dfrac{1}{4}$ $1\dfrac{5}{4}$
$-1\dfrac{3}{4}$ $-1\dfrac{3}{4}$
$\overline{\dfrac{2}{4}}$ $=$ $\overline{\dfrac{1}{2}}$

The fractions have a common denominator: 4.

$\dfrac{3}{4}$ cannot be subtracted from $\dfrac{1}{4}$.

Borrow (subtract) 1 from 2, and convert it to a fraction: $\dfrac{4}{4}$.

Add it to $\dfrac{1}{4}$ to arrive at $\dfrac{5}{4}$ $\times$ $\dfrac{5}{4}$ is equal to $1\dfrac{1}{4}$.

Subtract the fraction numerators: $\dfrac{5}{4} - \dfrac{3}{4}$.

Reduce the answer to its simplest terms.

RAPID PRACTICE 1-24   ## Subtracting Fractions

ESTIMATED COMPLETION TIME: 15 minutes   **ANSWERS ON:** page 47

DIRECTIONS: *Identify the lowest common denominator. Create an equivalent fraction. Reduce the answer to its lowest terms.*

Fraction	LCD	Answer	Fraction	LCD	Answer
1 $10\dfrac{1}{4}$ $-4\dfrac{5}{8}$			4 $1\dfrac{1}{2}$ $-\dfrac{1}{2}$		
2 $\dfrac{3}{5}$ $-\dfrac{1}{2}$			5 $1\dfrac{1}{6}$ $-\dfrac{3}{4}$		
3 $\dfrac{1}{8}$ $-\dfrac{1}{10}$					

Multiplying Fractions

- To multiply fractions, multiply the numerators straight across. Then multiply the denominators straight across.
- Reduce the answer to its simplest terms. The answer is the "product."

$$\frac{1}{2} \times \frac{1}{4} = \frac{1}{8} \qquad\qquad \frac{1}{4} \times \frac{1}{2} = \frac{1}{8}$$

$$\frac{1}{4} \times \frac{2}{3} = \frac{2}{12} = \frac{1}{6} \qquad\qquad \frac{2}{3} \times \frac{1}{4} = \frac{2}{12} = \frac{1}{6}$$

➤ The answer will be the same regardless of the order of the fractions.

RAPID PRACTICE 1-25 | Multiplying Fractions

ESTIMATED COMPLETION TIME 10 to 15 minutes   **ANSWERS ON:** page 47

DIRECTIONS: *Multiply the following fractions to find the product. Reduce the answer to its lowest terms.*

1. $\dfrac{1}{2} \times \dfrac{1}{250} =$ _____

2. $\dfrac{1}{2} \times \dfrac{3}{4} =$ _____

3. $\dfrac{9}{10} \times \dfrac{3}{5} =$ _____

4. $\dfrac{1}{3} \times \dfrac{1}{9} =$ _____

5. $\dfrac{2}{5} \times \dfrac{1}{6} =$ _____

> ▲ **Cultural Note**
>
> In some countries, the word **"of"** is used instead of *times* for multiplication of fractions. It might be simpler to understand *multiplication* of fractions by substituting the word *of* for *times*.
>
> For example, $\frac{1}{2}$ of 4 is 2, $\frac{1}{2}$ of $\frac{1}{4}$ is $\frac{1}{8}$, and $\frac{1}{4}$ of $\frac{1}{2}$ is $\frac{1}{8}$.

Cancellation and Multiplication of Fractions

Simplification of fractions is very helpful in reducing math errors. Canceling fractions is a method of simplifying fraction *multiplication* by reducing numerators and denominators diagonally in *front* of the equals sign (the left side of the equation) by a common factor.

➤ *Diagonal reduction* can be done only *before* the equals sign, *not* after it.

➤ Cancellation must be on a one-for-one basis: one numerator for one denominator.

Canceling when the numerators and denominators are the same

$$\frac{\cancel{1}}{3} \times \frac{1}{\cancel{2}} \times \frac{5}{7} = \frac{5}{21}$$

A numerator and denominator of 2 are the same. They cancel each other out.

Canceling when the numerators and denominators are not the same but have common factors

EXAMPLES

$$\frac{1}{\underset{5}{\cancel{15}}} \times \frac{\overset{1}{\cancel{3}}}{6} = \frac{1}{30}$$

A common factor of 3 and 15 is 3.

Select only *one* numerator for *each* denominator.

In multiplication of fractions, cancel diagonally on the left side of the equation. Then reduce the answer (the product).

Examine the differences between reduction and cancellation of fractions in the examples that follow:

EXAMPLES

Reduction	Cancellation
$\dfrac{\overset{3}{\cancel{6}}}{\underset{4}{\cancel{8}}} = \dfrac{3}{4}$	$\dfrac{\overset{1}{\cancel{6}}}{\underset{2}{\cancel{8}}} \times \dfrac{\overset{1}{\cancel{4}}}{\underset{2}{\cancel{12}}} = \dfrac{1}{4}$

Cancellation is used to simplify math during *multiplication* of fraction forms. *Cancellation occurs diagonally* with two or more fractions on the *left* side of the equation.

Reduction is *vertical*. Reduction is used in addition, subtraction, and simplification of fractions in *multiplication*.

➤ Cancellation is used in all dimensional analysis equations to cancel units.

EXAMPLES

$$1\frac{1}{3} \times \frac{2}{5} = \frac{4}{3} \times \frac{2}{5} = \frac{8}{15}$$

$$2\frac{5}{8} \times 2\frac{1}{7} = \frac{\overset{3}{\cancel{21}}}{8} \times \frac{15}{\underset{1}{\cancel{7}}} = \frac{45}{8} = 5\frac{5}{8}$$

Use cancellation to simplify the improper form of the fraction.

RAPID PRACTICE 1-26 ## Multiplication of Fractions

ESTIMATED COMPLETION TIME: 10 to 15 minutes   **ANSWERS ON:** page 47

DIRECTIONS: *Multiply the following fractions. Mixed fractions must be changed to improper fractions. Use cancellations to simplify the process. Reduce the answer to its lowest terms.*

1 $\dfrac{1}{4} \times 1\dfrac{1}{4} =$ _____   **3** $\dfrac{1}{5} \times 4\dfrac{1}{3} =$ _____

2 $2\dfrac{1}{2} \times \dfrac{1}{2} =$ _____   **4** $\dfrac{13}{5} \times \dfrac{5}{6} =$ _____

5 $3\frac{1}{6} \times 1\frac{1}{3} =$ _____

6 $\frac{5}{3} \times \frac{3}{2} =$ _____

7 $\frac{1}{6} \times 2\frac{1}{8} =$ _____

8 $\frac{100}{200} \times \frac{200}{250} =$ _____

9 $\frac{1}{2} \times \frac{6}{8} =$ _____

10 $\frac{4}{5} \times \frac{10}{12} =$ _____

Division of Fractions

To divide fractions, invert the dividing fraction, as shown in red in the examples below.

Proceed as for multiplication of fractions, using cancellation to simplify before multiplying.

Reduce the answer.

EXAMPLES

$$\frac{1}{3} \div \frac{1}{7} = \frac{1}{3} \times \frac{7}{1} = \frac{7}{3} = 2\frac{1}{3}$$

How many sevenths are there in $\frac{1}{3}$?

Answer: There are $2\frac{1}{3}$ sevenths in $\frac{1}{3}$.

$$\frac{1}{4} \div \frac{1}{8} = \frac{1}{4} \times \frac{8}{1} = \frac{2}{1} = 2$$

How many eighths are there in $\frac{1}{4}$?

Answer: There are 2 eighths in $\frac{1}{4}$.

➤ The most common error is to invert the dividend instead of the *dividing fraction,* the *divisor* (e.g., $\frac{1}{4} \div \frac{1}{8} = \frac{4}{1} \times \frac{1}{8} = \frac{1}{32}$).

Cancellation can be used to simplify during the multiplication process.

RAPID PRACTICE 1-27 Division of Fractions

ESTIMATED COMPLETION TIME: 10 minutes   **ANSWERS ON: PAGE 47**

DIRECTIONS: *Divide the following fractions* after *converting any mixed fractions to an improper fraction. Reduce the answer to its lowest terms.*

1 $\frac{1}{2} \div \frac{1}{6}$

2 $\frac{1}{3} \div \frac{1}{8}$

3 $\frac{2}{5} \div \frac{1}{4}$

4 $1\frac{1}{4} \div \frac{1}{4}$

5 $2\frac{1}{2} \div \frac{1}{2}$

Percentages

Percent means parts per 100. Percentages reflect the numerator of a fraction that has a denominator of 100. A percentage is the ratio of a number to 100. For example, $50\% = \frac{50}{100} \left(\frac{1}{2} \right)$ or $50:100$ or 0.5. $2\% = \frac{2}{100} \left(\frac{1}{50} \right)$ or $2:100$ or 0.02.

Changing a Fraction to a Percentage

To change a *fraction* to a *percentage, multiply* the fraction by 100 and add a percent sign to the answer, as shown in the examples that follow.

It is helpful to remember one easy example, such as 50% and its fraction and decimal equivalents ($\frac{1}{2}$ and 0.5) when you work with other percentage conversions.

EXAMPLES

$$\frac{1}{2} \times 100 = \frac{100}{2} = 50\% \qquad \frac{2}{3} \times 100 = \frac{200}{3} = 66\frac{2}{3}\%$$

Changing a Percentage to a Fraction

To change a percentage to a fraction, *divide* the percentage by a denominator of 100. Reduce the fraction. Eliminate the percent sign.

EXAMPLES

$$50\% = 50 \div 100 \quad \frac{50}{100} = \frac{1}{2} \qquad 75\% = 75 \div 100 \quad \frac{75}{100} = \frac{3}{4}$$

➤ A percentage is just another form of a fraction. It has a denominator of 100.

RAPID PRACTICE 1-28	Converting Fractions and Percentages

ESTIMATED COMPLETION TIME: 15 to 20 minutes   **ANSWERS ON:** page 47

DIRECTIONS: *Change the fractions to percentages. Round the answer to the nearest tenth. Change the percentages to a fraction. Reduce the answer to its lowest terms.*

Percentage	Fraction	Fraction	Percentage
1 $\frac{1}{3} \times 100 =$ _____		6 $\frac{1}{6} \times 100 =$ _____	
2 $\frac{3}{4} \times 100 =$ _____		7 $25\% =$ _____	
3 $10\% =$ _____		8 $15\% =$ _____	
4 $12\frac{1}{2}\% =$ _____		9 $\frac{5}{6} \times 100 =$ _____	
5 $\frac{1}{4} \times 100 =$ _____		10 $50\% =$ _____	

Changing a Decimal to a Percentage

- To change a decimal to a percentage, multiply the decimal by 100 and add a percent sign.
- Retain the leading zero and decimal point if there are numbers remaining after the decimal point (e.g., $0.003 = 0.3\%$). This lets the reader know a decimal will follow.
- Eliminate the decimal point and subsequent (trailing) zeros if there are no numbers higher than zero remaining after the decimal point (e.g., $0.590 = 59\%$). Examine the following examples. Note that the decimal point placement is the starting point when changing a decimal to a percentage.
- Check your answer by moving the decimal two places to the right.

EXAMPLES

$$0.3 = 30\% \qquad 0.03 = 3\% \qquad 0.003 = 0.3\% \qquad 0.125 = 12\frac{1}{2}\%$$

Remember: whenever percentages are involved, the number 100 is involved.

TEST TIP If you know that $25\% = 0.25$, it will help apply the decimal movement and direction to any other decimal or percent.

RAPID PRACTICE 1-29 Converting Decimals and Percentages by Moving Decimal Points

ESTIMATED COMPLETION TIME: 10 minutes   **ANSWERS ON:** page 47

DIRECTIONS: *Calculate the decimal or percentage. Check your answer by moving the decimal points two places to the left or right as needed.*

Decimal	Percentage		Percentage	Decimal
0.01	1%		10%	0.1
1	0.5	_____	5	0.0525	_____
2	0.05	_____	6	0.125	_____
3	5.5%	_____	7	300%	_____
4	35%	_____	8	75%	_____

Changing a Percentage to a Decimal

To change a percentage to a decimal, *divide* the percentage by 100 by moving the decimal point or implied decimal point two places to the left.

Insert zeros as placeholders and leading zeros where needed.

Remove the percent sign, and eliminate trailing zeros.

EXAMPLES

$$25\% = 0.25 \qquad 96\% = 0.96 \qquad 1.25\% = 0.0125 \qquad 5.9\% = 0.059$$

Note that 0.059 has a leading zero in front of the decimal point and a zero placeholder after the decimal point.

Converting Fractions, Decimals, and Percentages

ESTIMATED COMPLETION TIME: 15 minutes   **ANSWERS ON:** page 48

DIRECTIONS: *Examine the example in the first row. Fill in the table with the requested numbers. Simplify by changing the fraction denominator to a multiple of 10.*

TEST TIP   Make equivalent fraction have a denominator with a power of ten.

Fraction	Decimal	Percentage
$\dfrac{1}{4} = \dfrac{25}{100}$	0.25	25%
1 $\dfrac{1}{5}$	_____	_____
2 $\dfrac{3}{10}$	_____	_____
3 _____	_____	75%
4 _____	1.5	_____
5 _____	0.6	_____

Calculating the Percentage of a Whole Number

Change the percentage to a decimal by dividing by 100. Check your answer by moving the decimal points two places. Then multiply the result by the number.

EXAMPLES

200% of 35 $200 \div 100 = 2 \times 35 = 70$

5% of 20 $5 \div 100 = 0.05 \times 20 = 1$

➤ Trailing zeros are eliminated after decimals.

EXAMPLES

%	% to Decimal		Number		Result
5% of 25	0.05	×	25	=	1.25
20% of 80	0.2	×	80	=	16.~~0~~
125% of 50	1.25	×	50	=	62.5~~0~~

Constants

A constant is a number or quantity that does *not* change. It can be used to simplify such calculations as intravenous flow rates.

EXAMPLES

> To change minutes to hours, divide by the constant 60.
>
> To change pounds to kilograms, divide by the constant 2.2.
>
> Calculating percentages involves using the numerical constant 100.

Finding Unit Values and Totals

When performing calculations, comprehension is increased and the margin of error decreased if numbers can be *simplified*. If we buy more than one of something, we want to know the cost of each unit. Stores now assist us in comparing the value of similar products more quickly by posting the unit price on many items. If we pay $40 to fill our car's tank with gas, we usually are interested in the price *per* gallon: the unit price.

One of the common needs in medication math calculation is to find the value of *one part* of the whole of something. The math is very simple.

To find the unit value, divide the total by the number of units.

EXAMPLES

> What is the cost of *each tablet*?
>
> 10 tablets for $30 or $3 per unit (30 ÷ 10)
>
> How many dollars are earned *per hour*?
>
> $200 *every 8 hours* = $25.00 *each* hour ($200 ÷ 8)

TEST TIP   The unit and number in the question following "each" or "per" one unit become the *divisor*. The unit quantity in relation to another quantity expresses a *ratio* (e.g., $200 dollars per 8 hr; give 3 ounces each hr or per hr).

Drug concentrations are also expressed as ratios: for example, 100 milligrams per tablet, 10 grams per vial, or 15 milligrams per milliliter.

➤ Read slashes as the word "per". Write "per". Do not handwrite slashes because they can be misread as a number one (1). Write out the word "per". Refer to the ISMP list of Error-Prone Abbreviations, Symbols, and Dose Designations.

Finding the Total Value

Determine the unit value.

Multiply the unit value by the total quantity.

EXAMPLES

> Problem: 4 cups cost $1. How much will 16 cups cost?
>
> Solution: Each unit costs $0.25. 0.25 × 16 = $4.00 total cost.
>
> Problem: You earn $30 an hour. If you work 90 hr in 2 weeks, how much will you earn?
>
> Solution: $30 × 90 = $2700.

RAPID PRACTICE 1-31 Finding Unit and Total Values

ESTIMATED COMPLETION TIME: 15 minutes   ANSWERS ON: page 48

DIRECTIONS: *Examine the worked-out first problem and calculate the unit values requested.*

You worked 20 hours this week. This week's gross paycheck is $600. How many *dollars per hour* did you earn?

Answer: $\dfrac{\$600}{20\ hr} = \$30$ per hour (the question asks for dollars *per hour,* which indicates that the divisor will be *20 hours*)

1 Your car runs 300 miles on a tank of gas. The tank holds 12 gallons. How many miles per gallon does your car drive?

_____

2 You are on a diet that is limited to 80 grams (g) of carbohydrate daily. This amounts to 320 calories of carbohydrates. How many *calories* are there in each gram of carbohydrate?

_____

3 The patient has a water pitcher that contains 960 milliliters (mL) or 4 cups of water. How many mL of water per cup does the pitcher contain?

_____

4 Your computer has 6000 megabytes of memory storage. This equals 6 gigabytes. How many megabytes are there in 1 gigabyte?

_____

Equations

Equations describe an *equal* relationship between two mathematical expressions. The expressions on both sides of the equals sign are equivalent when solved. The equation is said to be *balanced.*

EXAMPLES

$$1 + 1 = 2 \qquad 3 - 2 = 1 \qquad \frac{3}{1} = 3 \qquad 4 \times 5 = 20 \qquad \frac{1}{2} \times \frac{1}{4} = \frac{1}{8}$$

$$\frac{1}{2} \div \frac{1}{4} = \frac{1}{\cancel{2}_1} \times \frac{\cancel{4}^2}{1} = 2$$

To further check comprehension, be sure that you can answer all of these medication math-related questions before taking the following chapter multiple-choice review and final practice. Review Chapter 1 for explanations and answers if needed.

ASK YOURSELF **Q & A**

MY ANSWER

1 How will I remember the difference for *less than* and *greater than* when I read the symbols? Why should these symbols be written out? Why is being able to read and interpret symbols in printed medication-related materials important?

2 How might trailing zeros (e.g., 2.0) be misinterpreted and result in a medication math error? How does a zero before a decimal point help prevent a math error?

3 Does a whole number multiplied or divided by 1 change its value?

4 Can you write your age as a whole number in fraction form that will equal itself? Can you create a fraction using your age that will equal the number 1?

5 How will I distinguish the following terms: factors, multipliers, multiples, and products? Can I find some factors and multiples of my age? The product of my age times 2?

6 Which is the base and which is the exponent of 5^2? Does $5^2 = 2^5$? What is the difference in the results of these two calculations?

7 Which number will be smaller: The square or the square root of the number 9?

8 How do reduction and cancellation help prevent math errors?

9 Can I write the fraction $\frac{1}{5}$ as a decimal and as a percent? Can I read 0.05 and write it as a fraction? What amount of error would result from misinterpreting 0.05 for 0.5 for a medication dose?

10 How can writing a slash for "per" result in a medication math error?

CHAPTER 1   MULTIPLE-CHOICE REVIEW

ESTIMATED COMPLETION TIME: 15 minutes   **ANSWERS ON:** page 48

DIRECTIONS: *Circle the correct answer.*

TEST TIP   *Change the percentage to a decimal first.* Then "read" the decimal.

1 Multiples of 50 are:
   a. 5, 10, 15   c. 5, 10, 20, 50
   b. 10, 20, 30, 40   d. 100, 150, 200

2 Factors of 30 include:
   a. 60, 90, 120   c. 3 and 0
   b. 3, 5, 8   d. 1, 10, 15

3 Common factors of 15 and 30 include:
   a. 1, 3, 5, 15   c. 3, 6, 10
   b. 10, 15, 30   d. 1, 2, 30

4 Five hundredths is written in decimal form as:

a. 0.5   c. 0.005
b. 0.05   d. 5.00

5 Identify 5% as a decimal.

a. 0.0005   c. 0.05
b. 0.005   d. 0.5

6 Which is a definition of cancellation of fractions?

a. Changing mixed whole numbers and fractions to improper fractions
b. Reducing fraction answers to the lowest terms
c. Diagonal reduction of fractions in fraction multiplication
d. Converting fractions to percentages

7 The square of 4 is:

a. 1   c. 4
b. 2   d. 16

8 The sequence for writing out 10^3 would be:

a. 10×3 c. $3 \times 3 \times 3$
b. 3×10 d. $10 \times 10 \times 10$

9 If a package of medicine cups costing $20 contains 40 cups, what is the unit value per cup?

a. $0.50   c. $20
b. $2.00   d. $80

10 Identify the improper fraction:

a. $\dfrac{1}{8}$ b. $\dfrac{6}{5}$ c. $2\dfrac{1}{3}$ d. $\dfrac{100}{200}$

11 The fraction $\dfrac{10}{15}$ can be reduced to which lowest terms?

a. $\dfrac{2}{3}$ b. $\dfrac{3}{5}$ c. $\dfrac{24}{30}$ d. $\dfrac{100}{150}$

12 Find the sum of $1\dfrac{1}{3}$ and $\dfrac{1}{5}$:

a. $1\dfrac{1}{15}$ b. $2\dfrac{1}{8}$ c. $1\dfrac{8}{15}$ d. $2\dfrac{2}{5}$

13 Interpret the symbol on a label of medicine in the following sentence: For children ≥ age 3 years, give 2 teaspoons of the medicine.

a. less than   c. less than or equal to
b. greater than   d. greater than or equal to

14 Identify the statement that describes a whole number that does not change in value.

a. a whole number divided by itself
b. a whole number divided or multiplied by 1
c. a whole number multiplied by itself
d. a whole number from which 1 is added or subtracted

15 Identify the multiplier in the problem 5×100:

a. 5   b. 20   c. 100   d. 500

16 The product of $\dfrac{1}{2}$ and 3 is:

a. $3\dfrac{1}{2}$ b. $\dfrac{1}{2}$ c. $1\dfrac{1}{2}$ d. 10

17 $\dfrac{1}{8} \div \dfrac{1}{2} =$

    a. $\dfrac{1}{16}$ **b.** $\dfrac{1}{4}$ **c.** $\dfrac{2}{16}$ **d.** $\dfrac{2}{8}$

18 Identify 2.5% as a fraction:

    a. $\dfrac{25}{100}$ **b.** $\dfrac{25}{1000}$ **c.** $\dfrac{2.5}{100}$ **d.** $\dfrac{0.025}{1000}$

19 If you were going to give one tenth of 1 milliliter of a certain amount of medication, how much would you give?

    a. 0.001   **b.** 0.01   **c.** 0.1   **d.** 1

20 A fraction equivalent to $\dfrac{6}{8}$ is:

    a. $\dfrac{2}{3}$ **b.** $\dfrac{3}{4}$ **c.** $\dfrac{8}{10}$ **d.** $\dfrac{8}{16}$

CHAPTER 1   FINAL PRACTICE

ESTIMATED COMPLETION TIME: 20 to 30 minutes   **ANSWERS ON:** page 48

DIRECTIONS: *Supply the answer in the space provided.*

TEST TIP   Answer the easiest questions first. The easier questions will boost your confidence and, it is hoped, increase relaxation and jog memory for more complex processes.

1 Find the lowest common denominator (LCD) in the following group of fractions: $\dfrac{10}{12} + \dfrac{1}{3} + \dfrac{1}{4} =$ _____

2 Write two equivalent fractions for $\dfrac{2}{3}$. _____

3 Use the whole number 350 to write a fraction that equals the number 1. _____

4 Write the *sum* of 9 and 4.6. _____

5 Write the *product* of 4 and 8. _____

6 Write all the *factors* of the number 12. _____

7 Label the numerator and denominator in $\dfrac{3}{4}$ _____

8 Change 0.025 to a fraction. _____

9 Write the *common factors* of the numbers 10 and 20. (Do not include 1.) _____

10 Write a multiple of both 6 and 8. _____

11 Write the *square* of 12. _____

12 Write the *square root* of 81. _____

13 Which number is the *base* in 10^8? _____

14 The nurse looks up an unfamiliar medication in a current pharmacology reference. It says that, for children <2 years, the physician should be consulted for dosage. Write out the meaning of the symbol. _____

15 Formulas for medications based on body surface area require that a square root be obtained. Write out the symbol that illustrates the square root of 7. _____

16 Fill in the meaning of the symbol (noted in red) found in many laboratory reports indicating that a total cholesterol level ≥200 is abnormal. _____

17 Add: $\dfrac{1}{2} + \dfrac{1}{6} + \dfrac{1}{8}$ _____

18 Subtract: $\dfrac{1}{5} - \dfrac{1}{8}$ _____

19 Find the product: $1\dfrac{1}{4} \times 2\dfrac{3}{7}$ _____

20 Divide: $\dfrac{2}{3} \div \dfrac{1}{6}$ _____

21 Change $\dfrac{1}{100}$ to a decimal _____ and a percentage. _____

22 There are 50 syringes in a package that costs $75. What is the unit value of a syringe? _____

23 Write the whole number 38 as a fraction *without* changing the value. _____

24 Write the whole number 44 with a decimal point in the *implied* decimal place for whole numbers. _____

25 Edit the trailing zeros in the following whole number to avoid misinterpretation: 750.00. _____

26 Divide 125.9 by 100 by moving the decimal place. _____

27 Multiply 9.75 by 1000 by moving the decimal place. _____

28 Round 0.893 to the *nearest* tenth. _____

29 Which number is the *multiplier* in $6 \times \dfrac{3}{4}$? _____

30 Write 10^4 out to illustrate the sequence you would use to calculate the result.

_____

31 Which is a decimal fraction: $\dfrac{1}{100}$ or $\dfrac{2}{3}$? _____

32 Which is larger: 0.042 or 0.36? _____

33 Write and solve an equation that reflects the product of 8 and 6. _____

34 The current pharmacology literature says, "Withhold the drug for a systolic blood pressure >180. Write out the meaning of the symbol. _____

35 Reduce the fraction to its lowest terms: $\dfrac{25}{80}$. _____

36 Find the greatest common factor for the numerator and denominator: $\dfrac{12}{20}$.

_____

37 Round 0.012 to the *nearest* hundredth. _____

38 Round 50.389 to the *nearest* whole number. _____

39 Write the decimal 0.5 as a fraction in simplest terms. _____

40 Write 3 *multiples* of the number 8. _____

41 Which number is the exponent in 10^6? _____

42 Write *4 divided by 6* as a fraction. _____

43 Which is greater: $\frac{1}{4}$ or $\frac{1}{16}$? _____

44 Which is smaller: $\frac{1}{6}$ or $\frac{1}{8}$? _____

45 Change $\frac{5}{100}$ to a decimal. _____

46 Multiply 0.1×4.67. _____

47 Divide 20 by 5.9. _____

48 Write the fraction $\frac{1}{100}$ as a percentage. _____

49 Change the improper fraction $\frac{25}{4}$ to a mixed fraction. _____

50 Change the mixed fraction $3\frac{3}{4}$ to an improper fraction. _____

CHAPTER 1   ANSWER KEY

RAPID PRACTICE 1-1 (p. 7)

1	c	**4**	c
2	d	**5**	a
3	b		

RAPID PRACTICE 1-2 (p. 8)

1	>	**4**	≥
2	<	**5**	≤
3	√		

RAPID PRACTICE 1-3 (p. 10)

1	a	**3**	a
2	a	**4**	d

RAPID PRACTICE 1-4 (p. 10)

1 Avoid errors. The decimal may be misread as the number one ("1").

2 125.5

3 $\frac{300}{1}$

4 $\frac{80}{1}$

5 $\frac{300}{300}$

RAPID PRACTICE 1-5 (p. 12)

1	2, 4	**4**	$8 \times 3 = 24$
2	3, 6, 9	**5**	2, 3, 4, 6
3	30		

RAPID PRACTICE 1-6 (p. 13)

1	50	**4**	2000
2	5	**5**	2.5
3	$\frac{1}{2}$		

RAPID PRACTICE 1-7 (p. 14)

1	d	**4**	b
2	d	**5**	a
3	c		

RAPID PRACTICE 1-8 (p. 14)

1 $7^2 = 7 \times 7 = 49$ **4** 12

2 Divisor = $\frac{1}{2}$ **5** 15

3 100

RAPID PRACTICE 1-9 (p. 16)

1	10^8		4	10×10
2	4		5	10
3	$2 \times 2 \times 2 \times 2 \times 2$			

RAPID PRACTICE 1-10 (p. 17)

	Number	÷ 10	÷ 100	÷ 1000
1	125	12.5	1.25	0.125
2	10	1	0.1	0.01
3	50	5	0.5	0.05

	Number	× 10	× 100	× 1000
4	0.25	2.5	25	250
5	0.5	5	50	500

RAPID PRACTICE 1-11 (p. 19)

1	$\dfrac{5}{10}$		4	$\dfrac{25}{100}$
2	$7\dfrac{628}{10,000}$		5	$\dfrac{8}{1000}$
3	$2\dfrac{76}{100}$			

RAPID PRACTICE 1-12 (p. 20)

1	0.07		4	0.8
2	0.6		5	0.48
3	0.078			

RAPID PRACTICE 1-13 (p. 20)

1	$1\dfrac{25}{100}$		4	$\dfrac{25}{100}$
2	$\dfrac{15}{1000}$		5	$\dfrac{5}{1000}$
3	$\dfrac{8}{10}$			

RAPID PRACTICE 1-14 (p. 21)

1	0.5		6	1.06
2	1.32		7	0.6
3	0.05		8	0.006
4	0.3		9	0.5
5	0.5		10	0.01

RAPID PRACTICE 1-15 (p. 21)

1	**a.** 1.3	2	**a.** 0.05	3	**a.** 1
	b. 0.3		**b.** 3.75		**b.** 3
	c. 0.1		**c.** 2.38		**c.** 2
	d. 1.9		**d.** 0.89		**d.** 2
	e. 0.8		**e.** 0.69		**e.** 11

RAPID PRACTICE 1-16 (p. 22)

1	9		4	0.25
2	0.1		5	0.5
3	0.8			

RAPID PRACTICE 1-17 (p. 24)

1	$250\overline{)200.}\;\;\;^{0.8}$		4	$5\overline{)20.}\;\;\;^{4.}$
2	$0.025\overline{)0.1}\;\;\;^{4}$		5	$25.\overline{)100.}\;\;\;^{4}$
3	$4\overline{)1.00}\;\;\;^{0.25}$			

RAPID PRACTICE 1-18 (p. 26)

1	d		4	b
2	b		5	d
3	b			

RAPID PRACTICE 1-19 (p. 27)

1	d		4	a
2	b		5	c
3	c			

RAPID PRACTICE 1-20 (p. 29)

1	18		4	50
2	30		5	200
3	12			

RAPID PRACTICE 1-21 (p. 29)

1	$\dfrac{2}{6}$		4	$\dfrac{9}{24}$
2	$\dfrac{4}{8}$		5	$\dfrac{12}{15}$
3	$\dfrac{6}{8}$			

RAPID PRACTICE 1-22 (p. 30)

	LCD	Equivalent Fractions	Greater Fraction
1	250	$\dfrac{1}{250} < \dfrac{20}{250}$	$\dfrac{4}{50}$
2	30	$\dfrac{24}{30} < \dfrac{25}{30}$	$\dfrac{5}{6}$
3	200	$\dfrac{2}{200} > \dfrac{1}{200}$	$\dfrac{1}{100}$
4	24	$\dfrac{3}{24} > \dfrac{2}{24}$	$\dfrac{1}{8}$

RAPID PRACTICE 1-23 (p. 31)

1	200	$\dfrac{1}{100} = \dfrac{2}{200} + \dfrac{1}{200} = \dfrac{3}{200}$
2	12	$\dfrac{8}{12} + \dfrac{3}{12} = \dfrac{11}{12}$
3	2	$\dfrac{1}{2} + \dfrac{1}{2} = \dfrac{2}{2} = 1$
4	24	$\dfrac{12}{24} + \dfrac{8}{24} = \dfrac{20}{24} = \dfrac{5}{6}$
5	4	$\dfrac{2}{4} + \dfrac{1}{4} = \dfrac{3}{4}$

RAPID PRACTICE 1-24 (p. 32)

	LCD	Answer
1	8	$9\frac{10}{8} - 4\frac{5}{8} = 5\frac{5}{8}$
2	10	$\frac{6}{10} - \frac{5}{10} = \frac{1}{10}$
3	40	$\frac{1}{8} - \frac{1}{10} = \frac{5}{40} - \frac{4}{40} = \frac{1}{40}$
4	2	$1\frac{1}{2} - \frac{1}{2} = 1$
5	12	$\frac{14}{12} - \frac{9}{12} = \frac{5}{12}$

RAPID PRACTICE 1-25 (p. 33)

1 $\frac{1}{500}$ 4 $\frac{1}{27}$

2 $\frac{3}{8}$ 5 $\frac{2}{30} = \frac{1}{15}$

3 $\frac{27}{50}$

RAPID PRACTICE 1-26 (p. 34)

1 $\frac{5}{16}$ $\left(\frac{1}{4} \times \frac{5}{4} = \frac{5}{16}\right)$

2 $\frac{5}{4} = 1\frac{1}{4}$ $\left(\frac{5}{2} \times \frac{1}{2} = \frac{5}{4} = 1\frac{1}{4}\right)$

3 $\frac{13}{15}$ $\left(\frac{1}{5} \times \frac{13}{3} = \frac{13}{15}\right)$

4 $2\frac{1}{6}$ $\left(\frac{13}{\frac{5}{1}} \times \frac{\frac{1}{5}}{6} = \frac{13}{6} = 2\frac{1}{6}\right)$

5 $\frac{38}{9} = 4\frac{2}{9}$ $\left(\frac{19}{\frac{6}{3}} \times \frac{\frac{2}{4}}{3} = \frac{38}{9} = 4\frac{2}{9}\right)$

6 $2\frac{1}{2}$ $\left(\frac{5}{\frac{3}{1}} \times \frac{\frac{1}{3}}{2} = \frac{5}{2} = 2\frac{1}{2}\right)$

7 $\frac{17}{48}$ $\left(\frac{1}{6} \times \frac{17}{8} = \frac{17}{48}\right)$

8 $\frac{2}{5}$ $\left(\frac{\frac{1}{100}}{\frac{200}{1}} \times \frac{\frac{1}{200}}{\frac{250}{5}} = \frac{2}{5}\right)$

9 $\frac{3}{8}$ $\left(\frac{\frac{1}{2}}{1} \times \frac{\frac{3}{6}}{8} = \frac{3}{8}\right)$

10 $\frac{2}{3}$ $\left(\frac{\frac{1}{4}}{\frac{5}{1}} \times \frac{\frac{2}{10}}{\frac{12}{3}} = \frac{2}{3}\right)$

RAPID PRACTICE 1-27 (p. 35)

1 3 $\left(\frac{\frac{1}{2}}{1} \times \frac{\frac{3}{6}}{1} = \frac{3}{1} = 3\right)$

2 $2\frac{2}{3}$ $\left(\frac{1}{3} \times \frac{8}{1} = \frac{8}{3} = 2\frac{2}{3}\right)$

3 $1\frac{3}{5}$ $\left(\frac{2}{5} \times \frac{4}{1} = \frac{8}{5} = 1\frac{3}{5}\right)$

4 5 $\left(\frac{5}{\frac{4}{1}} \times \frac{\frac{1}{4}}{1} = 5\right)$

5 5 $\left(\frac{5}{\frac{2}{1}} \times \frac{\frac{1}{2}}{1} = 5\right)$

RAPID PRACTICE 1-28 (p. 36)

1 33.3%

2 $75\% (3 \div 4 = 75\%)$

3 $\frac{1}{10} \left(10\% = \frac{\cancel{10}}{\cancel{10}0} = \frac{1}{10}\right)$

4 $\frac{1}{8}$

5 $25\% (1 \div 4 = 25\%)$

6 16.7%

7 $\frac{1}{4}$

8 $\frac{3}{20} \left(15\% = \frac{15}{100} = \frac{3}{20}\right)$

9 83.3%

10 $\frac{1}{2}$

RAPID PRACTICE 1-29 (p. 37)

1 50% 5 5.25%
2 5% 6 12.5%
3 0.055 7 3
4 0.35 8 0.75

RAPID PRACTICE 1-30 (p. 38)

	Fraction	Decimal	Percentage
1	$\dfrac{1}{5}$	0.2	20%
2	$\dfrac{3}{10}$	0.3	30%
3	$\dfrac{75}{100}$	0.75	75%
4	$1\dfrac{5}{10}$	1.5	150%
5	$\dfrac{6}{10}$	0.6	60%

RAPID PRACTICE 1-31 (p. 40)

1 $300 \div 12 = 25$ miles per gallon
2 $320 \div 80 = 4$ calories per gram of carbohydrate
3 $960 \div 4 = 240$ mL per cup
4 $6000 \div 6 = 1000$ megabytes per gigabyte

CHAPTER 1 MULTIPLE-CHOICE REVIEW (p. 41–43)

1 d
2 d
3 a
4 b
5 c
6 c
7 d
8 d
9 a
10 b
11 a
12 c
13 d

14 b
15 c
16 c
17 b
18 b
19 c
20 b

symbol in medical records. It may be misinterpreted. You will see symbols in printed materials.

Note: Do not handwrite this

CHAPTER 1 FINAL PRACTICE (p. 43–45)

1 12
2 $\dfrac{2}{3} = \dfrac{4}{6} = \dfrac{6}{9} = \dfrac{8}{12}$
3 $\dfrac{350}{350}$
4 $9 + 4.6 = 13.6$
5 $4 \times 8 = 32$
6 1, 2, 3, 4, 6, 12
7 Numerator = 3; Denominator = 4
8 $\dfrac{25}{1000} = \dfrac{1}{40}$
9 2, 5, 10
10 24
11 $12^2 = 12 \times 12 = 144$
12 $\sqrt{81} = 9$
13 10
14 For children *"less than"* two

15 $\sqrt{7}$
16 greater than or equal to
17 $\dfrac{12}{24} + \dfrac{4}{24} + \dfrac{3}{24} = \dfrac{19}{24}$
18 $\dfrac{8}{40} - \dfrac{5}{40} = \dfrac{3}{40}$
19 $\dfrac{5}{4} \times \dfrac{17}{7} = \dfrac{85}{28} = 3\dfrac{1}{28}$
20 $\dfrac{2}{\cancel{3}^{1}} \times \dfrac{\cancel{6}^{2}}{1} = 4$
21 0.01; 1%
22 $\dfrac{\$75}{50} = \$1.50$ per syringe
23 $\dfrac{38}{1}$
24 $44.\cancel{0} = 44$
25 $750.\cancel{00} = 750$
26 1.259 (1.2$\underset{\frown}{5}$9)
27 9750 (9.750.$\overset{\frown}{}$)
28 0.9
29 $\dfrac{3}{4}$
30 $10 \times 10 \times 10 \times 10 \; (= 10,000)$
31 $\dfrac{1}{100}$ (the denominator is a power of 10)
32 0.36
33 $8 \times 6 = 48$
34 greater than
35 $\dfrac{25}{80} = \dfrac{5}{16}$
36 4
37 0.01
38 50
39 $\dfrac{5}{10} = \dfrac{1}{2}$
40 16, 24, 32, . . .
41 6
42 $\dfrac{4}{6}$
43 $\dfrac{1}{4}$
44 $\dfrac{1}{8}$
45 0.05
46 0.467
47 3.39
48 $\dfrac{1}{100} = 1\%$
49 $6\dfrac{1}{4}$
50 $\dfrac{15}{4}$

Suggestions for Further Reading

http://www.khanacademy.org
http://www.basic-mathematics.com
http://aaamath.com/gwpg.html
http://math.com

Chapter 2 teaches the basic dimensional analysis method of solving equations. This method is used throughout the text to solve and verify medication dosage calculations.

2 Dimensional Analysis Method

OBJECTIVES

- Identify the three required elements needed to solve dimensional analysis equations.
- Set up dimensional analysis equations with the required elements.
- Analyze equation setups to determine if they will yield the desired answer.
- Estimate an approximate answer.
- Solve the equations.
- Evaluate the answers for accuracy.

ESTIMATED TIME TO COMPLETE CHAPTER: 2 hours

Dimensional analysis (DA) is a systematic mathematical method used in the medical sciences. It reflects an emphasis on factors, labels, and units of measurement. Competence with medication calculations is essential to provide safe patient care. Serious medication errors based on the wrong dosage do occur.

There are several advantages to using the DA method to solve medication dose problems:

- It is a simple organized system for setting up problems.
- It reduces dependence on memory.
- It can be used for all medication dosage problems.
- All of the calculations for a dosage can be entered in a single equation.
- Equations are always set up the same way allowing the nurse to easily identify an incorrect setup before calculations are carried out—a key factor in efficiency and reduction of errors.

This chapter focuses on analyzing, setting up, and solving basic DA equations. Examples and easy practice problems are provided in a "stepped" approach so that there is a clear understanding of the method. Once the method is mastered with simple problems, it can be expanded easily to solve more complex medication dosage problems. For students who have used DA in other courses, this chapter will require only a brief review.

VOCABULARY

Conversion Factor	A ratio written in fraction form that is used to convert one unit of measurement to an equivalent numerical amount in another unit of measurement, for example, $\dfrac{3\ ft}{1\ yard}; \dfrac{250\ mg}{1\ tablet}; \dfrac{1\ R.N.}{3\ CNA}; \dfrac{1\ g}{1000\ mg}; \dfrac{1000\ mL}{1\ liter}$
Dimensional Analysis (DA)	A practical scientific method used to solve mathematical equations with an emphasis on units of measurement to set up the equation. The method requires three elements: (1) desired answer units, (2) given quantity and units to convert, and (3) conversion factors.
Dimension	Unit of mass (or weight), volume, length, time, and so on, such as milligram (mass or weight), teaspoon (volume), liter (volume), meter (length), and minute (time).

Equation	Expression of an equal relationship between mathematical expressions on both sides of an equal sign, such as $2x = 4$, $3 \times 2 = 6$, and $\frac{10}{2} = 5$. When an equation is solved, the values on both sides of the equal sign have equivalent value.
Factors of Measurement	In DA, the data (numbers and units of measurement) that are entered in an equation in fraction form. In general, the word *factor* denotes anything that contributes to a result. The term has different meanings in different contexts.
Label	Descriptor of type, not necessarily a unit of dimension, such as 4 eggs, 4 dozen eggs, 1 tsp Benadryl, 100-mg tablets, 2 liters of 5% dextrose in water.
Numerical Orientation of a Fraction	Contents of the numerator (N) and denominator (D), such as $\frac{12\ \text{inches (N)}}{1\ \text{foot (D)}}$ and $\frac{1\ \text{foot (N)}}{12\ \text{inches (D)}}$.
Unit*	Descriptor of *dimension,* such as length, weight, and volume; for example, 2 inches ointment, 3 m height, 1 qt water, 250 mg antibiotic, 2 Tbsp Milk of Magnesia, and 6 kg body weight. In the first example, 2 is a quantity and inches is the unit of dimension. In the last example, 6 is a quantity and kilograms is the unit of dimension.

*The word *unit* has different meanings in different contexts. Other definitions will be provided later in the text when relevant to the topic.

Three Required Elements of All Dimensional Analysis (DA) Equations

1　Desired answer unit(s)

2　Given quantity and units to convert

3　One or more conversion factors

NOTE　The Dimensional Analysis Method takes a known quantity and units of measurement and multiplies by one or more conversion factors to solve an equation.

Setup of a Basic Equation Using the Dimensional Analysis (DA) Method

Analyze the following simple problem:

Problem: How many inches are in 2 feet? Conversion Factor: 12 inches = 1 foot.

EXAMPLES

➤ Identify the required elements *in this order:*

1　Desired answer unit(s): inches
2　Given quantity and units to be converted: 2 feet
3　A conversion factor: 12 inches = 1 foot (a factor that contains the desired answer units: inches, and the unit(s) to be converted: feet)

➤ *Only after* the first two required elements for the equation are identified in the problem are conversion factors selected that will convert the given units to the desired answer units. There is only one conversion factor needed in this basic problem.

After you have identified the three required elements, use the following systematic approach to enter them in the equation from left to right:

1　Write the desired answer unit(s) on the *left* as a reminder of the units needed in the answer.

2 Enter a conversion factor that contains the desired answer units (inches) in the numerator. It will be called the *Starting Factor.*

3 Enter the Given Quantity and Unit(s) (feet) to be converted on the *right.*

EXAMPLES

Desired Answer Units	= Starting Factor	× Given Quantity and Units to be Converted	= Answer
? inches	= $\dfrac{12 \text{ inches}}{1 \text{ foot}}$	× $\dfrac{2 \text{ feet}}{1}$	= x inches
Desired answer units (inches) are written on the left as a "reminder" of the units needed for the answer.	Enter the identified conversion factor that will convert the feet to inches with the desired answer units (12 inches) in the numerator to ensure correct placement in the answer. Enter the rest of the conversion factor in the denominator (1 foot), the unit to be canceled.	Enter the quantity and units to be converted in the numerator so it can be canceled diagonally. A number 1 is placed in the denominator to maintain alignment for the math. This reduces math errors.	

Cancellation: The unwanted unit (feet) is positioned diagonally to be canceled as in fraction multiplication.

$$? \text{ inches} = \frac{12 \text{ inches}}{1 \ \cancel{\text{foot}}} \times \frac{2 \ \cancel{\text{feet}}}{1} = x \text{ inches}$$

➤ Stop! Recheck the equation setup before doing any math. Are all unwanted units (feet) canceled so that only the desired answer units (inches) remain? This brief pause to recheck the setup prevents having to redo the entire problem. If the setup is wrong, the answer will be wrong.

If setup is correct:

➤ Stop again! Estimate an approximate answer. Should the answer be more or less than the given quantity? (If 1 foot = 12 in., then 2 feet would be twice as many inches [24].) Estimates reduce the chance of major math errors.

The math is the same as for fraction multiplication.

Desired Answer Units		Starting Factor	×	Given Quantity and Units	=	Answer
? inches	=	$\dfrac{12 \text{ inches}}{1 \ \cancel{\text{foot}}}$	×	$\dfrac{2 \ \cancel{\text{feet}}}{1}$	=	24 inches

EXAMPLES

Analysis: Inches are the desired answer unit of measurement. The unwanted unit (feet) has been entered *twice,* once in a denominator and second in a numerator. This permits cancellation. The number 1 is an important placeholder under the whole number 2 to keep the numerator (2 feet) in proper alignment for the math. This prevents errors. Ask yourself: Does only the desired answer unit remain? Does the estimate support the answer, 24 inches?

Evaluation: The answer unit, inches, matches the desired answer units. The estimate supports the answer, 24 inches. The answer is "yes" to both. The equation is complete.

➤ Review the elements, the setup instructions, and the equation once more before continuing.

➤ Placing the headings over your equations is strongly recommended as a visual aid to get a good start toward a correct setup.

FAQ *Why are the units canceled before multiplying?*

ANSWER This ensures a correct setup of the equation. Incorrect math setups pose problems for some students. DA permits a fast check of setup to ensure that only the desired answer units will remain in the answer. Analyzing the setup before multiplying is a timesaver.

---

1   What are the three main elements of a DA equation that must be identified before the setup? *(Use brief phrases.)*

   a. _____

   b. _____

   c. _____

➤ Remember: In DA, the placement of units, <u>not numbers</u>, guides the setup. The units are canceled *before* the math.

ASK YOURSELF

MY ANSWER

Examine the next example. The rest of the chapter will give brief practices for each phase of the setup.

EXAMPLES

How many ounces (oz) are in 5 pounds (lb)? Conversion factor: 16 oz = 1 lb.

Desired Answer Units	= Starting Factor × Given Quantity and Units (unwanted units)	= Answer
? ounces =	$\dfrac{16\ oz}{1\ \cancel{lb}}$ × $\dfrac{5\ \cancel{lb}}{1}$	= 80 oz

The final equation will be written like this:

$$? \text{ ounces: } \frac{16\ oz}{1\ \cancel{lb}} \times \frac{5\ \cancel{lb}}{1} = 80 \text{ oz in 5 lb}$$

Analysis: 5 lb needs to be converted to ounces. The three required elements are identified and entered. There is only one conversion factor which is placed as the starting factor. The math is not done until all unwanted units are canceled, the setup is checked to determine that only the desired answer units remain, and an estimate is made of the approximate answer.

Estimate: The answer will be a larger quantity than the given units. 5 × 16 is about 80.

Evaluation: The answer gives only the desired answer units (ounces). My estimate that the answer will be larger than the given 5 lb is correct. (Math check: 16 × 5 = 80.) My estimate supports the answer.

➤ Do not skip the check of the setup and the estimate before doing the math. Not only does it reduce errors, it also saves time of having to start all over again.

➤ Remember: In basic equations with only one conversion factor, the starting factor will also be the conversion factor.

Take a second look at the setups. In order to cancel undesired units, each set of undesired units (pounds) must appear *twice* in the final equation. They must be in a denominator and a numerator in order to be canceled.

FAQ *Does it matter in which order the data are entered in the equation?*

ANSWER A systematic sequential order is preferred. The method shown is designed to reduce errors. Identifying what is being asked is a logical time-saving approach to any type of question.

FAQ *Which are the most common types of errors?*

ANSWER Math errors and incorrect setup of the units will result in the wrong answer.

➤ Even if the setup is correct and even if both sides of the equation are equal, the answer may be wrong. Incorrect data entry and/or incorrect multiplication will yield a wrong answer. DA is one of the best methods of preventing a setup error, and the final math equality on both sides of the equation is very easy to prove. However, DA cannot prevent the nurse from making numerical entry and math errors. Careless handwriting that can be misread also contributes to errors.

EXAMPLES

INCORRECT EQUATION SETUP

How many yards are in 6 feet? Conversion factor: 3 feet = 1 yard.

Desired Answer Units	=	Starting Factor	×	Given Quantity and Units	=	Answer
yards	=	$\dfrac{3 \text{ feet}}{1 \text{ yard}}$	×	$\dfrac{6 \text{ feet}}{1}$	=	$\dfrac{18 \text{ feet squared}}{1 \text{ yard}}$

➤ Observe that this is an incorrect setup. The desired answer units (yards) should be in the numerator.

Analysis: A bad start. Because of the incorrect orientation of the starting factor, the unwanted feet cannot be canceled because they are both in a numerator. Incorrect orientation of units in the numerator or denominator leads to errors.

Evaluation: The answer does not make sense. If we had examined the units after cancelation, but before doing the math, we would not have done the math. This is how you know to recheck the setup.

How many yards are in 6 feet? Conversion factor: 3 feet = 1 yard.

Desired Answer Units	=	Starting Factor (with desired answer in numerator	×	Given Quantity and Units	=	Answer
yards	=	$\dfrac{1 \text{ yard}}{3 \text{ feet}}{1}$	×	$\dfrac{\overset{2}{\cancel{6 \text{ feet}}}}{1}$	=	2 yards

Conversion Factor Review

Conversion factors:

1 Are selected after the desired answer units and the given quantity and units are identified.

2 Must contain a *quantity* and a *unit of measurement* and/or a *label* (e.g., 12 inches = 1 foot, 250 mg per 1 tablet, 10 employees per 1 supervisor).

3 Are equivalent.

4 Are inserted in an equation in fraction form.

5 Do not change the value of the other units in the equation because they equal the number 1. (Multiplying numbers by 1 does not alter the value.)

6 Must be positioned (oriented) to match the desired answer units and permit cancellation of the unwanted units.

➤ Write out and read "per" for slashes. Slashes are widely used in printed drug labels and references. However, they may be mistaken for the number one (1).

RAPID PRACTICE 2-1   ## Correct Starting Factor Orientation

ESTIMATED COMPLETION TIME: 10 minutes   **ANSWERS ON:** page 68

DIRECTIONS: *Read the problem for the required elements. Place a circle around the correctly oriented starting factor (ensuring that numerator and denominator placement matches the desired answer units in the numerator and permits cancellation of the undesired units). Evaluate your setup. Review the previous examples if necessary.* **Do not** *carry out the math to solve the equation.*

1 How many ounces are in 6 pounds? Conversion factor: 16 oz = 1 lb.

Desired Answer Units	=	Starting Factor	Given Quantity and Units
? oz	=	$\dfrac{1\ lb}{16\ oz}$ *or* $\dfrac{16\ oz}{1\ lb}$	6 lb

➤ Circle the correct conversion factor placement.

2 How many eggs are in 10 dozen? Conversion factor: 12 eggs = 1 dozen.

Desired Answer Units	=	Starting Factor	Given Quantity and Units
? eggs	=	$\dfrac{1\ dozen}{12\ eggs}$ *or* $\dfrac{12\ eggs}{1\ dozen}$	10 dozen

➤ Circle the correct conversion factor placement.

3 How many quarts are in 10 gal? Conversion factor: 4 qt = 1 gal.

Desired Answer Units	=	Starting Factor	Given Quantity and Units
? quarts	=	$\dfrac{4\ qt}{1\ gal}$ *or* $\dfrac{1\ gal}{4\ qt}$	10 gal

➤ Circle the correct conversion factor placement.

4 How many seconds are in 30 minutes? Conversion factor: 60 seconds = 1 minute.

Desired Answer Units	=	Starting Factor		Given Quantity and Units
? seconds	=	$\dfrac{1\ \text{min}}{60\ \text{sec}}$ *or* $\dfrac{60\ \text{sec}}{1\ \text{min}}$		30 min

➤ Circle the correct conversion factor placement.

5 How many kilometers are in 5 miles? Conversion factor: 1 km = 0.6 mile.

Desired Answer Units	=	Starting Factor		Given Quantity and Units
? km	=	$\dfrac{0.6\ \text{mi}}{1\ \text{km}}$ *or* $\dfrac{1\ \text{km}}{0.6\ \text{mi}}$		5 mi

➤ Circle the correct conversion factor placement.

RAPID PRACTICE 2-2 | Basic Equation Setup

ESTIMATED COMPLETION TIME: 15 minutes   **ANSWERS ON:** page 68

DIRECTIONS: *Fill in the equation in the space provided, as illustrated in problem 1.* **Do not** *solve the equation. Use the following conversion factors: 3 feet = 1 yard, 4 cups = 1 quart, 1 yard = approximately 1 meter, 12 dozen = 1 gross, 1 eurodollar = approximately $1.40 U.S. dollars.*

1 How many dozen are in 2 gross?

Desired Answer Units	=	Starting Factor	×	Given Quantity and Units

2 If you have $500, how many eurodollars can you buy?

Desired Answer Units	=	Starting Factor	×	Given Quantity and Units

3 Approximately how many yards are in 50 meters?

Desired Answer Units	=	Starting Factor	×	Given Quantity and Units

4 How many feet are in 8 yards?

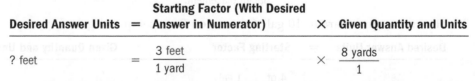

Desired Answer Units	=	Starting Factor (With Desired Answer in Numerator)	×	Given Quantity and Units
? feet	=	$\dfrac{3\ \text{feet}}{1\ \text{yard}}$	×	$\dfrac{8\ \text{yards}}{1}$

Since the denominator unit (yard) is repeated in the next numerator (yards), it can be canceled.

5 How many quarts are in 8 cups?

Desired Answer Units	=	Starting Factor	×	Given Quantity and Units

Conversions for Dimensional Analysis Calculations

Two kinds of conversions are commonly used as factors for DA calculations:

1   Conversion factors within the same dimension, such as 12 eggs = 1 dozen (quantity), 4 qt = 1 gal (volume), or 1000 milligrams (mg) = 1 gram (g) (weight or mass)

2   Conversions factors within different dimensions (ratios), such as 10 pills per day (10 pills per 1 day), 250 mg per tablet (250 mg in 1 tablet), 1 g per capsule (1 gram [g] in 1 capsule), 10 workers per 1 supervisor, $12 per hr, or 10 tickets per 2 free passes.

➤   Both types of conversion factors are equivalents and entered the same way in equations.

RAPID PRACTICE 2-3	Identifying Correct Equation Setup

ESTIMATED COMPLETION TIME: 5 to 10 minutes   **ANSWERS ON:** page 68

DIRECTIONS: *Identify the required elements in the problem statement. Focus on the setup. Correct the incorrect setup. Do not solve the equation. You will see that you do not need to be familiar with the terminology to analyze these setups.*

1   The patient takes 10 tablets per day. How many tablets will the patient need for 7 days? _____

Desired Answer Units	=	Starting Factor(s)	×	Given Quantity and Units
? tablets	=	$\dfrac{10 \text{ tablets}}{1 \text{ day}}$	×	$\dfrac{7 \text{ days}}{1}$

   a.   Is the DA setup correct? _____
   b.   If it is incorrect, correct it.

   c.   Will the answer be larger or smaller than the units to be converted? _____

2   If there are approximately 2.5 centimeters (cm) in 1 inch (in), how many centimeters are there in 50 inches?

Desired Answer Units	=	Starting Factor	×	Given Quantity and Units
? cm	=	$\dfrac{2.5 \text{ cm}}{1 \text{ in}}$	×	$\dfrac{50 \text{ in}}{1}$

   a.   Is the DA setup correct? _____
   b.   If it is incorrect, correct it.

   c.   Estimate: Will the numerical answer be larger or smaller than the units to be converted? _____

3   The average baby weighs 7 pounds (lb) at birth. There are 2.2 lb in 1 kg. How many kilograms does the average baby weigh? _____

Desired Answer Units	=	Starting Factor	×	Given Quantity and Units
? kg	=	$\dfrac{2.2 \text{ lb}}{1 \text{ kg}}$	×	$\dfrac{7 \text{ lb}}{1}$

   a.   Is the DA setup correct? _____
   b.   If it is incorrect, correct it.

   c.   Estimate: Will the numerical answer be larger or smaller than the units to be converted? _____

4 A bottle contains 2500 milliliters (mL) of fluid. There are 1000 mL in 1 liter (L). How many liters are in the bottle? _____

Desired Answer Units	=	Starting Factor	×	Given Quantity and Units
? L	=	$\dfrac{1000 \text{ mL}}{1 \text{ L}}$	×	$\dfrac{2500 \text{ mL}}{1}$

a. Is the DA setup correct? _____
b. If it is incorrect, correct it.

c. Will the numerical answer be larger or smaller than the units to be converted? _____

5 There are 1000 milligrams (mg) in 1 gram (g). If you have 5.5 grams, how many milligrams do you have? _____

Desired Answer Units	=	Starting Factor(s)	×	Given Quantity and Units
? mg	=	$\dfrac{1000 \text{ mg}}{1 \text{ g}}$	×	$\dfrac{5.5 \text{ g}}{1}$

a. Is the DA setup correct? _____
b. If it is incorrect, correct it.

c. Will the numerical answer be larger or smaller than the units to be converted? _____

FAQ *Why practice the DA method with problems that can easily be calculated mentally?*

ANSWER The goal is to practice this systematic method with simple problems and to plant it in long-term memory so that the setup can be recalled for solutions to more complex calculations. Some problems call for more entries. If you can set up simple problems, you will be able to apply the technique to more complex problems.

CLINICAL RELEVANCE

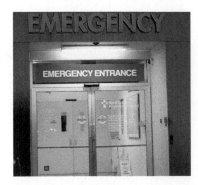

Many medications ordered do not require calculations for administration, but some do. The nurse needs to demonstrate competency with a calculation method and be able to apply this method to a variety of medication applications correctly.

➤ Even when a calculator is used, the nurse must understand the math process well enough to enter the data correctly.

➤ Frail and at-risk populations may require fractional doses, which involve calculations of a small dose from a large amount on hand.

➤ Almost all intravenous solutions require some calculations.

➤ It is critical to check your calculations, and ask yourself, "Does my answer make sense?" prior to the administration of each medication.

Basic DA Equations Practice

ESTIMATED COMPLETION TIME: 20 minutes   **ANSWERS ON:** page 68

DIRECTIONS: *Set up equations 2 to 5 as shown in the first problem. Identify the required elements. Enter them in the equation from left to right. Cancel undesired units. Check that only the desired answer units will remain. Estimate the answer, then solve the equation. Check answer with estimate.*

   Conversion factors: 32 ounces (oz) = 1 quart (qt), 1000 megabytes (MB) = 1 gigabyte (GB), 4 liters (L) = approximately 1 gallon (gal), 5 CNAs per 2 LPNs, $20 = 1 hr pay.

1 You have 3 quarts of milk. How many ounces do you have?

Desired Answer Unit	=	Starting Factor	×	Given Quantity and Units	=	Answer
? oz	=	$\dfrac{32\ oz}{1\ \cancel{qt}}$	×	$\dfrac{3\ \cancel{qt}}{1}$	=	96 oz

2 The hospital has 40 CNA employees. How many LPN slots are there?

Desired Answer Unit	=	Starting Factor	×	Given Quantity and Units	=	Answer

3 Your computer backup storage device holds 4 gigabytes (GB). How many megabytes (MB) is this?

Desired Answer Unit	=	Starting Factor	×	Given Quantity and Units	=	Answer

4 Your salary is $20 per hr. You earned $500. How many hours did you work?

Desired Answer Unit	=	Starting Factor	×	Given Quantity and Units	=	Answer

5 You buy 40 liters (L) of gas for your car in Mexico. About how many gallons (gal) did you buy?

Desired Answer Unit	=	Starting Factor	×	Given Quantity and Units	=	Answer

Problems That Call for More Than One Conversion Factor

The process is the same as for one conversion factor. Note: Extra space is made after the starting factor to permit additional conversion factors.

EXAMPLES

How many seconds (s) are in 5 hours?

Conversion factors: 60 seconds = 1 minute
                     60 minutes = 1 hour

Desired Answer Units = Starting Factor ×	Given Quantity and Units and Conversion Factor(s) =	Estimate, Multiply, Evaluate
seconds $= \dfrac{60 \text{ s}}{1 \text{ min}}$	$\times \dfrac{60 \text{ min}}{1 \text{ hr}} \times \dfrac{5 \text{ hr}}{1}$	= 18,000 seconds

Plan to cancel minutes,
then hours

The final equation will be written like this:

seconds $= \dfrac{60 \text{ s}}{1 \text{ min}} \times \dfrac{60 \text{ min}}{1 \text{ hr}} \times \dfrac{5 \text{ hr}}{1}$ = 18,000 seconds in 5 hr

Analysis: There are two conversion factors to get from seconds to hours.
1   To get from seconds to minutes (in the Starting Factor)
2   To get from minutes to hours (following the Starting Factor)

The selected Starting Factor is a conversion factor with seconds in the numerator to match the desired answer units. It is accompanied by 1 *minute* in the denominator. Positioning 60 *minutes* in the *numerator* of the next conversion factor permits *sequential cancellation* of the unwanted minutes. 5 hr must be placed in the next numerator so that hr can be canceled diagonally. 5 hr is treated like a whole number as a *numerator* with an *implied* denominator of 1.

In order to cancel the unwanted units, minutes and hours had to appear *twice* in the final calculation, once in a numerator and once in a denominator.

The rest of the process is the same as for basic equations. Recheck the setup. Cancel all the unwanted units. Be sure that only the desired answer units (seconds) remain. Make a rough estimate of the answer (5 × 60 = 300 × 60 = 18,000). Complete the multiplication. Comparison with the estimate is the final step.

Evaluation: All of the required elements are in the equation. Only seconds remain in the answer. The estimate of 18,000 seconds supports the answer. You would probably use a calculator for large numbers.

➤ *Always* enter calculator data *twice* to verify the answer.

RAPID PRACTICE 2-5	DA Equations With Two Conversion Factors

ESTIMATED COMPLETION TIME: 30 minutes   **ANSWERS ON:** page 68

DIRECTIONS: *Circle A or B to indicate the correct setup of the equations for the following problems; then solve the equation using the correct setup as shown in Example 1. Label the answer. Remember to cancel all unwanted units before doing math.*

1   How many millimeters (mm) are in 10 inches? Conversion factors: 2.5 centimeters (cm) = 1 inch, and 10 mm = 1 cm.

Desired Answer Unit				×		=	
A. ? millimeters	=	$\dfrac{1\ cm}{10\ mm}$	$\times\ \dfrac{1\ inch}{2.5\ cm}$	×	$\dfrac{10\ inches}{1}$	=	Answer
B. ? millimeters	=	$\dfrac{10\ mm}{1\ cm}$	$\times\ \dfrac{2.5\ cm}{1\ inch}$	×	$\dfrac{10\ inches}{1}$	=	Answer

DA equation:

Evaluate your choice. Is the desired answer unit the only remaining unit?

2   How many grams (g) are in 4000 micrograms (mcg)? Conversion factors: 1000 mg = 1 g, and 1000 mcg = 1 mg.

Desired Answer Unit				×		=	
A. ? grams	=	$\dfrac{1\ g}{1000\ mg}$	$\times\ \dfrac{1000\ mcg}{1\ mg}$	×	$\dfrac{4000\ mcg}{1}$	=	Answer
B. ? grams	=	$\dfrac{1\ g}{1000\ mg}$	$\times\ \dfrac{1\ mg}{1000\ mcg}$	×	$\dfrac{4000\ mcg}{1}$	=	Answer

DA equation:

Evaluate your choice. Is the desired answer unit the only remaining unit or most common?

3   Approximately how many weeks are in 4 years? Conversion factors: 12 months = 1 year, and 4 weeks = 1 month.

Desired Answer Unit				×		=	
A. ? weeks	=	$\dfrac{4\ weeks}{1\ month}$	$\times\ \dfrac{1\ year}{12\ months}$	×	$\dfrac{4\ years}{1}$	=	Answer
B. ? weeks	=	$\dfrac{4\ weeks}{1\ month}$	$\times\ \dfrac{12\ months}{1\ year}$	×	$\dfrac{4\ years}{1}$	=	Answer

DA equation:

$$weeks = \frac{4\ weeks}{1\ \cancel{month}} \times \frac{12\ \cancel{months}}{1\ \cancel{year}} \times 4\ \cancel{years} = 192\ weeks$$

Evaluate your choice. Is the desired answer unit the only remaining unit?

4 How many inches are in 20 yards? Conversion factors: 12 inches = 1 foot, and 3 feet = 1 yard.

Desired Answer Unit				$\times$		$=$	

A. ? inches $= \dfrac{1 \text{ yard}}{3 \text{ feet}} \times \dfrac{1 \text{ foot}}{12 \text{ inches}} \times \dfrac{20 \text{ yards}}{1} =$ Answer

B. ? inches $= \dfrac{12 \text{ inches}}{1 \text{ foot}} \times \dfrac{3 \text{ feet}}{1 \text{ yard}} \times \dfrac{20 \text{ yards}}{1} =$ Answer

DA equation:

Evaluate your choice. Is the desired answer unit the only remaining unit?

5 How many cups in 5 qt? Conversion factors: 2 cups = 1 pt, and 2 pt = 1 qt.

Desired Answer Unit				$\times$		$=$	

A. ? cups $= \dfrac{2 \text{ cups}}{1 \text{ pt}} \times \dfrac{2 \text{ pt}}{1 \text{ qt}} \times \dfrac{5 \text{ qt}}{1} =$ 20 cups

B. ? cups $= \dfrac{1 \text{ pt}}{2 \text{ cups}} \times \dfrac{2 \text{ pt}}{1 \text{ qt}} \times \dfrac{5 \text{ qt}}{1} =$

DA equation:

Evaluate your choice. Is the desired answer unit the only remaining unit? Did the setup permit sequential cancellation?

FAQ *Which are the most common errors when using two or more conversion factors?*

ANSWER Assuming that the desired answer unit is entered correctly, the second conversion formula may be positioned incorrectly. The second conversion formula numerator must cancel the denominator of a previous conversion formula. Also, the numbers may be transposed if the writer is not focused. Finally, each *undesired unit* must be entered *two* times, once in a denominator and once in a numerator.

RAPID PRACTICE 2-6   DA Equations With One or Two Conversion Factors

ESTIMATED COMPLETION TIME: 30 minutes   **ANSWERS ON:** page 68

DIRECTIONS: *Identify the required elements. Solve the equations using the 4-column systematic approach presented in this chapter. Allow space for an extra conversion factor if needed. Evaluate your equation. Even if you can solve the equations mentally, the benefit of this practice is to reinforce a solid method of verification for more complex problems using DA.*

1 How many inches are in 25 millimeters (mm)? Conversion factors: 10 mm = 1 cm, and 2.5 cm = 1 inch.

DA equation:

2 How many pounds (lb) are in 80 kilograms (kg)? Conversion factor: 2.2 lb = 1 kg.

DA equation:

3 How many hours are in 7200 seconds? Conversion factors: 60 seconds = 1 minute, and 60 minutes = 1 hour.

DA equation:

4 A patient has to take 1 capsule 3 times a day. How many capsules will the patient need for a 2-week prescription? Conversion factors: 3 capsules = 1 day, and 7 days = 1 week.

DA equation:

5 How many pints are in 5 gallons (gal)? Conversion factors: 2 pt = 1 qt, and 4 qt = 1 gal.

DA equation:

CHAPTER 2   MULTIPLE-CHOICE REVIEW

ESTIMATED COMPLETION TIME: 20 minutes   **ANSWERS ON:** page 68

DIRECTIONS: *Circle the number of the correct choice.*

1 Which DA equation is correct for solving the following question?

Question: How many kilobytes (KB) are in 2 gigabytes (GB)?
Conversion factors: 1000 kilobytes (KB) = 1 megabyte (MB), and 1000 MB = 1 GB.
Circle the letter of the correct conversion formula.

a. ? kilobytes $= \dfrac{1000\ GB}{1\ MB} \quad \dfrac{1\ GB}{1000\ MB} \times \dfrac{2\ GB}{1}$

b. ? kilobytes $= \dfrac{1\ MB}{1000\ KB} \quad \dfrac{1\ GB}{1000\ MB} \times \dfrac{2\ GB}{1}$

c. ? kilobytes $= \dfrac{1000\ KB}{1\ MB} \quad \dfrac{1000\ MB}{1\ GB} \times \dfrac{2\ GB}{1}$

d. ? kilobytes $= \dfrac{1000\ MB}{1\ GB} \quad \dfrac{25000\ KB}{1\ MB} \times \dfrac{2\ GB}{1}$

2 Which of the following choices reflects the *correct* setup for a DA equation?

Question: How many micrograms are in 0.5 grams (g)?
Conversion formulas: 1000 mcg = 1 mg, and 1000 mg = 1 g.
Circle the letter of the correct choice.

a. ? grams $= \dfrac{1000\ mcg}{1\ mg} \times \dfrac{0.5\ g}{1000\ mg} \times \dfrac{1000\ mcg}{1}$

b. ? micrograms $= \dfrac{1\ mg}{1000\ mcg} \times \dfrac{1000\ mg}{0.5\ g} \times \dfrac{0.5\ g}{1}$

c. ? milligrams $= \dfrac{0.5\ g}{1000\ mg} \times \dfrac{1\ mg}{1000\ mcg} \times \dfrac{0.5\ g}{1}$

d. ? micrograms $= \dfrac{1000\ mcg}{1\ mg} \times \dfrac{1000\ mg}{1\ g} \times \dfrac{0.5\ g}{1}$

3 The *final* evaluation of a DA equation should include which of the following critical steps?

a. Ensuring the desired answer units are the only remaining units
b. Checking the conversion factor(s) for correct placement in the numerator and denominator
c. Estimating the answer
d. Identifying the known quantity

4 What is the *first* step in analyzing a problem to solve a DA equation?

a. Identify the given units and quantities.
b. Estimate the answer.
c. Identify the desired answer units.
d. Set up the equation.

5 Two types of conversion factors are as follows:

a. Data and factors to be entered
b. Units and fractions
c. Those that contain the same dimensions and those that contain different dimensions
d. Fraction equivalents and decimal equivalents

6 Which of the following is a key process that *guides* the setup of DA equations?

a. Placement of units
b. Placement of numbers
c. Multiplication of units
d. Multiplication of numbers

7 Solving an equation using DA requires which of the following processes?

a. Cancellation of units followed by multiplication
b. Multiplication of units followed by cancellation
c. Cancellation of desired answer units
d. Division of desired and undesired units

8 Which of the following statements is true?

a. The Starting Factor contains the given quantity and units supplied by the manufacturer.
b. Conversion factors are selected after the desired answer and given quantity and units are identified.
c. An estimate of an approximate answer is made before cancellation of units.
d. The unwanted units are canceled after the math is carried out.

9 The analysis of the DA equation setup to ensure that all unwanted units are canceled should take place at which step of the process?

a. After entering the first conversion fraction
b. When entering the original factors
c. After all the data are entered but before multiplication of quantities
d. After all the data are entered and after the multiplication of quantities

10 Which conversion factor setup is correct for the following question?

Question: How many yards are in 72 inches?
Conversion factors: 12 inches = 1 foot, and 3 feet = 1 yard.
Circle the letter of the correct choice.

a. ? yards $= \dfrac{72 \text{ inches}}{1 \text{ foot}} \times \dfrac{3 \text{ feet}}{1 \text{ yard}} \times \dfrac{72 \text{ inches}}{1}$

b. ? yards $= \dfrac{1 \text{ yard}}{3 \text{ feet}} \times \dfrac{1 \text{ foot}}{12 \text{ inches}} \times \dfrac{72 \text{ inches}}{1}$

c. ? yards $= \dfrac{12 \text{ inches}}{1 \text{ foot}} \times \dfrac{3 \text{ feet}}{1 \text{ yard}} \times \dfrac{72 \text{ inches}}{1}$

d. ? yards $= \dfrac{1 \text{ yard}}{72 \text{ inches}} \times \dfrac{3 \text{ feet}}{12 \text{ inches}} \times \dfrac{72 \text{ inches}}{1}$

CHAPTER 2   FINAL PRACTICE

ESTIMATED COMPLETION TIME: 1 to 2 hours   **ANSWERS ON:** page 68

DIRECTIONS: *Set up and solve the following problems using the four-step DA method even if you can obtain the answer with mental arithmetic. Label all data. Evaluate your equations.*

1 Write the three required *elements* of dimensional analysis equations.

a. _____

b. _____

c. _____

2 How many millimeters are in 1 inch? Conversion factors: 10 mm = 1 cm, and 2.5 cm = 1 inch. _____

DA equation:

3 How many inches are in 50 yards? Conversion factors: 12 inches = 1 foot, and 3 feet = 1 yard. _____

DA equation:

4 How many kilometers are in 50 miles to the nearest tenth? Conversion factor: 1 km = 0.6 mile. _____

DA equation:

5 How many syringes can be bought for $100? Conversion factor: Each syringe costs $8. How much money will be left over? _____

DA equation:

6 How many eggs are in 10 dozen? Conversion factor: 12 eggs = 1 dozen. _____

DA equation:

7 How many pounds are in 60 kg? Conversion factor: 2.2 lb = 1 kg. _____

DA equation:

8 How many meters are in 30 yards? Conversion factor: 1 m = 1.09 yards. Round to the nearest tenth. _____

DA equation:

➤ Use two conversion factors in a DA-style equation for the next 12 questions.

9 How many nurses will be needed for a new 480-bed hospital? Conversion factor: 1 nurse per 12 beds. Round answer to nearest whole number. _____

DA equation:

10 How many liters are in 8 gal? Conversion factors: 1 L = 1 qt, and 4 qt = 1 gal. _____

DA equation:

11 How many inches are in 10 yards? Conversion factors: 12 inches = 1 foot, and 3 feet = 1 yard. _____

DA equation:

12 How many tablespoonfuls are in a cup of fluid? Conversion factors: 2 Tbsp = 1 oz, and 8 oz = 1 cup. _____

DA equation:

13 How many cups are in 2 qt? Conversion factors: 2 cups = 1 pt, and
2 pt = 1 qt. _____

DA equation:

14 How many hours are in 1800 seconds (s)? Conversion factors:
60 seconds = 1 minute, and 60 minutes = 1 hour. _____

DA equation:

15 How many micrograms (mcg) are in 2 grams (g) of sugar? Conversion
factors: 1000 mcg = 1 mg, and 1000 mg = 1 g. _____

DA equation:

16 How many centimeters are in a foot? Conversion factors: 2.5 cm = 1 inch,
and 12 inches = 1 foot. _____

DA equation:

17 How many milliliters are in 3 Tbsp of milk? Conversion factors: 5 mL = 1 tsp,
and 3 tsp = 1 Tbsp. _____

DA equation:

18 How many nurse assistants are needed for a 300-bed hospital? Conversion
factors: 1 nurse per 10 beds, and 2 nurse assistants for each nurse. _____

DA equation:

19 How many inches are in a meter (m)? Conversion factors: 2.5 cm = 1 inch,
and 100 cm = 1 m. _____

DA equation:

20 How many prescriptions (Rx) can be bought with an insurance policy that has
a $2000 limit? Conversion factor: $50 average cost per prescription. _____

DA equation:

CHAPTER 2 ANSWER KEY

RAPID PRACTICE 2-1 (p. 55)

1 $\dfrac{16 \text{ oz}}{1 \text{ lb}}$

2 $\dfrac{12 \text{ eggs}}{1 \text{ dozen}}$

3 $\dfrac{4 \text{ qt}}{1 \text{ gal}}$

4 $\dfrac{60 \text{ sec}}{1 \text{ min}}$

5 $\dfrac{1 \text{ km}}{0.6 \text{ mi}}$

➤ Note that all the starting factors in these problems are conversion factors.

RAPID PRACTICE 2-2 (p. 56)

Desired Answer Units	Starting Factors	Given Quantity Units
2 yards:	$\dfrac{1 \text{ yard}}{1 \text{ meter}}$	$\dfrac{50 \text{ meters}}{1}$
3 quarts:	$\dfrac{1 \text{ quart}}{4 \text{ cups}}$	$\dfrac{8 \text{ cups}}{1}$
4 eurodollars:	$\dfrac{1 \text{ eurodollar}}{\$1.40}$	$\dfrac{\$500}{1}$
5 dozen:	$\dfrac{12 \text{ dozen}}{1 \text{ gross}}$	$\dfrac{2 \text{ gross}}{1}$

➤ Note that original numbers and units to be converted do not have a denominator and are placed in the numerator position with an implied denominator of 1. This helps prevent multiplication errors.

RAPID PRACTICE 2-3 (p. 57)

1 **a.** Yes
  b. N/A
  c. Larger

2 **a.** Yes
  b. N/A
  c. Larger

3 **a.** No
  b. $\dfrac{1 \text{ kg}}{2.2 \text{ lb}}$
  c. Smaller

4 **a.** No
  b. $\dfrac{1 \text{ L}}{1000 \text{ mL}}$
  c. Smaller

5 **a.** Yes
  b. N/A
  c. Larger

RAPID PRACTICE 2-4 (p. 59)

2 LPNs : $\dfrac{2 \text{ LPNs}}{5 \text{ CNAs}} \times \dfrac{40 \text{ CNAs}}{1} = \dfrac{2 \text{ LPNs}}{1} \times \dfrac{8}{1} = 16 \text{ LPNs}$

3 megabytes $= \dfrac{1000 \text{ megabytes}}{1 \text{ gigabyte}} \times \dfrac{4 \text{ gigabytes}}{1}$
    $= 4000 \text{ megabytes}$

4 hours : $\dfrac{1 \text{ hour}}{2 \text{ 0 dollars}} \times \dfrac{500 \text{ dollars}}{1}$
    $= \dfrac{1 \text{ hour}}{2} \times \dfrac{50}{2} = 25 \text{ hours}$

5 gallons : $\dfrac{1 \text{ gallon}}{4 \text{ liters}} \times \dfrac{40 \text{ liters}}{1} = \dfrac{1}{1} \times \dfrac{10}{1} = 10 \text{ gallons}$

RAPID PRACTICE 2-5 (p. 61)

1 B mm : $\dfrac{10 \text{ mm}}{1 \text{ cm}} \times \dfrac{2.5 \text{ cm}}{1 \text{ inch}} \times \dfrac{10 \text{ inches}}{1} = 250 \text{ mm}$

2 B grams $= \dfrac{1 \text{ g}}{1000 \text{ mg}} \times \dfrac{1 \text{ mg}}{1000 \text{ mcg}} \times \dfrac{4000 \text{ mcg}}{1}$
    $= \dfrac{4}{1000} = 0.004 \text{ g}$

3 B weeks $= \dfrac{4 \text{ weeks}}{1 \text{ month}} \times \dfrac{12 \text{ months}}{1 \text{ year}} \times \dfrac{4 \text{ years}}{1}$
    $= 192 \text{ weeks}$

4 B inches $= \dfrac{12 \text{ inches}}{1 \text{ foot}} \times \dfrac{3 \text{ feet}}{1 \text{ yard}} \times \dfrac{20 \text{ yards}}{1}$
    $= 720 \text{ inches}$

5 A cups : $\dfrac{2 \text{ cups}}{1 \text{ pint}} \times \dfrac{2 \text{ pints}}{1 \text{ quart}} \times \dfrac{5 \text{ quarts}}{1} = 20 \text{ cups}$

RAPID PRACTICE 2-6 (p. 62)

1 inches : $\dfrac{1 \text{ inch}}{2.5 \text{ cm}} \times \dfrac{1 \text{ cm}}{10 \text{ mm}} \times \dfrac{25 \text{ mm}}{1} = 1 \text{ inch}$

2 lbs : $\dfrac{2.2 \text{ lbs}}{1 \text{ kg}} \times \dfrac{80 \text{ kg}}{1} = 176 \text{ lbs}$

3 hours : $\dfrac{1 \text{ hour}}{60 \text{ min}} \times \dfrac{1 \text{ min}}{60 \text{ s}} \times \dfrac{7200 \text{ s}}{1} = 2 \text{ hours}$

4 capsules $= \dfrac{3 \text{ capsules}}{1 \text{ day}} \times \dfrac{7 \text{ days}}{1 \text{ week}} \times \dfrac{2 \text{ weeks}}{1}$
    $= 42 \text{ capsules for 2 weeks}$

5 pints : $\dfrac{2 \text{ pints}}{1 \text{ qt}} \times \dfrac{4 \text{ qts}}{1 \text{ gallon}} \times \dfrac{5 \text{ gallons}}{1} = 40 \text{ pints}$

CHAPTER 2 MULTIPLE-CHOICE REVIEW (p. 63)

1	c	6	a
2	d	7	a
3	a	8	b
4	c	9	c
5	c	10	b

CHAPTER 2 FINAL PRACTICE (p. 65)

1 **a.** Desired answer units
  b. Given quantity and units (factors to convert)
  c. Conversion factors

2 $\text{mm} = \dfrac{10 \text{ mm}}{1 \text{ cm}} \times \dfrac{2.5 \text{ cm}}{1 \text{ inch}} \times \dfrac{1 \text{ inch}}{1}$
$= 25 \text{ mm (millimeters)}$

Comment: 2.5 cm is an approximate equivalent. There are 2.54 cm in an inch.

3 $\text{inches} = \dfrac{12 \text{ in}}{1 \text{ foot}} \times \dfrac{3 \text{ feet}}{1 \text{ yard}} \times \dfrac{50 \text{ yards}}{1}$
$= 1800 \text{ inches}$

4 $\text{km} = \dfrac{1 \text{ km}}{0.6 \text{ miles}} \times \dfrac{50 \text{ miles}}{1} = 83.3 \text{ km}$

5 $\text{syringes} = \dfrac{1 \text{ syringe}}{8 \text{ dollars}} \times \dfrac{100 \text{ dollars}}{1}$
$= 12.5 \text{ syringes}$
(12 syringes with \$4 remaining)

6 $\text{eggs} = \dfrac{12 \text{ eggs}}{1 \text{ dozen}} \times \dfrac{10 \text{ dozen}}{1} = 120 \text{ eggs}$

7 $\text{lbs} = \dfrac{2.2 \text{ lb}}{1 \text{ kg}} \times \dfrac{60 \text{ kg}}{1} = 132 \text{ lb}$

8 $\text{meters} = \dfrac{1 \text{ meter}}{1.09 \text{ yards}} \times \dfrac{30 \text{ yards}}{1} = 27.5 \text{ meters}$

9 $\text{Nurses} = \dfrac{1 \text{ nurse}}{12 \text{ beds}} \times \dfrac{480 \text{ beds}}{1}$
$= \dfrac{1 \text{ nurse}}{1} \times \dfrac{4}{1} = 40 \text{ nurses}$

10 $\text{liters} = \dfrac{1 \text{ liter}}{1 \text{ qt}} \times \dfrac{4 \text{ qt}}{1 \text{ gallon}} \times \dfrac{8 \text{ gallons}}{1}$
$= 32 \text{ liters (L)}$

11 $\text{inches} = \dfrac{12 \text{ inches}}{1 \text{ foot}} \times \dfrac{3 \text{ feet}}{1 \text{ yard}} \times \dfrac{10 \text{ yards}}{1}$
$= 360 \text{ inches}$

12 $\text{tablespoons} = \dfrac{2 \text{ tbs}}{1 \text{ oz}} \times \dfrac{8 \text{ oz}}{1 \text{ cup}} \times \dfrac{1 \text{ cup}}{1}$
$= 16 \text{ Tbsp (tablespoons)}$

13 $\text{cups} = \dfrac{2 \text{ cups}}{1 \text{ pt}} \times \dfrac{2 \text{ pt}}{1 \text{ qt}} \times \dfrac{2 \text{ qt}}{1} = 8 \text{ cups}$

14 $\text{hours} = \dfrac{1 \text{ hr}}{60 \text{ minutes}} \times \dfrac{1 \text{ minute}}{60 \text{ s}} \times \dfrac{1800 \text{ s}}{1}$
$= \dfrac{18}{36} = \dfrac{1}{2} \text{ hour}$

15 $\text{mcg} = \dfrac{1000 \text{ mcg}}{1 \text{ mg}} \times \dfrac{1000 \text{ mg}}{1 \text{ gram}} \times \dfrac{2 \text{ grams}}{1}$
$= 2,000,000 \text{ mcg (micrograms)}$

Note: A meter is a little longer than a yard (36 in).

16 $\text{cm} = \dfrac{2.5 \text{ cm}}{1 \text{ inch}} \times \dfrac{12 \text{ inches}}{1 \text{ ft}} \times \dfrac{1 \text{ ft}}{1}$
$= 30 \text{ cm (centimeters)}$

17 $\text{mL} = \dfrac{5 \text{ mL}}{1 \text{ tsp}} \times \dfrac{3 \text{ tsp}}{1 \text{ Tbsp}} \times \dfrac{3 \text{ Tbsp}}{1}$
$= 45 \text{ mL (milliliters)}$

18 $\text{NA} = \dfrac{2 \text{ NA}}{1 \text{ RN}} \times \dfrac{1 \text{ RN}}{10 \text{ beds}} \times \dfrac{\overset{30}{300 \text{ beds}}}{\underset{1}{1}}$
$= 60 \text{ NA}$

19 $\text{inches} = \dfrac{1 \text{ inch}}{2.5 \text{ cm}} \times \dfrac{100 \text{ cm}}{1 \text{ meter}} \times \dfrac{1 \text{ meter}}{1}$
$= 40 \text{ inches}$

20 $\text{Rx} = \dfrac{1 \text{ Rx}}{50 \text{ dollars}} \times \dfrac{2000 \text{ dollars}}{1}$
$= \dfrac{1 \text{ Rx}}{1} \times \dfrac{40}{1} = 40 \text{ Rx}$

Suggestions for Further Reading

http://www.pinellas.wateratlas.usf.edu/education/curriculum/Pinellas/
production/pdf/MiddleSchool/16-dimensional_analysis_s.pdf
http://www.purplemath.com/modules/units2.htm
http://study.com/academy/lesson/unit-conversion-and-dimensional analysis.html

Chapter 3 focuses on the units of measurement currently used for medications. Medications are primarily ordered and supplied in metric system measurements, a system used in most parts of the world. DA-style equations are useful for verifying conversions and solving metric-equivalent medication dose problems.

PART II

Metric System and Medication Calculations

3 Metric Units and Conversions

Metric measurements have replaced the imprecise English apothecary system.* The metric system is logical, precise, and easy to work with because it's a standardized decimal measurement system using multiples (powers) of 10, similar to our monetary structure, which is also based on a decimal structure.

It has been adopted by most countries as the standard for weights and measurements. Known as the International System of Units (SI), it is the modern form of the former French metric system. It is required for admission to the European Union. Resistance to change and the expense involved to educate and convert have slowed the U.S. "metrication" progress, except in the scientific community.

This chapter focuses on understanding and interpreting the metric measurements used in medication orders, health records, on medication labels, in laboratory reports, and nursing practice. It also includes examples of household measurements and the metric-household equivalents for home care practice for patient discharge and home-care teaching. Teaspoons and tablespoons vary in size and capacity, which can cause dangerous variations in dosages of medications.

Metric Equivalent Chart

Weight	Volume
1000 mcg (micrograms) = 1 mg (milligram)	1000 mL (milliliter) = 1 L (liter)
1000 mg = 1 g (gram)	
1000 g = 1 kg (kilogram)	

	Length
lb to kg conversion	10 mm (millimeters) = 1 centimeter (cm)
2.2 lb (pound) = 1 kg	100 cm = 1 meter (m)
inch to cm conversion	1000 mm = 1 meter (m)
1 inch = 2.5 cm (approximate)	

---

*Refer to Appendix E for the apothecary system.

VOCABULARY

Base Units	Three base units are commonly used for metric measurement of medications to indicate weight (or mass), volume, and length: **gram** (g), **liter** (L), and **meter** (m). The abbreviation for *liter* is capitalized, *L,* to avoid confusion with the number 1.
Household System of Measurement	Utensils used in the home, such as cups, teaspoons, tablespoons, and droppers. Their use can create a safety risk for measuring medication doses because of inconsistent capacities.
ISMP	Institute for Safe Medication Practices (ISMP), a nonprofit organization that educates the health care community and consumers about safe medication practices.
Metric System	A popular name for the International System of Units (SI). Modified and adopted for uniform measurement in most countries, now recommended for all medication doses in the U.S. by TJC and by ISMP.
SI Units	International System of Units (SI units) in the metric system refer to a dimension, such as weight (or mass), volume, and length. Examples of metric units of measurement include kilogram (kg), microgram (mcg), milligram (mg), gram (g), liter (L), and meter (m).
TJC	The Joint Commission (TJC), a national nonprofit independent agency dedicated to improved quality of health care through the provision of accreditation and certification to health care organizations with an emphasis on high standards and patient safety including medication administration safety.

Metric Measurements: Base Units

Three *base* units are commonly used in medicine. Two are used mainly for medication doses (gram and liter) and one (meter) is used occasionally for topical medications.

➤ Memorize the three base units.

Base Units

Dimension	Metric Base Unit	Approximate Household System Equivalent
Weight (or mass)	gram (g)	About $\frac{1}{30}$ ounce dry weight
Volume	liter (L)	About 4 measuring cups, a little more than a quart
Length	meter (m)	About 39 inches, a little more than a yard

The abbreviation for the base unit liter is capitalized (L) to avoid misreading as the number 1. The base units abbreviations for gram (g) and meter (m) are written in lowercase letters. No other abbreviations are authorized.

---

1 What are the three base units of metric measurement used for medications and their abbreviations?

ASK YOURSELF **Q & A**

MY ANSWER

_____

Metric Units Number Line

The following metric units number line illustrates the relationship of the values for selected metric prefixes.

Prefix	Abbreviation		Value
kilo-	k		1000
hecto-	h		100
deka-	da		10
			0 (zero)
deci-	d		0.1
centi-	c		0.01
milli-	m		0.001
micro-	mc		0.000001

Metric Prefixes

Four prefixes are commonly used for medication dose calculations:
- centi- (meaning hundredth)
- milli- (meaning thousandth)
- micro- (meaning millionth)
- kilo- (meaning a thousand times)
- A fifth prefix, deci- (meaning tenth), is used in laboratory reports.

➤ Memorize the prefixes and their meanings.

Study Table 3-1, and note the numerical values and relationships. Metric prefixes are combined with bases to create new quantities, as shown in the examples in the table.

TABLE 3-1 Metric Measurements, Prefixes, Values, and Meaning

Prefix	Multiplier	Exponential Power of 10	Meaning	Examples	Meaning
micro- (mc)	.000001	10^{-6}	millionth part of	microgram (mcg)	one millionth of a gram
milli- (m)	.001	10^{-3}	thousandth part of	milliliter (mL)	one thousandth of a liter
				milligram (mg)	one thousandth of a gram
centi- (c)	.01	10^{-2}	hundredth part of	centimeter (cm)	one hundredth of a meter
deci- (d)	.1	10^{-1}	tenth part of	deciliter (dL)	one tenth of a liter
kilo- (k)	1000	10^{3}	1000 times	kilogram (kg)	one thousand grams

Note: The prefix value never changes when combined with a base unit (e.g., the prefix *milli* [m] = .001).
1 mm = 0.001 (one thousandth of a meter).
1 mL = 0.001 (one thousandth of a liter).
1 mg = 0.001 (one thousandth of a gram).

Q & A	**ASK YOURSELF**	1	What are the numerical values of the prefixes *m, c, d,* and *k*?
	MY ANSWER		_____

- For review, write out the five prefixes and three base units used for medication administration. Learn them in preparation for analyzing medication orders.

Prefixes and Abbreviations	**Base Units and Abbreviations**
1 _____	1 _____
2 _____	2 _____
3 _____	3 _____
4 _____	
5 _____	

RAPID PRACTICE 3-1   Metric Units and Abbreviations

ESTIMATED COMPLETION TIME: 10 minutes   **ANSWERS ON:** page 96

DIRECTIONS: *Write the metric name and abbreviation in the space provided.*

1 Write the name and abbreviation for the base unit of weight, or mass. _____

2 Write the name for the base unit *m.* _____

3 Write the name and abbreviation for the base unit of length. _____

4 Write the name for the prefix *m.* _____

5 Write the name and abbreviation for the prefix that means $\dfrac{1}{1000}$. _____

6 Write the name and abbreviation for the prefix that means $\dfrac{1}{100}$. _____

7 Write the name and abbreviation for the prefix that means $\dfrac{1}{1,000,000}$. _____

8 Write the name and abbreviation for the prefix that means $\dfrac{1}{10}$. _____

9 Write the name and abbreviation for the prefix that means 1000 times. _____

10 Write the name and abbreviation for the base unit of volume. _____

Writing Metric Units Correctly

Study the examples and note the correct order of writing as follows:

1 Numeral or numerals
2 Space
3 Prefix
4 Base unit

The following are examples of correctly written metric quantities: 100 mg, 1000 mL, 10 L, 250 cm, 2500 mcg, and 150 kg.

EXAMPLES

CLINICAL RELEVANCE

AVOID THE RISK OF MEDICATION ERRORS

- Do not write an *m* to look like a *w* or a *u*.
- Capitalize *L* for *liter*.
- Metric abbreviations are case sensitive.
- Do not close up a *c* so that *cm* looks like *am*.
- Use commas to group numbers with more than three consecutive zeros in groups of three from right to left.
- Do not make up your own metric abbreviations
- Do not pluralize metric abbreviations.
- Use the prefix micro- rather than the Greek letter mu (μ) in handwritten medical records. A handwritten μg (microgram) can be mistaken for mg (milligram). May use abbreviation mcg or write out "microgram."

Guide to Metric Notation	Examples
Abbreviations are always used when accompanied by a number. The number, followed by a space, precedes the abbreviation.	10 mg, 2 g, 5 L Metric terms are written out when unaccompanied by a number, as illustrated in the following sentence: "Write out grams and milligrams."
When the number of units following the slash meaning *per* is 1, the number 1 may be omitted from the abbreviation. It is implied.	40 mg per liter, not 40 mg per 1 liter
Metric *abbreviations* are always singular. They are *not* plural.	*Milligrams* is abbreviated *mg*. *Liters* is abbreviated *L*. Write *mg*, not *mgs; g*, not *gs*; and *L*, not *Ls*.
There is no period after metric abbreviations except when they fall at the end of a sentence.	Give 2 mg, not 3 mg. He drank 2 L of water, followed by 1 L.

Slashes appear in many drug and laboratory references. The nurse must be able to interpret them. Do not write them. They have been mistaken for the number one (1). The word "per" is to be written out instead of a slash. Refer to the ISMP list of symbols that lead to medication errors on p. 114.

RAPID PRACTICE 3-2   Metric Measurements

ESTIMATED COMPLETION TIME 5 to 10 minutes   **ANSWERS ON:** page 96

DIRECTIONS: *Write the metric measurement in the space provided.*

1   Which prefix shown in Table 3-1 equals $\frac{1}{100}$ of the base unit? _____

2   Write the names and abbreviations for the three base units in the metric system. _____ ; _____ ; _____.

3   If a laboratory report indicated that a blood sugar level was 80 mg/dL, how would that quantity be written out and read aloud? _____

4   Which prefix shown in Table 3-1 equals 1000 times the base unit? _____

5   Write out the name and abbreviation for the base unit that is capitalized so that it will not be confused with the number 1. _____ ; _____

RAPID PRACTICE 3-3 | Metric Abbreviations

ESTIMATED COMPLETION TIME: 3 minutes   **ANSWERS ON:** page 96

DIRECTIONS: *Circle the recommended abbreviation for the metric units of measurement.*

1 Milligrams
- **a.** mgm
- **b.** mg
- **c.** Mgs
- **d.** mcg

2 Milliliters
- **a.** m
- **b.** mL
- **c.** mg
- **d.** mLs

3 Liters
- **a.** L
- **b.** l
- **c.** ls
- **d.** Ls

4 Grams
- **a.** gr
- **b.** gms
- **c.** G
- **d.** g

5 Micrograms
- **a.** μg
- **b.** mg
- **c.** mcg
- **d.** mc

RAPID PRACTICE 3-4 | Metric Measurements

ESTIMATED COMPLETION TIME: 5 minutes   **ANSWERS ON:** page 96

DIRECTIONS: *Write the recommended abbreviation for the metric unit in the space provided.*

1 Milliliter _____   **4** Kilogram _____

2 Milligram _____   **5** Millimeter _____

3 Microgram _____

---

1 Are there 100 or 1000 cm in a meter?

_____

2 Are there 100 or 1000 mg in a gram?

_____

3 Are there 10 or 100 dL in a liter?

_____

ASK YOURSELF Q & A

MY ANSWER

RAPID PRACTICE 3-5	Metric Base Units

ESTIMATED COMPLETION TIME: 5 minutes   **ANSWERS ON:** page 96

DIRECTIONS: *Write the metric base units in the correct form in the space provided.*

1 Which metric base unit abbreviation would be added to the prefix *m* in a measurement of drug weight? _____

2 Which metric base unit abbreviation would be added to the prefix *m* in a measurement of fluids consumed? _____

3 Which metric base unit abbreviation would be added to the prefix *k* in a measurement of current weight? _____

4 Which metric base unit abbreviation presented in this chapter must be capitalized? _____

5 Which metric base unit abbreviation would be added to the prefix *c* in a measurement of the length of a scar? _____

Q & A   **ASK YOURSELF**   1   The average American consumes about 3700 mg (3.7 g) of sodium per day. Intake should be about 1 tsp table salt a day (2300 mg, or 2.3 g) of sodium. Approximately how many grams of sodium do you consume on an average day?

     MY ANSWER   _____

➤ To accelerate mastery of the metric system, begin to THINK METRIC. Read the labels on food, beverages, medicines, and vitamins to speed up the learning of the uses of *g* and *mg*.

Equivalent Metric Measurements of Weight (Mass)

Memorize: 1000 mcg = 1 mg   1000 mg = 1 g   1000 g = 1 kg

CLINICAL RELEVANCE

- In clinical agencies, the kilogram is used for weight reporting and dose calculations. At birth the average baby weighs 3200 g, or 3.2 kg (approximately 7 lb). Low-birth-weight infants are those who weigh ≤2500 g (2.5 kg, or 5.5 lb) at birth.
- Many drug doses are ordered and adjusted on the basis of kilogram weight. Oral medications contain large ranges of doses in milligrams, such as 0.5 mg, 50 mg, 100 mg, 250 mg, or 500 mg. Doses of some oral medications are very small, such as those found in Synthroid (0.175 mg, or 175 mcg). The smaller the dose, the greater the risk of harm should a medication error occur.

RAPID PRACTICE 3-6 **Metric Unit Identification**

ESTIMATED COMPLETION TIME: 3 minutes   **ANSWERS ON:** page 96

DIRECTIONS: *Circle the metric unit(s) dose on the front of each of the labels, as shown in problem 1.*

1

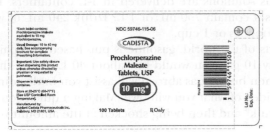

2

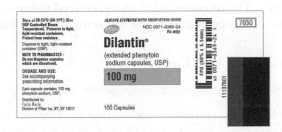

3

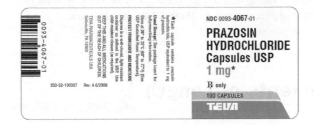

4   Some medications, particularly antibiotics, are supplied in grams.

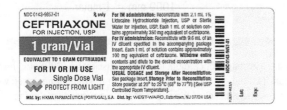

5

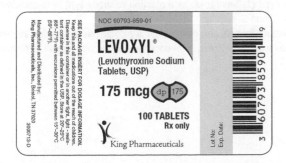

Equivalent Metric Measurements of Volume

Memorize: 1000 mL = 1 L

The volume of a liter is slightly greater than a quart (1 L = 1.06 qt, 1 qt = 0.9 L). Many intravenous solutions are delivered in 1-L containers. Examine a water or soda bottle. Does it contain 750 mL or 1 L? Drink 240 mL of water several times a day instead of 8 ounces or 1 cup.

In many parts of the world, gasoline is purchased and paid for by the liter. If you normally buy 10 gal, you would buy about 40 L. While this conversion is not exact, using it when buying gas abroad will assist you in deciding how much to buy and give you an idea of what you will owe. Making a quick conversion is safer than saying, "fill the tank" and then being shocked at the amount you owe.

➤ The abbreviation for cubic centimeter (cc) is often written to indicate milliliters (mL). The recommended and preferred abbreviation for milliliter is mL because cc has been misread as two zeros (00), resulting in medication errors.

➤ *Interpret* 1 cc as 1 mL. *Write* 1 mL.

CLINICAL RELEVANCE

In clinical agencies, liquids are usually ordered and supplied in milliliters and liters. When calculating liquid dose problems, the answer should be in milliliters. A special calibrated medicine teaspoon holds 5 mL of fluid. Plastic liquid medicine cups, referred to as *ounce cups,* hold 30 mL, which is approximately 1 oz. **Think *30 mL* for an ounce.**

Equivalent Metric Measurements of Length

Memorize:
10 mm = 1 cm
100 cm = 1 meter
1000 mm = 1 meter

CLINICAL RELEVANCE

- When you are assisting with cardiopulmonary resuscitation (CPR), it is helpful to know that fully dilated pupils (10 mm, or 1 cm) can indicate that the patient has been without oxygen for more than 4 minutes. Assessment of the pupils of the eye provides a clue as to a patient's response to CPR.
- The pinpoint pupil (1-2 mm) may be a reaction to strong light or to certain narcotics or other medications (Figure 3-1).
- Familiarity with millimeters and centimeters is also helpful in gauging the length of specified areas, such as wounds or scars, or in documenting the application of ointments in the clinical setting.

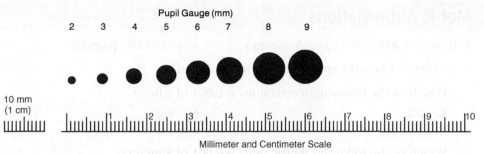

FIGURE 3-1 Pupil gauge in millimeters.

ASK YOURSELF **Q & A**

1 What is the width of a friend's, family member's, or friendly pet's eye pupil in millimeters? (Caution: Do not place the ruler on the eye or face.)

MY ANSWER

_____

2 Do you have any arm scars, freckles, or skin lesions you can measure in millimeters and/or centimeters? If so, what is the length?

_____

3 What is your height in centimeters? Multiply your height in inches by 2.5 (2.5 cm = approximately 1 inch).

_____

4 If you had to put 10 mm of ointment on a wound, how many centimeters would you need?

_____

- Once you have established some personal landmarks in millimeters and centimeters, you can estimate the size of skin lesions at the bedside by comparing them with your own landmarks without searching for a ruler.
- Topical prescription ointments usually supply paper tape rulers when exact measurements are needed.
- Note that some ointments such as nitroglycerin may be prescribed and measured in inches. A paper tape ruler is supplied.

CLINICAL RELEVANCE

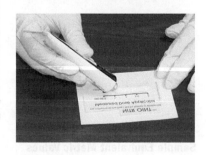

Metric Abbreviations

ESTIMATED COMPLETION TIME: 5 minutes   **ANSWERS ON:** page 96

DIRECTIONS: *Circle the correct units of measurement.*

1 Which of the following metric units is 0.001 of a liter?
   a. mL   **c.** mg
   b. kL   **d.** 1 L

2 Which of the following metric units is 0.001 of a meter?
   a. millimeter   **c.** milligram
   b. centimeter   **d.** kilometer

3 Which of the following metric units is a measure of mass or weight?
   a. g   **c.** L
   b. m   **d.** cc or mL

4 The three *base* units of measurement, noted correctly, in the metric system are
   a. c, k, m   **c.** cm, mL, g
   b. g, l, m   **d.** g, L, m

5 Which of the following metric units is a measure of liquid volume?
   a. mg   **c.** mL
   b. cm   **d.** mcg

Q & A   **ASK YOURSELF**   1   What is the recommended abbreviation for the unit *microgram?*

          MY ANSWER   _____

➤ Metric measurements do *not* require *conversions* within the system. The prefixes *c, m,* and *k* denote the *equivalent* amount in powers of 10.

Metric Equivalents

Weight (Mass)	Volume	Length
1000 mcg = 1 mg	1000 mL = 1 L	1000 mm = 1 m
1000 mg = 1 g		100 cm = 1 m
1000 g = 1 kg		10 mm = 1 cm

After you learn the major equivalent values, you can infer equivalent values for quarters, halves, and one and a half. You can obtain metric equivalents by moving the decimal place.

Sample Equivalent Metric Values

Row	Length	Volume	Volume	Weight	Weight	Weight	Weight	Weight	Weight
A	10 mm	500 mL	1000 mL	1000 mcg	250 mg	500 mg	1000 mg	1500 mg	1000 g
B	1 cm	0.5 L	1 L	1 mg	0.25 g	0.5 g	1 g	1.5 g	1 kg

➤ Do not confuse micrograms with milligrams. Note the difference in value between 1 mcg and 1 mg. The metric system uses only decimals for numbers less than 1. Note the leading zeros in front of decimals and the elimination of trailing zeros after numbers.

Use the examples in the table above to answer the following questions:

1   Can you identify the base unit in each abbreviation?

_____

2   Can you identify the numerical value (e.g., $\frac{1}{10}$ or $\frac{1}{1000}$) of the prefix (e.g., *milli-, centi-, micro-,* or *kilo-*) when you read them in an abbreviation?

_____

3   Can you distinguish when to read *m* as *meter* and when to read *m* as *milli-*? One is a prefix, and the other is a base. Which would be placed on the left and which would be placed on the right?

_____

4   Which dimension (weight or volume) does milliliter measure?

_____

Converting Milligrams to Grams and Grams to Milligrams

Grams and milligrams are the units most frequently encountered in the administration of tablets and capsules.

Equivalent amounts within units of the metric system are established by moving decimal places to confirm your math.

Conversion factor: 1000 mg = 1 g.

Verifying metric equivalents by moving decimals

➤ To change milligrams to grams, divide milligrams by 1000.

➤ To change grams to milligrams, multiply grams by 1000.

Divide milligrams by 1000 by moving the decimal place (implied or existing) three places to the left: 2500 mg = 2.5 g

Multiply grams by 1000 by moving the decimal place (implied or existing) three places to the right: 2.5 g = 2500 mg

EXAMPLES

How many milligrams are in 1.5 grams?

Conversion factor: 1000 mg = 1 g

Step 1	:	Step 2	×	Step 3	=	Answer
Desired Answer Units	:	Starting Factor	×	Given Quantity and Units	=	× Units
mg	:	$\dfrac{1000 \text{ mg}}{1 \text{ g}}$	×	$\dfrac{1.5 \text{ g}}{1}$	=	1500 mg
				Cancel units.		
				Stop and check setup.		

The final equation will be written like this:

mg	:	$\dfrac{1000 \text{ mg}}{1 \text{ g}}$	×	$\dfrac{1.5 \text{ g}}{1}$	=	1500 mg in 1.5 g

Analysis: The simple equation contains the desired answer units and the given information. The selected Starting Factor is in the correct orientation. The given unwanted units, grams, are canceled. A number 1 is placed as a denominator under 1.5 g to hold the 1.5 g in the numerator position. This maintains alignment and helps prevent multiplication errors.

Evaluation: Only mg remain in the answer. My estimate that the number would be 1.5 times 1000 is supported by the answer. (Math check: 1000 × 1.5 = 1500). The equation is balanced.

Refer to Chapter 2 for a more extensive review of DA equations.

FAQ   *How can I decide whether to divide or multiply in order to move the decimal point to the left or the right of a number for metric equivalents?*

ANSWER   The (memorized) equivalent formula (e.g., 1000 mg = 1 g) reveals the direction in which to move the decimal point. Converting milligrams to grams requires division. Converting grams to milligrams requires multiplication. Write out the relevant conversion formulas when taking a test so that they are in front of you for reference until the conversions become automatic.

RAPID PRACTICE 3-8 — Milligram and Gram Equivalents

ESTIMATED COMPLETION TIME: 10 to 20 minutes   ANSWERS ON: page 96

DIRECTIONS: *Fill in the equivalent amount. Insert leading zeros and eliminate trailing zeros. Label the answer using correct notation.*

Grams	Milligrams		Milligrams	Grams
1 2	_____		6 60	_____
2 0.04	_____		7 500	_____
3 0.6	_____		8 1500	_____
4 0.25	_____		9 2000	_____
5 0.125	_____		10 250	_____

RAPID PRACTICE 3-9 — Converting Milligrams to Grams

ESTIMATED COMPLETION TIME: 10 to 15 minutes   ANSWERS ON: page 96

DIRECTIONS: *Determine the metric equivalent dose and move the decimal places accordingly. Insert leading zeros and remove trailing zeros from the answer. Confirm your answer with a DA equation.*

1   The physician ordered 2.5 g of a medication. What is the equivalent dose in milligrams? _____

DA equation:

2   The physician ordered 60 mg of a medication. What is the equivalent dose in grams? _____

DA equation:

3 The physician ordered 0.15 g of a medication. What is the equivalent dose in milligrams? _____

DA equation:

4 The physician ordered 4 g of a medication. What is the equivalent dose in milligrams? _____

DA equation:

5 The physician ordered 500 mg of a medication. What is the equivalent dose in grams? _____

DA equation:

FAQ   *Why verify these decimal movements with a DA-style equation?*

ANSWER   Both methods require practice. Moving decimals gives an estimate. Mastery of a verification method for backup proof of any calculation is essential. If a nurse practices and masters DA with some simple equations, the more complex conversions requiring DA will be simple also.

RAPID PRACTICE 3-10   Metric Equivalents

ESTIMATED COMPLETION TIME: 5 minutes   **ANSWERS ON:** page 96

DIRECTIONS: *Circle the correct metric equivalent for the amount presented.*

1 Ordered: 50 mg
   a. 0.05 g   **b.** 50 g   **c.** 500 g   **d.** 5000 g

2 Ordered: 400 mg
   a. 0.04 g   **b.** 0.4 g   **c.** 40 g   **d.** 4000 g

3 Ordered: 1.6 g
   a. 1600 mg   **b.** 160 mg   **c.** 1.6 mg   **d.** 0.016 mg

4 Ordered: 0.2 g
   a. 0.002 mg   **b.** 0.02 mg   **c.** 200 mg   **d.** 2000 mg

5 Ordered: 0.04 g
   a. 0.004 mg   **b.** 0.04 mg   **c.** 4 mg   **d.** 40 mg

Examining Micrograms

The metric equivalents of micrograms are as follows:

$$1000 \text{ mcg} = 1 \text{ mg}$$

$$1{,}000{,}000 \text{ mcg} = 1 \text{ g}$$

Milligrams and grams are among the most common measurements in medications. Of the two, milligrams are used more frequently. In order to avoid errors, it is advisable to avoid using decimals and to select an equivalent that can be stated in whole numbers.

Micrograms are very small units. Microgram and milligram conversions are needed for intravenous calculations and occasionally for very small doses of powerful medications. Just as with milligrams and grams, it is helpful to examine the prefix to determine the equivalent units.

➤ To change micrograms to equivalent milligrams, divide micrograms by 1000.

➤ To change milligrams to equivalent micrograms, multiply milligrams by 1000.

RAPID PRACTICE 3-11 | Converting Micrograms, Milligrams, and Grams

ESTIMATED COMPLETION TIME: 10 minutes   **ANSWERS ON:** page 96

DIRECTIONS: *Fill in the equivalent metric measure in the spaces provided by moving decimal points.*

MILLIGRAMS TO MICROGRAMS		MILLIGRAMS TO GRAMS		MICROGRAMS TO MILLIGRAMS	
mg	mcg	mg	g	mcg	mg
1 0.5	_____	6 600	_____	11 2500	_____
2 2	_____	7 _____	0.001	12 20,000	_____
3 0.15	_____	8 _____	0.03	13 1500	_____
4 0.6	_____	9 _____	0.4	14 300	_____
5 1.8	_____	10 5000	_____	15 5000	_____

➤ Write numbers, commas, and decimals neatly, to avoid errors.

CLINICAL RELEVANCE

As with mastering arithmetic, mastery of the metric system frees precious time for other priorities, such as

- Patient and medical record assessments
- Patient and family communications
- Medication preparation and administration
- Clinical theory
- Patient treatments
- Documentation in the patient record

RAPID PRACTICE 3-12	Identification of Metric Units

ESTIMATED COMPLETION TIME: 10 minutes   **ANSWERS ON:** page 97

DIRECTIONS: *Fill in the full word or approved abbreviation for the metric units in the space provided.*

	Approved Abbreviation			Full Word
1 kilometer	_____		**6** mg	_____
2 deciliter	_____		**7** mcg	_____
3 kilogram	_____		**8** cm	_____
4 liter	_____		**9** mm	_____
5 meter	_____		**10** mL	_____

RAPID PRACTICE 3-13	Metric Equivalents

ESTIMATED COMPLETION TIME: 10 minutes   **ANSWERS ON:** page 97

DIRECTIONS: *Convert to equivalent metric units by moving decimal places.*

1 1 g = _____ mg		**6** 2.5 g = _____ mg
2 1 kg = _____ g		**7** 1 g = _____ mcg
3 500 mg = _____ g		**8** 1 cm = _____ mm
4 1 L = _____ mL		**9** 1 mg = _____ mcg
5 2500 mg = _____ g		**10** 500 mcg = _____ mg

Milliequivalents (mEq)

FAQ   *What is a milliequivalent (mEq), and what is the difference between a milliequivalent and a milligram (mg)?*

ANSWER   The milliequivalent is another way of expressing the contents of a medication in solution. A milliequivalent is the number of grams of solute in 1 mL of solution. Milligrams are a measure of *weight*.

Solutions of electrolytes, such as potassium, sodium, and magnesium, are usually ordered and supplied in numbers of mEq/mL or mEq/L. The medication label may also state the amount of milligrams of drug contained in the product.

➤ Milligrams and milliequivalents are not equivalent.

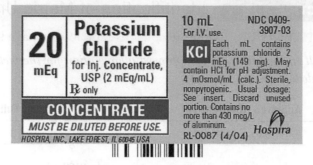

FIGURE 3-2 Potassium chloride label.

CLINICAL RELEVANCE

Many intravenous solutions contain electrolytes. The sample medication label in Figure 3-2 includes both milliequivalents and milligrams. In small print, the label lists 2 mEq (149 mg).

➤ When interpreting the label shown in Figure 3-2, it is important for the nurse to recognize that 2 mEq *cannot be substituted for* 149 mg in dose calculations.

Other Medication Measurement Systems

Household Measurements

Most people are familiar with household (kitchen) measurement terms. It is important to realize that household utensils are usually not calibrated precisely. There are small and large teaspoons and tablespoons, cups, and glasses. Medicines taken at home should be taken with metric-calibrated droppers, measuring teaspoons, and cups. Patients and their families need instruction about the use of precisely calibrated measuring devices before being discharged from the hospital. (Refer to Table 3-2.)

Apothecary System

The imprecise older apothecary system of weights and measures has been replaced by the metric system for medication measurements. Refer to Appendix E for a brief explanation. Refer to The Joint Commission recommendations for apothecary units' future inclusion in the Official "Do Not Use" list on p. 111.

Compare the metric and household systems in Table 3-2.

TABLE 3-2 Comparison of Metric and Household Liquid Measurements Used for Medications

Metric	Household
1 mL	20 drops
5 mL	1 teaspoon (tsp)
15 mL	1 tablespoon (tbs) (3 tsp) (½ oz)
30 mL	2 tablespoons (1 oz)
240 mL	1 measuring cup (8 oz)
500 mL	1 pint (16 oz)
1000 mL (1 L)	1 quart (32 oz)
4 L	1 gallon (gal) (4 quarts)

Note: All household equivalents are approximate.
Use metric for medications.

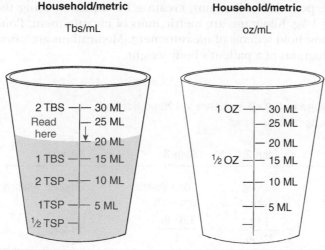

FIGURE 3-3 Household and metric liquid measuring containers. (From Brown M, Mulholland J: *Drug calculations: ratio and proportion problems for clinical practice,* ed 11, St Louis, 2020, Elsevier.)

Interpret 1 cc (cubic centimeter) = 1 mL (milliliter)

Write 1 mL

The handwritten abbreviation cc can easily misread as two zeros (00), resulting in a medication error. Example: When written poorly, 1 cc might be interpreted to read 100. When giving this as a medication, the patient might receive 100 times the dose that was ordered.

CLINICAL RELEVANCE

Household and metric liquid measuring containers

➤ Syringes, calibrated medicine cups, and calibrated droppers are used in clinical practice to prepare small amounts of liquid doses (Figure 3-3).

ASK YOURSELF

MY ANSWER

1 If an order calls for 1 tsp of cough medicine, how many milliliters will the nurse prepare?

2 If an order calls for 1 tbs of a laxative, how many calibrated teaspoons will the nurse prepare?

3 If an order calls for $\frac{1}{2}$ oz of an antacid, how many milliliters will the nurse prepare?

Converting pounds to kilograms

➤ Review the required elements of a DA equation

- Desired answer units
- Conversion factors
- Given quantity and units to be converted

To change pounds to kilograms, create a DA equation using the conversion factor 2.2 lb = 1 kg. Kilograms are metric units of measurement. Pounds are units used in the household systems of measurement. Medications are often ordered on the basis of kilograms of a patient's body weight.

EXAMPLES

✴ Communication

A sample communication to clarify an order would be:

"This is Bob Green, RN from fourth-floor east. May I please speak to Dr. X? Hello, Dr. X. I have an order for patient Mary Smith for ferrous sulfate grains v po daily written by you. The medication is available as ferrous sulfate 324 mg. Would you please clarify the dosage and frequency you would like to have given?"

The clarification order is repeated back to the doctor and documented as a telephone physician's order. Telephone orders are taken only when absolutely necessary and require a physician signature within a specified time period, usually 24 to 48 hours.

How many kilograms (kg) are equivalent to 120 pounds (lb)?
Conversion factor: 2.2 lb = 1 kg

Step 1	:	Step 2	×	Step 3	=	Answer
Desired Answer Units	:	Starting Factor	×	Given Quantity and Units	=	Estimate, Multiply, Evaluate
kg	:	$\dfrac{1\ kg}{2.2\ \cancel{lb}}$	×	$\dfrac{120\ \cancel{lb}}{1}$	=	54.5 kg

The final equation will be written like this:

kg	:	$\dfrac{1\ kg}{2.2\ \cancel{lb}}$	×	$\dfrac{120\ \cancel{lb}}{1}$	=	54.5 kg in 120 lb

Analysis: This simple equivalent equation contains the required elements in the correct orientation.

Evaluation: My rough estimate of 60 lb (120 ÷ 2) is supported by the answer. (Math check: 120 ÷ 2.2 = 54.5.) The equation is balanced.

➤ Estimates can help prevent major math errors. The estimate needs verification.

Q & A **ASK YOURSELF**

1 A 150-lb adult weighs 68.2 kg (150 lb ÷ 2.2 rounded to the nearest tenth). What is your weight in kilograms to the nearest tenth? (Divide your weight in pounds by 2.2.)

MY ANSWER _____

RAPID PRACTICE 3-14 ## Metric and Household Equivalents

ESTIMATED COMPLETION TIME: 5 minutes   **ANSWERS ON:** page 97

DIRECTIONS: *Using Table 3-2, supply the correct approximate metric or household equivalent.*

1 How many milliliters are there in an 8 oz cup? _____

2 How many milliliters are in 2 tsp? _____

3 How many milliliters are in half an ounce? _____

4 How many milliliters are in a tablespoon? _____

5 How many mL are in 2 tbs? _____

➤ Use metric. Clarify any unclear orders with the prescribers and/or the pharmacist.

➤ Document the clarification in the medical record.

Key Points About the Measurement Systems

- The metric system uses Arabic numerals and decimals.
- The metric system basic unit for weight (mass) is the gram.
- Use only approved abbreviations to avoid misinterpretation.
- The metric system measures *liquids* in milliliters and liters.
- Household measurements have many implications for patient discharge teaching. Kitchen utensils are not calibrated for medicines.
- A teaspoon order for medication doses must be calibrated for 5-mL capacity.
- A tablespoon order is for 15 mL (3 calibrated tsp) or $\frac{1}{2}$ of a calibrated medication 30-mL cup.
- An ounce is 30 mL (2 measuring tbs). Teach patients to use equipment supplied with the medication or calibrated ounce measurement cups at home. Do not substitute liquor "shot" glasses for ounce cups at home.
- The milliliter is the preferred metric unit for liquid measurements. The abbreviation *mL* has been used interchangeably with *cc* (the abbreviation for cubic centimeters) by some prescribers. Write mL. Do not write cc.
- A liter is a little more than a quart. Liters are used in clinical agencies. Quarts are not.
- If the l in lb is written next to the number without a space (e.g., 2.2 lb), it may be misread as the number 1.
- Think metric, but be prepared to see occasional orders that are unclear. Verify the equivalent measurement with the pharmacy or the prescriber. Never guess.
- Knowing the value of the difference between a microgram, a milligram, and a gram is critical.
- Knowing that a milliequivalent is not a milligram is critical.
- Hospital policy may require that the prescriber be contacted for use of nonmetric terms and unapproved abbreviations.

Nurses must learn the metric system in order to read and interpret the orders written by health care prescribers, medication labels, and medical literature. Nurses must master and become comfortable using the metric units employed to administer medications. A nurse who has committed the relevant metric system terminology and values to memory and understands the system will never have to say, "I thought *mg* and *mcg* were the same thing," after administering a dosage that was a thousand-fold (thousand-times) error.

CLINICAL RELEVANCE

Examples of errors in the clinical setting include the following:*
- Giving 10 mL of a liquid drug instead of 10 mg
- Converting 1 g to 100 mg instead of 1000 mg, a ten-fold error
- Giving 20 mg instead of 200 mg for a 0.2 g order, a ten-fold error
- Reading 100U as 1000 because *units* was not spelled out or a space was not left between the number and the *U*, or the *U* was closed and looked like a zero, resulting in a ten-fold overdose
- Reading 7.5 mg as 75 mg because the decimal was not seen
- Reading 100 mEq as 100 mg, two very different measurements

*For more examples of errors refer to Appendix D.

➤ Table 3-3 lists some recommendations on how to avoid metric abbreviation errors.

➤ For the TJC "Do Not Use" list, refer to p. 111.

➤ For the ISMP list of Error-Prone Abbreviations, Symbols, and Dose Designations, refer to pp. 111–114.

TABLE 3-3	Metric Abbreviations That May Generate Errors		
Unit	Abbreviation to Use	Abbreviations to Avoid	Potential Errors
milliliter(s)	mL	cc (cubic centimeter), ccs, mls	Misread when written poorly; *L* for *liter* capitalized to prevent misreading as the number 1; metric abbreviations not pluralized
gram(s)	g	gm, gms, gs, G, Gs	Misread when poorly written; should not be capitalized or pluralized
microgram(s)	mcg	μg, μgs, μ	Misread as *mg* (milligram) or zero (0)
milligram(s)	mg	mgm, mgms	Misread as microgram
Units	Write out Units (do not abbreviate)	U,* u*	Misread as zero (0)
International Units	Write out Interna-tional Units (do not abbreviate)	IU*	Misread as the number 10

*Metric units included in TJC's "Do Not Use" list since January 1, 2004. Their use has been banned in clinical agency handwritten medical records. Refer to pp. 111–114 for the complete TJC's "Do Not Use" list and the ISMP list of error-prone abbreviations.

CHAPTER 3 MULTIPLE-CHOICE REVIEW

ESTIMATED COMPLETION TIME: 10-20 minutes   **ANSWERS ON:** page 97

DIRECTIONS: *Circle the correct answer. Verify your math answers with a DA equation.*

1 Select the correct equivalent for 0.5 L.

   a. 50 mL   **c.** 0.5 mL
   b. 500 mL   **d.** 5000 mL

2 Select the correct equivalent for 50 mg.

   a. 5 g   **c.** 0.05 g
   b. 0.5 g   **d.** 0.005 g

3 Select the correct equivalent for 0.2 g:

   a. 2000 mg   **c.** 2 mg
   b. 20 mg   **d.** 200 mg

4 Select the correct equivalent for 0.003 g.

   a. 3 mcg   **c.** 30 mg
   b. 3 mg   **d.** 300 mg

5 Select the correct equivalent for 100 mg.

   a. 1 g   **c.** 0.1 g
   b. 10 g   **d.** 0.05 g

6 The correct abbreviations for metric prefixes are

   a. L, m, g   **c.** mg, mL, cc
   b. m, c, k, mc   **d.** mm, cm, mg, kg

7 Which is the appropriate way to write *units* in the medical record?

  a. Units   **c.** u

  b. U   **d.** U's

8 Select the correct equivalent for 0.25 g.

  a. 2500 mg   **c.** 25 mg

  b. 250 mg   **d.** 2.5 mg

9 Select the correct equivalent for 3 kg.

  a. 1 g   **c.** 3000 g

  b. 3 g   **d.** 30,000 g

10 Select the correct equivalent for 3500 g.

  a. 3.5 kg   **c.** 3500 kg

  b. 350 kg   **d.** 35 kg

CHAPTER 3   FINAL PRACTICE

ESTIMATED COMPLETION TIME: 15 to 20 minutes   **ANSWERS ON:** page 97

1 Write out the three approved base units and the five prefixes, as well as their abbreviations, covered in this chapter.

Base Unit	Abbreviation	Prefix	Abbreviation
a. _____	_____	d. _____	_____
b. _____	_____	e. _____	_____
c. _____	_____	f. _____	_____
		g. _____	_____
		h. _____	_____

2 How many teaspoons are in 2 calibrated tablespoons? _____

DA equation:

3 If you were giving medications in home care, how many milliliters would you prepare for 3 tsp? _____

DA equation:

4 How many pounds are in a kilogram? _____

5 How many grams are in 250,000 mcg? _____

DA equation:

6 How many milliliters are in 1.5 oz of medication? _____

DA equation:

7 If you drank 0.25 L, how many milliliters would you have consumed? _____

DA equation:

8

8.4% SODIUM BICARBONATE

Approx. mL

5 10 15 20 25 30 35 40 45 50

50 mL Single-dose   NDC 0409-3495-16

8.4% SODIUM BICARBONATE

Injection, USP

50 mEq (1 mEq/mL)   ℞ only   Hospira

For I.V. use. Usual dosage: See insert. Sterile, nonpyrogenic.
Discard unused portion.
2 mOsmol/mL (calc.).   pH 8.0 (7.5 to 8.5).   RL-2033 (2/07)

(01) 0 030409 349516 6

Hospira, Inc., Lake Forest, IL 60045 USA

How many milliequivalents (mEq) of sodium bicarbonate are contained
per milliliter (mL) in this vial? _____

9 The physician ordered 0.15 g of a medication. How many milligrams would
be the equivalent? _____ Use the DA method to back up your answer.
Label all work.

DA equation:

10 How many grams are in a kilogram? _____

11 The physician ordered 400 mg of a medication. How many grams would be
the equivalent? _____ Use the DA method to back up your answer. Label
all work.

DA equation:

12 How many medication tablespoons are in 2 ounces? _____

DA equation:

13   * ▶

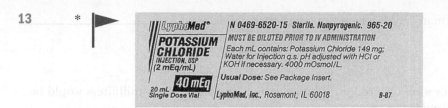

   a. How many milligrams per milliliter of potassium chloride are noted on the label shown above? _____

   b. How many milliequivalents per milliliter of potassium chloride are noted on the label? _____

14 The physician ordered 0.1 g of a medication. How many milligrams would be the equivalent? _____

   DA equation:

15 The physician ordered 0.2 mg of a medication. How many micrograms would be the equivalent? _____

   DA equation:

16 A baby weighs 1.5 kg. How many grams would be the equivalent? _____

   DA equation:

17 If a scar measured 15 mm, how many centimeters would be the equivalent? _____ Use the appropriate conversion formula and DA style method to solve.

   DA equation:

18 How many milligrams are in a medication that contains 1500 mcg? _____

   DA equation:

---

*This red flag is a visual reminder that this drug is on the ISMP high-alert drug list, which means it has a heightened risk to cause harm when used in error. Refer to Appendix B.

19 How many milliliters are in a half-liter (0.5 L)? _____

20 If 2 tbs were ordered for a home-care patient, how many milliliters would be prepared? _____

DA equation:

| CHAPTER 3 | ANSWER KEY |

RAPID PRACTICE 3-1 (p. 75)

1	gram	g		6	centi-	c
2	meter			7	micro-	mc
3	meter	m		8	deci-	d
4	milli-			9	kilo-	k
5	milli-	m		10	liter	L

RAPID PRACTICE 3-2 (p. 76)

1 centi- (c)
2 g = gram; L = liter; m = meter
3 80 milligrams per deciliter
4 kilo- (k)
5 Liter, L

RAPID PRACTICE 3-3 (p. 77)

1	b		4	d
2	b		5	c
3	a			

Note: Metric unit abbreviations are not pluralized.

RAPID PRACTICE 3-4 (p. 77)

1	mL		4	kg
2	mg		5	mm
3	mcg			

RAPID PRACTICE 3-5 (p. 78)

1	g = gram		4	L = liter
2	L = liter		5	m = meter
3	g = gram			

RAPID PRACTICE 3-6 (p. 79)

2 100 mg (milligram)
3 1 mg (milligram)
4 1 g (gram)
5 175 mcg (microgram) (0.175 mg) (milligram)

RAPID PRACTICE 3-7 (p. 82)

1	a		4	d
2	a		5	c
3	a			

RAPID PRACTICE 3-8 (p. 84)

1	2 g = 2000 mg		6	60 mg = 0.06 g
2	0.04 g = 40 mg		7	500 mg = 0.5 g
3	0.6 g = 600 mg		8	1500 mg = 1.5 g
4	0.25 g = 250 mg		9	2000 mg = 2 g
5	0.125 g = 125 mg		10	250 mg = 0.25 g

RAPID PRACTICE 3-9 (p. 84)

1 $mg = \dfrac{1000 \text{ mg}}{1 \text{ g}} \times \dfrac{2.5 \text{ g}}{1} = 2500 \text{ mg}$

2 $g = \dfrac{1 \text{ g}}{1000 \text{ mg}} \times \dfrac{60 \text{ mg}}{1} = 0.06 \text{ g}$

3 $mg = \dfrac{1000 \text{ mg}}{1 \text{ g}} \times \dfrac{0.15 \text{ g}}{1} = 150 \text{ mg}$

4 $mg = \dfrac{1000 \text{ mg}}{1 \text{ g}} \times \dfrac{4 \text{ g}}{1} = 4000 \text{ mg}$

5 $g = \dfrac{1 \text{ g}}{\overset{}{\underset{2}{1000 \text{ mg}}}} \times \dfrac{\overset{1}{500 \text{ mg}}}{1} = 0.5 \text{ g}$

Note: Reduce large numbers to make the calculations easier.

RAPID PRACTICE 3-10 (p. 85)

1	a		4	c
2	b		5	d
3	a			

RAPID PRACTICE 3-11 (p. 86)

	mcg		mg and g		mg
1	500 mcg	6	0.6 g	11	2.5 mg
2	2000 mcg	7	1 mg	12	20 mg
3	150 mcg	8	30 mg	13	1.5 mg
4	600 mcg	9	400 mg	14	0.3 mg
5	1800 mcg	10	5 g	15	5 mg

RAPID PRACTICE 3-12 (p. 87)

1	km	5	m	8	centimeter
2	dL	6	milligram	9	millimeter
3	kg	7	microgram	10	milliliter
4	L				

RAPID PRACTICE 3-13 (p. 87)

1	1000 mg	6	2500 mg
2	1000 g	7	1,000,000 mcg
3	0.5 g	8	10 mm
4	1000 mL	9	1000 mcg
5	2.5 g	10	0.5 mg

RAPID PRACTICE 3-14 (p. 90)

1	240 mL	3	15 mL	5	30 mL
2	10 mL	4	15 mL		

CHAPTER 3 MULTIPLE-CHOICE REVIEW (p. 92)

1	b	5	c	8	b
2	c	6	b	9	c
3	d	7	a	10	a
4	b				

CHAPTER 3 FINAL PRACTICE (p. 93)

1.
   a. meter = m
   b. liter = L
   c. gram = g
   d. kilo- = k
   e. centi- = c
   f. deci- = d
   g. milli- = m
   h. micro- = mc

2. $tsp = \dfrac{3\ tsp}{1\ \cancel{tbs}} \times \dfrac{2\ \cancel{tbs}}{1} = 6\ tsp$

3. $mL = \dfrac{5\ mL}{1\ \cancel{tsp}} \times \dfrac{3\ \cancel{tsp}}{1} = 15\ mL$

4. 2.2 lbs

5. $g = \dfrac{1\ g}{1000\ \cancel{mg}} \times \dfrac{1\ \cancel{mg}}{1000\ \cancel{mcg}} \times \dfrac{250,000\ \cancel{mcg}}{1}$
   $= 0.25\ g$

6. $mL = \dfrac{30\ mL}{1\ \cancel{oz}} \times \dfrac{1.5\ \cancel{oz}}{1} = 45\ mL$

7. $mL = \dfrac{1000\ mL}{1\ \cancel{L}} \times \dfrac{0.25\ \cancel{L}}{1} = 250\ mL$

8. 1 mEq/mL

9. $mg = \dfrac{1000\ mg}{1\ \cancel{g}} \times \dfrac{0.15\ \cancel{g}}{1} = 150\ mg$

Note: The first numerator, mg, matches the described answer units, mg. Only mg remains in the answer.

10. 1000 g

11. $g = \dfrac{1\ g}{1000\ \cancel{mg}} \times \dfrac{400\ \cancel{mg}}{1} = 0.4\ g$

12. $tbs = \dfrac{2\ tbs}{1\ \cancel{oz}} \times \dfrac{2\ \cancel{oz}}{1} = 4\ tbs$

13.
   a. 149 mg per mL
   b. 2 mEq per mL

Note: Potassium chloride is a high-alert medication (see Appendix B).

14. $mg = \dfrac{1000\ mg}{1\ \cancel{g}} \times \dfrac{0.1\ \cancel{g}}{1} = 100\ mg$

15. $mcg = \dfrac{1000\ mcg}{1\ \cancel{mg}} \times \dfrac{0.2\ \cancel{mg}}{1} = 200\ mcg$

16. $g = \dfrac{1000\ g}{1\ \cancel{kg}} \times \dfrac{1.5\ \cancel{kg}}{1} = 1500\ g$

17. $cm = \dfrac{\overset{1}{\cancel{100}}\ cm}{1\ \cancel{m}} \times \dfrac{1\ \cancel{m}}{\underset{10}{1000\ \cancel{mm}}} \times \dfrac{15\ \cancel{mm}}{1}$
    $= \dfrac{15}{10} = 1.5\ cm$

Note: Notice the diagonal direction of the cancelled units.

18. $mg = \dfrac{1\ mg}{10\cancel{00}\ \cancel{mcg}} \times \dfrac{15\cancel{00}\ \cancel{mcg}}{1} = 1.5\ mg$

19. $mL = \dfrac{1000\ mL}{1\ \cancel{L}} \times \dfrac{0.5\ \cancel{L}}{1} = 500\ mL$

20. $mL = \dfrac{15\ mL}{1\ \cancel{tbs}} \times \dfrac{2\ \cancel{tbs}}{1} = 30\ mL$

Suggestions for Further Reading

www.ismp.org
www.jointcommission.org
www.mathforum.org/library

⊖volve   For additional practice problems, refer to the Conversions and Equivalents section of the Elsevier's Interactive Drug Calculation Application, Version 1 on Evolve.

Chapter 4 incorporates the material that has been learned in Chapters 1 through 3—arithmetic, metric units, mental math, and dimensional analysis—and applies that knowledge to interpretation of medication orders, drug labels, and health records.

4 Patient Records, Medication Orders, and Medication Labels

OBJECTIVES

- Interpret medication orders and labels correctly.
- Identify abbreviations that cannot be used for handwritten medical records.
- Identify abbreviations that can lead to medication errors.
- Utilize The Joint Commission (TJC) and Institute for Safe Medication Practices (ISMP) medication-related recommendations.
- Interpret time using the 24-hour clock.
- Interpret Medication Administration Records (MARs and eMARS).
- Describe medication-related nurse actions that can lead to medication errors.
- Identify patients' rights.

ESTIMATED TIME TO COMPLETE CHAPTER: 2 hours

Health care records now come in a variety of formats. Some facilities continue to have hard copy, and even handwritten records. Most acute care facilities have eliminated paper and have gone to an electronic health care record. Many have some paper and some electronic, a hybrid health care record. Nurses must be able to work with a variety of health care records while maintaining accuracy and ensuring error-free medication administration.

Physicians and other health care providers may order medication and treatments on the Physician's Orders or Health Care Provider Orders page by one of the following methods:

1 Entering the orders directly into the patient's electronic health record (via a computer), or

2 Handwriting the orders in the patient's medical record (a paper chart)

Medication orders are either handwritten or directly entered into the computer by the prescriber. The pharmacy uses these orders to formulate the patient's database that generates the medication administration record (MAR) that nurses use to administer the medications. The MAR can be a hard copy, or if it is electronic it is sometimes known as an eMAR. The nurse must check the complete written order against the MAR and the label on the medication supplied. If there is any question regarding the order, the prescriber or the pharmacist must be contacted. The following are just a few examples of the types of questions that may be raised that would require further clarification of a medication order:

- Dose was unusually high or low compared with the usual dose or safe dosage range (SDR)
- Drug would generally be contraindicated for the patient's condition
- Patient states that he or she has an allergy to the drug
- Drug is not compatible with other medications the patient is currently taking
- Patient is not physically able to take the medication by the route it was ordered
- Drug is not available in the strength that was ordered

- Handwriting is unclear, or nurse is unsure what order says
- Drug is not available

The pharmacy most often dispenses unit-dose (single-serving) packages labeled in metric system measurements. The pharmacy delivers the medications to the nursing unit in one of two ways:

1   A wide variety of medications are placed in a locked cabinet that contains many drawers and compartments that are controlled by a central computer. It serves as a "mini-pharmacy" so that most of the commonly used drugs are readily accessible to the nurse without having to make a trip to the pharmacy to obtain them. The computer is programmed to know its contents, and also contains the database of all of the patients and their current medication orders. Every time the nurse needs to give a medication, the patient's name is entered, and the patient's medication profile is accessed requiring specific selection by the nurse. The cabinet then unlocks the drawer(s) that contain the correct medication and correct dosage. The computer issues a warning or may even deny access to the drug if it is not ordered or is not within the correct time frame.

2   Unit-dose medications are placed in individually labeled patient drawers that are kept in a locked medication cart. Generally the pharmacy only places enough doses in the patient drawer for a 24-hour period, and they are generally restocked every 24 hours at a set time every day. This minimizes the chance of large overdoses.

There is potential for error in each step of the medication process: the medication order, the medication record, the supplied medication and its label, and the preparation and administration. The nurse who administers the medication is legally responsible to administer the right drug, the right dosage, to the right patient, via the right route, at the right time, and to document it correctly. The nurse should know the patient, the patient's diagnosis, the appropriate (as well as inappropriate) drugs for use with the diagnosis, and the safe dosage ranges. The nurse can be held legally responsible for medications given, even if the order was in error or the dose supplied by the pharmacy was in error if it is determined that the nurse should have been able to recognize that the patient should not have received it. The nurse provides the final protection for the patient in the medication chain.

VOCABULARY

Adverse Drug Event (ADE)	A medication-related event that causes harm to a patient. Can be caused by improper label, prescription, dispensing, administration, among other factors. Refer to http://www.psqh.com/novdec06/librarian.html.
Drug Form	The composition of a drug: liquid or solid; tablet, capsule, or suppository, etc.
Drug Route	The body location where the drug will be administered, e.g., mouth, nasogastric (nose to stomach), vein, muscle, subcutaneous tissue, rectum, or vagina.
FDA	Food and Drug Administration, the federal agency responsible for approving tested drugs for consumer use in the United States.
Generic Drug	*Official* name used for a drug by all companies that produce it. For example, there are many brands and trade names for *acetaminophen,* the *generic* name for Tylenol. *Acetaminophen* is the official name. Tylenol is a brand name.
	Generic drugs are identical or bioequivalent to brand-name drugs in dosage form, safety, strength, route of administration, quality, performance, and intended use.
⚑ High-Alert Medications	High-alert medications are medications that have been identified by the Institute for Safe Medication Practices (ISMP) as those that can cause significant harm to patients when used in error. The icon is a visual reminder to help you become familiar with some of these medications. Refer to the ISMP's list of high-alert medications in Appendix B as you work through the text and prepare patient care plans.

Continued

VOCABULARY—cont'd

MAR	Medication Administration Record, the official record of all medications ordered for and received by each patient during an inpatient visit. It is maintained by nurses. Each page may reflect one or more hospital days.
NKA	No known allergies.
NKDA	No known drug allergies.
OTC Drug	Drug sold and purchased "over the counter" in drugstores, grocery stores, and health food stores without a prescription. Some were formerly required to be dispensed only by prescription and have been released from that requirement by the FDA.
Patent	Official permission from the U.S. Patent Trade Office to market a drug exclusively for 20 years from the time of application. The patent period compensates the first company to market a drug for the costs of drug research and development. After the patent period expires, other manufacturers may apply to sell the generic form of the drug and must meet the same standards as the original company.
Sentinel Event	An unexpected occurrence involving death or serious physical or psychological injury, or the risk thereof. Includes among other, severe adverse drug events (ADE). Refer to www.jointcommission.org/SentinelEvents.
Trade Name	Name assigned to a product by its manufacturer. The symbol ® or ™ written as a superscript after a trade name indicates that the manufacturer has officially registered that name for the product with the U.S. Patent Trade Office. If a trade name is listed on the label, the generic name must also be listed.
24-Hour Clock	System for telling time that begins with 0001 (1 minute after midnight) and ends with 2400 (midnight). Also known as the international clock or military time.
	The 24-hour clock system is used internationally and has been adopted in the United States by many agencies to avoid potential confusion caused by duplication of AM and PM hours (a 12-hour clock).
Unit Dose	Single serving size of a drug (e.g., 250 mg per tablet, 250 mg per 5 mL).
Unit-Dose Packaging	Unit-dose packaging of single servings functions as a safety net. It helps limit the amount of overdose and/or waste that might occur. Refer to Figure 4-3.
Usual Dose	Manufacturer's recommendation for the average dose strength (concentration) that usually achieves the desired therapeutic effect for the target population (e.g., "for adults with fever, 1-2 tablets every 4-6 hours, not to exceed 6 tablets in 24 hours"). Based on clinical trials, the usual dose is often specified by the patient's weight and occasionally by body surface area or age.

Q & A   **ASK YOURSELF**

1   What is the difference between a trade-name product and a generic product and why must the nurse know the difference?

MY ANSWER   _____

2   What are some examples of drug forms?

_____

3   How may unit-dose packaging help prevent a medication error?

_____

4   What is the abbreviation for the medication administration record maintained by the nurses?

_____

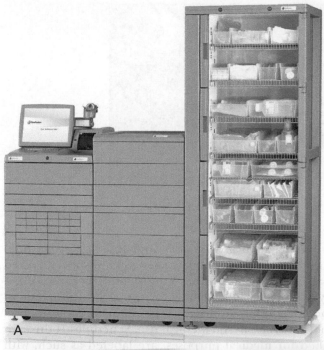

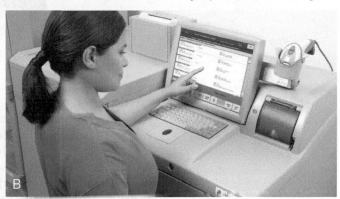

FIGURE 4-1 Completing the seven right of medication administration using the Pyxis MedStation®. **A,** Pyxis MedStation®. **B,** The nurse enters personal security codes or scans a fingerprint to gain access to confidential patient information. The nurse then selects the patient's name and the appropriate medication. **C,** The appropriate drawer(s) are opened and the nurse takes the needed medication. **D,** The nurse scans the medication. If the medication selected is not the correct drug or the correct dosage, the scan will cause the computer to issue a warning stating the reason. (From Becton, Dickinson, and Company, Franklin Lakes, NJ.)

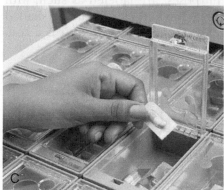

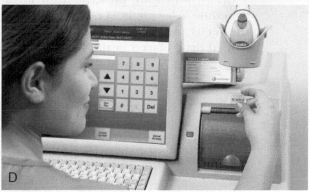

Nurses are now able to enter their medications prior to logging in the Pyxis. They can do this from their assigned computer in an often quieter environment. This reduces the number of mistakes and time at the Pyxis.

Medication Storage and Security

Medications for institutional use are stored in locked cabinets, carts, and drawers (Figure 4-1).

Bar codes are increasingly used to reduce medication errors. The pharmacy enters the patient's drug information, records, and medication orders into a computer. Each dose is bar-coded in the pharmacy. The nurse uses a handheld scanner to scan the drug and the patient's wrist bracelet (Figure 4-2). The computer checks that it is the right medication for the right patient. Unit-dose medications supplied by the pharmacy also reduce medication errors.

To complete the **Nine Rights of Medication Administration** the nurse enters the patient room, and uses at least two methods of identifying the correct patient, i.e., verbal identification and armband scanning identification. The computer will state whether the scan was successful, which indicates that the (1) right drug was scanned, (2) in the right dosage, (3) for the right patient, (4) in the right route, and (5) within the right time frame. The nurse must then ascertain whether the drug is being given for the (6) right reason (based on assesment), (7) that patient receives education about the medication, (8) the patient is offered the right to refuse and (9) administration (or refusal) is documented.

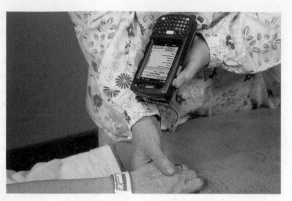

FIGURE 4-2 Bar code reader.

Controlled (scheduled) drugs such as narcotics, opiates, and some non-narcotic drugs such as tranquilizers and anti-anxiety agents, have special locked storage, dispensing, disposal, and documentation requirements because of potential risk for abuse. They are placed in **schedules** by the Drug Enforcement Administration (DEA). Schedule I refers to drugs at the highest risk for abuse, such as crack cocaine and heroin and have no medical use. Schedules II through V drugs, which are prescribed for medical purposes, are labeled as such, with Schedule V having least potential for abuse. Note the C II classification (shaded in green) for morphine on the label below. The C II indicates that it is a controlled drug placed by the DEA on Schedule II.

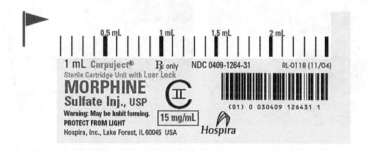

➤ Check your agency storage, disposal, and documentation policies for these high-alert medications.

Medication Forms and Packaging

Medications are supplied in a variety of solid and liquid forms, including granules, tablets, capsules, suppositories, and various liquid preparations. The physician's order must specify the form of the medication. A single medication may be prepared in several forms and marketed and packaged in several single and/or multi-dose sizes. Multidose sizes are convenient for pharmacy and home use (Figure 4-3). At most clinical facilities, the pharmacy packages smaller single-serving-size amounts from the multidose containers to reduce medication errors (Figure 4-4).

Since medications are supplied in a variety of forms to meet patients' needs, it is important to select the form that matches the health care provider's order. This is done by matching the order to the medication label. The orders for medication forms are abbreviated. There is a trend to reduce and/or eliminate abbreviations in medical records.

Refer to Vocabulary in this chapter and Appendix B for a list of high-alert medications.

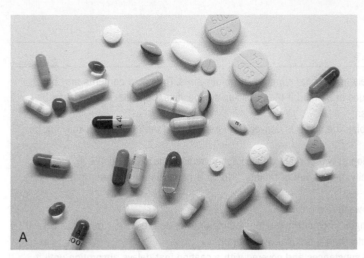

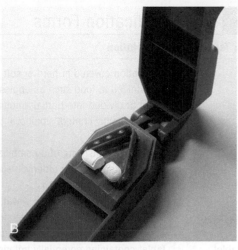

FIGURE 4-3 A, Oral medications come in a variety of forms. **B,** Single-patient use pill cutter for scored tablets.

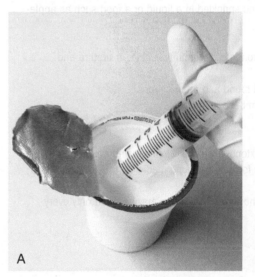

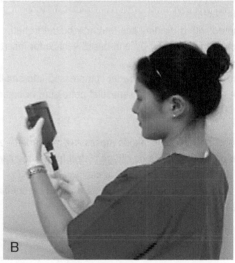

FIGURE 4-4 A, Drawing up liquid medicine in an oral syringe from a unit dose package. **B,** Drawing up liquid oral medicine from a bottle.

Solid Medication Forms

Table 4-1 lists solid medication abbreviations, terms, and forms. Since the nurse must be able to interpret the abbreviations and terms, the contents of Table 4-1 should be memorized.

➤ A single medication may be available as a tablet, a capsule, a gelcap, and an enteric-coated tablet. When there is a choice, the prescriber orders the specific type that is most appropriate for the patient.

➤ Never crush gelcaps, enteric-coated, or other long-acting or slow-release medications.

➤ Only scored tablets are to be cut.

TABLE 4-1	Solid Medication Forms
Abbreviation or Term	**Description**
cap: capsule	Medication covered in hard or soft gelatin. They are supplied in various sizes. The entire contents may be sprinkled in food such as applesauce or a liquid if the physician so specifies. Capsules should never be cut or divided into partial amounts.
caplet	Smooth, lightly coated, small oval tablet. The name is derived from capsule and tablet. It may or may not be scored.
compound	Medication consisting of a combination of two or more drugs. Each ingredient may be available in one or more strengths. The order will specify the number of tablets. If there is more than one strength, the order will specify the strength.
cr: cream	Medication contained within a water-washable base.
DS: double-strength	Dosage of medication is double strength. Does not mean long-acting or extended-release. However, a DS pill probably will be given less frequently than a "regular" counterpart.
enteric-coated tablet (Always write out.)	Tablet containing potentially irritating substances and covered with a coating that delays absorption until it reaches the intestine. This protects the oral, esophageal, and gastric mucosa. Should not be crushed, cut, or chewed. *Enteric* should be written out to avoid misunderstanding.
gelcap, soft-gel	Capsule cover made of a soft gelatin for ease of swallowing.
oral dissolving tablet (ODT)	Tablet that dissolves in the mouth and does not need to be taken with water.
powders and granules	Pulverized fragments of solid medication, to be measured and sprinkled in a liquid or a food such as applesauce or cereal.
scored tablet	Tablets scored with a dividing line that may be cut in half.
supp: suppository	Medication distributed in a glycerin-based vehicle for insertion into the rectum, vagina, or urethra and absorbed systemically.
tab: tablet	Medication combined with a powder compressed into small round and other shapes.
ung: ointment	Medication contained within a semisolid petroleum or cream base.

Medications that delay absorption

CD: controlled-dose	Terms reflecting the use of various processing methods to extend or delay the release and absorption of the medication. They need to be differentiated from a regular form of the same medicine. These medications should not be chewed, crushed, or cut.
CR: controlled release (sustained action)	
LA: long-acting	A regular medication may be ordered, for example, every 4 hours. An XR version may be given only every 12 or 24 hours.
SR: slow-release	
XL: extra-long-acting	
XR: extended-release	

Q & A	**ASK YOURSELF**	1	How is DS different from medications marked XL, XR, CD, and LA?
	MY ANSWER		_____

RAPID PRACTICE 4-1	Solid Medication Forms

ESTIMATED COMPLETION TIME: 5 to 10 minutes   **ANSWERS ON:** page 151

DIRECTIONS: *Study the abbreviations in Table 4-1. Supply the abbreviation that may be seen in the prescriber's orders for the following types of medication.*

1 enteric _____   6 suppository _____

2 long-acting _____   7 controlled dose _____

3 tablet _____   8 ointment _____

4 extra-long-acting _____   9 extended-release _____

5 double-strength _____   10 capsule _____

RAPID PRACTICE 4-2	Solid Medication Forms

ESTIMATED COMPLETION TIME: 5 to 10 minutes   **ANSWERS ON:** page 151

DIRECTIONS: *Study the abbreviations in Table 4-1. Give the requested information pertaining to oral medication forms. Use brief phrases.*

1 Name the only oral medication form that may be *cut* in order to give a half-dosage. _____

2 What is the name for a medication that contains more than one drug, will be ordered by the *quantity* to be given, and may include the strength of each medication within the form supplied? _____

3 Give five abbreviations for *longer-acting* oral medications that would be given less often than a regular medication. _____

4 Name two solid medication forms that should never be chewed, crushed, or cut. _____

5 What is the abbreviation for the kind of oral medication that is packaged in a soft or hard gelatin covering? _____

Liquid Medication Forms

Liquid medication forms are packaged in small prefilled unit-dose-serving containers and larger stock bottles, such as the containers seen for multidose home prescriptions. The liquids are supplied and administered through a variety of routes to the patient in an amount of *milliliters*.

Liquid drug forms are administered using specially calibrated equipment: cups; teaspoons; needles attached to tubing; syringes with needles; needle-less oral syringes; droppers for the mouth, eye, or ear; or tubes for the stomach and intestine. See Figure 4-5 for some examples of oral liquid medication equipment.

Doses of oral liquid medications such as milk of magnesia (MOM) can be supplied in small single-dose packages or larger multidose bottles. As stated in Chapter 3, 5 mL and 15 mL are the equivalents of 1 calibrated teaspoon and 1 calibrated tablespoon, respectively. The manufacturer attempts to provide the usual drug dose for the target population within those two measurements because they are reasonable volumes to swallow.

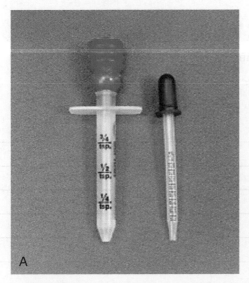
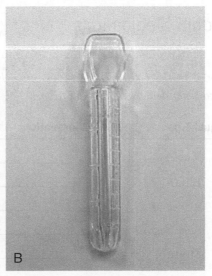

FIGURE 4-5 A, Calibrated medicine droppers. **B,** Calibrated medicine spoon.

Abbreviations appear in most patients' orders and medication records. They may be handwritten or printed. Memorize the abbreviations in Table 4-2.

➤ Manufacturer-supplied equipment provides precise dose measurement.

TABLE 4-2	Liquid Medication Forms
Abbreviation: Term	**Form**
aq: aqueous	Medication supplied in a water-based solution
elix: elixir	Liquid medication sweetened with alcohol (e.g., phenobarbital elixir)
emul: emulsion	A mixture of two liquids, such as oil and water, that normally do not mix
fld: fluid	Of liquid composition
gtt	gtt is an old abbreviation derived from Latin, meaning "drop." Recognize it but do not write it. Write out "drop(s)."
mixt: mixture	Compound medicine consisting of more than one liquid medication
sol: solution	Water-based liquid medication
susp: suspension	Solid particles mixed in liquid that must be gently but thoroughly mixed immediately before administration; should not be shaken vigorously

➤ Liquid forms such as elixirs and suspensions cannot be distinguished without reading the label.

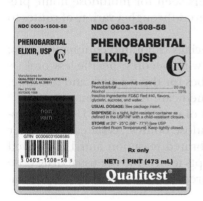
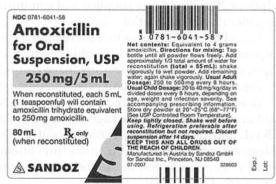

RAPID PRACTICE 4-3	Liquid Medications

ESTIMATED COMPLETION TIME: 5 to 10 minutes   **ANSWERS ON:** page 151

DIRECTIONS: *Using Table 4-2, supply the abbreviations requested if approved. If recommended, write out the term.*

	Liquid Type	**Abbreviation**
1	Solution	_____
2	Elixir	_____
3	Aqueous	_____
4	Suspension	_____
5	Mixture	_____

1   Which of the oral liquid drug forms contains alcohol?

_____

2   Which of the liquid drug forms must be gently and thoroughly mixed before administration?

_____

_____

Medication Routes

Medication routes can be divided into two types:
- Nonparenteral (noninjectable)
- Parenteral (injectable)

➤ The nurse may *not* substitute a different route for the one ordered. Only the prescriber can write and change the medication order.

Nonparenteral routes through which medications are delivered include the following:
- Oral
  - Mouth
  - Buccal and sublingual
- Nasogastric
- Enteric (intestinal)
- Eye and ear
- Gastric
- Rectal
- Skin (topical)
- Vaginal

Several abbreviations are used in medication orders to describe specific nonparenteral routes of administration (Table 4-3). Some of these abbreviations are derived from Latin and Greek. The abbreviations must be learned even though the trend is to write more of them out in English to avoid misinterpretation.

➤ Refer to pp. 111-114 for the ISMP list of error-prone abbreviations and symbols.

 Mnemonic

Associate *O* with *oral* and *N* with *nothing* or *no*. (*NPO* is the abbreviation for the Latin phrase *non per os*, meaning "*nothing by mouth*.")

TABLE 4-3	Nonparenteral Medication Route
Abbreviation or Term	**Route**
Ear and eye (write out)	Right ear or eye
Ear and eye (write out)	Left ear or eye
Ear and eye (write out)	Both ears or eyes
buccal (bucc)	To be dissolved in the cheek, not swallowed
enteric (write out)	Administered through a tube or port to the small intestine
GT	Gastrostomy tube; given through a tube or port directly to the stomach
MDI	Metered dose inhaler
NG (T)	Nasogastric; given through a tube inserted in the nose to the stomach
NPO	Nothing by mouth
PO	Given by mouth
Rectal	Write "per rectum"; do not write "PR" or "R"
SL, subl	Sublingual, meaning "under the tongue"; to be dissolved, not swallowed
Top	Topical, meaning "applied to the skin" (e.g., ointments and lotions)
Vag	Given per vagina

Q & A	ASK YOURSELF	1	What is the difference between NPO and PO?
	MY ANSWER		_____
		2	What is the difference between the buccal and sublingual routes?
			_____

FAQ　　*What kind of problem can occur from administering medication via the wrong route?*

ANSWER　　A student nurse did not interpret the route GT for a medication. The patient was acutely ill and had a gastric tube as well as a tracheostomy tube. The student administered the medication without supervision into the tracheostomy tube. The tracheostomy tube is an airway tube, and the liquid medication went into the patient's lungs. The student must seek supervision when performing unfamiliar procedures.

RAPID PRACTICE 4-4　Nonparenteral Routes

ESTIMATED COMPLETION TIME: 5 to 10 minutes　　　**ANSWERS ON:** page 151

DIRECTIONS: *Study the nonparenteral routes. Supply the abbreviation for the route in the space provided. If an abbreviation is not recommended, be sure to write out the term.*

1　topical _____
2　nothing by mouth _____
3　cheek _____
4　left ear _____
5　gastric tube _____

6　nasogastric _____
7　metered dose inhaler _____
8　vaginal _____
9　sublingual _____
10　by mouth _____

Q & A	ASK YOURSELF	1	What cue will help you remember that *PO* means "by mouth"?
	MY ANSWER		_____
		2	How will you distinguish *subl* and *subcut*?
			_____
		3	How will you distinguish *GT* and *NGT*?
			_____

The routes listed in Table 4-4 are for parenteral, or injectable, medications. Parenteral medications are administered under the skin into soft tissue, muscle, vein, or spinal cord. Memorize the abbreviations and terms in the table.

4　Why should the route for rectal medications be spelled out rather than abbreviated with the letter *R?*
_____

5　How will you distinguish *IV, IVP,* and *IVPB?*
_____

6　What is the abbreviation for the intramuscular route?
_____

7   What is the abbreviation for the intradermal route?

_____

MY ANSWER

8   What is the abbreviation for metered dose *inhaler*?

_____

9   What kind of solution is PN?

_____

TABLE 4-4 Parenteral Medication Route

Abbreviation or Term	Route
epidural	Injected into the epidural space, in the lumbar region
hypo	Hypodermic; injected under the skin; refers to subcutaneous and intramuscular routes
ID	Intradermal; given under the skin in the layer just below epidermis (e.g., skin test)*
IM	Intramuscular, intramuscularly; given into the muscle layer, usually the gluteal muscles, the thigh, or the deltoid
intrathecal	Given into the spinal canal
IV	Intravenous, intravenously; given into vein
IVPB	Intravenous piggyback; given into vein via a small container attached to an established intravenous line
subcut†	Subcutaneous, subcutaneously; given beneath the skin, usually into the fat layer of abdomen, upper arm, or thigh
PN	Parenteral nutrition; nutritional feedings per intravenous line into a large vein

*Do not confuse ID route with the word "identify."
†Do not write SC or Subq for subcutaneous.

Frequency and Times of Medication Administration

Table 4-5 lists abbreviations for terms that denote the frequency and times of medication administration. Memorize the abbreviations in the table.

➤ "Give with food" and "Give after meals" are usually orders for medications that irritate the gastric mucosa.

Refer to the TJC "Do Not Use" list on p. 111.
Refer to the ISMP List of Error-Prone Abbreviations, Symbols, and Dose Designations on pp. 111–114.

➤ "Give 1 hour before meals" and "Give 2 hours after meals" are orders for medications that have reduced absorption if given with food.

> ✳ *Mnemonic*
> tid (three times daily)—"tricycle"
> bid (two times daily)—"bicycle"

---

1   How will you remember to distinguish the abbreviations for *before* and *after* meals?

_____

ASK YOURSELF **Q & A**

MY ANSWER

TABLE 4-5	Medication Frequency and Time
Abbreviation or Term	**Meaning**
ā or a	Before
p̄	After
c̄	With (e.g., with meals)
s̄	Without
ac	Before meals
pc	After meals
ad lib	Give as desired; pertains to fluids and activity, *not* to medication
bid	Two times a day
tid	Three times a day
qid	Four times a day
on call	Give the medication when the x-ray department or the operating room (OR) calls for the patient
prn	As needed
q	Each, every
qh	Every hour
q2h	Every 2 hours
q4h	Every 4 hours
q6h	Every 6 hours
q8h	Every 8 hours
q12h	Every 12 hours
qhs	Every night at bedtime
stat	Immediately and only one dose

Q & A   **ASK YOURSELF**

1 What is the error on the TJC list, Table 4-6 that can occur with abbreviations beginning with a "Q"?

MY ANSWER _____

2 What error can occur with the abbreviation for International Unit?

_____

3 To which kind of specific orders and documentation must the TJC official "Do Not Use" list apply? (see footnote of table, page 111)

_____

4 What does the ISMP List, Table 4-7, recommend about writing of drug names and doses? Numerical doses and unit of measure?

_____

5 What does the ISMP list state about periods following mg or mL abbreviations?

_____

➤ If a medication order contains an abbreviation that has been banned or may be misinterpreted, clarify it with the prescriber. Refer to TJC "Do Not Use" list on p. 111 and the ISMP list of error-prone abbreviations on pp. 111–114.

TABLE 4-6	The Joint Commission Official "Do Not Use" List*	

Do Not Use	Potential Problem	Use Instead
U (unit)	Mistaken for "0" (zero), the number 4 (four) or "cc"	Write "unit"
IU (International Unit)	Mistaken for IV (intravenous) or the number 10 (ten)	Write "International Unit"
Q.D., QD, q.d., qd (daily)	Mistaken for each other	Write "daily"
Q.O.D., QOD, q.o.d., qod (every other day)	Period after the Q mistaken for "I" and the "O" mistaken for "I"	Write "every other day"
Trailing zero (X.0 mg)†	Decimal point is missed	Write X mg
Lack of leading zero (.X mg)		Write 0.X mg
MS	Can mean morphine sulfate or magnesium sulfate	Write "morphine sulfate"
MSO_4 and $MgSO_4$	Confused for one another	Write "magnesium sulfate"

ADDITIONAL ABBREVIATIONS, ACRONYMS, AND SYMBOLS (FOR POSSIBLE FUTURE INCLUSION IN THE OFFICIAL "DO NOT USE" LIST)		
Do Not Use	**Potential Problem**	**Use Instead**
> (greater than)	Misinterpreted as the number "7" (seven) or the letter "L"	Write "greater than"
< (less than)	Confused for one another	Write "less than"
Abbreviations for drug names	Misinterpreted due to similar abbreviations for multiple drugs	Write drug names in full
Apothecary units	Unfamiliar to many practitioners Confused with metric units	Use metric units
@	Mistaken for the number "2" (two)	Write "at"
cc	Mistaken for U (units) when poorly written	Write "mL" or "ml" or "milliliters" ("mL" is preferred)
μg	Mistaken for mg (milligrams) resulting in 1000-fold overdose	Write "mcg" or "micrograms"

Copyright The Joint Commission, 2010. Reprinted with permission.

*Applies to all orders and all medication-related documentation that is handwritten (including free-text computer entry) or on pre-printed forms.

†**Exception:** A "trailing zero" may be used only where required to demonstrate the level of precision of the value being reported, such as for laboratory results, imaging studies that report size of lesions, or catheter/tube sizes. It may not be used in medication orders or other medication-related documentation.

TABLE 4-7	Error-Prone Abbreviations, Symbols, and Dose Designations

The abbreviations, symbols, and dose designations in the **Table** below were reported to ISMP through the ISMP National Medication Errors Reporting Program (ISMP MERP) and have been misinterpreted and involved in harmful or potentially harmful medication errors. These abbreviations, symbols, and dose designations should **NEVER** be used when communicating medical information verbally, electronically, and/or in handwritten applications. This includes internal communications; verbal, handwritten, or electronic prescriptions; handwritten and computer-generated medication labels; drug storage bin labels; medication administration records; and screens associated with pharmacy and prescriber computer order entry systems, automated dispensing cabinets, smart infusion pumps, and other medication-related technologies.

In the **Table**, error-prone abbreviations, symbols, and dose designations that are included on The Joint Commission's "**Do Not Use**" list (Information Management standard IM.02.02.01) are identified with a double asterisk (**) and must be included on an organization's "**Do Not Use**" list. Error-prone abbreviations, symbols, and dose designations that are relevant mostly in handwritten communications of medication information are highlighted with a dagger (†).

Error-Prone Abbreviations, Symbols, and Dose Designations	Intended Meaning	Misinterpretation	Best Practice
Abbreviations for Doses/Measurement Units			
cc	Cubic centimeters	Mistaken as u (units)	Use mL
IU**	International unit(s)	Mistaken as IV (intravenous) or the number 10	Use unit(s) (International units can be expressed as units alone)
l	Liter	Lowercase letter l mistaken as the number 1	Use L (UPPERCASE) for liter
ml	Milliliter		Use mL (lowercase m, UPPERCASE L) for milliliter

Continued

TABLE 4-7	Error-Prone Abbreviations, Symbols, and Dose Designations—cont'd		
Error-Prone Abbreviations, Symbols, and Dose Designations	Intended Meaning	Misinterpretation	Best Practice
MM or M	Million	Mistaken as thousand	Use million
M or K	Thousand	Mistaken as million	Use thousand
		Mhas beenusedtoabbreviate both million and thousand (M is the Roman numeral for thousand)	
Ng or ng	Nanogram	Mistaken as mg Mistaken as nasogastric	Use nanogram or nanog
U or u**	Unit(s)	Mistaken as zero or the number 4, causing a 10-fold overdose or greater (e.g., 4U seen as 40 or 4u seen as 44) Mistaken as cc, leading to administering volume instead of units (e.g., 4u seen as 4cc)	Use unit(s)
µg	Microgram	Mistaken as mg	Use mcg
Abbreviations for Route of Administration			
AD, AS, AU	Right ear, left ear, each ear	Mistaken as OD, OS, OU (right eye, left eye, each eye)	Use right ear, left ear, or each ear
IN	Intranasal	Mistaken as IM or IV	Use NAS (all UPPERCASE letters) or intranasal
IT	Intrathecal	Mistaken as intratracheal, intratumor, intra-tympanic, or inhalation therapy	Use intrathecal
OD, OS, OU	Right eye, left eye, each eye	Mistaken as AD, AS, AU (right ear, left ear, each ear)	Use right eye, left eye, or each eye
Per os	By mouth, orally	The os was mistaken as left eye (OS, oculus sinister)	Use PO, by mouth, or orally
SC, SQ, sq, or sub q	Subcutaneous(ly)	SC and sc mistaken as SL or sl (sublingual) SQ mistaken as "5 every" The q in sub q has been mistaken as "every"	Use SUBQ (all UPPERCASE letters, without spaces or periods between letters) or subcutaneous(ly)
Abbreviations for Frequency/Instructions for Use			
HS	Half-strength	Mistaken as bedtime	Use half-strength
hs	At bedtime, hours of sleep	Mistaken as half-strength	Use HS (all UPPERCASE letters) for bedtime
o.d. or OD	Once daily	Mistaken as right eye (OD, oculus dexter), leading to oral liquid medications administered in the eye	Use daily
Q.D., QD, q.d., or qd**	Every day	Mistaken as q.i.d., especially if the period after the q or the tail of a handwritten q is misunderstood as the letter i	Use daily
Qhs	Nightly at bedtime	Mistaken as qhr (every hour)	Use nightly or HS for bedtime
Qn	Nightly or at bedtime	Mistaken as qh (every hour)	Use nightly or HS for bedtime
Q.O.D., QOD, q.o.d., or qod**	Every other day	Mistaken as qd (daily) or qid (four times daily), especially if the "o" is poorly written	Use every other day
q1d	Daily	Mistaken as qid (four times daily)	Use daily
q6PM, etc.	Every evening at 6 PM	Mistaken as every 6 hours	Use daily at 6 PM or 6 PM daily

TABLE 4-7	**Error-Prone Abbreviations, Symbols, and Dose Designations—cont'd**			
Error-Prone Abbreviations, Symbols, and Dose Designations	**Intended Meaning**	**Misinterpretation**	**Best Practice**	
SSRI	Sliding scale regular insulin	Mistaken as selective-serotonin reuptake inhibitor	Use sliding scale (insulin)	
SSI	Sliding scale insulin	Mistaken as Strong Solution of Iodine (Lugol's)		
TIW or tiw	3 times a week	Mistaken as 3 times a day or twice in a week	Use 3 times weekly	
BIW or biw	2 times a week	Mistaken as 2 times a day	Use 2 times weekly	
UD	As directed (ut dictum)	Mistaken as unit dose (e.g., an order for "dilTIAZem infusion UD" was mistakenly administered as a unit [bolus] dose)	Use as directed	

Miscellaneous Abbreviations Associated with Medication Use

BBA	Baby boy A (twin)	B in BBA mistaken as twin B rather than gender (boy)	When assigning identifiers to newborns, use the mother's last name, the baby's gender (boy or girl), and a distinguishing identifier for all multiples (e.g., Smith girl A, Smith girl B)
BGB	Baby girl B (twin)	B at end of BGB mistaken as gender (boy) not twin B	
D/C	Discharge or discontinue	Premature discontinuation of medications when D/C (intended to mean discharge) on a medication list was misinterpreted as discontinued	Use discharge and discontinue or stop
IJ	Injection	Mistaken as IV or intrajugular	Use injection
OJ	Orange juice	Mistaken as OD or OS (right or left eye); drugs meant to be diluted in orange juice may be given in the eye	Use orange juice
Period following abbreviations (e.g., mg., mL.)†	mg or mL	Unnecessary period mistaken as the number 1, especially if written poorly	Use mg, mL, etc., without a terminal period

Drug Name Abbreviations

To prevent confusion, avoid abbreviating drug names entirely. Exceptions may be made for multi-ingredient drug formulations, including vitamins, when there are electronic drug name field space constraints; however, drug name abbreviations should NEVER be used for any medications on the *ISMP List of High-Alert Medications* (in Acute Care Settings [www.ismp.org/node/103], Community/Ambulatory Settings [www.ismp.org/node/129], and Long-Term Care Settings [www.ismp.org/node/130]). Examples of drug name abbreviations involved in serious medication errors include:

Antiretroviral medications (e.g., DOR, TAF, TDF)	DOR: doravirine TAF: tenofovir alafenamide TDF: tenofovir disoproxil fumarate	DOR: Dovato (dolutegravir and lamiVUDine) TAF: tenofovir disoproxil fumarate TDF: tenofovir alafenamide	Use complete drug names
APAP	acetaminophen	Not recognized as acetaminophen	Use complete drug name
ARA A	vidarabine	Mistaken as cytarabine ("ARA C")	Use complete drug name
AT II and AT III	AT II: angiotensin II (Giapreza) AT III: antithrombin III (Thrombate III)	AT II (angiotensin II) mistaken as AT III (antithrombin III) AT III (antithrombin III) mistaken as AT II (angiotensin II)	Use complete drug names
AZT	zidovudine (Retrovir)	Mistaken as azithromycin, azaTHIOprine, or aztreonam	Use complete drug name

Continued

TABLE 4-7	Error-Prone Abbreviations, Symbols, and Dose Designations—cont'd		
Error-Prone Abbreviations, Symbols, and Dose Designations	**Intended Meaning**	**Misinterpretation**	**Best Practice**
CPZ	Compazine (prochlorperazine)	Mistaken as chlorpro**MAZINE**	Use complete drug name
DTO	diluted tincture of opium or deodorized tincture of opium (Paregoric)	Mistaken as tincture of opium	Use complete drug name
HCT	hydrocortisone	Mistaken as hydro**CHLORO**thiazide	Use complete drug name
HCTZ	hydro**CHLORO**thiazide	Mistaken as hydrocortisone (e.g., seen as HCT250 mg)	Use complete drug name
MgSO4**	magnesium sulfate	Mistaken as morphine sulfate	Use complete drug name
MS, MSO4**	morphine sulfate	Mistakenasmagnesiumsulfate	Use complete drug name
MTX	methotrexate	Mistaken as mito**XANTRONE**	Use complete drug name
Na at the beginning of a drug name (e.g., Na bicarbonate)	Sodium bicarbonate	Mistaken as no bicarbonate	Use complete drug name
NoAC	novel/new oral anticoagulant	Mistaken as no anticoagulant	Use complete drug name
OXY	oxytocin	Mistaken as oxy**CODONE**, Oxy**CONTIN**	Use complete drug name
PCA	procainamide	Mistaken as patient-controlled analgesia	Use complete drug name
PIT	Pitocin (oxytocin)	Mistakenas Pitressin, a discontinued brand of vasopressin still referred to as PIT	Use complete drug name
PNV	prenatal vitamins	Mistaken as penicillin VK	Use complete drug name
PTU	propylthiouracil	Mistaken as Purinethol (mercaptopurine)	Use complete drug name
T3	Tylenol with codeine No. 3	Mistaken as liothyronine, which is sometimes referred to as T3	Use complete drug name
TAC or tac	triamcinolone or tacrolimus	Mistaken as tetracaine, Adrenalin, and cocaine; or as Taxotere, Adriamycin, and cyclophosphamide	Use complete drug names Avoid drug regimen or protocol acronyms that may have a dual meaning or may be confused with other common acronyms, even if defined in an order set
TNK	TNKase	Mistaken as TPA	Use complete drug name
TPA or tPA	tissue plasminogen activator, Activase (alteplase)	Mistaken as TNK (TNKase, tenecteplase), TXA (tranexamic acid), or less often as another tissue plasminogen activator, Retavase (retaplase)	Use complete drug names
TXA	tranexamic acid	Mistaken as TPA (tissue plasminogen activator)	Use complete drug name
ZnSO4	zinc sulfate	Mistaken as morphine sulfate	Use complete drug name

TABLE 4-7	Error-Prone Abbreviations, Symbols, and Dose Designations—cont'd		
Error-Prone Abbreviations, Symbols, and Dose Designations	**Intended Meaning**	**Misinterpretation**	**Best Practice**
Stemmed/Coined Drug Names			
Nitro drip	nitroglycerin infusion	Mistaken as nitroprusside infusion	Use complete drug name
IV vanc	Intravenous vancomycin	Mistaken as Invanz	Use complete drug name
Levo	levofloxacin	Mistaken as Levophed (norepinephrine)	Use complete drug name
Neo	Neo-Synephrine, a well known but discontinued brand of phenylephrine	Mistaken as neostigmine	Use complete drug name
Coined names for compounded products (e.g., magic mouth-wash, banana bag, GI cocktail, half and half, pink lady)	Specific ingredients compounded together	Mistaken ingredients	Use complete drug/product names for all ingredients Coined names for compounded products should only be used if the contents are standardized and readily available for reference to prescribers, pharmacists, and nurses
Number embedded in drug name (not part of the official name) (e.g., 5-fluorouracil, 6-mercaptopurine)	fluorouracil mercaptopurine	Embedded number mistaken as the dose or number of tablets/capsules to be administered	Use complete drug names, without an embedded number if the number is not part of the official drug name
Dose Designations and Other Information			
1/2 tablet	Half tablet	1 or 2 tablets	Use text (half tablet) or reduced font-size fractions (½ tablet)
Doses expressed as Roman numerals (e.g., V)	5	Mistaken as the designated letter (e.g., the letter V) or the wrong numeral (e.g., 10 instead of 5)	Use only Arabic numerals (e.g., 1, 2, 3) to express doses
Lack of a leading zero before a decimal point (e.g., .5 mg)**	0.5 mg	Mistaken as 5 mg if the decimal point is not seen	Use a leading zero before a decimal point when the dose is less than one measurement unit
Trailing zero after a decimal point (e.g., 1.0 mg)**	1 mg	Mistaken as 10 mg if the decimal point is not seen	Do not use trailing zeros for doses expressed in whole numbers

Continued

TABLE 4-7	Error-Prone Abbreviations, Symbols, and Dose Designations—cont'd

Error-Prone Abbreviations, Symbols, and Dose Designations	Intended Meaning	Misinterpretation	Best Practice
Ratio expression of a strength of a single-entity injectable drug product (e.g., EPINEPHrine 1:1,000; 1:10,000; 1:100,000)	1:1,000: contains 1 mg/mL 1:10,000: contains 0.1 mg/mL 1:100,000: contains 0.01 mg/mL	Mistaken as the wrong strength	Express the strength in terms of quantity per total volume (e.g., **EPINEPH**rine 1 mg per 10 mL) **Exception:** combination local anesthetics (e.g., lidocaine 1% and **EPINEPH**rine 1:100,000)
Drug name and dose run together (problematic for drug names that end in the letter l [e.g., propranolol20 mg; TEGretol300 mg])	propranolol 20 mg **TEG**retol 300 mg	Mistaken as propranolol 120 mg Mistaken as **TEG**retol 1300 mg	Place adequate space between the drug name, dose, and unit of measure
Numerical dose and unit of measure run together (e.g., 10mg, 10Units)	10 mg 10 mL	The m in mg, or U in Units, has been mistaken as one or two zeros when flush against the dose (e.g., 10mg, 10Units), risking a 10- to 100- fold overdose	Place adequate space between the dose and unit of measure
Large doses without properly placed commas (e.g., 100000 units; 1000000 units)	100,000 units	100000 has been mistaken as 10,000 or 1,000,000	Use commas for dosing units ator- above 1,000 oruse words such as 100 thousand or 1 million to improve readability
	1,000,000 units	1000000 has been mistaken as 100,000	**Note:** Usecommastoseparate digits only in the US; commas are used in place of decimal points in some other countries

Symbols

ʒ or	Dram	Symbol for dram mistaken as the number 3	Use the metric system
♏†	Minim	Symbol for minim mistaken as mL	
x1	Administer once	Administer for 1 day	Use explicit words (e.g., for 1 dose)
> and <	More than and less than	Mistaken as opposite of intended	Use more than or less than
		Mistakenly have used the incorrect symbol	
		< mistaken as the number 4 when hand-written (e.g., <10 misread as 40)	

TABLE 4-7	Error-Prone Abbreviations, Symbols, and Dose Designations—cont'd

Error-Prone Abbreviations, Symbols, and Dose Designations	Intended Meaning	Misinterpretation	Best Practice
↑ and ↓[†]	Increase and decrease	Mistaken as opposite of intended	Use increase and decrease
		Mistakenly have used the incorrect symbol	
		↑ mistaken as the letter T, leading to misinterpretation as the start of a drug name, or mistaken as the numbers 4 or 7	
/ (slash mark)[†]	Separates two doses or indicates per	Mistaken as the number 1 (e.g., 25 units/10 units misread as 25 units and 110 units)	Use per rather than a slash mark to separate doses
@[†]	At	Mistaken as the number 2	Use at
&[†]	And	Mistaken as the number 2	Use and
+[†]	Plus or and	Mistaken as the number 4	Use plus, and, or in addition to
°	Hour	Mistaken as a zero (e.g., q2° seen as q20)	Use hr, h, or hour
⌀ or ∅[†]	Zero, null sign	Mistaken as the numbers 4, 6, 8, and 9	Use 0 or zero, or do or ribo intent using whole words
#	Pound(s)	Mistaken as a number sign	Use the metric system (kg or g) rather than pounds
			Use lb if referring to pounds

Apothecary or Household Abbreviations

Explicit apothecary or household measurements may **ONLY** be safely used to express the directions for mixing dry ingredients to prepare topical products (e.g., dissolve 2 capfuls of granules per gallon of warm water to prepare a magnesium sulfate soaking aid). Otherwise, metric system measurements should be used.

gr	Grain(s)	Mistaken as gram	Use the metric system (e.g., mcg, g)
dr	Dram(s)	Mistaken as doctor	Use the metric system (e.g., mL)
min	Minim(s)	Mistaken as minutes	Use the metric system (e.g., mL)
oz	Ounce(s)	Mistaken as zero or O_2	Use the metric system (e.g., mL)
tsp	Teaspoon(s)	Mistaken as tablespoon(s)	Use the metric system (e.g., mL)
tbsp or Tbsp	Tablespoon(s)	Mistaken as teaspoon(s)	Use the metric system (e.g., mL)

Common Abbreviations with Contradictory Meanings	Contradictory Meanings		Correction

For additional information and tables from Neil Davis (MedAbbrev.com) containing additional examples of abbreviations with contradictory or ambiguous meanings, please visit: www.ismp.org/ext/638.

B	Breast, brain, or bladder		Use breast, brain, or bladder
C	Cerebral, coronary, or carotid		Use cerebral, coronary, or carotid
D or d	Day or dose		Use day or dose
	(e.g., parameter-based dosing formulas using D or d [mg/kg/d] could be interpreted as either day or dose [mg/kg/day or mg/kg/dose]; or x3d could be interpreted as either 3 days or 3 doses)		

Continued

TABLE 4-7　Error-Prone Abbreviations, Symbols, and Dose Designations—cont'd

Common Abbreviations with Contradictory Meanings	Contradictory Meanings	Correction
H	Hand or hip	Use hand or hip
I	Impaired or improvement	Use impaired or improvement
L	Liver or lung	Use liver or lung
N	No or normal	Use no or normal
P	Pancreas, prostate, preeclampsia, or psychosis	Use pancreas, prostate, preeclampsia, or psychosis
S	Special or standard	Use special or standard
SS or ss	Single strength, sliding scale (insulin), signs and symptoms, or ½ (apothecary) SS has also been mistaken as the number 55	Use single strength, sliding scale, signs and symptoms, or one-half or ½

While the abbreviations, symbols, and dose designations in the **Table** should **NEVER** be used, not allowing the use of **ANY** abbreviations is exceedingly unlikely. Therefore, the person who uses an organization-approved abbreviation must take responsibility for making sure that it is properly interpreted. If an uncommon or ambiguous abbreviation is used, and it should be defined by the writer or sender. Where uncertainty exists, clarification with the person who used the abbreviation is required.

**On The Joint Commission's "Do Not Use" list
†Relevant mostly in handwritten medication information

RAPID PRACTICE 4-5　Abbreviations for Time and Frequency

ESTIMATED COMPLETION TIME: 10 to 15 minutes　　　　**ANSWERS ON:** page 151

DIRECTIONS: *Study the terms and abbreviations for frequency and time on p. 110. Write in the term or abbreviation requested in the space provided. If an abbreviation is listed as not recommended, write out the term.*

1　ac _____

2　stat _____

3　prn _____

4　s̄ _____

5　four times a day _____

6　as needed _____

7　bid _____

8　with _____

9　NPO _____

10　each, every _____

11　every 2 hours _____

12　q4h _____

13 pc _____

14 three times daily _____

15 without _____

16 c̄ _____

17 every 12 hours _____

18 ad lib _____

19 before meals _____

20 subcutaneously _____

RAPID PRACTICE 4-6   Terminology for Time and Frequency

ESTIMATED COMPLETION TIME: 5 minutes   **ANSWERS ON:** page 151

DIRECTIONS: *Answer the following questions pertaining to abbreviations for times of medication administration in brief phrases.*

1   If you were going to administer two medications, one four times a day (within 12 hours) and the other q4h (within 24 hours), how many doses would you give of each? four times a day: _____ q4h: _____

2   What commonly used words that begin with *t* and *b* will you use to distinguish the abbreviations for three times a day (tid) and two times a day (bid)? _____

3   What would be the *total times* a day a patient would receive a medication q4h?
    _____

4   How would you interpret the following orders?

    a. Give Tears No More 2 drops in each eye bid prn itching or burning.
        _____

    b. Give antacid Mylanta 1 oz. tid ac. _____
        _____

    c. Whom would you consult if you were unfamiliar with these abbreviations?
        _____

5   What abbreviation would be used if the physician's order indicated to take acetaminophen only *when needed?* _____

---

1 Why would it be very important for the nurse to differentiate the meaning of *ad lib* and *prn* in medication orders? _____	**ASK YOURSELF** **Q & A** **MY ANSWER**

FAQ   *Why are orders written for four times a day versus q6h?*

ANSWER   Many medications, such as a cough medicine, may be given totally within waking hours, such as 0900, 1300, 1700, and 2100. The patient will not have to be disturbed during sleep. Other medications, such as some antibiotics, need to have a more stable blood level concentration to be effective and/or safe and are ordered at equal intervals around the clock, such as q6h, q4h, or q8h.

RAPID PRACTICE 4-7	Abbreviations for Form, Route, and Time

ESTIMATED COMPLETION TIME: 10 minutes   **ANSWERS ON:** page 151

DIRECTIONS: *Write the medical abbreviation in the space provided.*

1 as needed _____   6 fluid _____

2 intramuscular _____   7 solution _____

3 elixir _____   8 apply to the skin _____

4 immediately _____   9 nothing by mouth _____

5 fluid extract _____   10 suspension _____

DIRECTIONS: *Write the meaning in the space provided.*

11 prn _____   16 MDI _____

12 bucc _____   17 on call x-ray _____

13 ad lib _____   18 NPO _____

14 IVPB _____   19 ID _____

15 bid _____   20 q6h _____

➤ Look up unfamiliar abbreviations. Contact the prescriber when a banned or unclear abbreviation is used. Do not guess. Document the clarification.

RAPID PRACTICE 4-8	Abbreviations—Additional Review

ESTIMATED COMPLETION TIME: 5 to 10 minutes   **ANSWERS ON:** page 151

DIRECTIONS: *Write the correct term in the space provided.*

1 bid _____   11 q8h _____

2 q6h _____   12 qhs _____

3 stat _____   13 PO _____

4 IM _____   14 sol _____

5 ac _____   15 NGT _____

6 pc _____   16 SL _____

7 prn _____   17 elix _____

8 tid _____   18 q4h _____

9 NPO _____   19 DS _____

10 GT _____   20 qh _____

➤ Memorize these two important abbreviations seen on medication records:
  • NKDA, no known *drug* allergies
  • NKA, no known allergies

➤ These are not interchangeable.

The 24-Hour Clock

Most health care agencies use the 24-hour clock (Figure 4-6). The 24-hour clock runs sequentially from 0001, one minute after midnight, to 2400, midnight. Each hour is written in increments of 100. It is written with four digits: the first two for hours and the second two for minutes.* No number is repeated.

The system is computer compatible and helps avoid the confusion of duplication of numbers (e.g., 1 AM, 1 PM; 12 AM, 12 PM; etc.) in the traditional AM/PM time.

- At 2400 hours, midnight, the clock is reset to 0000 for counting purposes only so that 0001 will be 1 minute after midnight. Examine the illustration below of the clock at midnight.
- The AM clock begins at midnight, 2400 hours (12:00 AM), and ends at 1159 hours (11:59 AM).
- The PM clock begins at noon, 1200 hours (12:00 PM), and ends at 2359 hours (11:59 PM).
- Observe the chart again: The major difference from traditional time begins at 1300 hours, or 1 PM. This is when duplication is avoided. Focus on the PM hours.

Note: 24-hour time is always stated in hundreds (e.g., "twelve hundred"). Do not say "one thousand two hundred."

---

*Seconds may be designated as follows: 1830:20 (6:30 PM and 20 seconds).

12-hr Clock	24-hr Clock	12-hr Clock	24-hr Clock
Midnight 12:00 AM	0000	Noon 12:00 PM	1200
1:00 AM	0100	1:00 PM	1300
2:00 AM	0200	2:00 PM	1400
3:00 AM	0300	3:00 PM	1500
4:00 AM	0400	4:00 PM	1600
5:00 AM	0500	5:00 PM	1700
6:00 AM	0600	6:00 PM	1800
7:00 AM	0700	7:00 PM	1900
8:00 AM	0800	8:00 PM	2000
9:00 AM	0900	9:00 PM	2100
10:00 AM	1000	10:00 PM	2200
11:00 AM	1100	11:00 PM	2300

A

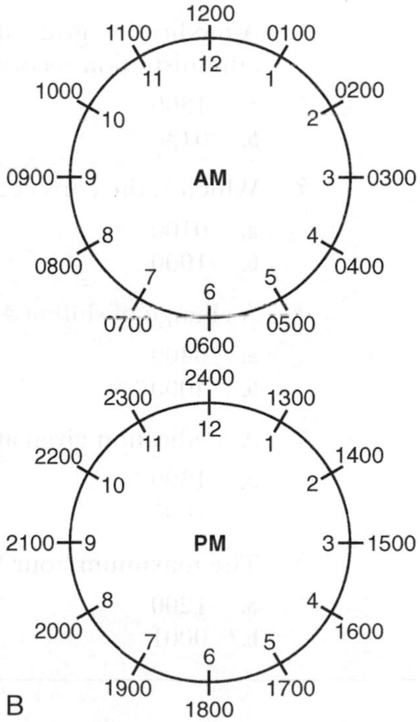

B

FIGURE 4-6 **A,** Comparison of the 12-hour clock and the 24-hour clock. The 24-hour clock does not use colons or AM and PM. Adding or subtracting 1200 is the constant that converts PM hours between the two systems. **B,** Comparison of the times used on a 12-hour clock and the corresponding time used on a 24-hour clock.

Q & A   ASK YOURSELF

1   Can you describe an acute problem that might arise if there was confusion about carrying out an urgent order at "2" as opposed to the clarity of 1400 or 0200 hours?

MY ANSWER   _____

2   If you were going to set your timer for a TV show at noon, would you set it for 12:00 AM or 12:00 PM? Would 1200 or 2400 hours be more helpful?

_____

Remember:

PM Hours	AM Hours
12:00 PM = noon = 1200 hours	12:00 AM = *midnight* = *2400* hours and resets to 0000 hours
1:00 PM = 1300 hours	1:00 AM = 0100 hours

RAPID PRACTICE 4-9   **The 24-Hour Clock**

ESTIMATED COMPLETION TIME: 10 to 20 minutes   **ANSWERS ON:** page 151

DIRECTIONS: *Analyze the question to determine whether AM or PM hours are to be identified. Calculate the time using mental arithmetic. Circle the correct answer.*

1   A medication given at 1:30 AM would be written in the medication administration record (MAR) as
   a. 1300   **c.** 1030
   b. 0130   **d.** 01:30

2   Which is the correct 24-hour clock designation for 1:10 AM?
   a. 0100   **c.** 0110
   b. 1000   **d.** 2110

3   A change of shift at 4 PM would be noted on the MAR as
   a. 0400   **c.** 1400
   b. 4000   **d.** 1600

4   A medication given at 1 PM would be charted in international time as
   a. 1300   **c.** 0001
   b. 1000   **d.** 0100

5   The maximum hour for the 24-hour clock is
   a. 1200   **c.** 2400
   b. 0001   **d.** 2459

Q & A   ASK YOURSELF

1   At what time, in 24-hour terms, do you usually wake up, eat dinner, and go to bed?

MY ANSWER   _____

Write all your appointments from now on in 24-hour clock terms, and in a few days the time will become automatic for you.

Medication Orders

The following terms and abbreviations may be seen in medication orders and prescriptions:

Abbreviation	Meaning	Example
Rx	Prescription	Rx Sig aspirin 325 mg q4h prn
Sig	Take	Sig aspirin 325 mg q4h prn
TO	Telephone order	TO Dr. Smith
VO	Verbal order	VO Dr. Smith

Complete medication orders

In order to be *complete*, a medication order *must be legible* and contain the following elements:

- Patient's name
- Date and time ordered
- Medication name
- Form
- Total amount in strength to be given
- Route
- Frequency schedule
- Additional instructions if needed
- Signature

Sample physician's order sheet

Directions: *See if you can read and translate the orders. Check your interpretation on the next page.*

GILROY HOSPITAL	
Smith, John Q. D.O.B. 03/27/1955 Patient ID: 345987123 Allergies: NKDA	

Date/Time	Health Care Prescriber Orders
01/05/2018	Amoxicillin 500 mg 1 cap PO q 8h × 10d
0900	Lispro 10 units subcut. ac & at bedtime if FSBG >150 mg/dL
	Tylenol 325 mg 2 tab PO q4h prn headache
	Phenergan supp 25 mg per rectum q8h PRN N/V
	MOM 30 mL PO at bedtime prn constipation
	01/05/2018 William Smith MD
01/07/2018	DC amoxicillin
1000	Bactrim DS 1 tab PO stat and bid × 5d
	Prednisone 10 mg PO tid. Give c̄ food
	01/07/2018 William Smith MD
01/08/2018	NPO p MN
1800	DC Lispro
	01/08/2018 TO Jane Jones CRNA/Susan Brown RN
01/09/2018	Atropine 0.4 mg IM on call OR
0700	*01/09/2018 TO Jane Jones CRNA/Cal Pearce RN*

Interpretation

GILROY HOSPITAL
Morimoto, Amy D.O.B. 03/27/1955 Patient ID: 345987123 Allergies: No Known Drug Allergies

Date/Time	Health Care Prescriber Orders
01/05/2022	Amoxicillin 500 mg 1 capsule by mouth every 8 hours for 10 days
0900	Lispro 10 units subcutaneous injection before meals and at bedtime if fingerstick blood glucose is greater than 150 mg per deciliter
	Tylenol 325 mg 2 tablets by mouth every 4 hours as needed for headache
	Phenergan suppository 25 mg per rectum every 8 hours as needed for nausea and/or vomiting
	Milk of Magnesia 30 mL by mouth at bedtime as needed for constipation
	01/05/2018 William Smith MD
01/07/2022	Discontinue amoxicillin
1000	Bactrim Double Strength 1 tablet by mouth immediately and then twice a day for 5 days
	Prednisone 10 mg by mouth. Give with food.
	01/07/2018 William Smith MD
01/08/2022	Nothing by mouth after midnight
1800	Discontinue Lispro
	01/08/2018 Telephone order received from Jane Jones Certified Registered Nurse Anesthetist received by Susan Brown Registered Nurse
01/09/2022	Atropine 0.4 mg intramuscular injection when receive call from the operating room
0700	*01/09/2022 Telephone order received from Jane Jones Certified Registered Nurse Anesthetist received by Cal Pearce Registered Nurse*

➤ Consult a current drug reference text, glossary, or the pharmacy for interpretation of unfamiliar abbreviations such as ASA (aspirin) or MOM (Milk of Magnesia).

➤ The nurse cannot give medications more often or earlier than ordered because a nurse does not have prescribing rights. The prescriber must always be contacted if there is a need to revise the order, such as a need for a prn pain or nausea medication before the prescribed interval.

➤ When orders are handwritten, capitalization, periods, and decimal guidelines are often obscured or ignored. Be very careful with interpretation of handwritten orders.

Interpreting Medication Orders and Medication Labels

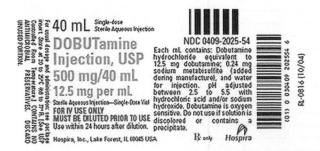

Compare the two labels above. These are "look alike–sound alike" drugs that have a high risk for medication error. They use the TALL MAN lettering to draw attention to the differences of the two drugs in order to reduce the chance for error.

Medication labels must be read carefully and compared with the prescriber's order before preparing a medication. Many drug names look and sound alike, for example, Flonase and FluMist; dopamine and dobutamine; prednisone and prednisolone; digoxin and digitoxin; phentermine and phentolamine; and Norcet and Nordette, to name a few. Analyze the contents, abbreviations, and *differences* among the labels for solid and liquid medications shown in this section.

Most of the information on a medication label is self-explanatory if one understands metric measurements and abbreviations. The unit dose concentration is usually specified in milligrams per tablet or capsule for *solid* forms and micrograms or milligrams per milliliter(s) for *liquid* forms.

➤ Key pieces of information are used in all medication calculations:

1 Ordered dose
2 Drug concentration (on the label)

➤ Misreading a label can result in a medication error. Accurate medication administration is the responsibility of the nurse.

The nurse focuses on the order in the medical record and on the label.

EXAMPLES

Order: ampicillin 250 mg cap PO qid

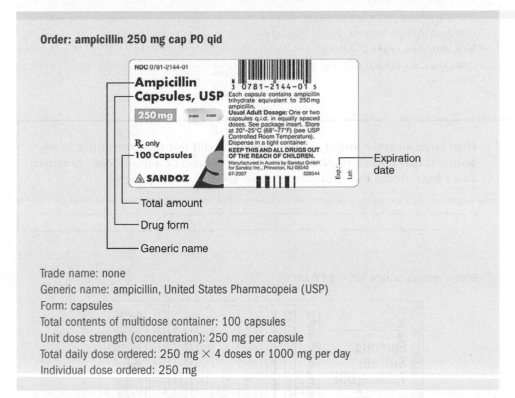

Trade name: none
Generic name: ampicillin, United States Pharmacopeia (USP)
Form: capsules
Total contents of multidose container: 100 capsules
Unit dose strength (concentration): 250 mg per capsule
Total daily dose ordered: 250 mg × 4 doses or 1000 mg per day
Individual dose ordered: 250 mg

Note that the drug is contained in capsules. Oral solid drugs are usually placed in some type of *capsule* or *tablet*. Read the cautions; the expiration date; the usual dose, if mentioned; and storage directions, if any. The nurse seldom has access to the multidose container in large institutions. The pharmacy dispenses the individual doses from the multidose containers. The *label* must match the medication *order*, either the trade name or the generic name.

FAQ   *What should the nurse do if the name of the drug on the order is not the same as the name on the label?*

ANSWER   Check carefully to see whether the ordered name is the generic equivalent of the name on the label. The order may be written with either the trade or the generic name. Look in a drug reference. Then call the pharmacy if you are uncertain.

EXAMPLES

Order: Tegretol susp 100 mg PO qid c̄ food for a patient with seizures

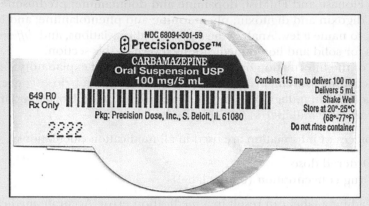

Trade name: Tegretol®

Generic name: carbamazepine USP

Form: liquid suspension

Total contents of multidose container: 450 mL

Unit dose strength (concentration): 100 mg per 5 mL

Total daily dose ordered: 400 mg

Individual dose ordered: 100 mg

Route: oral

Q & A   ASK YOURSELF   1   How large an error would a nurse make who did not read the entire label, assumed that it was a single-dose container instead of a multidose container, and administered the entire contents of 450 mL to the patient?

MY ANSWER   _____

EXAMPLES

Order: ferrous sulfate 325 mg PO bid pc

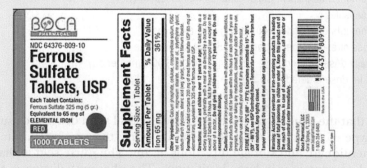

Trade name: none

Generic name: ferrous sulfate (USP)

Form: tablets

Total contents of multidose container: 1000 tablets

Total daily dose ordered: 650 mg

Individual dose ordered: 325 mg

Unit dose strength (concentration): 325 mg per tablet. Note the apothecary measurement of grains (5 gr). Focus on the metric measurement (mg). Do not use the apothecary measurement.

Order: Septra DS 1 tablet PO daily

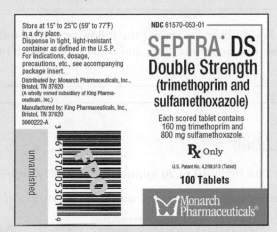

Trade name: Septra®

Generic name: trimethoprim and sulfamethoxazole

Total contents of multidose container: 100 tablets

Form: scored tablet compound drug

Unit dose strength (concentration): double-strength (DS) compound containing two drugs; 160 mg trimethoprim and 800 mg sulfamethoxazole. (If a medication has *DS* on the label, it is available in at least one other strength: regular. It is important to read the order and label carefully to find a match for dosage in a regular-strength or a DS order.)

Route: oral*

---

*When the route is not mentioned on the label of an unfamiliar medication, check the route with a current reference or pharmacy.

Compound medications can be ordered by the quantity (i.e., the number of tablets or capsules, e.g., Septra DS 1 capsule daily). Compound medications are combined in one capsule.

➤ Tablets can be administered through various routes.

Order: Nitroglycerin 0.6 mg SL q 5 min × 3 prn angina (chest pain). Call MD if relief is not obtained.

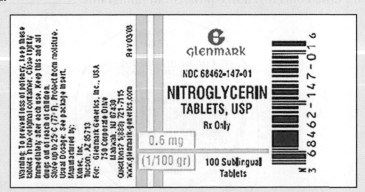

Trade name: none

Generic name: nitroglycerin

Total contents of multidose container: 100 tablets

Form: tablet

Unit dose strength (concentration): 0.6 mg per tablet

Route: sublingual SL (or subl)

➤ Sublingual (SL) tablets must be held under the tongue until they are absorbed. They are not to be swallowed nor crushed.

Q & A **ASK YOURSELF**	**1**	What are the key differences among the following terms: total contents, total daily dose, dose ordered, unit dose, and usual dose? (Give brief answers.)
MY ANSWER		_____

RAPID PRACTICE 4-10   Interpreting Labels

ESTIMATED COMPLETION TIME: 10 to 20 minutes   **ANSWERS ON:** page 152

DIRECTIONS: *Examine the labels provided, and write the requested information.*

1

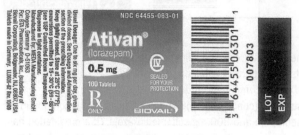

   a.   Generic name: _____
   b.   Total number of tablets in container: _____
   c.   Unit dose concentration per tablet: _____

2

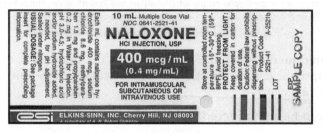

   a.   Single- or multiple-dose vial? _____
   b.   Unit dose concentration in micrograms: _____
   c.   Unit dose concentration equivalent in milligrams: _____

3

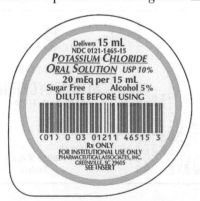

   a.   Generic name: _____
   b.   Unit dose concentration: _____

4

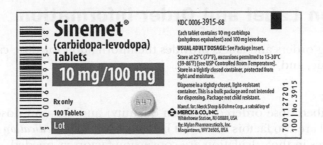

a. Trade name: _____

b. Number of drugs contained in the tablet: _____

c. Generic names and doses within the compound: _____

5   * ⚑

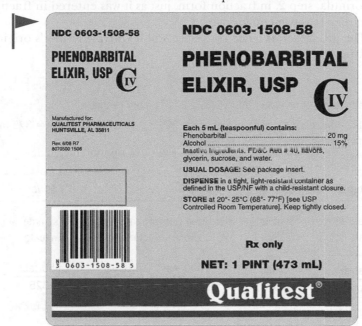

_____

*High alert if prescribed for a pediatric patient.

a. Form of medication: _____

b. Unit dose concentration: _____

c. What percent alcohol is contained in this medicine? _____

Note: **The red flag icon used throughout this text is a visual reminder of high-alert medications that may cause significant harm if used in error. See Appendix B.**

1	What is the *amount* of difference between a microgram and a milligram?	**ASK YOURSELF**
	_____	MY ANSWER

Calculating Dose Based on Label and Order Information

Interpreting orders and labels provides the information for dose calculation, mental arithmetic, and/or DA equations.

Remember:

The prescribed dose ordered (a given quantity) and the unit dose concentration on the label are two factors that must be entered in *every medication dose* calculation. Other entries in the calculation are conversion factors as needed.

- The desired answer unit will almost always contain tablets, capsules, or milliliters.
- The drug concentration often will be placed in the first conversion formula, step 2, in fraction form, just as it was entered in fraction form in earlier DA-style equations.
- The given factors to be converted will be the prescriber's original ordered drug and quantity.

EXAMPLES

Ordered: (a dose) of aspirin (ASA) 0.65 g PO q 4 h prn headache.

Available: Unit dose concentration on label: 325 mg per tablet (1 tablet = 325 mg)
How many tablets will you give (per dose)?
Conversion factor: 1000 mg = 1 g.

	Step 1	=	Step 2	×	Step 3			=	Answer	
?	Desired Answer Units	=	Starting Factor	×	Given Quantity and Conversion Factor(s)			=	Estimate, Multiply, Evaluate	
?	$\dfrac{\text{tablets}}{\text{dose}}$	=	$\dfrac{1 \text{ tab}}{325 \text{ mg}}$	×	$\dfrac{1000 \text{ mg}}{1 \text{ g}}$	×	$\dfrac{0.65 \text{ g}}{\text{dose}}$	=	$\dfrac{650 \text{ tabs}}{325}$ =	$\dfrac{2 \text{ tabs}}{\text{per dose}}$

Answer: 2 tabs per dose

Analysis: The starting factor must contain "tablets in the numerator." This will be found on the medication label (see below) as will the concentration (325 mg) per tablet. The accompanying 325-mg concentration must be entered in the denominator as shown. They "go together."

The rest of the desired answer "per dose" will need to appear in a later denominator to match the desired answer position.

The ordered units (g) do not match the units in the container on hand (mg). A conversion factor changes grams to milligrams (1000 mg = 1 g).

➤ The medication may be ordered every 4 hours but you only give one dose at a time!

Evaluation: Only tablets per dose remain. The estimate of two tablets supports the answer. (Math check: 100 × 0.65 ÷ 325 = 2.) The equation is balanced.

Note: Equations for medications need to differentiate orders per dose, per day, per hr, etc.

Note: The equation entry pattern from left to right—the label concentration, conversion factor if needed, and the order—works well with oral and injectable medication orders.

Reminder: The goal of DA is to multiply a known quantity (the ordered dose) by one or more conversion factors to solve an equation.

Q & A **ASK YOURSELF** 1 What are the additional factors that may need to be added if the units ordered and supplied do not match?

MY ANSWER _____

Some unofficial abbreviations for medications will be seen with clinical experience, for example:
- Aspirin (ASA for its chemical name: acetylsalicylic acid)
- Penicillin (PCN)
- Codeine (Cod)

➤ These are given so often that they are frequenrtly abbreviated. There have been recommendations to ban the use of abbreviations for names of medicines.

FAQ   *Why isn't the medication administered in milligrams?*

ANSWER   When all the calculations are completed, the correct amount of medication is given in the form of solids or liquids (e.g., 1 or 2 tablets or capsules or a number of milliliters).

Drug/Form	Drug/Form	Drug/Form	Drug/Form
1 mg/1 tablet	1 mg/2 capsules	1 mg/1 suppository	1 mg/1000 mL

RAPID PRACTICE 4-11   Order and Label Interpretation for DA Equations

ESTIMATED COMPLETION TIME: 20 to 30 minutes   **ANSWERS ON:** page 152

DIRECTIONS: *Examine the example shown in problem 1. Read the order and the label to obtain the answers. Be sure you can read the abbreviations in the order.*

1   Ordered: aspirin tab 0.65 g PO tid and at bedtime for a patient with joint pain.

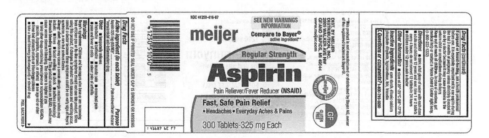

a.   Identify desired answer units: <u>tablet</u>

b.   Identify the unit dose metric concentration: <u>325 mg per tablet</u>

c.   Identify the factor(s) to be converted: <u>0.65</u>

d.   State the given conversion factor needed: <u>1000 mg = 1 g</u>

e.   How often should the medication be administered? <u>3 times a day and at bedtime</u>

f.   What is the ordered dose equivalent in mg? <u>650 mg</u>

2 **Ordered:** cephalexin cap 0.5 g PO q6h × 5 days for a patient with an infection.

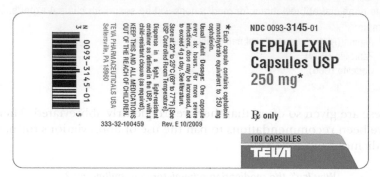

a. Identify desired answer units. _____

b. Identify the unit-dose concentration to be entered in a DA equation. ____

c. Identify the given factors to be converted. _____

d. State the conversion factor needed. _____

e. What is the total daily dose ordered? _____

f. What is the ordered dose equivalent in milligrams? _____

3 **Ordered:** azithromycin susp 0.2 g PO q24h for a patient with an upper respiratory infection.

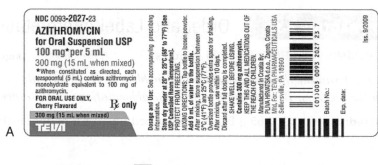

a. What is the generic name? _____

b. What is the form? _____

c. What is the unit dose strength of the medication you would select? _____

d. What are the given factors to be converted? _____

e. What conversion factor would convert the given quantity to the dose supplied? _____

4 **Ordered:** morphine sulfate 15 mg IM stat for pain.

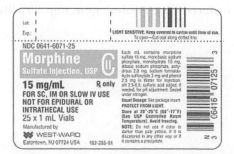

a. Identify desired answer units. _____

b. Identify the unit dose concentration to be entered in a DA equation.

_____

c. What is the route ordered? _____

d. When is the drug to be administered? _____

e. Three routes by which the label states the drug can be administered:

_____

➤ Morphine (see #4) has a C II (Schedule II) printed on the label. This means that it is regulated under the Controlled Substances Act, which is enforced by the Drug Enforcement Agency (DEA). There are five classifications or schedules for these drugs. Schedule II drugs have a high potential for abuse but are permitted by prescription for medical use. Schedule II drugs include barbiturates, Percodan, and methylphenidate (Ritalin) as well as other medications.

➤ Do not abbreviate morphine sulfate as MS. It has been mistaken for magnesium sulfate.

➤ Remember that liquid medications are delivered in milliliters. Solid drugs are supplied in many forms, including tablets, capsules, powders, and suppositories.

5 **Ordered:** cephalexin susp 0.25 g PO q6h × 10 days for a child discharged with an infection.

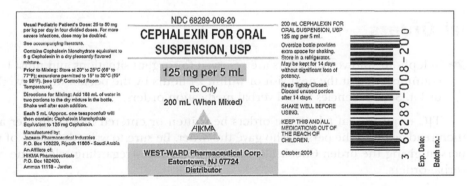

a. Identify the desired answer units. _____

b. Identify the unit dose concentration to be entered in a DA equation. ____

c. Identify the given factors to be converted. _____

d. State the given conversion factor needed. _____

e. What is the total daily dose ordered? _____

f. What is the ordered dose equivalent in milligrams? _____

---

1 Morphine is a powerful opioid narcotic. What would probably happen to a patient if the nurse gave the total contents instead of the unit dose strength?

ASK YOURSELF **Q & A**

_____ **MY ANSWER**

For reinforcement, the next time you are in a pharmacy section of a store, spend 5 or 10 minutes browsing the cold, cough, and headache medication section and examine the labels. Note the variety of forms and strengths on the labels. Look for the registered sign ®, the generic name, the total dose, and the unit dose on the container. Stores sell drugs in multidose containers so that the customer does not have to return hourly or daily for refills.

 ASK YOURSELF   **1**   What are the *sources* of the two key pieces of information that must be entered in all DA equations for medications?

MY ANSWER   _____

Orders for Two or More Medications to Be Combined

Examine this sample order:

$$9/9/18 \quad 1800 \left\{ \begin{array}{l} \text{morphine 10 mg} \\ \text{Vistaril 25 mg} \end{array} \right\} \text{IM stat and q4h prn pain TO Dr. John Smith,}$$
Jane Nurse, RN

Translation:
9/9/18, 6 PM. Give morphine 10 mg and Vistaril 25 mg together, intramuscular route, immediately and every 4 hours as needed for pain, telephone order, Dr. John Smith per Jane Nurse, RN.

Telephone and Verbal Orders

✴ *Communication*

➤ It is safer to read back and restate numbers individually, such as "three five zero milligrams" as opposed to "350 mg."

➤ Telephone and verbal orders are reserved for urgent situations and must be countersigned at the next visit or within 24 hours by the person who gave the order. Some agencies forbid verbal medication orders.

TJC requires that telephone orders be written or entered in a computer and then read again to the person who gave the order. Be sure to write the name of the person giving the order. Check TJC and agency policies regarding telephone and verbal orders.

Examples of Orders That Must Be Clarified

EXAMPLES   **Order: Tylenol (acetaminophen) 650 mg PO 2 tablets q4h fever over 38° C.**

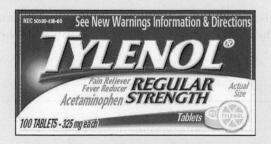

➤ The prescriber wrote "2 tablets." The medication is supplied as 325 mg per tablet. Does the order mean 2 tablets of 650 mg, 2 tablets of 325 mg, or 4 tablets of 325 mg? Guidelines require the total dose to be written. This order is confusing and could result in a toxic overdose. Most medicines are supplied in more than one strength. The prescriber cannot second guess which strength the pharmacy will supply. The nurse cannot guess what dose the prescriber meant.

➤ Clarify unclear dose orders, such as total dose desired, with the *prescriber*.

The order should read: Tylenol (acetaminophen) tab 650 mg PO q4h fever over 38° C. The nurse will calculate the number of tablets to give depending on the strength supplied.

EXAMPLES

Order: Children's Tylenol 1 tsp q4h.

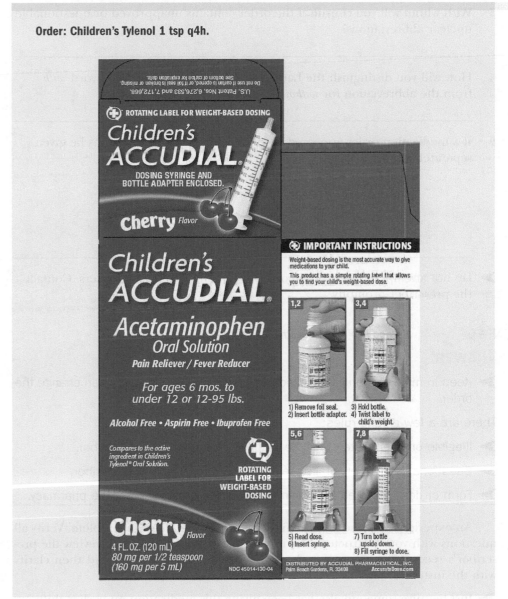

➤ The dose strength and form need to be specified.

The order should read: Children's acetaminophen susp 160 mg PO q4h.

RAPID PRACTICE 4-12	Review of Abbreviations Used for Medication Orders

ESTIMATED COMPLETION TIME: 15 minutes   **ANSWERS ON:** page 152

DIRECTIONS: *Use brief phrases to describe the hazards of the following types of abbreviations.*

1   What do you think may be some of the safety hazards of TO and VO?

    _____

2   How can handwritten abbreviations, numbers, decimals, and slashes result in medication errors?

    _____

3   With whom will you consult if the order contains unapproved or questionable unclear abbreviations?

    _____

4   How will you distinguish the Latin-derived abbreviation for the word *with* from the abbreviation for *without*?

    _____

5   If a medication order appeared as follows, would the medications be given separately or together?

        [Morphine sulfate 10 mg]
        [Atropine 0.4 mg]   } IM stat

    _____

➤ Do not attempt to interpret incorrectly written or confusing orders. Contact the prescriber promptly.

FAQ	*How do I go about questioning orders?*
ANSWER	

➤ Keep in mind that *only* the prescriber or designated physician can change the order.

There are a few ground rules:

➤ Illegible or incomplete order: be prepared to contact the prescriber.

➤ Questionable dose or total dose unspecified: contact the prescriber.

➤ Form or dose supplied is a mismatch with the order: contact the pharmacy.

An experienced nurse may not find the order illegible or incomplete. Verify all questions with your instructor after investigation. Students need to review the prescriber's recent progress notes, check a current drug reference, and then clarify with the instructor.

➤ Just because someone else has been giving this medication on earlier shifts does not mean that it is right. Decide whether the pharmacy or the prescriber is the appropriate first contact.

➤ Document all clarifications in the patient's record.

✳ Communication

"This is Rose Quartz, RN at General Hospital, Unit 4 A. I'm calling Dr. Doe to clarify a medication order written by Dr. John Doe for patient Mark Smith, aged 60, admitted with appendicitis in room 222." (Read the whole order.) "Please confirm the order for _____ (dose, medication, route, times, etc.). The telephone number here is _____." One more sentence may be added regarding the reason for clarification, for example, "The patient is allergic to _____," "The patient is having difficulty swallowing solids," or "The patient had only been receiving half that dose in the past."

Medication Administration Records

The MAR is the official record of all the medications given to the patient. It is maintained by the nurses. The forms are usually computerized in large agencies, but some smaller agencies may use handwritten records (Figures 4-7 and 4-8). The MAR must match the original medication orders.

Janelle Espinoza
ID 13254444
Age: 84 Rm 250-B

Adm. 06/01/2022

Pacific Hills Skilled
Nursing Facility

Allergies
Penicillin (PCN); Aspirin (ASA)

Today's Date: *6/03/2022*

Date Ordered	Medication Dose Rte, Freq	Start Date	Stop Date	1st shift 2400–0659	2nd shift 0700–1459	3rd shift 1500–2359
6/01/22	Lasix 20mg po daily AM	6/01			(0930) Xray JP 1130 JP	
6/01/22	Humalog 75/25 mix 20 units subcut daily 15 min before bkst	6/01		0630 MS	PA	
6/01/22	Digoxin 0.25mg PO daily	6/01			P=76 0930 JP	
6/01/22	Minocin 100mg PO q12h	6/01	6/05	0600 MS		1800 LG

Handwritten MARs may be seen in smaller clinical agencies. They also may be seen on admission until pharmacy computerizes the admission orders. Medications that are withheld typically have the time due encircled with a brief reason for the omission such as NPO, Xray, Lab, or See notes. Some medications such as antibiotics and control drugs have an automatic stop date based on each agency's policy. Take special care with interpretation of handwritten medications, numbers, decimal points, and zeros. Also be aware that these records have been hand-copied from prescriber order sheets. Any copying increases the risk for error.

PRN and ONE-TIME-ONLY MEDICATIONS

6/01/22	Morphine 4mg IV q2h prn pain	1400 LJ			

Signature	Init.	Signature	Init.
Mary Smith, RN	MS		
John Pauli, RN	JP		
Louise Gray, RN	LG		

FIGURE 4-7 Example of a handwritten medical administration record (MAR).

Patient ID stamp William Smythe 523469 Room 572-A	MEDICATION ADMINISTRATION RECORD ST. LOUISE HOSPITAL		ALLERGIES: **Penicillin**	

DATE START STOP	MEDICATION DOSAGE, ROUTE ADMINISTRATION TIME	8/3/2021 07:00 to 14:59	8/3/2021 15:00 to 22:59	8/4/2021 23:00 to 06:59
	Ord. 08-01-2021 5% Lactated Ringer's Sol. 1000 mL IV TKO at 20 mL/hr continuous			
	Ord. 08-01-2021 losartan (Cozaar) tablet 50 mg once daily AM and HS Hold for systolic BP less than 130 Call MD	0900 BP=		2100 BP=
	Ord. 08-01-2021 Insulin glargine (Lantus) 20 units subcut. daily at 8 AM Give on time Record on insulin MAR Do not mix with other insulins or medications	0800 Document on Insulin MAR		
	Ord. 08-02-2021 norfloxacin (Noroxin) 400 mg q12h × 3 days STOP 8-05-2021 after 6 doses Take with glass water 1 hr before or 2 hr after meals	1000		2200

This type of a 24-hour printed MAR for routine scheduled medications can be computer or pharmacy generated. It mentions some administration priorities and includes both the generic and the trade name to reduce chance of error. Separate MARs may be used for one-time-only and prn orders (refer to p.136) and certain drugs such as heparin and insulin, which require coagulation or blood glucose assessment prior to administration.

SIGNATURES (FIRST & LAST NAME)	INITIALS	SIGNATURES (FIRST & LAST NAME)	INITIALS	SITE CODES	MEDICATIONS NOT GIVEN
				LU - L Gluteus	NPO - NPO
				RU - R Gluteus	RF - Refused
				LT - L Thigh	WH - Withheld
				RT - R Thigh	
				LA - L Abdomen	
				RA - R Abdomen	
				LV - L Ventrogluteal	
				RV - R Ventrogluteal	
				LM - L Arm	
				RM - R Arm	
				LD - L Deltoid	
				RD - R Deltoid	

A

FIGURE 4-8 A, Example of an electronically generated medical administration record (MAR).

The data should be entered as *soon as possible* after the medications have been administered so that no other personnel will mistakenly think a medication was not given and give it again. A medication that is ordered but not given for any reason, including refusal by patient, must also be noted on the MAR. The codes for abbreviations on the MAR differ among departments and institutions, but they are similar enough that they are self-explanatory or can be understood after only a few minutes of consultation with the staff.

PRN Medication Administration Record

**** PRN ****			
ACETAMINOPHEN 650 MG SUPP 650 MG PER RECTUM Q4H PRN PAIN DO NOT GIVE > 4000 MG APAP/24H Start: 9/23 Stop:			
50% DEXTROSE 50 ML IV PRN BS <70 Start: 9/23 Stop:			
PURALUBE NP OPTH OINT (LACRI-LUBE) 1.00 BID PRN BOTH EYES Start: 9/23 Stop:			
POTASSIUM CL 10 MEQ ER TAB (KLOR-CON) 20 MEQ PO PRN MAY GIVE Q8H X 3 FOR K=3-3.4 OR Q12H X 2 FOR K=3.5-3.8 Start: 9/23 Stop:			

RN/LPN SIGNATURE & INIT: _____

B

C

FIGURE 4-8 cont'd
B, Example of an electronically generated medication administration record for PRN medications. **C,** Screen shot from eMAR.

ASK YOURSELF   **Q & A**

1   Refer to the ISMP's list of high-alert medications in Appendix B. Are there any drugs there that you recognize? How many on the list pertain to oral drugs?

MY ANSWER

_____

2   What are some of the recommendations made at the top of the list for reducing errors with these medications?

_____

Spaces in rows are avoided as each medication order is entered to prevent overlooked medication order errors.

RAPID PRACTICE 4-13 Interpreting MARs

ESTIMATED COMPLETION TIME: 10 to 15 minutes   **ANSWERS ON:** page 152

DIRECTIONS: *Refer to the handwritten MAR in Figure 4-7 to answer these questions.*

1 What are the patient's medication allergies? _____

2 Which drug was withheld because the patient was in x-ray? _____

3 At what time will a new MAR be used? _____

4 When is the next dose of morphine for pain available for the patient if needed? _____

5 Which medication must be given before breakfast? _____

DIRECTIONS: *Read the computerized MARs in Figure 4-8, A and B, and answer the following questions.*

6 Which medication order for a tablet is based on a bedside physical assessment? (See Figure 4-8, *A*.) _____

7 Which prn medication is given per rectum? (See Figure 4-8, *B*.) _____

8 The prn ophthalmic ointment route states to instill the ointment in both eyes. Is this an appropriate order? _____

9 Does the patient have medication allergies? (See Figure 4-8, *A*.) _____

10 How often may the patient have acetaminophen if needed? _____

CLINICAL RELEVANCE

You must witness patients taking their medications in order to document on the MAR that they were administered. Often, when administration is unsupervised, medications have been found in the bedding or have gone back to the kitchen on a food tray. Check your agency's policy for any exceptions to this rule.

The Nine Rights of Medication Administration

Meeting the patient's basic rights to quality medical care and a safe clinical environment makes sense to everyone and is an accreditation requirement of TJC. The process of guaranteeing this involves several steps that must be followed consistently to be permanently embedded in practice. The means to ensure safe and effective medication administration is addressed throughout the text. Think of *yourself* as a patient as you read the seven basic rights regarding medication administration.

Nine Basic Rights

1	Right patient	6	Right reason for the drug (based on assessment)
2	Right drug	7	Right patient education
3	Right dose	8	Right to refuse treatment
4	Right time	9	Right documentation (of administration or refusal)
5	Right route		

1 **Right Patient** TJC requires that at least two methods be used to identify the patient for medications and treatments. You may identify the patient by checking the wristband identification number or birth date and asking the patient to state his or her full name. A patient who is hard of hearing or confused may respond to a wrong name. A room number or bed number does not constitute a valid identification. Medication errors have occurred from relying on room and bed numbers as means of identifying patients. The trend is to scan the patient's ID bracelet with a bar code scanner as one method of identifying the patient.

> ✳ **Communication**
>
> "What is your name?" is best. Asking, "Are you Mr. Smith?" may yield a "Yes" answer from a confused or hard-of-hearing patient. You need to check the full first and last names.

2 **Right Drug** Name the drug and dose you are administering. Ask the patient and family about allergies or problems with medications. The stress on admission may cause patients to forget some of these details. Mention the class and purpose of the drug. Many patients do not know their medications by name.

CLINICAL RELEVANCE

Suppose the nurse fails to communicate to the patient and/or close family member the name of the medication that has been prepared; the patient has an allergy to it but was too distracted or ill to recall this on admission or does not recognize it by the generic name. It is not noted on the MAR. The nurse gives the medication. The patient has a severe adverse drug reaction (ADE).

---

1 Do you think that giving a "look-alike" drug to a patient instead of the ordered drug because the spelling was very similar would constitute a valid legal defense (e.g., AndroGel, which is testosterone, for Amphojel, an antacid)?

ASK YOURSELF

_____ **MY ANSWER**

---

3 **Right Dose** The dose prepared must be the same as the _ordered_ dose. The ordered dose may involve giving 1 to 2 tablets or 1 to 2 unit-dose servings of an injectable or oral liquid. When the dose to be administered exceeds 1 to 2 portions of the unit-dose serving, withhold the medication and promptly recheck the order. Clarify the order with the prescriber. Remember that the unit dose is the usual average dose ordered.

➤ Beware of reading decimals incorrectly.

➤ Look up unfamiliar drugs and unusual doses in current drug references.

4 **Right Time** Medications generally should be given within 30 minutes of the designated time. Check your agency policies. The need to give medications on time can present delivery difficulties if the institution schedules all daytime medications at the same time for all patients, for example, at 0900, 1300, 1700, and 2100.

➤ Some priority medications must be given very promptly:

- Stat and emergency medications
- Medications for acute pain or nausea and powerful intravenous medications
- Medications to be taken with meals or before or after meals, such as insulin and other antidiabetic agents

If the nurse is delivering many medications to a group of patients, the delivery schedule must be prioritized. Safe prioritization can be achieved through experience and study.

➤ Ask for help when the medication work load is too heavy to deliver medications in a timely manner.

5   **Right Route** Many medications are packaged in several forms: solids and liquid, oral and injectable, or for intravenous or intramuscular injection. The name will be the same, but the forms and routes may differ.

Compare the ordered route with the fine print on the label. Students in particular need to ask for help from the appropriate source when they meet the unfamiliar.

CLINICAL RELEVANCE

A student who had never seen very large capsules or a suppository was observed walking down the hall with a large capsule in a paper cup held in a latex-gloved hand. An RN inquired about the need for the glove, since the capsule was observed to be the only medication on hand.

"I'm giving the patient a suppository. It's a laxative," the student informed the nurse. The patient had a laxative ordered that was supplied as a large capsule to be taken orally. The student had never taken a laxative and assumed that all laxatives were administered rectally. The student also thought, as a result of recent study of medication routes, that medications pertaining to bowels were probably suppositories and that this large capsule was a suppository. The student made two faulty assumptions.

The *route* was not specified in the order. Occasionally, the provider may omit writing the PO route when the medication is a tablet or capsule. This is an error. The front of labels specifies tablets or capsules, but the oral route is not always mentioned on the label. All other routes are specified on the label. Suppository labels contain the words *suppository* and *the route*. It is understandable that some very large pills and capsules might seem too large to swallow, but giving them rectally would not be effective or wise. The form (suppository) of a drug and the route (rectal) must be specified in the order and on the label.

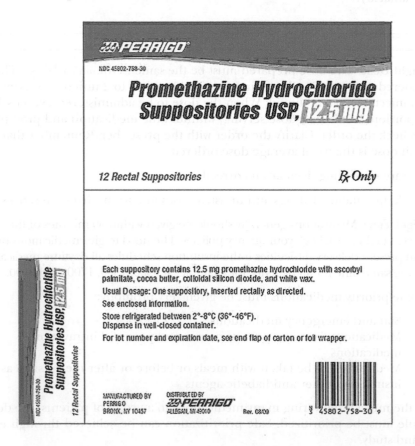

6 **Right Reason for the Drug** (based on assessment) It is the responsibility of the nurse to assess the patient for the appropriateness of administering the medication.

Consider a patient who has round the clock pain medication ordered. The nures assesses the patient, finds them difficult to arouse, BP 90/60 (lower than usual 130/80), respirations 10/minute. Giving this patient additional pain medication could be very dangerous and further slow the patient's respiratory rate and BP.

7 **Right Patient Education** The nurse should be providing education regarding the need for every medication given and the potential side effects the patient should watch for and report.

8 **Right to Refuse Treatment** All patients have the right to refuse a medication. The nurse should attempt to educate the patient as to the reasons it is beneficial, but ultimately it is the patient's choice. Promptly report and document the refusal and the reason given for the refusal. Be sure to include an assessment of the patient's mental status.

9 **Right Documentation** (of administration or refusal) Prompt documentation on the correct MAR prevents duplication errors. Serious errors can occur when another nurse gives the medication again because the first nurse did not record it in the right record or in a timely manner.

➤ Document soon *after* medication is given, never *before* it is given. Include drugs that had to be held, omitted, or refused.

➤ Remember the cliché, "If it wasn't documented, it wasn't done."

FDA-required labeling changes

A few drugs, such as epinephrine, isoproterenol, and neostigmine, were previously labeled in ratios rather than in mg/mL, which at times resulted in medication dosing errors that sometimes caused severe harm to a patient.

As of May 1, 2016, these drugs are no longer labeled as a ratio, but are now expressed in mg/mL to avoid confusion and to help reduce dosing errors.

Before	Now
Epinepherine 1:1000	Epinepherine 1 mg/mL
Epinepherine 1:10,000	Epinepherine 0.1 mg/mL

Epinepherine is frequently given in emergency situations to treat anaphylaxis (severe allergic reactions). When the medication was expressed in terms of a ratio, providers needed to calculate the dosage differently than most other drugs, which are expressed in mg/mL. In an emergency situation, calculating the dosage of a medication expressed in entirely different terms (such as 1:10,000) can increase the chances of error. Standardizing the units to mg/mL will reduce the chances for an error being made.

| RAPID PRACTICE 4-14 | Seven Basic Rights of Medication Administration |

ESTIMATED COMPLETION TIME: 5 to 10 minutes   **ANSWERS ON:** page 152

DIRECTIONS: *Match the nurse action to the letter that corresponds to the appropriate basic patient right.*

Patient's Basic Rights

a.	Right patient	**e.**	Right time
b.	Right drug	**f.**	Right documentation
c.	Right dose	**g.**	Right to refuse treatment
d.	Right route		

1 Check wrist identification band with full written name. _____

2 Instruct the patient to hold a sublingual tablet under the tongue until dissolved. _____

3 Record medication administration promptly on the MAR. _____

4 The patient refuses to swallow the ordered medications. _____

5 Compare the order and name of the drug on the label three times before administering it. _____

6 Recalculate and question an order that exceeds 2 times the unit dose supplied by the manufacturer and pharmacy. _____

7 Give the stat medication within 10 minutes after order is received. _____

8 Write out the nine rights of medication administration in abbreviated form.

a _____   f _____

b _____   g _____

c _____   h _____

d _____   i _____

e _____

| CHAPTER 4 | MULTIPLE-CHOICE REVIEW |

ESTIMATED COMPLETION TIME: 10 to 15 minutes   **ANSWERS ON:** page 152

DIRECTION: *Circle the correct answer. Consult Chapter 2 if necessary.*

1 What is the correct interpretation for the following abbreviations: *tid ac?*
   a. Twice a day after meals and periodically
   b. Twice a day before meals and periodically
   c. Three times a day before meals
   d. Three times a day after meals

2 How would you interpret the following order: NPO p midnight?
   a. May not eat after 1200
   b. Nothing by mouth after 2400 hours
   c. No physical activity after midnight
   d. Do not wake after midnight

3 Which is the correct interpretation for the following physician's order: Amphojel 15 mL po tid pc and hs?
   a. Amphojel 15 mL 3 times a day by mouth after meals and at bedtime
   b. Amphojel 15 mg twice a day before meals and at bedtime
   c. Amphojel 15 mL twice a day before meals and at bedtime
   d. Amphojel 15 mL 4 times a day after meals and at bedtime

4 If a medicine was ordered PO and the patient had a GT, what action would the nurse take?

   a. Mix the PO medicine with liquid and place in the gastric tube.

   b. Clarify the route with the physician who wrote the order.

   c. Give the medicine PO as ordered.

   d. Clarify the route with another, more experienced nurse on duty.

5 What would be the appropriate interpretation for the following order: morphine sulfate 10 mg IM stat?

   a. Give morphine sulfate 10 mg IM when needed

   b. Give morphine sulfate 10 mg IM as desired

   c. Give morphine sulfate 10 mg on call to x-ray

   d. Give morphine sulfate 10 mg IM immediately

6 How would you interpret the following 24-hour time in standard time: 0001 and 1425?

   a. 1 AM and 4:25 PM

   b. 1 PM and 2:25 AM

   c. 12:01 AM and 2:25 PM

   d. 12:01 PM and 2:25 AM

7 What would be an appropriate schedule for the following order: 8 oz H_2O q6h?

   a. 0800, 1400, 2000, and 0200

   b. 0900, 1300, 1700, and 2100

   c. 0900, 1300, 1700, 2100, 0100, and 0500

   d. 0800, 1200, 1800, and 2400

8 How many times a day is a q4h medicine given?

   a. 4

   b. 6

   c. 8

   d. 12

9 Which is the correct interpretation for the following physician's order: ampicillin 500 mg IM stat and q8h?

   a. Ampicillin 500 mg intramuscular whenever necessary and three times a day

   b. Ampicillin 500 mg intramuscular immediately and every 8 hours

   c. Ampicillin 500 mg intravenously and every 8 hours

   d. Ampicillin 500 mg intramuscularly at discharge and every 8 hours

10 How should a suspension be prepared for administration?

   a. Shake well until completely dissolved.

   b. Shake vigorously until completely dissolved.

   c. Administer as supplied without shaking.

   d. Shake gently until completely dissolved.

DIRECTIONS: *For problems 11 to 20, read the labels supplied to obtain the answer. Use mental arithmetic to calculate a dose if requested. Circle the correct answer.*

11 Whom should the nurse consult if a handwritten medication order is incomplete or unclear?

   a. The prescriber

   b. A nurse who gave the medication during the preceding shift

   c. A drug reference

   d. The pharmacy

12 Ordered: gemfibrozil tablet 0.6 g PO bid 30 minutes ac for a patient with hypercholesterolemia.

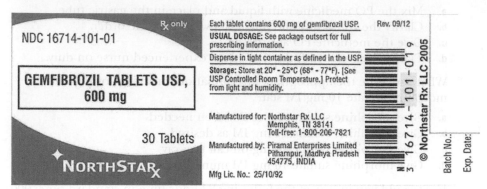

How many tablets would the nurse administer to the patient?

a. $\frac{1}{2}$ tablet

b. 1 tablet

c. 2 tablets

d. 4 tablets

13 Ordered: metformin tablets 1 g PO bid with meals for a patient with Type 2 diabetes.

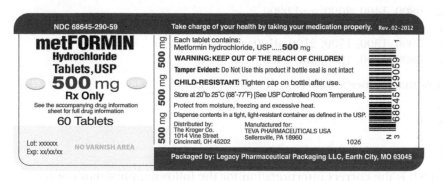

What is the information from the label that would need to be entered in a complete DA equation to calculate the dose?

a. The total amount supplied in the container, the unit dose supplied, and a conversion formula

b. The generic name of the drug

c. The unit dose concentration supplied

d. The ordered dose

14 Ordered: Synthroid 0.05 mg for a patient with hypothyroidism.

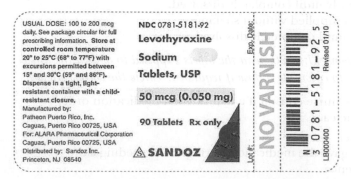

The unit dose concentration is

a. 100 tablets

b. 50 mcg per tab

c. 0.5 mg per tab

d. 50 mg per tab

15 **Ordered:** epinephrine 0.3 mg IM stat for a patient who is having a severe
allergic reaction.

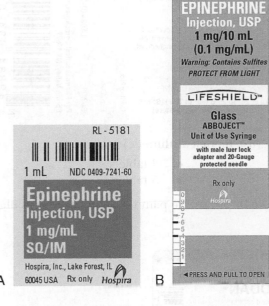

Which medication and dose would you select and prepare?

a. Label B, 0.03 mL
b. Label A, 0.3 mL
c. Label B, 3 mL
d. Label A, 3.3 mL

16 **Ordered:** erythromycin 250-mg tablet PO q8h for a patient with an infection.

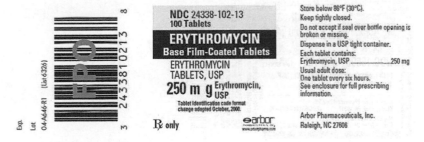

What is the form of this drug?

a. Milligrams
b. Film-coated tablets
c. Capsules
d. Double-strength tablets

17 **Ordered:** dexamethasone tablets 500 mcg PO daily in AM for a patient with an inflammatory disorder.

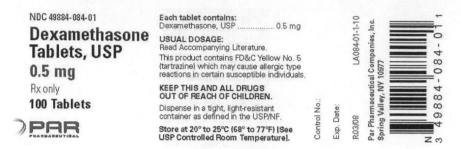

The nurse would administer (use mental arithmetic)

a. 1 tablet   **c.** 3 tablets
b. 2 tablets   **d.** 5 tablets

18 **Ordered:** Percodan 1 tab PO q4h prn severe pain for a patient who is allergic to aspirin.

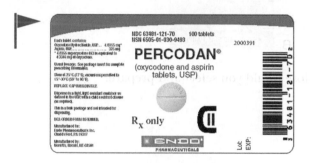

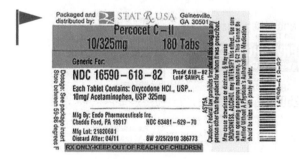

Which action should the nurse take?

a. Give the Percodan as ordered by the prescriber.
b. Give the Percocet because the patient is allergic to aspirin.
c. Withhold the medication and contact the prescriber.
d. Withhold the medication until the prescriber visits the patient.

Always check doses for compound medications such as Percocet and Percodan. They may be offered in different strengths.

19 Ordered: digoxin 62.5 mcg PO for a child with heart failure.

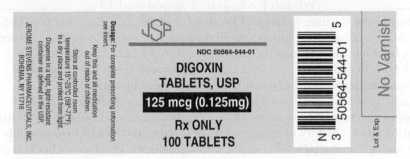

   a. You would give 1 tablet.

   b. You would give $\frac{1}{2}$ tablet.

   c. You would hold this tablet and clarify with the physician.

   d. You would give two tablets.

20 Ordered: cimetidine 0.8 g PO at bedtime daily for an adult with a gastric ulcer.

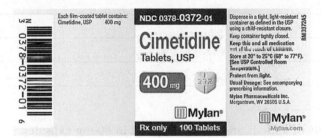

What would be the appropriate complete nurse interpretation?

   a. Give 1 tablet daily at bedtime.

   b. Give 2 tablets daily at bedtime.

   c. Give $\frac{1}{2}$ tablet daily at bedtime.

   d. Hold the medication and notify the prescriber.

CHAPTER 4   FINAL PRACTICE

ESTIMATED COMPLETION TIME: 10 to 20 minutes   **ANSWERS ON:** page 152

DIRECTIONS: *As you read the following paragraph, write out the definition of each italicized abbreviation in the space provided. Reread the paragraph as often as necessary to become comfortable with the abbreviations.*

A patient was admitted to the hospital in a diabetic coma. X-rays and laboratory tests were ordered **1** _____ *(stat).* The vital signs were assessed **2** _____ *(qh)* and **3** _____ *(prn).* All of the medications were given **4** _____ *(IV)* because the patient was **5** _____ *(NPO).* Patients who are in a coma cannot swallow **6** _____ *(PO)* medications. Oral medications and feedings may go into their airways. The patient's mental status was slow to respond to treatment. Feedings were administered via **7** _____ *(TPN)* with a tube inserted into the subclavian vein. Later, as the patient began to be more alert, a **8** _____ *(NG)* tube was inserted to deliver liquid food and medications with the patient in an upright position. Insulin was discontinued **9** _____ *(IV)* and given **10** _____ *(subcut).* The patient still had difficulty swallowing for a while but eventually graduated to sips and chips: sips of water and chips of ice. Because that was tolerated well, the **11** _____ *(NG).* tube was removed and small **12** _____ *(PO)* soft feedings were introduced **13** _____ *(q2h)* during the daytime hours and fluids **14** _____ *(ad lib).* The nurse always assessed the patient's mental status and ability to swallow before giving a feeding. Medications for pain were given **15** _____ *(IM q4h prn).* Rectal **16** _____ *(supp)* were given for complaints of nausea. Medications for coexisting problems were now given **17** _____ *(PO),* such as **18** _____ *(elix* and *susp bid)* because they were easy to swallow **19** _____ *(s̄)* choking incidents. The patient had a history of angina and chest pain attacks and now was able to take nitroglycerine pills **20** _____ *(subl).* The nurse checked at each visit to find out how many the patient had taken because the physician needed to be called if more than a maximum of 3 tablets, 5 minutes apart, did not provide relief. The nurse knew that all chest pain signals a heart attack unless proven otherwise. The patient did not suffer any adverse drug events (ADE) during hospitalization and was discharged in 10 days.

DIRECTIONS: *For questions 21 to 29, state the Nine Rights of Medication Administration.*

21 _____   **26** _____

22 _____   **27** _____

23 _____   **28** _____

24 _____   **29** _____

25 _____

30 Ordered: 0.1 g PO daily of a medication. It is supplied in 50-mg capsules.

How many capsules will you give? _____

31 **Ordered:** erythromycin delayed-release 0.5 g capsules PO twice daily for a patient with an infection.

NDC 0074-6301-13
100 Capsules

ERYTHROMYCIN
Delayed-release
Capsules, USP

250 mg

℞ only

3 00746 30113 4

Exp.
Lot
02-8497-3/R6

Do not accept if seal over bottle opening is broken or missing.
Protect from moisture and excessive heat.
Store below 86°F (30°C).
Dispense in a USP tight container.
Each capsule contains:
Erythromycin, 250 mg
Usual adult dose:
One capsule every six hours.
See enclosure for full prescribing information.
Each maroon and clear capsule contains yellow and pink particles and bears the ⬡ and Abbo-Code ER for product identification.
©Abbott
Abbott Laboratories
North Chicago,
IL 60064, U.S.A.

a. What is the generic name of this medication? _____
b. What is the total daily dose in grams and milligrams? _____
c. What is the unit dose concentration? _____
d. How many capsules will you give per dose? _____

32 a. Write the two required pieces of information from the medication order and the label that must be entered in all medication dose calculations.

_____

_____

b. Write the variable piece or pieces of information that may need to be entered in medication dose calculations. _____

RAPID PRACTICE 4-1 (p. 104)

1	enteric coated	6	supp
2	LA	7	CD
3	tab	8	UNG
4	XL	9	XR
5	DS	10	cap

RAPID PRACTICE 4-2 (p. 105)

1 scored tablet
2 compound
3 XR; XL; SR; CD; LA
4 enteric-coated tablet; capsules
5 cap

RAPID PRACTICE 4-3 (p. 106)

1	sol.	4	susp.
2	elix.	5	mixt.
3	aq.		

RAPID PRACTICE 4-4 (p. 108)

1	top	6	NG
2	NPO	7	MDI
3	bucc	8	vag
4	left ear	9	SL
5	GT	10	PO

RAPID PRACTICE 4-5 (p. 118)

1 before meals
2 immediately (and only one dose)
3 as needed
4 without
5 qid
6 prn
7 twice a day
8 c̄
9 nothing by mouth
10 q
11 q2h
12 every 4 hours
13 after meals
14 tid
15 s̄
16 with (as "with meals")
17 q12h
18 give as desired (pertaining to fluids or activity)
19 ac
20 subcut or written out subcutaneously

RAPID PRACTICE 4-6 (p. 119)

1 4; 6
2 T = tricycle; B = bicycle (3 wheels)   (2 wheels)
3 q4h = 6 times a day
4 **a.** Give "Tears No More" 2 (two) drops in each eye twice a day as needed for itching or burning
   b. Give Mylanta antacid 1 (one) ounce three times a day before meals
   c. Pharmacy
5 PRN

RAPID PRACTICE 4-7 (p. 120)

1	prn	6	fld
2	IM	7	sol
3	elix	8	top
4	stat	9	NPO
5	fld ext	10	susp

11 as needed; when necessary
12 cheek (to be dissolved, not swallowed)
13 as desired (for fluids, activity)
14 intravenous piggyback*
15 two times daily
16 metered dose inhaler
17 Give medication when X-ray calls for the patient.
18 nothing by mouth
19 intradermal
20 every 6 hours

*Do not use the abbreviation IVP for medication routes. IVP is an IV renal function test.

RAPID PRACTICE 4-8 (p. 120)

1	two times daily	10	gastrostomy tube
2	every six hours	11	every eight hours
3	immediately (for only one dose)	12	every night at bedtime
4	intramuscular	13	oral, by mouth
5	before meals	14	solution
6	after meals	15	nasogastric tube
7	as needed, when necessary	16	sublingual
8	three times daily	17	elixir
9	nothing by mouth	18	every four hours
		19	double strength
		20	every hour

RAPID PRACTICE 4-9 (p. 122)

1	b	4	a
2	c	5	c
3	d		

RAPID PRACTICE 4-10 (p. 128)

1 **a.** lorazepam
   b. 100 tab
   c. 0.5 mg
2 **a.** multiple dose vial
   b. 400 mcg per mL
   c. 0.4 mg per mL
3 **a.** potassium chloride
   b. 20 mEq per 15 mL
4 **a.** Sinemet
   b. 2 (it is a compound drug)
   c. carbidopa 10 mg, levodopa 100 mg
5 **a.** Elixir
   b. 20 mg per 5 mL
   c. 15%

RAPID PRACTICE 4-11 (p. 131)

2 **a.** capsules
   b. 250 mg per capsule
   c. 0.5 g
   d. 1000 mg = 1 gram
   e. 2 g or 2000 mg (q6h = 4 times in 24 hrs)
   f. 0.5 g = 0.500. = 500 mg
3 **a.** azithromycin
   b. suspension
   c. 200 mg per 5 mL—label B (0.2 g = 200 mg)
   d. 0.2 g
   e. 1000 mg = 1 gram
4 **a.** mL
   b. 15 mg per mL
   c. intramuscular
   d. immediately
   e. intramuscular, subcutaneous, intravenous
5 **a.** mL
   b. 125 mg per 5 mL
   c. 0.25 g
   d. 1000 mg = 1 g
   e. 1 g (0.25 g × 4 doses) = 1 gram per day
   f. 0.250 g = 250 mg

RAPID PRACTICE 4-12 (p. 136)

1 medication errors due to misinterpretation, forgetting, not hearing, etc.
2 They may look like other numbers such as 1 and 0.
3 the prescriber
4 with = $\bar{c}$; without = $\bar{s}$
5 Prepare and mix medications together; deliver immediately by intramuscular route.

RAPID PRACTICE 4-13 (p. 140)

1 penicillin; ASA (aspirin)
2 Lasix. Document the clarification. Report to nurse supervisor.
3 2400
4 1600
5 Humalog

6 losartan (Cozaar). Blood pressure assessment is needed.
7 acetaminophen
8 This is an appropriate order as it writes out where the ointment is to be instilled instead of using outdated abbreviations which are on the TJC "Official Do Not Use List", or the ISMP Error-Prone Abbreviations, Symbols and Dosage Designations.
9 NKDA–No
10 every 4 hours

RAPID PRACTICE 4-14 (p. 144)

1 a
2 d
3 f
4 g
5 b
6 c
7 e
8 **a** Right patient
   b Right drug
   c Right dose
   d Right time
   e Right route
   f Right reason for the drug
   g Right patient education
   h Right to refuse treatment
   i Right documentation

CHAPTER 4 MULTIPLE-CHOICE REVIEW (p. 144)

1 c
2 b
3 a
4 b
5 d
6 c
7 a
8 b
9 b
10 d
11 a
12 b
13 c
14 b
15 b
16 b
17 a
18 c
19 b (scored tablet)
20 b

CHAPTER 4 FINAL PRACTICE (p. 149)

1 immediately
2 every hour
3 as needed
4 intravenously
5 nothing by mouth
6 by mouth
7 total parenteral nutrition
8 nasogastric
9 intravenously
10 subcutaneously
11 nasogastric
12 by mouth
13 every 2 hours
14 as desired
15 intramuscularly every 4 hours as needed
16 suppositories
17 by mouth
18 elixirs and suspensions two times daily
19 without
20 sublingually
21 right patient

22 right drug
23 right dose
24 right time
25 right route
26 right documentation
27 right to refuse
28 right patient education
29 right reason
30 2 capsules

$$\frac{\text{capsules}}{\text{dose}} = \frac{1 \text{ capsule}}{\cancel{50 \text{ mg}}} \times \frac{\overset{20}{\cancel{1000 \text{ mg}}}}{1 \text{ g}} \times \frac{0.1 \cancel{\text{ g}}}{\text{dose}}$$

$$= \frac{2 \text{ capsules}}{\text{dose}}$$

31 **a.** erythromycin
b. 0.5 g × 2 = 1 g per day or 1000 mg per day
c. 250 mg per capsule
d. 2 tablets per dose

$$\frac{\text{capsule}}{\text{dose}} = \frac{1 \text{ capsule}}{\cancel{250 \text{ mg}}} \times \frac{\overset{4}{\cancel{1000 \text{ mg}}}}{1 \cancel{\text{ g}}} \times \frac{0.5 \cancel{\text{ g}}}{\text{dose}}$$

$$= \frac{2 \text{ capsules}}{\text{dose}}$$

32 **a.** the ordered dose; the unit dose concentration
b. one or more conversion formulas

Suggestions for Further Reading

Lilley LL, Collins SR, Snyder JS: Pharmacology and the nursing process, ed 9,
    St Louis, 2020, Mosby.
http://www.justice.gov/dea/druginfo
http://www.fda.gov/Drugs
http://www.ismp.org/
http://www.jointcommission.org/
www.fda.gov/Safety/MedWatch

Chapter 5 introduces a large variety of metric oral medication problems using dimensional analysis to calculate and verify results.

22. right drug
23. right dose
24. right time
25. right route
26. right documentation
27. right to refuse
28. right patient education
   right reason
29. 2 capsules.

$$\text{capsules} = \frac{1 \text{ capsule}}{50 \text{ mg}} \times \frac{1000 \text{ mg}}{1 \text{ g}} \times \frac{0.1 \text{ g}}{\text{dose}}$$

$$= \frac{\overset{1}{\cancel{2}} \text{ capsules}}{\text{dose}}$$

31. a. erythromycin
   b. $0.5 \text{ g} \times 2 = 1 \text{ g per day or } 1000 \text{ mg per day}$
   c. 250 mg per capsule
   d. 2 tablets per dose

$$\text{capsules} = \frac{1 \text{ capsule}}{250 \text{ mg}} \times \frac{1000 \text{ mg}}{1 \text{ g}} \times \frac{0.5 \text{ g}}{\text{dose}}$$

$$= \frac{2 \text{ capsules}}{\text{dose}}$$

32. a. the ordered dose, the unit dose concentration
   b. one or more conversion formulas

Suggestions for Further Reading

Lilley LL, Collins SR, Snyder JS. Pharmacology and the nursing process, ed 9. St. Louis, 2020, Mosby.

http://www.justice.gov/dea/druginfo
http://www.fda.gov/Drugs
http://www.ismp.org/
http://www.jointcommission.org/
www.fda.gov/Safety/MedWatch

Chapter 5 introduces a large variety of parenteral medication problems using dimensional analysis to calculate and verify results.

PART III

Reconstituted Medications

5 Oral Medications

OBJECTIVES

- Estimate, calculate, and evaluate a variety of solid and liquid medication doses.
- Calculate dosages for liquid medications to the nearest tenth of a milliliter.
- Measure oral liquids in a calibrated measuring cup.
- Measure syringe volumes in 3- and 5-mL syringes.
- Calculate and evaluate safe dose ranges (SDRs) for medication doses.

ESTIMATED TIME TO COMPLETE CHAPTER: 2 hours

Giving medications orally is generally safe, convenient, and relatively economical. Most medications are available in an oral form by tablet, capsule, lozenge, or liquid. The rate of absorption can vary based on the gastric environment produced by digestive enzymes, food, other medications, and liver function. The drugs are absorbed by the gastrointestinal tract, generally in the small intestine.

This chapter builds on prior knowledge to solve many basic and complex medication problems using dimensional analysis (DA), with an emphasis on estimation of answers before completing the calculations and evaluating the final answer by comparing it to the estimation.

VOCABULARY

Calibration	Set of graduations that indicate capacity or size in standard units of measure. Measuring devices for precise doses of medications have calibrations, such as the lines on a measuring cup or a syringe.
Concentration, Liquid	Ratio of a specific amount of drug in a specified amount of solution; for example, 10 mg per mL or 5 mg per 5 mL.
Concentration, Solid	Ratio of a specific amount of drug contained in the solid drug form supplied; for example, 50 mg per cap. The concentration of a medication, solid or liquid, is always found on the label.
Fractional, Partial, or Divided Doses	Total dose for the day divided by a frequency schedule.
Precise	Having sharply defined, accurate limits based on a standard. For example, syringes, special medication droppers, and teaspoons have precise capacities. Household equipment does not.
Ratio	The relationship between two quantities.
Safe Dose Range (SDR)	Manufacturer's dosage guidelines for minimum and maximum safe medication doses based on laboratory and clinical trials of therapeutic effectiveness. For example, the SDR for aspirin for adults is 325 to 650 mg q4h. The nurse must interpret and apply this information to a medication order with consideration of the patient's age, weight, and medical condition.

| RAPID PRACTICE 5-1 | Oral Solid Dosage Calculations |

ESTIMATED COMPLETION TIME: 10 to 20 minutes   **ANSWERS ON:** page 198

DIRECTIONS: *Convert the dose ordered to the desired dose using estimation and mental arithmetic. Verify your answer with calculations.*

	Ordered	Dose Concentration Supplied	Amount to Give
1	350 mcg	0.175 mg per tab scored	
2	0.5 mg	0.25 mg per cap	
3	250 mg	0.5 g per tab scored	
4	1 g	500 mg per cap	
5	0.25 mg	0.125 mg per tab scored	
6	2.5 g	1000 mg per tab scored	
7	0.5 mg	0.25 mg per tab scored	
8	150 mg	0.1 g per tab scored	
9	0.1 mg	0.2 mg per tab scored	
10	125 mg	250 mg per tab scored	

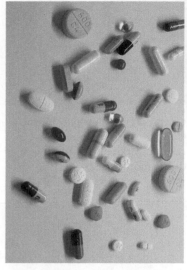

Examples of oral tablets (both scored and unscored) and capsules.

➤ To avoid major math errors, make it a habit to estimate the approximate dose before doing the calculations.

➤ Always recheck orders that exceed one to two times the unit dose supplied.

➤ Administering three tablets is a red flag to the nurse that the dose may exceed the recommended range.

EXAMPLES

Ordered: 250 mg.

Available: dose concentration 125 mg per cap.

The nurse can see at a glance that the order is about *twice* the amount on hand. If the numbers do not divide evenly, an *approximate* amount of the unit dose is estimated.

| RAPID PRACTICE 5-2 | Oral Solid Dose Calculations Using Estimation and DA Equations |

ESTIMATED COMPLETION TIME: 30 to 60 minutes   **ANSWERS ON:** page 198

DIRECTIONS: *Review the metric equivalents in Chapter 4. Study worked-out problem 1, and solve problems 2-5. Estimate answers by moving decimals for needed conversions, and <u>verify</u> with a DA equation. Evaluate answers: Is the equation balanced? Does the estimate support the answer? It would be helpful to write out the four steps of the DA equation before proceeding to problem 2.*

➤ Remember that the unit concentration supplied (on the label) and the dose ordered by the prescriber must be part of every medication dose calculation.

1   **Ordered:** 0.5 g tab PO daily. **Label:** dose concentration 250 mg per tab.
   a.   Metric conversion factor needed: 1000 mg = 1 g
   b.   Estimated dose: 0.5 g = 500 mg; 500 mg = 2 × 250 mg, or 2 tab

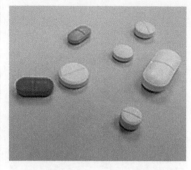

Only scored tablets may be cut. Cutting unscored tablets can result in uneven distribution of drug amounts.

c. Amount of tablets to administer:
DA equation:

$$? \frac{\text{tab}}{\text{dose}} = \frac{1 \text{ tab}}{\underset{1}{\cancel{250 \text{ mg}}}} \times \frac{\overset{4}{\cancel{1000 \text{ mg}}}}{1 \cancel{\text{ g}}} \times \frac{0.5 \cancel{\text{ g}}}{\text{dose}} = \frac{2 \text{ tab}}{\text{dose}}$$

d. Evaluation: The equation is balanced. The estimate supports the answer.

2 **Ordered:** 0.25 g tab PO daily. **Label:** dose concentration 125 mg per tab scored.

a. Metric conversion factor needed: _____
b. Estimated dose: _____
c. Amount of tablets to administer:
DA equation:

d. Evaluation: _____

3 **Ordered:** 0.1 g tab PO daily. **Label:** dose concentration 0.05 g per tab.

a. Metric conversion factor needed: _____
b. Estimated dose: _____
c. Amount of tablets to administer:
DA equation:

d. Evaluation: _____

4 **Ordered:** 0.175 mg tab PO daily. **Label:** dose concentration 350 mcg per tab scored.

a. Metric conversion factor needed: _____
b. Estimated dose: _____
c. Amount of tablets to administer:
DA equation:

d. Evaluation: _____

5 **Ordered:** 0.2 g cap PO at bedtime. **Label:** dose concentration 100 mg per cap.

a. Metric conversion factor needed: _____
b. Estimated dose: _____
c. Amount of capsules to administer:
DA equation:

d. Evaluation: _____

6 **Ordered:** 0.25 g cap PO tid. **Label:** dose concentration 125 mg per cap.

a. Metric conversion factor needed: _____
b. Estimated dose: _____
c. Amount of capsules to administer:
DA equation:

d. Evaluation: _____

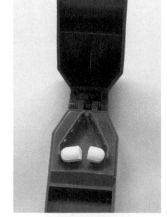

Pill cutter to cut scored tablets. Each patient must have his or her own pill cutter.

7 Ordered: 20 mEq tab PO bid. **Label:** dose concentration 10 mEq per tab.

   a. Metric conversion factor needed: _____

   b. Estimated dose: _____

   c. Amount of tablets to administer:
     DA equation:

   d. Evaluation: _____

8 Ordered: 0.1 mg tab PO daily. **Label:** dose concentration 50 mcg per tab.

   a. Metric conversion factor needed: _____

   b. Estimated dose: _____

   c. Amount of tablets to administer:
     DA equation:

   d. Evaluation: _____

9 Ordered: 75 mcg tab PO daily. **Label:** dose concentration 50 mcg per tab scored.

   a. Metric conversion factor needed: _____

   b. Estimated dose: _____

   c. Amount of tablets to administer:
     DA equation:

   d. Evaluation: _____

10 Ordered: 250 mg cap PO at bedtime. **Label:** dose concentration 0.25 g per cap.

   a. Metric conversion factor needed: _____

   b. Estimated dose: _____

   c. Amount of capsules to administer:
     DA equation:

   d. Evaluation: _____

---

1 What are the two pieces of information obtained from the order and label that must be entered in every dose calculation?

ASK YOURSELF **Q & A**

_____   _____   **MY ANSWER**

Metric Conversions by Moving Decimal Places

When a problem calls for converting micrograms to grams or grams to micrograms, beginners enter *two* conversion factors in a DA equation: micrograms to milligrams and milligrams to grams, or grams to milligrams and milligrams to micrograms.

Microgram–milligram conversions are frequently encountered in dose calculations. Microgram–gram conversions are occasionally needed in calculations of intravenous doses. Medication errors can occur when the prescriber writes an order in micrograms and the nurse mistakes it for milligrams or vice versa.

Microgram–gram conversions can be reduced to one step if desired by using the conversion factor 1,000,000 mcg = 1 g, since *micro-* means one millionth of the base unit, or by moving the decimal place six places to the right or left.

EXAMPLES

Conversion factor: 1,000,000 mcg = 1 g.

➤ To convert grams to micrograms, multiply by 1,000,000.

➤ To convert micrograms to grams, divide by 1,000,000.

Ordered		Equivalent	Decimal Movement
0.5 g	=	500,000 mcg	decimal moved six places to the right
250,000 mcg	=	0.25 0000 g	implied decimal moved six places to the left
0.004 g	=	4000 mcg	decimal moved six places to the right

TEST TIP If you are comfortable with milligram conversions (milligrams to micrograms and milligrams to grams), use a stepped approach for microgram–gram conversions. First, change the ordered amount to milligrams and then to micrograms.

➤ Converting micrograms to grams and grams to micrograms involves two steps—1000 mcg = 1 mg, and 1000 mg = 1 g—for a total of six decimal place movements. It is expedient to study the relationships among the mcg/mg/g conversions at one time.

RAPID PRACTICE 5-3 Converting Microgram, Milligram, and Gram Equivalents

ESTIMATED COMPLETION TIME: 5 to 10 minutes   ANSWERS ON: page 199

DIRECTIONS: *Convert the ordered units to milligram, microgram, or gram equivalents.*

Ordered	Milligrams	Micrograms or Grams
1 0.3 g	300 mg	300,000 mcg
2 300,000 mcg	_____	_____ g
3 25,000 mcg	_____	_____ g
4 80,000 mcg	_____	_____ g
5 0.1 g	_____	_____ mcg

RAPID PRACTICE 5-4	Decimal Conversions

ESTIMATED COMPLETION TIME: 10 to 15 minutes   **ANSWERS ON:** page 199

DIRECTIONS: *Fill in the equivalent units.*

Needed Conversion	Answer	Needed Conversion	Answer
1 350 mcg = ? mg	_____	**6** 0.05 g = ? mg	_____
2 50,000 mcg = ? g	_____	**7** 0.004 g = ? mcg	_____
3 0.3 g = ? mg	_____	**8** 0.5 mg = ? mcg	_____
4 500 mg = ? g	_____	**9** 200 mcg = ? mg	_____
5 2200 mg = ? g	_____	**10** 15,000 mcg = ? g	_____

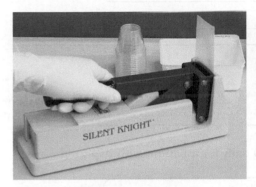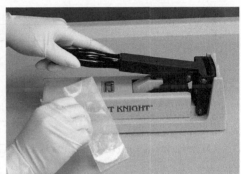

Tablet-crushing system that contains disposable pouches to prevent cross-contamination with other crushed medications

RAPID PRACTICE 5-5	Oral Medication Practice

ESTIMATED COMPLETION TIME: 30 minutes   **ANSWERS ON:** page 199

DIRECTIONS: *Study the medication order and the unit dose supplied. Estimate the answer and verify it with a DA equation. Evaluate the answer. Is the equation balanced? Does the estimate support the answer?*

➤ The desired answer unit is usually found in the available unit dose concentration. How is the ordered drug supplied: in tablets, capsules, or milliliters? That unit will be the desired answer unit for these kinds of problems.

➤ To prevent medication errors, always tell the patient and or family the name and dose of the medication being given and recheck when there's a question. Recognize that generics are often substituted for brand names.

1 Ordered: Oxycodone 60 mg PO stat for a patient with pain.

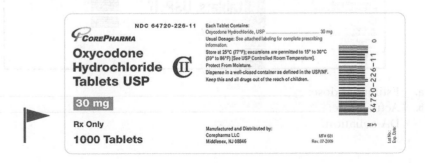

> **✴ Communication**
>
> Nurse: "Mr. Jones, I have your blood pressure medication, lopressor, ____ mg. Do you take this at home?"
> Mr. Jones: "I take blood pressure medication but I can't remember the name or how much."
> Nurse: "It has another name, metoprolol."
> Mr. Jones: "That's what I take at home, but it's a different color."
>   The nurse holds the medication and rechecks the order because a different color of the same medication indicates a different dosage. If there is nothing on the record to indicate why the dosage would be changed, the prescriber needs to be contacted promptly.

    a. Estimated dose: _____

    b. Actual dose: _____

        DA equation:

    c. Evaluation: _____

2 **Ordered:** clorazepate dipotassium tablets 15 mg PO tid for a patient with chronic anxiety.

    a. Estimated dose: _____

    b. Actual dose: _____

        DA equation:

    c. Evaluation: _____

3 **Ordered:** metoprolol tablets 0.1 g PO daily for a patient with hypertension.

    a. Estimated dose: _____

    b. Actual dose: _____

        DA equation:

    c. Evaluation: _____

4 **Ordered:** alprazolam tablets 1 mg PO prn at bedtime for a patient with anxiety.

    a. Estimated dose: _____

    b. Actual dose: _____

        DA equation:

    c. Evaluation: _____

5 **Ordered:** Biaxin 0.25 g PO daily for a patient with an infection.

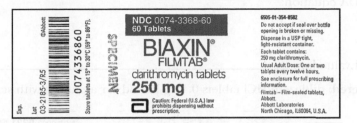

   a. Estimated dose: _____

   b. Actual dose: _____
      DA equation:

   c. Evaluation: _____

RAPID PRACTICE 5-6   Additional Oral Medication Practice

ESTIMATED COMPLETION TIME: 20 minutes   **ANSWERS ON:** page 199

DIRECTIONS: *Estimate answer and verify with DA equation. Evaluate the answer. Supply needed conversion factors.*

1 **Ordered:** methocarbamol tablets 1000 mg PO tid for a patient with recurrent muscle spasms.

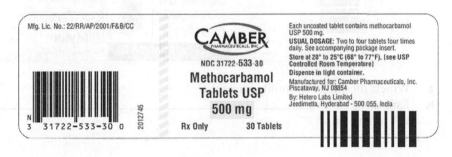

   a. Estimated dose: _____
      DA equation:

   b. Evaluation: _____

2 **Ordered:** enalapril maleate tablets 5 mg PO daily for a patient with hypertension.

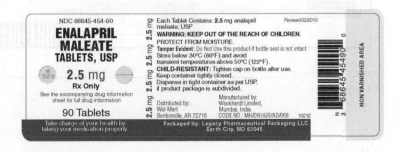

a. Estimated dose: _____

DA equation:

b. Evaluation: _____

3   **Ordered:** diltiazem HCl tablets 0.12 g PO tid for a patient with stable angina.

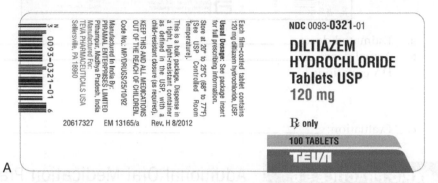

A

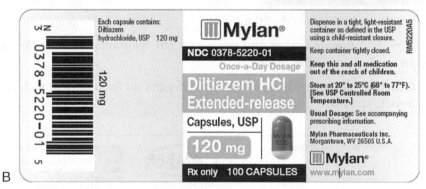

B

a. Which medication would you select?

b. Estimated dose: _____

DA equation:

c. Evaluation: _____

4   **Ordered:** zidovudine capsules 0.3 g PO bid for a patient who is HIV positive.

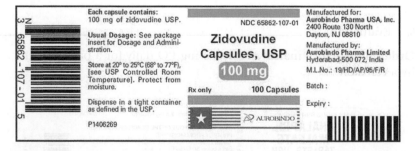

a. Estimated dose: _____

DA equation:

b. Evaluation: _____

5 **Ordered:** alprazolam tablet 0.5 mg PO q12h for a patient with anxiety.

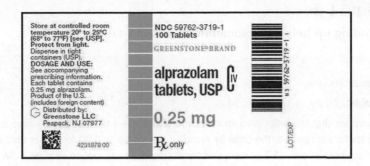

a. Estimated dose: _____

DA equation:

b. Evaluation: _____

Estimating Liquid Dose Medication Orders

Liquids may be supplied in a variety of containers. As with all dose calculations, the ordered dose and the drug concentration noted on the label must be included in the calculation. Liquid medications *ordered* and *supplied* in milligrams may require a calculation if the dose is supplied in more than 1 mL of solution. The estimate of the answer can be made right away if the metric units are matched. Compare the result with your estimate.

Estimating is a critical thinking skill versus "guessing," which is not and leads to wrong answers.

Estimating liquid doses

Ordered: Drug A 350 mg PO daily.

Available: Dose concentration supplied: 250 mg per 5 mL.

The dose ordered and the drug supplied are in the same terms (milligrams). It is easy to see that the dose *ordered* (350 mg) will be *more than one* but *less than two* times the unit dose concentration supplied (250 mg in 5 mL, less than 2 × 5 mL).

EXAMPLES

Misinterpretation

Loss of focus may cause the nurse to reverse the order with the concentration supplied.

➤ Avoid distractions. Focus on the order in relation to the strength on hand.

Rounding numbers to simplify estimations of a liquid dose

➤ Rounding up helps the estimation in some instances.

EXAMPLES

Ordered: 300 mg.

Available: 75 mg in 1 mL of liquid.

It is obvious that the order calls for *much more* than the unit dose per milliliter supplied. The nurse might approximate the dose by rounding the 75 up to 100 for easier division, giving a rough estimate of around 3 or more unit doses. The exact calculation requires a DA equation.

EXAMPLES

Examine the following order:

Ordered: 200 mg liquid.

Available: 80 mg per 5 mL concentration.

The terms are the same: milligrams. It is obvious that the order for 200 mg exceeds two times the dose (80 mg) per volume on hand. Thus, *the estimate is that more than 10 mL will be given.* Follow the estimate with an exact calculation in a DA equation. Compare the result with the estimate.

➤ Your calculation rounding is based on the calibration (nearest measurable dose) of the equipment you are using.

RAPID PRACTICE 5-7

Metric Conversions and Estimating Answers for Liquid Medications

ESTIMATED COMPLETION TIME: 10 minutes   **ANSWERS ON:** page 200

DIRECTIONS: *Examine the order and the label concentration. Follow the example in problem 1 to estimate the dose to be administered to the nearest milliliter or number of tablets.*

	Dose Ordered	Concentration Available	Conversion	Give Same, More, or Less of Available Dose per Volume	Estimated Amount
1	0.25 g	250 mg per mL	0.25 g = 250 mg	Same	1 mL
2	5000 mcg	2.5 mg per mL	_____	_____	_____
3	200 mg	0.1 g per mL	_____	_____	_____
4	0.1 g	300 mg per mL	_____	_____	_____
5	750 mg	0.5 g per mL	_____	_____	_____

Liquid unit dose concentrations are often written with a slash (e.g., 100 mg/5 mL). The slash mark (/) appears in printed drug literature for drug concentrations. It should *not be handwritten* in a patient's medical record. The slash can be misinterpreted as the number 1 if it occurs next to a number. For example, 100 mg/5 mL could be read as 100 mg per 15 mL instead of 5 mL. Write *per* instead of using the slash: 100 mg **per** 5 mL. The slash is clearly seen in printed materials.

➤ With oral liquid metric measurements, the final question is usually: How many milliliters should be given?

Setting Up DA-Style Equations

Review: The process required is to multiply a given quantity by one or more conversion factors to solve an equation. The process is the same for a liquid as for a solid.
- The given quantity in medication calculations is the *prescribed order.*
- The first entry in the equation is the *dose concentration on the label with the desired answer in the numerator.*

When ordered dose and available unit concentration match

Ordered: diazepam 10 mg at bedtime for a patient with anxiety.

Available: Unit dose concentration (on label): diazepam 20 mg per 5 mL.

How many milliliters (mL) (per dose implied) will you give?

?	Step 1	=	Step 2	×	Step 3	=	Answer
?	Desired Answer Units	=	Starting Factor	×	Given Quantity and Conversion Factor(s)	=	Estimate, Multiply, Evaluate
?	$\dfrac{mL}{dose}$	=	$\dfrac{5\ mL}{20\ mg}$	×	$\dfrac{\overset{1}{\cancel{10\ mg}}}{dose}$	=	$\dfrac{5}{2} = \dfrac{2.5\ mL}{per\ dose}$

(Step 2 denominator: $\underset{2}{\cancel{20\ mg}}$)

Analysis: This simple equation contains the ordered dose and the unit dose information from the medication label (5 mL per 20 mg or 20 mg per 5 mL). The unit dose information is selected for the Starting Factor and oriented to match up the desired answer units (mL) in the numerator. Per dose is related to the order as well as the answer. No other conversion factors are needed because the order and the label are both mg units. The nurse needs to calculate the individual dose to be given.

Evaluation: Only mL per dose remain in the answer. The estimate to give ½ of the available 5 mL unit dose supports the answer (math check: 50/20 = 2.5). The equation is balanced.

FAQ *What is the most common error seen with liquid dose calculations?*

ANSWER Sometimes the amount of drug is confused with the amount of solution. For example, *10 mg per 5 mL* means there are 10 mg of drug in *each 5 mL* of solution. The nurse needs to stay focused when doing the math.

When the ordered units do not match the available units

Metric equivalent conversion factor(s) are necessary when the ordered units do not match the available dose concentration. If another conversion is necessary, make room for it before entering the ordered dose.

EXAMPLES

Ordered: 1 mg of a medicine.

Available: Dose concentration 500 mcg per 2 mL.

Conversion factor: 1000 mcg = 1 mg.

How many milliliters will you give (per dose)?

?	Step 1	=	Step 2	×	Step 3	=	Answer
?	Desired Answer Units	=	Starting Factor	×	Given Quantity and Conversion Factor(s)	=	Estimate, Multiply, Evaluate

$$? \quad \frac{mL}{dose} = \frac{2\ mL}{\overset{1}{\underset{}{500\ mcg}}} \times \frac{\overset{2}{1000\ mcg}}{1\ mg} \times \frac{1\ mg}{dose} = 4\ mL\ per\ dose$$

Analysis: The available dose concentration stated on the label has a numerator and a denominator. This is a conversion factor that can be inverted without changing the value. For every 2 mL there are 500 mcg and in every 500 mcg there are 2 mL. Once again, the selected Starting Factor *matches up* to the desired answer, permitting sequential cancellation.

Evaluation: The ordered information, the unit dose information on the label, and a conversion factor were entered in the correct orientation. An estimate that the answer would be about double the unit dose of 2 mL was made after all the data were entered. The estimate supported the answer (math check: 2000 ÷ 500 = 4). The equation is balanced.

➤ TIP: The math is very simple if the units and numbers are cancelled.

Q & A **ASK YOURSELF**

1   As you look at the previous example, which *three* key pieces of data are entered in the equation?

MY ANSWER   _____

2   If the units supplied and the units ordered were in the same measurement terms, milligrams, which entry in step 3 could be eliminated?

_____

Usual Unit Doses

➤ Most solid doses ordered are $\frac{1}{2}$ to 2 times the supplied unit dose, such as $\frac{1}{2}$ to 2 tablets or 1 or 2 capsules.

➤ With liquids, check current drug references for the usual dose; the amount can vary.

CLINICAL RELEVANCE

Sometimes a very frail person—a baby or an adult with a very low weight, or a person with a very serious illness—will receive a fractional dose (a very small amount of the unit dose), or because an illness is so aggressive or the person is larger than average, an unusually large dose will be ordered.

➤ If there is a question on an order, hold the medication, recheck the order, then a current drug reference and promptly clarify unusual doses with the prescriber if there is a question.

FAQ *Why are DA equations required when the answer can be calculated more simply?*

ANSWER Safe dose calculations require that the nurse has a solid back-up method for verification and for more complex problems. With repetition and practice, the nurse will find it easy to quickly and independently confirm calculations. It is unsafe to rely on peers who may make a calculation error.

➤ The nurse who administers the medication is legally responsible to verify a safe medication dose and be able to calculate medication dosages accurately.

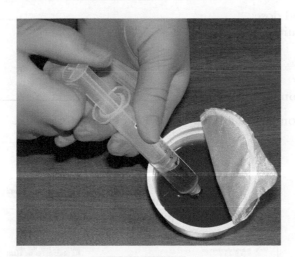

Many oral medications come in unit dose packages. The patient may drink from the cup, or a partial dose may be drawn up with a syringe or measured in a calibrated medicine cup.

Oral Liquid Doses Using DA

ESTIMATED COMPLETION TIME: 20 to 30 minutes   **ANSWERS ON:** page 200

DIRECTIONS: *Estimate, calculate, and evaluate the following ordered doses using DA.*

1 **Ordered:** diphenhydramine oral solution 15 mL PO at bedtime for a patient with allergic rhinitis.

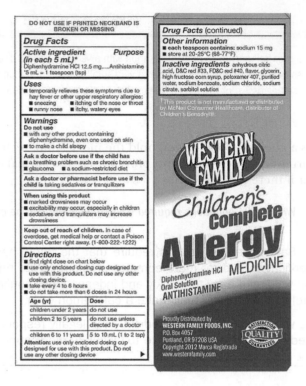

a. Estimated dose: _____

DA equation:

b. Evaluation: _____

2 **Ordered:** promethazine syrup 10 mg PO q6h prn for cough.

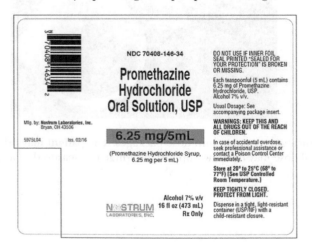

a. Estimated dose: _____

DA equation:

b. Evaluation: _____

3 **Ordered:** Quadrapax elixir 40.5 mg PO twice daily for seizure control.

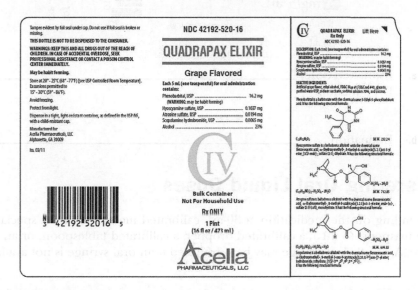

a. Estimated dose: _____

DA equation:

b. Evaluation: _____

4 **Ordered:** cefixime oral susp. 0.4 g PO q12h for a patient with otitis media.

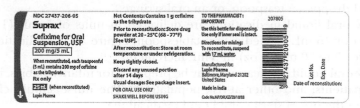

a. Estimated dose: _____

DA equation:

b. Evaluation: _____

5 **Ordered:** ondansetron hydrochloride solution 6 mg PO q8h prn to prevent chemotherapy-induced nausea and vomiting in a patient with cancer.

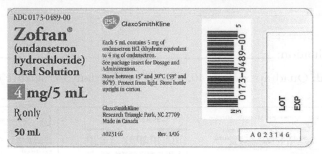

a. Estimated dose: _____

DA equation:

b. Evaluation: _____

Equipment for Administering Oral Liquid Doses

Depending on the medication, a 30-mL calibrated medicine cup, a special medicine teaspoon (5 mL), a calibrated dropper, a calibrated tablespoon, or an oral syringe. A needle-less syringe may be substituted if an oral syringe is not available.

Selecting the implement for oral liquid medications

The implement used to deliver an oral liquid unit dose is selected according to:

1 The amount of liquid to be administered

2 The ability of the patient to drink from a nipple or cup or to swallow from a medication spoon or dropper

Choosing the appropriate implement is not always age-related. Often, the medication is packaged with the equipment to be used, such as a medicine cup, a calibrated dropper, a teaspoon, or an oral syringe.

Many oral liquid medications are delivered in units of 5 mL (1 medication teaspoon) or 15 mL (1 medication tablespoon; Figure 5-1). Medication cups may be used for 5 to 30 mL (1 oz) in 5-mL increments.

Sterile oral liquid medications may be prepared for infants, babies, immunosuppressed patients, and other at-risk populations. The nurse should check agency policies on the use of sterile oral liquid medications.

➤ Nurses do not use household implements because they vary greatly in capacity.

➤ Patients must be instructed to use calibrated measuring devices if they will be discharged on liquid oral medications.

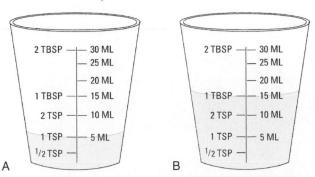

FIGURE 5-1 Medication cups. **A,** Filled to 5 mL. **B,** Filled to 15 mL.

Measuring Liquids

Measuring oral milliliter doses that call for more or less than the calibrated lines on the cup

Measuring oral doses may require the use of a syringe for more precise dosing if the dose is not a multiple of 5 mL. The metric measurements on the medication cups are calibrated in multiples of 5 mL (see Figure 5-1).

Oral Syringes

Oral syringes have milliliter marks on one side, and some have household *teaspoon* marks on the other (Figure 5-2). Their tips may be off center. Some of them are capped.

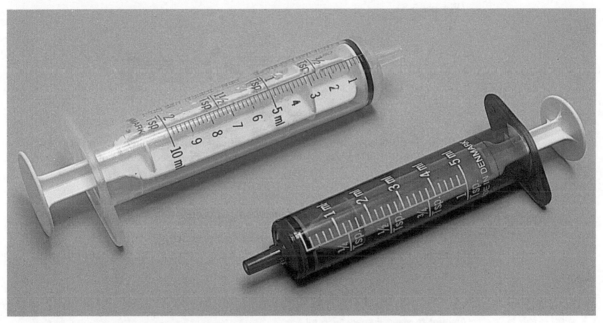

FIGURE 5-2 Oral syringes calibrated in 0.2 mL (two tenths). (From Willihnganz M, Gurevitz S, Clayton B: *Clayton's Basic pharmacology for nurses,* ed 18, St Louis, 2020, Elsevier.)

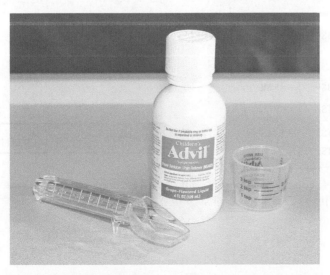

Liquid medications can be measured in a variety of methods.

Oral Syringes Versus Injectable Syringes

Only oral syringes should be used to give oral medications. Injectable (parenteral) syringes should never be used to give oral medications.

CLINICAL RELEVANCE

➤ Oral syringes are not to be used for injections. Do not confuse oral syringes with parenteral syringes. Oral syringes have milliliter calibrations and may have teaspoon or tablespoon marks as well. Their tips do not fit needles. They are *not sterile*. Errors have been caused by jamming needles onto oral syringes. The needles do not fit properly and can fall off during "injection."

➤ Remember to use special calibrated medication teaspoons, droppers, or oral syringes if they are needed.

➤ The exact amount ordered to the nearest tenth of a mL should be measured (Figure 5-3).

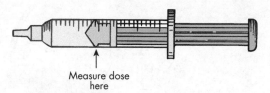

Measure dose
here

FIGURE 5-3 Reading a measured amount of medication in a syringe. (From Perry AG, Potter PA, Ostendorf WR: *Clinical nursing skills and techniques,* ed. 9, St. Louis, 2018, Mosby.)

FAQ   *May the whole dose be prepared in a syringe and inserted in the cup?*

ANSWER   Yes, oral liquid doses need to be drawn to the nearest tenth of a milliliter. Select the oral syringe that will provide the nearest measurable dose.

EXAMPLES

Amount to give: Prepare 17.5 mL.

Procedure: Pour to 15 mL and add 2.5 mL with a syringe (Figure 5-4).

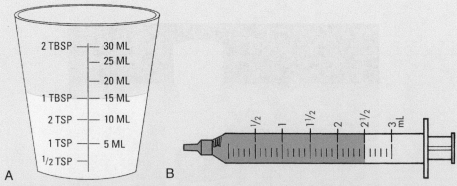

FIGURE 5-4 Total dose will be 17.5 mL. **A,** 15 mL prepared in medicine cup. **B,** 2.5 mL precise remainder added with syringe.

EXAMPLES

Amount to give: 12.4 mL.

Procedure: Pour to 10-mL calibration and add 2.4 mL with a 3-mL syringe.

Amount to give: 19 mL.

Procedure: Pour to 15-mL calibration and add 4 mL with a 5-mL syringe.

Review the steps

➤ Pour the nearest measurable dose in a 30-mL medicine cup; when the dose is *not* a multiple of 5, pour the liquid to the *nearest* 5-mL calibration that is *less* than the dose.

➤ *Add* the precise additional amount needed to the *nearest tenth* of a milliliter with a syringe. The top center of the fluid is read at eye level (Figure 5-5).

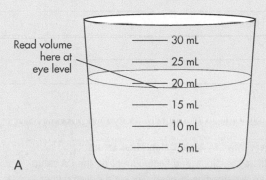

Read volume here at eye level

- 30 mL
- 25 mL
- 20 mL
- 15 mL
- 10 mL
- 5 mL

A

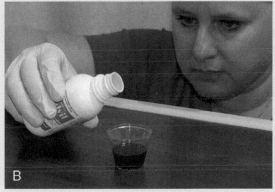

B

FIGURE 5-5 A, Pour the desired volume of liquid so that base of meniscus is level with line on scale. **B,** Hold cup at eye level to confirm volume poured.

CLINICAL RELEVANCE

➤ Be sure to remove and discard cap from prefilled oral syringes.

➤ Failure to do so could cause aspiration or choking.

➤ Avoid drawing excess amounts of medication.

RAPID PRACTICE 5-9 — Measuring Liquid Doses with 30-mL Medicine Cup and Syringe

ESTIMATED COMPLETION TIME: 10 minutes   **ANSWERS ON:** page 200

DIRECTIONS: *Given the amount to prepare, state the nearest measurable amount to place in the 30-mL medicine cup and the amount to place in the syringe, and state whether a 3-mL or a 5-mL syringe is needed.*

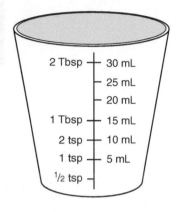

2 Tbsp — 30 mL
— 25 mL
— 20 mL
1 Tbsp — 15 mL
2 tsp — 10 mL
1 tsp — 5 mL
½ tsp —

Amount to Prepare	Amount to Place in Cup	Amount to Place in Syringe	Syringe Size (3-mL or 5-mL)
1 6.5 mL	_____	_____	_____
2 9 mL	_____	_____	_____
3 27.4 mL	_____	_____	_____
4 17 mL	_____	_____	_____
5 14 mL	_____	_____	_____

CLINICAL RELEVANCE

Patient Safety: Seven Ways to Avoid Calculation Errors

1. Know the metric conversions, and keep current on the DA setup.
2. Focus strictly on the situation at hand. Screen out distractions.
3. Make a habit of estimating a reasonable answer, if possible, before performing final calculations.
4. Write neatly and watch placement of decimals.
5. Evaluate equation and answers using a systematic method.
6. Consult an *appropriate* source for assistance when needed.
7. Keep the patient and/or family informed about the medication and the dose that you plan to administer. They may provide the final protection from an error.

RAPID PRACTICE 5-10 — Liquid Doses

ESTIMATED COMPLETION TIME: 20 to 30 minutes   **ANSWERS ON:** page 200

DIRECTIONS: *Estimate, calculate, and evaluate the liquid dose problems to the nearest tenth of a milliliter.*

✷ Communication

Nurse: "I have your liquid antibiotic erythromycin, Mrs. R."
Patient: "Would you please get me some grapefruit or orange juice to kill the taste?"
Nurse (returns with orange juice or some other alternative): "Would either of these work for you? As long as you're taking this medication, please don't take any grapefruit juice. It can cause very serious problems such as kidney damage. Orange juice is fine though. Do you have any questions?"

1 **Ordered:** 45 mg. Supplied dose concentration: 25 mg per 10 mL.

   a. Estimated dose: _____
      DA equation:

   b. Evaluation: _____

2 **Ordered:** 75 mg. Supplied dose concentration: 50 mg per mL.

   a. Estimated dose: _____
      DA equation:

   b. Evaluation: _____

3 **Ordered:** 20 mg. Supplied dose concentration: 5 mg per 5 mL.

   a. Estimated dose: _____
      DA equation:

   b. Evaluation: _____

4 **Ordered:** 35 mg. Supplied dose concentration: 15 mg per 2 mL.

   a. Estimated dose: _____
      DA equation:

   b. Evaluation: _____

5 **Ordered:** 125 mg. Supplied dose concentration: 75 mg per 8 mL.

   a. Estimated dose: _____
      DA equation:

   b. Evaluation: _____

RAPID PRACTICE 5-11   Calculating and Measuring Liquid Dose Orders

ESTIMATED COMPLETION TIME: 30 minutes   **ANSWERS ON:** page 201

DIRECTIONS: *Identify and enter all the required elements in the DA equation.
Estimate the answer, solve to the nearest tenth of a milliliter, and evaluate the
equation. Shade in the medicine cup to the nearest 5 mL, and draw a vertical line
through the calibrated line of the syringe for the remainder of the dose.*

1 **Ordered:** lithium citrate syrup 0.6 g PO tid for a patient with bipolar disorder.

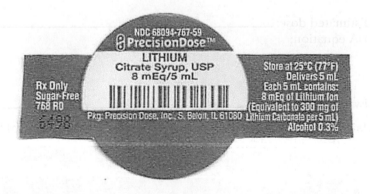

   a. Estimated dose: _____
      DA equation:

   b. Evaluation: _____

Shade in the dose in mL for the medicine cup.

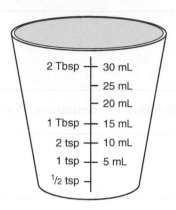

2 **Ordered:** oxycodone HCl oral solution 32.5 mg PO stat for patient with severe pain.

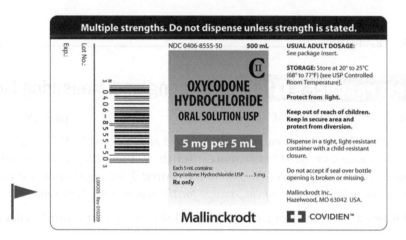

a. Estimated dose: _____
   DA equation:

b. Evaluation: _____

Shade in the dose in mL for the medicine cup and draw a vertical line through the calibrated line of the syringe.

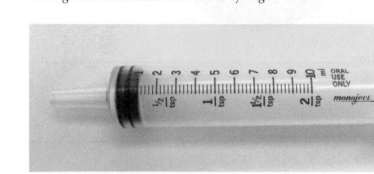

3 **Ordered:** Zithromax oral suspension 0.5 g PO once daily for a patient with an infection.

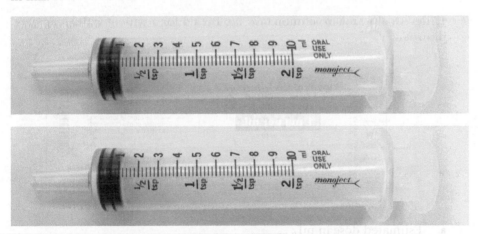

a. Estimated dose: _____

DA equation:

b. Evaluation: _____

Draw a vertical line through the calibrated lines of the syringes for the dose in mL.

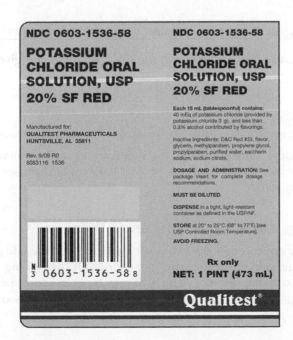

4 **Ordered:** potassium chloride solution 25 mEq PO daily 20% sugar-free solution.

NDC 0603-1536-58	NDC 0603-1536-58
POTASSIUM CHLORIDE ORAL SOLUTION, USP 20% SF RED	**POTASSIUM CHLORIDE ORAL SOLUTION, USP 20% SF RED**

Each 15 mL (tablespoonful) contains:
40 mEq of potassium chloride (provided by potassium chloride 3 g), and less than 0.3% alcohol contributed by flavorings.

Manufactured for:
QUALITEST PHARMACEUTICALS
HUNTSVILLE, AL 35811

Rev. 9/09 R0
8083116 1536

Inactive Ingredients: D&C Red #33, flavor, glycerin, methylparaben, propylene glycol, propylparaben, purified water, saccharin sodium, sodium citrate.

DOSAGE AND ADMINISTRATION: See package insert for complete dosage recommendations.

MUST BE DILUTED.

DISPENSE in a tight, light-resistant container as defined in the USP/NF.

STORE at 20° to 25°C (68° to 77°F) [see USP Controlled Room Temperature].

AVOID FREEZING.

Rx only
NET: 1 PINT (473 mL)

Qualitest®

N 3 0603-1536-58 8

a. Estimated dose: _____
DA equation:

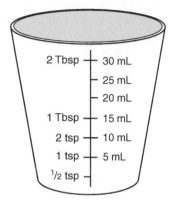

b. Evaluation: _____

Draw a vertical line through the calibrated line of the syringe for the dose in mL.

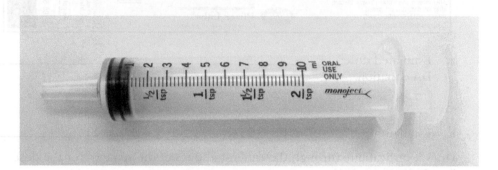

5 **Ordered:** alprazolam solution 0.75 mg PO tid for a patient with an anxiety disorder.

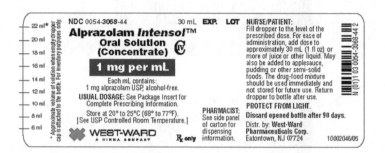

a. Estimated dose in mL: _____
b. Enclosed dropper dose in mL: _____

c. Evaluation: <u>(Does your estimate agree with the dropper?)</u>

➤ Teach the patient to use the enclosed dropper when you give the medicine. Assess patient vision.

Safe Dose Ranges (SDRs)

Verifying safe dose ranges (SDRs) for medications and estimating doses for all medications are two techniques that protect patients and nurses from medication dose calculation errors.

Calculating safe dose ranges (SDRs)

Medications are approved by the FDA with guidelines for the safe amount to administer to the target audience, for example, "For adult use, 20 mg per day" or "Safe dose range 10 to 20 mg per day." The SDR may be even more specific for powerful drugs, for drugs that are supplied in various dose strengths or for intravenous routes, and for at-risk populations, such as infants, children, and frail adults (e.g., 1 to 2 mg per kg body weight per day).

The nurse must compare the prescribed order with the SDR in current pharmacologic references or drug package inserts to be sure that the order is within the SDR for a given dose and target population.

The SDR guidelines are usually for a 24-hour day. If the total dose cannot safely be administered on a once-a-day basis, the recommendation will include the *frequency schedule:* the number of times at which the total daily dose should be *divided* into individual doses.

The arithmetic to calculate the SDR is very simple:

- Calculate the low safe dose.
- Calculate the high safe dose.
- Evaluate the order in relation to the SDR and frequency schedule.
- Decision: *Hold* the medication and contact the prescriber if the order is not within the SDR or frequency, or *give* the medication because the order is within the SDR and frequency.

Three kinds of SDRs are commonly seen:

1 Simple range

2 Divided doses

3 Simple or divided based on weight

SDR With Simple Ranges

EXAMPLES

Ordered: Drug A 10 mg tid.

SDR: 10–30 mg per day.

Order: 10 mg $\times$ 3 doses $=$ 30 mg per day

10 mg is the *low safe dose* for 24 hours. 30 mg is the *maximum safe dose* for 24 hours.

Evaluation: It can be seen at a glance that this order is within the SDR for the total daily dose.

➤ Take care to avoid confusing the SDR amount with the ordered amount. It is easier to avoid error if the SDR is placed above the order.

SDR With Divided Doses

EXAMPLES

Ordered: Drug B 10 mg tid.

SDR: 30 mg per day in 2 or 3 divided doses.

The phrase *divided doses* indicates that the entire daily dose cannot be given safely at one time. 30 mg per day must be divided into individual servings:

$$\text{in 2 servings: } \frac{30}{2} = 15 \text{ mg per dose}$$

$$\text{or into 3 servings: } \frac{30}{3} = 10 \text{ mg per dose}$$

SDR: 30 mg per day in 2 or 3 divided doses.

Order: 10 $\times$ 3 or 30 mg a day total in 3 divided doses.

Evaluation: The order falls within SDR for both total daily dose and frequency.

Safe and Unsafe Orders

EXAMPLES

Safe Order	Unsafe Order
Ordered: Drug A 75 mg per day	**Ordered:** Drug B 200 mg per day
SDR: 50-100 mg per day	**SDR:** 50-100 mg per day
Order: 75 mg per day	**Order:** 200 mg per day
Evaluation: Safe to give.	**Evaluation:** Hold medication and contact prescriber promptly. Order exceeds maximum therapeutic dose.

SDR With Range Based on Weight

EXAMPLES

Ordered: Drug A 150 mg 4 times daily.

Patient's weight: 88 lb.

SDR: 10-20 mg per kg per day in 3 or 4 divided doses.

Conversion factor: 1 kg = 2.2 lb

?	Step 1	=	Step 2	×	Step 3	=	Answer
?	Desired Answer Units	=	Starting Factor	×	Given Quantity and Conversion Factor(s) (Quantity and Units)	=	Estimate, Multiply, Evaluate

The final equations will be written like this:

$$? \quad \frac{mg}{day} \quad = \quad \frac{10\ mg}{\cancel{kg} \times day} \quad \times \quad \frac{1\ \cancel{kg}}{\underset{1}{\cancel{2.2\ lb}}} \times \frac{\overset{40}{\cancel{88\ lb}}}{1} \quad = \quad \begin{array}{l}\text{400 mg per day}\\ \text{Low safe dose}\end{array}$$

$$? \quad \frac{mg}{day} \quad = \quad \frac{20\ mg}{\cancel{kg} \times day} \quad \times \quad \frac{1\ \cancel{kg}}{\underset{1}{\cancel{2.2\ lb}}} \times \frac{\overset{40}{\cancel{88\ lb}}}{1} \quad = \quad \begin{array}{l}\text{800 mg per day}\\ \text{High safe dose}\end{array}$$

Analysis: For starting factor, we chose the SDR because it contains the desired answer and oriented it so that the desired answer units are in the numerator *to match the desired answer position.*

➤ Note that a triple factor mg per kg per day is placed with the first unit mg in the numerator and kg × day in the denominator. Remember this setup for more complex equations.

A number 1 in the denominator of 88 lb helps maintain correct alignment for numerators and denominators to avoid errors during multiplication. It does *not* change the answer.

➤ Before multiplication, recheck the setup: After all unwanted units were cancelled, are the only units remaining the same as those identified initially for the desired answer?

Evaluation: The order for 150 mg 4 times a day for a total of 600 mg is within the safe dose range and matches the frequency.

➤ Frequency is as important as dose. If given less often than recommended, the drug will not be therapeutic. If given too frequently, too much drug may be given, which can cause serious damage. The equation answers give only the desired answer units (mg per day).

My estimate is that the kg will be about $\frac{1}{2}$ the pound weight, supports the answer. (Math check: 10 × 40 = 400 and 20 × 40 = 800.) The equation is balanced. The order is safe to give.

FAQ *How do I know when to contact the prescriber?*

ANSWER The prescriber must be contacted:

- If the order is incomplete or contains TJC "Do Not Use" abbreviations (see p. 111).
- If the total daily dose ordered is below or above SDR.
- If the frequency schedule does not match the recommended schedule.
- When an allergy to the drug or interaction with another drug might occur.

Clarify the order with the prescriber promptly and document the clarification.

| **RAPID PRACTICE 5-12** | Safe Dose Range and Milligrams per Kilogram of Body Weight Calculator Practice |

ESTIMATED COMPLETION TIME: 20 minutes   **ANSWERS ON:** page 202

DIRECTIONS: *Fill in the estimated weight, actual weight, and SDR in the spaces provided. Follow the example given for problem 1. Move decimal places to change the metric units to milligrams if necessary. Use a calculator to convert pounds to kilograms and calculate the SDR.*

➤ *Estimation helps prevent major math errors. It must be followed with exact math calculation. Enter your calculations twice.*

Safe Dosage Range (SDR)	Patient's Weight (lb)	Estimated Weight (kg) to the Nearest Whole Number	Actual Weight (kg) to the Nearest Tenth	Total SDR to Nearest Tenth
1 10–20 mg per kg per day	66	33 (66 ÷ 2)	30 (66 ÷ 2.2)	10 × 30 = 300 mg per day 20 × 30 = 600 mg per day SDR = 300–600 mg per day
2 10–20 mg per kg per day in 3 divided doses	200	_____	_____	_____
3 0.2–0.5 g per kg per day	44	_____	_____	_____
4 0.25–1.5 mg per kg per day	150	_____	_____	_____
5 2–5 mcg per kg per day	180	_____	_____	_____

CLINICAL RELEVANCE

The SDR is particularly needed for unfamiliar medications and medications that represent a fraction of the unit dose or more than two times the unit dose. SDR checks are also needed for frail patients, immunocompromised patients, patients in the intensive care unit, and pediatric populations.

FAQ *What is a common math error with kilogram weight-based dosing?*

ANSWER Multiplying the number of pounds by 2.2 instead of dividing the number of pounds by 2.2 is a common mistake, which may lead to a fourfold error.

Evaluation of Medication Orders According to SDR

ESTIMATED COMPLETION TIME: 25 minutes   **ANSWERS ON:** page 202

DIRECTIONS: *Examine the example given for problem 1. Compare the frequency and total daily dose ordered with the SDR guidelines for problems 2 to 5. Evaluate the findings and make a decision to hold the medication, clarify the order promptly with the prescriber and document the clarification, or give the medication because the order is a safe dose. Use a calculator to calculate the SDR.*

1   **Ordered:** Drug Y, 0.5 g PO tid.

   SDR: 25–50 mg per kg per day in 3 divided doses.

   a.   Patient's weight: 100 lb. Estimated kilograms: 50 (nearest whole number). Actual kilograms: 45.5 (nearest tenth).
   b.   SDR low and high dose based on actual kilogram weight.

   25 mg × 45.5 kg = 1137.5 mg per day = Low safe dose

   50 mg × 45.5 kg = 2 × 1137.5, or 2275 mg per day = High (maximum) safe dose

   Conversion of order using decimal movement: 0.5 g = 500 mg tid = 1500 mg ordered per day

   SDR: 1137.5–2275 mg per day divided in 3 doses.

   c.   Daily dose ordered: 1500 mg
   d.   Evaluation: Within SDR and recommended frequency (circle one)? (Yes) or *No*
   e.   Decision: Order is within SDR and safe to give.

2   **Ordered:** Drug Y, 50 mg PO q6h.

   SDR: 2–4 mg per kg per day in 4 divided doses.

   a.   Patient's weight: 120 lb. Estimated weight in kilograms: _____. Actual weight in kilograms: _____.
   b.   SDR low and high dose based on actual kilogram weight: _____
   c.   Daily dose ordered: _____
   d.   Evaluation: Within SDR and recommended frequency (circle one)? *Yes* or *No*
   e.   Decision: _____

3   **Ordered:** Drug Y, 25 mg PO bid.

   SDR: 5–10 mg per kg per day in 2–3 divided doses.

   a.   Patient's weight: 60 lb. Estimated weight in kilograms: _____. Actual weight in kilograms: _____.
   b.   SDR low and high dose based on actual kilogram weight: _____
   c.   Daily dose ordered: _____
   d.   Evaluation: Within SDR and recommended frequency (circle one)? *Yes* or *No*
   e.   Decision: _____

4   **Ordered:** Drug Y, 50 mg PO q4h.

   SDR: 1–2 mg per kg per day in 4–6 divided doses.

   a.   Patient's weight: 160 lb. Estimated weight in kilograms: _____. Actual weight in kilograms: _____.
   b.   SDR low and high dose based on actual kilogram weight: _____
   c.   Daily dose ordered: _____
   d.   Evaluation: Within SDR and recommended frequency (circle one)? *Yes* or *No*
   e.   Decision: _____

5 **Ordered:** Drug Y, 0.25 g PO tid.

SDR: 10–20 mg per kg per day in 2–3 divided doses.

a. Patient's weight: 100 lb. Estimated weight in kilograms: _____. Actual weight in kilograms: _____ .

b. SDR low and high dose based on actual kilogram weight: _____

c. Daily dose ordered: _____

d. Evaluation: Within SDR and recommended frequency (circle one)? *Yes* or *No*

e. Decision: _____

---

1 What are three instances in which the medication ordered needs to be clarified with the prescriber?

ASK YOURSELF **Q & A**

_____

MY ANSWER

2 Why is documentation of the clarification important for the patient and the nurse?

_____

FAQ *Are low or high doses outside of the SDR ever administered?*

ANSWER

➤ Yes, but only the prescriber can make the decision. Beginning practitioners should hold the medication and clarify the order with the prescriber promptly. They should research the reason by reviewing the medical record and patient history as to why the dose might be low (subtherapeutic) or high (supratherapeutic). Always recheck the order and the label first. Document and report contacts with the prescriber and actions promptly.

CLINICAL RELEVANCE

Even if the medication order falls within SDR guidelines in the literature, the nursing assessments of the patient's record and of the patient may generate a decision to hold the medication pending clarification with the prescriber. Medication-related nursing assessments may disclose that one or more medications are unsafe for the patient at that point in time. For example, a change in the patient's mental status may render the patient unable to swallow food or fluids. This condition would necessitate a new order for a changed route of administration. Nausea and vomiting are also good reasons to withhold oral medications. If the medication is a critical one, such as a heart medication, the prescriber needs to be informed immediately.

➤ Interactions cited in the literature with one or more drugs already being administered would be another reason to hold the medication and clarify the order with the prescriber.

FAQ *How do I know whom to contact when there is a question about a medication order?*

ANSWER The decision comes with experience. There are three good sources: the prescriber, the pharmacist, and a recent drug reference or drug information insert. The source to select depends upon the nature of the question. Here are some general guidelines:

➤ If the medication order is illegible, unclear, or incomplete, contact the prescriber.

➤ If the problem is with the amount of the *dose,* check a drug reference or a pharmacist first and then the prescriber if necessary.

➤ If the medication *supplied* is in question, contact the pharmacist.

➤ Students should hold the medication, analyze the problem, use the references to determine the SDR and/or contact the pharmacist if appropriate, determine independently which action would be best, and promptly contact the instructor to confer regarding the decision, particularly if the prescriber is to be contacted.

RAPID PRACTICE 5-14	Calculating Safe Doses With DA Verification

ESTIMATED COMPLETION TIME: 25 minutes   **ANSWERS ON:** page 202

DIRECTIONS: *Examine and analyze the example in problem 1. Then complete problems 2 to 5, working out each step of the problem in order. If the decision is to hold the medication, stop calculations.*

1 **Ordered:** digoxin (Lanoxin) pediatric elixir 0.1 mg PO daily for an adult patient with heart failure.

   SDR for adult maintenance: 50–300 mcg per day.

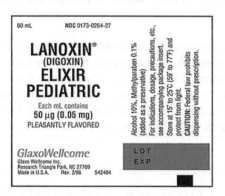

➤ Note that the label uses *μg* for *mcg*. Write mcg.*

   a. Unit dose available: 50 mcg per mL, or 0.05 mg per mL.
   b. Order within SDR (circle one)? *Yes* or *No.* SDR is 50–300 mcg per day and the order (0.1 mg) is 100 mcg.
   c. Estimated dose if safe to give: More than 1 mL would be given, two times the unit dose.
   d. Actual dose to be given: 2 mL
   DA equation:

$$? \frac{mL}{dose} = \frac{1\ mL}{0.05\ \cancel{mg}} \times \frac{0.1\ \cancel{mg}}{dose} = 2\ mL\ per\ dose\ (answer)$$

   e. Evaluation: The estimate supports the answer. The equation is balanced.

   Note: No math for conversions are necessary because the conversion is given on the label.

---
*μg can be misread as mg.

2 **Ordered:** lithium citrate syrup 0.6 g PO bid daily for a patient with a bipolar disorder.

SDR: 900–1200 mg daily in 2–3 divided doses.

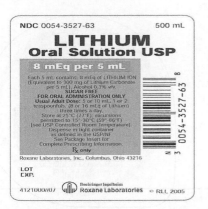

a. Unit dose available in mEq per mL: _____ ; mg per mL: _____

b. Order within SDR (circle one)? *Yes* or *No*

c. Estimated dose if safe to give: _____

d. Actual dose: _____
   DA equation:

e. Evaluation: _____

Shade in the dose in mL for the medicine cup.

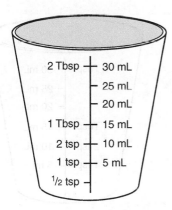

➤ Remember that the estimate cannot be made until the measurement units are *the same.*

3 **Ordered:** potassium chloride solution 45 mEq PO stat for a patient with hypokalemia.

SDR for adult for potassium depletion: 40–100 mEq PO daily.

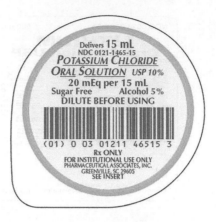

a. Unit dose available in mEq per mL: _____

b. Order within SDR (circle one)? *Yes* or *No*

c. Estimated dose if safe to give: _____

d. Actual dose: _____

DA equation:

e. Evaluation: _____

Shade in the dose in mL for the medicine cup and draw a vertical line through the calibrated line of the syringe to the nearest measurable dose.

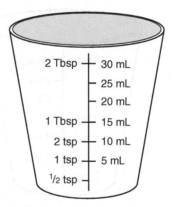

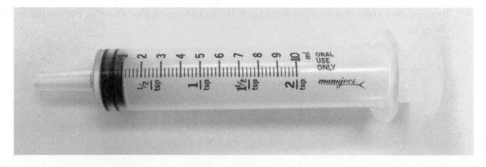

Check carefully for dilution directions.

4 **Ordered:** loperamide hydrochloride oral susp. 2 mg PO after each loose stool up to six times daily. The patient has already received a 4-mg initial dose.

SDR: 4 mg initially, then 2 mg after each loose stool, not to exceed 16 mg per day.

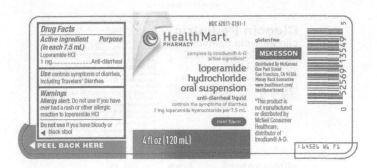

a. Unit dose available in mg per mL: _____
b. Order within SDR (circle one)? *Yes* or *No*
c. Estimated dose if safe to give: _____
d. Actual dose: _____
    DA equation:

e. Evaluation: _____

Shade in the dose in mL for the medicine cup.

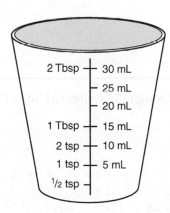

5 **Ordered:** clindamycin palmitate HCl solution 120 mg PO q8h.

SDR for a child: 10–25 mg per kg per day equally divided doses every 6–8 hours.

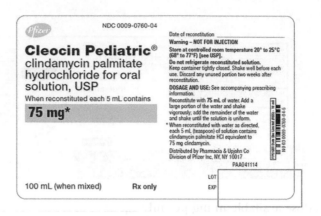

Child's weight: 53 lb. Estimated weight in kilograms (nearest whole number): _____. Actual weight in kilograms (nearest tenth): _____.

a. Unit dose available in mg per mL: _____

b. Order within SDR (circle one)? *Yes* or *No.*

c. Estimated dose if safe to give: _____

d. Actual dose: _____
DA equation:

e. Evaluation: _____

Draw a vertical line through the calibrated line of the syringe as applicable.

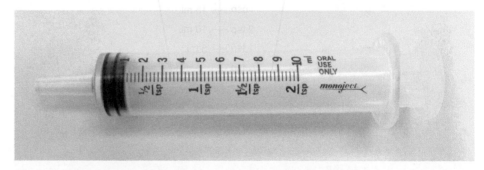

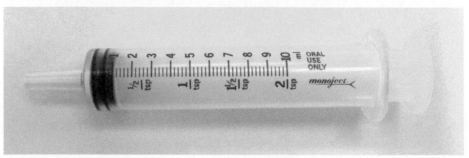

ESTIMATED COMPLETION TIME: 10 minutes   **ANSWERS ON:** page 203

DIRECTIONS: *Select the best answer.*

1 Which is the correct conversion for 50 mg to grams?
- **a.** 0.005 g
- **b.** 0.05 g
- **c.** 0.5 g
- **d.** 500 g

2 Select the appropriate measuring device and volumes when preparing an oral medication of 24 mL to be administered in a 30-mL calibrated medicine cup.
- **a.** Pour to 25 mL in the measuring cup and remove 1 mL.
- **b.** Pour to 20 mL in the measuring cup and administer 4 mL with a 3-mL syringe.
- **c.** Pour to approximately 24 mL, just short of the 25-mL line.
- **d.** Pour to 20 mL in the cup and add 4 mL with a 5-mL syringe.

3 One of the most important safety nets a nurse can use for catching major calculation errors is
- **a.** Performing metric conversions
- **b.** Estimating answers
- **c.** Using a calculator
- **d.** Carrying a math text to clinical

4 The SDR for 10–30 mg per kg per day for a patient weighing 44 lb is
- **a.** 300 mg per day
- **b.** 440–1320 mg/day
- **c.** 200–600 mg per kg per day
- **d.** 200–600 mg per day

5 Which of the following conversions is correct?
- **a.** 0.5 g = 50 mg
- **b.** 10,000 mcg = 20 mg
- **c.** 0.25 g = 250 mg
- **d.** 120 mg = 1.2 g

6 Which is the correct conversion for 25,000 mcg to grams?
- **a.** 250 g
- **b.** 25 g
- **c.** 0.25 g
- **d.** 0.025 g

7 Which of the following pairs of units will need to have the decimal moved six places?
- **a.** Grams to micrograms
- **b.** Grams to milligrams
- **c.** Micrograms to milligrams
- **d.** Milliequivalents to milliliters

8 The recommended way to write large numbers in the metric system for ease of reading, as in one hundred thousand micrograms, is
- **a.** With commas: 100,000
- **b.** With decimal points: 100.000
- **c.** With spaces: 100 000
- **d.** Without spaces or inserts: 100000

9 If 25 mg per kg per day is ordered in two divided doses and kg = 10, what will each dose be?
- **a.** 50 mg
- **b.** 100 mg
- **c.** 125 mg
- **d.** 250 mg

10 Milligram–gram conversions require movement of how many decimal places?
- **a.** Three places
- **b.** Five places
- **c.** Six places
- **d.** 1 million places

ESTIMATED COMPLETION TIME: 40 to 50 minutes   **ANSWERS ON:** page 203

DIRECTIONS: *Evaluate the order and SDR. If safe to give, estimate and approximate dose. Verify the estimate with a DA-style equation. Evaluate the answer. Use a calculator to determine kg weights and SDR. Write the answers in the space provided.*

1 **Ordered:** carbamazepine chewable tablets 0.2 g PO bid for *initial* treatment for a patient with seizures.

  SDR: 200 mg bid to start; may be increased by 200 mg per day in divided doses.

NDC 0078-0492-05   Rx only

Tegretol® 100 mg

carbamazepine USP

Chewable Tablets

100 tablets
PHARMACIST: Dispense with Medication Guide
attached or provided separately.

Ⴑ NOVARTIS

  a. SDR comparison with order: _____
  b. Decision: _____
  c. Estimate: _____
  d. Amount to give: _____
     DA equation:

  e. Evaluation: _____

2 **Ordered:** potassium chloride elixir 30 mEq PO daily for a patient taking diuretics.

  SDR: 20–40 mEq per day.

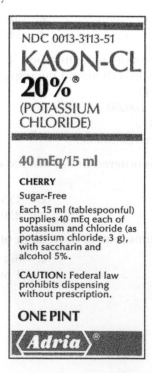

NDC 0013-3113-51

KAON-CL
20%®
(POTASSIUM
CHLORIDE)

40 mEq/15 ml

CHERRY

Sugar-Free

Each 15 ml (tablespoonful)
supplies 40 mEq each of
potassium and chloride (as
potassium chloride, 3 g),
with saccharin and
alcohol 5%.

CAUTION: Federal law
prohibits dispensing
without prescription.

ONE PINT

❮Adria❯®

a. SDR comparison with order: _____
b. Decision: _____
c. Estimate: _____
d. Amount to give: _____
    DA equation:

e. Evaluation: _____

Shade in the dose in mL for the medicine cup and draw a vertical line through the calibrated line of the syringe as applicable.

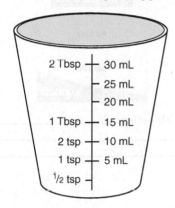

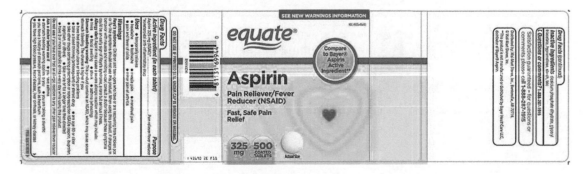

3 Ordered: aspirin 0.65 g PO q4h prn for pain for a 22-year-old patient with a sprained ankle.

SDR (adult): (Consult label.)

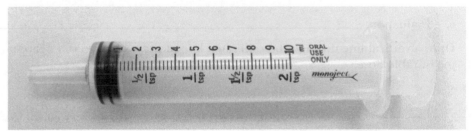

a. SDR comparison with order: _____
b. Decision: _____
c. Estimate of number of tablets to be given: _____ More or less than unit dose? _____
d. Actual number of tablets to be given: _____
    DA equation:

e. Evaluation: _____

4 **Ordered:** ondansetron hydrochloride oral solution 14 mg PO 1 hr preoperatively stat to prevent postoperative nausea and vomiting.

SDR: 8–16 mg per dose 1 hr before surgery.

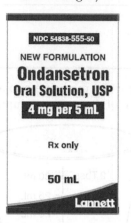

NDC 54838-555-50

NEW FORMULATION

Ondansetron
Oral Solution, USP

4 mg per 5 mL

Rx only

50 mL

Lannett

a. SDR comparison with order: _____

b. Decision: _____

c. Estimate: _____

d. Amount to give: _____
    DA equation:

e. Evaluation: _____

Draw a vertical line through the calibrated line of the syringe to the nearest measurable dose.

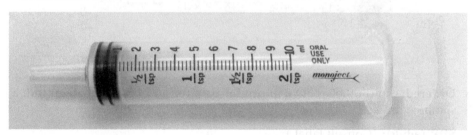

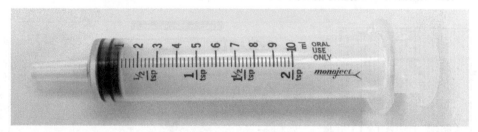

5 Ordered: tramadol HCl* tablets 0.15 g PO q12h for a patient with chronic back pain.

SDR: 50–400 mg per day in 2 divided doses.

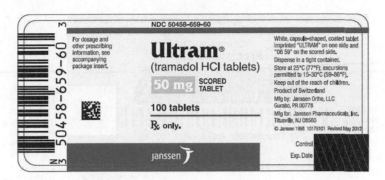

a. SDR comparison with order: _____

b. Decision: _____

c. Estimate: _____

d. Amount to give: _____
   DA equation:

e. Evaluation: _____

6 Ordered: raloxifene HCl tablet 0.06 g PO bid daily for an adult patient with osteoporosis.

SDR (adult): 60 mg once daily.

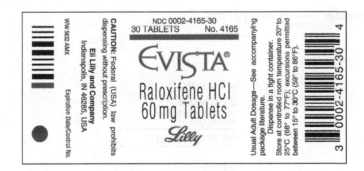

a. SDR comparison with order: _____

b. Decision: _____

c. Estimate: _____

d. Amount to give: _____
   DA equation:

e. Evaluation: _____

_____

*High alert if given to a patient more than 75 years of age.

7 Ordered: acetaminophen oral suspension 0.65 g PO q6h for a patient with a fever who cannot swallow tablets.

SDR (adult): 325–650 mg q4–6h up to 4 g per day.

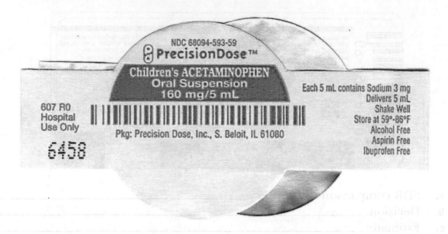

a. SDR comparison with order: _____

b. Decision: _____

c. Estimated dose: _____

d. Amount to give: _____
    DA equation:

e. Evaluation: _____

8 Ordered: levothyroxine tablets 0.1 mg PO daily for a patient with hypothyroidism.

Maintenance: 75–125 mcg per day.

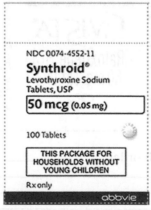

a. SDR comparison with order: _____

b. Decision: _____

c. Estimate: _____

d. Amount to give: _____
    DA equation:

e. Evaluation: _____

9 **Ordered:** valproic acid oral solution 300 mg PO bid starting dose for a patient with a seizure disorder. Patient weight: 50 kg.

SDR: 10–15 mg per kg per day in 2 or 3 divided doses.

Directions: Immediately before use, dilute the medication with distilled water, acidified tap water, or juice.

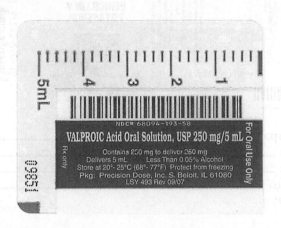

a. SDR comparison with order: _____

b. Decision: _____

c. Estimate: _____

d. Amount to prepare before dilution: _____
   DA equation:

e. How many packages will you need? _____

f. Evaluation: _____

Draw a vertical line through the calibrated line of the syringe as applicable.

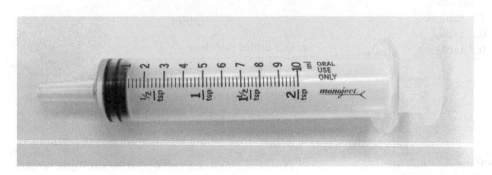

10 **Ordered:** penicillin V potassium tabs* 0.25 g PO q8h × 10 days for a patient with streptococcal infection.

SDR: 125-250 mg q6-8h × 10 days.

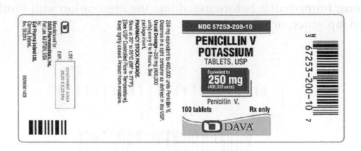

a. SDR comparison with order: _____

b. Decision: _____

c. Estimate: _____

d. Amount to give: _____
   DA equation:

e. Evaluation: _____
_____

*Be sure to reassess for allergies to antibiotics and to the specific drug—penicillin, in this case. If there is a problem, hold the drug and contact the prescriber.

CHAPTER 5 | ANSWER KEY

RAPID PRACTICE 5-1 (p. 157)

1 2 tablets **6** 2.5 tablets
2 2 capsules **7** 2 tablets
3 0.5 tablet **8** 1.5 tablets
4 2 capsules **9** 0.5 tablet
5 2 tablets **10** 0.5 tablet

RAPID PRACTICE 5-2 (p. 157)

2 a. 1000 mg = 1 g
   b. 2 tablets (250 = 2 × 125)
   c. 2 tablets per dose

$$? \, \frac{\text{tablet}}{\text{dose}} = \frac{1 \text{ tablet}}{125 \text{ mg}} \times \frac{\overset{8}{\cancel{1000 \text{ mg}}}}{1 \text{ g}} \times \frac{0.25 \text{ g}}{\text{dose}}$$
$$= \frac{2 \text{ tablets}}{\text{dose}}$$

   d. Equation is balanced. Answer equals estimate.

3 a. No conversion formula needed
   b. 2 tablets (0.1 = 2 × 0.05)
   c. 2 tablets per dose

$$? \, \frac{\text{tablet}}{\text{dose}} = \frac{1 \text{ tablet}}{\underset{1}{\cancel{0.05 \text{ g}}}} \times \frac{\overset{2}{\cancel{0.1 \text{ g}}}}{\text{dose}} = \frac{2 \text{ tablets}}{\text{dose}}$$

   d. Equation is balanced. Answer equals estimate.

4 a. 1000 mcg = 1 mg
   b. 0.175 mg = 175 mcg = $\frac{1}{2}$ of 350 mcg
      $= \frac{1}{2}$ tablet
   c. 0.5 tablet per dose

$$? \, \frac{\text{tablet}}{\text{dose}} = \frac{1 \text{ tablet}}{350 \text{ mcg}} \times \frac{1000 \text{ mcg}}{1 \text{ mg}} \times \frac{0.175 \text{ mg}}{\text{dose}}$$
$$= \frac{175}{350} = \frac{0.5 \text{ tablet}}{\text{dose}}$$

   d. Equation is balanced. Answer equals estimate.

   Note: If you use a calculator to multiply larger numbers, verify the result by reentering the factors a second time.

5 a. 1000 mg = 1 g
   b. 0.2 g = 200 mg; 2 capsules (200 = 2 × 100)
   c. 2 capsules per dose

$$? \, \frac{\text{capsule}}{\text{dose}} = \frac{1 \text{ capsule}}{\underset{1}{\cancel{100 \text{ mg}}}} \times \frac{\overset{10}{\cancel{1000 \text{ mg}}}}{1 \text{ g}} \times \frac{0.2 \text{ g}}{\text{dose}}$$
$$= \frac{2 \text{ capsules}}{\text{dose}}$$

   d. Equation is balanced. Answer equals estimate.

6   **a.** 1000 mg = 1 g
    b. 0.25 = 2 × 0.125; 2 capsules
    c. 2 capsules per dose

$$? \frac{\text{capsule}}{\text{dose}} = \frac{1 \text{ capsule}}{\underset{1}{\cancel{125 \text{ mg}}}} \times \frac{\overset{8}{\cancel{1000 \text{ mg}}}}{1 \cancel{\text{g}}} \times \frac{0.25 \cancel{\text{g}}}{\text{dose}}$$

$$= \frac{2 \text{ capsules}}{\text{dose}}$$

    d. Equation is balanced. Answer equals estimate.

7   **a.** No conversion formula needed
    b. 2 tablets (20 = 2 × 10)
    c. 2 tablets per dose

$$\frac{\text{tablet}}{\text{dose}} = \frac{1 \text{ tablet}}{\underset{1}{\cancel{10 \text{ mEq}}}} \times \frac{\overset{2}{\cancel{20 \text{ mEq}}}}{\text{dose}} = \frac{2 \text{ tablets}}{\text{dose}}$$

    d. Equation is balanced. Answer equals estimate.

8   **a.** 1000 mcg = 1 mg
    b. 0.1 mg = 100 mcg = 2 × 50 mcg; 2 tablets
    c. 2 tablets (100 = 50 × 2)

$$? \frac{\text{tablet}}{\text{dose}} = \frac{1 \text{ tablet}}{\underset{1}{\cancel{50 \text{ mcg}}}} \times \frac{\overset{20}{\cancel{1000 \text{ mcg}}}}{1 \cancel{\text{mg}}} \times \frac{0.1 \cancel{\text{mg}}}{\text{dose}}$$

$$= \frac{2 \text{ tablets}}{\text{dose}}$$

    d. Equation is balanced. Answer equals estimate.

9   **a.** No conversion formula needed
    b. $1\frac{1}{2}$ tablets ($75 = 1\frac{1}{2} \times 50$)
    c. 1.5 tablets per dose

$$? \frac{\text{tablet}}{\text{dose}} = \frac{1 \text{ tablet}}{\underset{2}{\cancel{50 \text{ mcg}}}} \times \frac{\overset{3}{\cancel{75 \text{ mcg}}}}{\text{dose}} = \frac{1.5 \text{ tablets}}{\text{dose}}$$

    d. Equation is balanced. Answer equals estimate.

10   **a.** 1000 mg = 1 g
    b. 250 mg = 0.25 g; 1 capsule
    c. 1 capsule per dose

$$? \frac{\text{capsule}}{\text{dose}} = \frac{1 \text{ capsule}}{0.25 \cancel{\text{g}}} \times \frac{1 \cancel{\text{g}}}{\underset{4}{\cancel{1000 \text{ mg}}}} \times \frac{\overset{1}{\cancel{250 \text{ mg}}}}{\text{dose}}$$

$$= \frac{1}{1} = \frac{1 \text{ capsule}}{\text{dose}}$$

    d. Equation is balanced. Answer equals estimate.

RAPID PRACTICE 5-3 (p. 160)

2   300 mg   0.3 g
3   25 mg   0.025 g
4   80 mg   0.08 g
5   100 mg   100,000 mcg

RAPID PRACTICE 5-4 (p. 161)

1 0.35 mg   **6** 50 mg
2 0.05 g   **7** 4000 mcg
3 300 mg   **8** 500 mcg
4 0.5 g   **9** 0.2 mg
5 2.2 g   **10** 0.015 g

RAPID PRACTICE 5-5 (p. 161)

1   **a.** 60 mg = 30 mg × 2
    b. 2 tablets per dose

$$? \frac{\text{tablet}}{\text{dose}} = \frac{1 \text{ tablet}}{\underset{1}{\cancel{30 \text{ mg}}}} \times \frac{\overset{2}{\cancel{60 \text{ mg}}}}{\text{dose}} = \frac{2 \text{ tablets}}{\text{dose}}$$

    c. Equation is balanced. Estimate equals answer.

2   **a.** 15 mg = 7.5 mg × 2 tabs
    b. 2 tablets per dose

$$? \frac{\text{tablet}}{\text{dose}} = \frac{1 \text{ tablet}}{\underset{1}{\cancel{7.5 \text{ mg}}}} \times \frac{\overset{2}{\cancel{15 \text{ mg}}}}{\text{dose}} = \frac{2 \text{ tablets}}{\text{dose}}$$

    c. Equation is balanced. Estimate equals answer.

3   **a.** 0.1 g = 100 mg; 50 × 2 = 100
    b. 2 tablets per dose

$$? \frac{\text{tablet}}{\text{dose}} = \frac{1 \text{ tablet}}{\underset{1}{\cancel{50 \text{ mg}}}} \times \frac{\overset{20}{\cancel{1000 \text{ mg}}}}{1 \cancel{\text{g}}} \times \frac{0.1 \cancel{\text{g}}}{\text{dose}}$$

$$= \frac{2 \text{ tablets}}{\text{dose}}$$

    c. Equation is balanced. Estimate equals answer.

4   **a.** 1 mg = 2 × 0.5 mg
    b. 2 tablets per dose

$$? \frac{\text{tablet}}{\text{dose}} = \frac{1 \text{ tablet}}{0.5 \cancel{\text{mg}}} \times \frac{1 \cancel{\text{mg}}}{\text{dose}} = \frac{2 \text{ tablets}}{\text{dose}}$$

    c. Equation is balanced. Estimate equals answer.

5   **a.** 0.25 g = 250 mg
    b. 1 tablet per dose

$$? \frac{\text{tablet}}{\text{dose}} = \frac{1 \text{ tablet}}{\underset{1}{\cancel{250 \text{ mg}}}} \times \frac{\overset{4}{\cancel{1000 \text{ mg}}}}{1 \cancel{\text{g}}} \times \frac{0.25 \cancel{\text{g}}}{\text{dose}}$$

$$= \frac{1 \text{ tablet}}{\text{dose}}$$

    c. Equation is balanced. Estimate equals answer.

RAPID PRACTICE 5-6 (p. 163)

1   **a.** 500 mg per tablet; 500 mg × 2 tablets = 1000 mg; 2 tablets

$$? \frac{\text{tablet}}{\text{dose}} = \frac{1 \text{ tablet}}{\underset{1}{\cancel{500 \text{ mg}}}} \times \frac{\overset{2}{\cancel{1000 \text{ mg}}}}{\text{dose}} = \frac{2 \text{ tablets}}{\text{dose}}$$

    b. Equation is balanced. Answer equals estimate.

2 **a.** 5 mg = 2.5 mg × 2 tablets

$$? \frac{\text{tablet}}{\text{dose}} = \frac{1 \text{ tablet}}{\underset{1}{\cancel{2.5 \text{ mg}}}} \times \frac{\overset{2}{\cancel{5 \text{ mg}}}}{\text{dose}} = \frac{2 \text{ tablets}}{\text{dose}}$$

b. Equation is balanced. Answer equals estimate.

3 **a.** Would select label A—The order does not state extended release.

b. 0.12 g = 120 mg; 1 tablet

$$? \frac{\text{tablet}}{\text{dose}} = \frac{1 \text{ tablet}}{120 \cancel{\text{ mg}}} \times \frac{1000 \cancel{\text{ mg}}}{1 \cancel{\text{ g}}} \times \frac{0.12 \cancel{\text{ g}}}{\text{dose}}$$
$$= \frac{120}{120} = \frac{1 \text{ tablet}}{\text{dose}}$$

c. Equation is balanced. Answer equals estimate.

4 **a.** 0.3 g = 300 mg; 3 capsules

$$? \frac{\text{capsule}}{\text{dose}} = \frac{1 \text{ capsule}}{\underset{1}{\cancel{100 \text{ mg}}}} \times \frac{\overset{10}{\cancel{1000 \text{ mg}}}}{1 \cancel{\text{ g}}} \times \frac{0.3 \cancel{\text{ g}}}{\text{dose}}$$
$$= \frac{3 \text{ capsules}}{\text{dose}}$$

b. Equation is balanced. Answer equals estimate.

5 **a.** 0.25 mg × 2 = 0.5 mg; 2 tablets

$$? \frac{\text{tablet}}{\text{dose}} = \frac{1 \text{ tablet}}{\underset{1}{\cancel{0.25 \text{ mg}}}} \times \frac{\overset{2}{\cancel{0.5 \text{ mg}}}}{\text{dose}} = \frac{2 \text{ tablets}}{\text{dose}}$$

b. Equation is balanced. Answer equals estimate.

RAPID PRACTICE 5-7 (p. 166)

2 5000 mcg = 5 mg   more   2 mL
3 200 mg = 0.2 g   more   2 mL
4 0.1 g = 100 mg   less   0.3 mL
5 750 mg = 0.75 g   more   1.5 mL

RAPID PRACTICE 5-8 (p. 170)

1 **a.** Give slightly more than 5 mL (15 mg is more than 12.5 mg)

$$? \frac{\text{mL}}{\text{dose}} = \frac{5 \text{ mL}}{12.5 \cancel{\text{ mg}}} \times \frac{15 \cancel{\text{ mg}}}{\text{dose}} = \frac{75}{12.5} = \frac{6 \text{ mL}}{\text{dose}}$$

b. Equation is balanced. Estimate supports answer.

2 **a.** Give about $1\frac{1}{2}$ times the 5 mL supplied

$$? \frac{\text{mL}}{\text{dose}} = \frac{5 \text{ mL}}{6.25 \cancel{\text{ mg}}} \times \frac{10 \cancel{\text{ mg}}}{\text{dose}} = \frac{8 \text{ mL}}{\text{dose}}$$

b. Equation is balanced. Estimate supports answer.

3 **a.** Give about $2\frac{1}{2}$ times the unit dose (5 mL) supplied, or about $12\frac{1}{2}$ mL.

$$? \frac{\text{mL}}{\text{dose}} = \frac{5 \text{ mL}}{16.2 \cancel{\text{ mg}}} \times \frac{40.5 \cancel{\text{ mg}}}{\text{dose}}$$
$$= \frac{202.5}{16.2} = 12.5 \text{ mL}$$

b. Equation is balanced. Estimate supports answer.

4 **a.** (0.4 g = 400 mg) Give 10 mL (2 × the unit dose supplied)

$$\frac{\text{mL}}{\text{dose}} = \frac{5 \text{ mL}}{\underset{1}{\cancel{200 \text{ mg}}}} \times \frac{\overset{5}{\cancel{1000 \text{ mg}}}}{1 \cancel{\text{ g}}} \times \frac{0.4 \cancel{\text{ g}}}{\text{dose}} = \frac{10 \text{ mL}}{\text{dose}}$$

b. The estimate supports the answer. The equation is balanced.

5 **a.** Give about $1\frac{1}{2} \times 5$ mL (7.5 mL).

$$? \frac{\text{mL}}{\text{dose}} = \frac{5 \text{ mL}}{\underset{2}{\cancel{4 \text{ mg}}}} \times \frac{\overset{3}{\cancel{6 \text{ mg}}}}{\text{dose}} = \frac{15}{2} = \frac{7.5 \text{ mL}}{\text{dose}}$$

b. Equation is balanced. Estimate supports answer.

RAPID PRACTICE 5-9 (p. 176)

	Amount to Prepare	Place in Cup	Place in Syringe	Syringe Size
1	6.5 mL	5	1.5	3
2	9 mL	5	4	5
3	27.4 mL	25	2.4	3
4	17 mL	15	2	3
5	14 mL	10	4	5

RAPID PRACTICE 5-10 (p. 176)

1 **a.** Give slightly less than 20 mL.

$$\frac{\text{mL}}{\text{dose}} = \frac{10 \text{ mL}}{\underset{5}{\cancel{25 \text{ mg}}}} \times \frac{\overset{9}{\cancel{45 \text{ mg}}}}{\text{dose}} = \frac{90}{5} = \frac{18 \text{ mL}}{\text{dose}}$$

b. Equation is balanced. Estimate supports answer.

2 **a.** Give $1\frac{1}{2}$ times the available unit dose of 1 mL or 1.5 mL

$$? \frac{\text{mL}}{\text{dose}} = \frac{1 \text{ mL}}{\underset{2}{\cancel{50 \text{ mg}}}} \times \frac{\overset{3}{\cancel{75 \text{ mg}}}}{\text{dose}} = \frac{1.5 \text{ mL}}{\text{dose}}$$

b. Equation is balanced. Estimate equals answer.

3 **a.** Give 4 × 5 mL (20 mL).

$$? \frac{\text{mL}}{\text{dose}} = \frac{\overset{1}{\cancel{5}} \text{ mL}}{\underset{1}{\cancel{5 \text{ mg}}}} \times \frac{20 \cancel{\text{ mg}}}{\text{dose}} = \frac{20 \text{ mL}}{\text{dose}}$$

b. Equation is balanced. Answer equals estimate.

4 **a.** Give slightly more than 4 mL.

$$? \frac{mL}{dose} = \frac{2\ mL}{\underset{3}{\cancel{15\ mg}}} \times \frac{\overset{7}{\cancel{35\ mg}}}{dose} = \frac{14}{3} = \frac{4.7\ mL}{dose}$$

b. Equation is balanced. Estimate supports answer.

5 **a.** Give more than 8 mL but less than 16 mL.

$$? \frac{mL}{dose} = \frac{8\ mL}{\underset{3}{\cancel{75\ mg}}} \times \frac{\overset{5}{\cancel{125\ mg}}}{dose} = \frac{40}{3} = \frac{13.3\ mL}{dose}$$

b. Equation is balanced. Estimate supports answer.

RAPID PRACTICE 5-11 (p. 177)

1 **a.** 0.6 g = 600 mg; Give about 2 × the unit dose of 5 mL

$$? \frac{mL}{dose} = \frac{5\ mL}{\underset{3}{\cancel{300\ mg}}} \times \frac{\overset{10}{\cancel{1000\ mg}}}{1\ \cancel{g}} \times \frac{0.6\ \cancel{g}}{dose}$$

$$= \frac{30}{3} = \frac{10\ mL}{dose}$$

b. The answer equals the estimate. The equation is balanced.

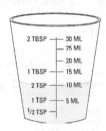

2 **a.** Give slightly more than 30 mL.

$$? \frac{mL}{dose} = \frac{\overset{1}{\cancel{5}}\ mL}{\underset{1}{\cancel{5}\ \cancel{mg}}} \times \frac{32.5\ \cancel{mg}}{dose} = \frac{162.5}{5}$$

$$= 32.5\ mL\ per\ dose$$

b. Equation is balanced. Estimate supports answer.

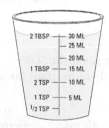

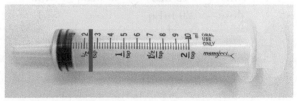

3 **a.** 0.5 g = 500 mg. Give about $2\frac{1}{2}$ times the 5 mL unit dose (slightly more than 10 mL).

$$? \frac{mL}{dose} = \frac{5\ mL}{\underset{1}{\cancel{200\ mg}}} \times \frac{\overset{5}{\cancel{1000\ mg}}}{1\ \cancel{g}} \times \frac{0.5\ \cancel{g}}{dose}$$

$$= \frac{12.5\ mL}{dose}$$

b. The estimate supports the answer. The equation is balanced.

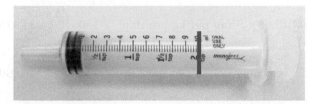

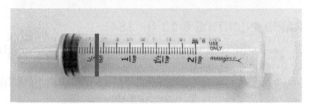

4 **a.** Give less than 15 mL but more than 7.5 mL.

$$\frac{mL}{dose} = \frac{15\ mL}{\underset{8}{\cancel{40\ mEq}}} \times \frac{\overset{5}{\cancel{25\ mEq}}}{dose} = \frac{75}{8}$$

$$= 9.37,\ rounded\ to\ \frac{9.4\ mL}{dose}$$

b. Equation is balanced. Estimate supports answer.

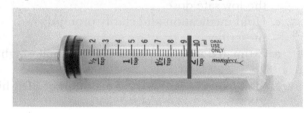

5 **a.** Give about $\frac{3}{4}$ of a mL

b. $? \dfrac{mL}{dose} = \dfrac{mL}{1\ \cancel{mg}} \times \dfrac{0.75\ \cancel{mg}}{dose}$

$$= \frac{0.75\ mL}{dose}\ from\ dropper\ provided$$

c. Equation is balanced. The answer is the same as the estimate.

RAPID PRACTICE 5-12 (p. 183)

SDR		Patient's Weight (lb)	Estimated Weight (kg) to the Nearest Whole Number	Actual Weight (kg) to the Nearest Tenth	Total SDR to Nearest Tenth
2	10-20 mg per kg per day in 3 divided doses	200	100	90.9	$10 \times 90.9 = 909$ mg per day $20 \times 90.9 = 1818$ mg per day SDR = 909-1818 mg per day
3	0.2-0.5 g per kg per day	44	22	20	$0.2 \times 20 = 4$ g per day $0.5 \times 20 = 10$ g per day SDR = 4-10 g per day
4	0.25-1.5 mg per kg per day	150	75	68.2	$0.25 \times 68.2 = 17.1$ mg per day $1.5 \times 68.2 = 102.3$ mg per day SDR = 17.1-102.3 mg per day
5	2-5 mcg per kg per day	180	90	81.8	$2 \times 81.8 = 163.6$ mcg per day $5 \times 81.8 = 409$ mcg per day SDR = 163.6-409 mcg per day

RAPID PRACTICE 5-13 (p. 184)

2   **a.** Estimated weight in kg = 60 kg; actual weight in kg = 54.5 kg
  b. SDR low, $2 \times 54.5 = 109$ mg per day; SDR high, $4 \times 54.5 = 218$ mg per day
  c. 50 mg $\times$ 4 = 200 mg
  d. Yes
  e. Order within SDR and safe to give.

3   **a.** Estimated weight in kg = 30 kg; actual weight in kg = 27.3 kg
  b. SDR low, $5 \times 27.3 = 136.5$ mg per day; SDR high, $10 \times 27.3 = 273$ mg per day
  c. 25 mg $\times$ 2 = 50 mg
  d. No. The ordered dose is significantly less than the low safe dose.
  e. Hold medication and clarify promptly with prescriber.

4   **a.** Estimated weight in kg = 80 kg; actual weight in kg = 72.7 kg
  b. SDR low, $1 \times 72.7 = 72.7$ mg per day; SDR high, $2 \times 72.7 = 145.4$ mg per day*
  c. 50 mg $\times$ 6 = 300 mg
  d. No. The ordered dose exceeds the high safe dose.
  e. Hold medication and clarify promptly with prescriber.

5   **a.** Estimated weight in kg = 50 kg; actual weight in kg = 45.5 kg
  b. SDR low, $10 \times 45.5 = 455$ mg per day; SDR high, $20 \times 45.5 = 910$ mg per day
  c. 250 mg $\times$ 3 = 750 mg (0.25 g = 250 mg)
  d. Yes
  e. Order within SDR and safe to give.

---
*SDR is usually seen in printed drug literature with a slash for "per." Do not use slashes in patient records. Estimated kg weight can prevent major math errors. Follow up with verification of actual DA weight.

RAPID PRACTICE 5-14 (p. 186)

2   **a.** 300 mg per 5 mL; 8 mEq per 5 mL (Tip: Examine orders and labels carefully!)
  b. Yes. Order is within SDR.
  c. Give 2 times the unit dose volume of 5 mL (10 mL).
  d. 10 mL per dose

$$\frac{?\ mL}{dose} = \frac{5\ mL}{\underset{3}{\cancel{300\ mg}}} \times \frac{\overset{10}{\cancel{1000\ mg}}}{1\ \cancel{g}} \times \frac{0.6\ \cancel{g}}{dose}$$

$$= \frac{30}{3} = \frac{10\ mL}{dose}$$

  e. Equation is balanced. Estimate supports answer.

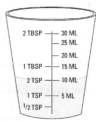

3   **a.** 20 mEq per 15 mL
  b. Yes. Order is within SDR
  c. Give slightly more than 30 mL
  d. 16.9 mL

$$\frac{?\ mL}{dose} = \frac{15\ mL}{\underset{4}{\cancel{20\ mEq}}} \times \frac{\overset{9}{\cancel{45\ mEq}}}{dose} = \frac{135}{4}$$

$$= 33.75 = 33.8\ mL$$

e. Equation is balanced. Estimate supports answer.

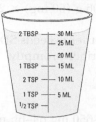

1	b	**6**	d
2	d	**7**	a
3	b	**8**	a
4	d	**9**	c
5	c	**10**	a

CHAPTER 5 FINAL PRACTICE (p. 192)

1 **a.** SDR: 200 mg bid to start.
   Order: 0.2 g (200 mg) bid.
   b. Safe to give
   c. 2 tablets = 100 mg × 2 = 200 mg = 2 tablets
   d. 2 tablets

$$? \frac{\text{tab}}{\text{dose}} = \frac{1 \text{ tab}}{\cancel{100 \text{ mg}}} \times \frac{\overset{10}{\cancel{1000 \text{ mg}}}}{1 \cancel{\text{ g}}} \times \frac{0.2 \cancel{\text{ g}}}{1}$$

$$= \frac{2 \text{ tabs}}{\text{dose}}$$

e. Equation is balanced. Estimate equals answer.

2 **a.** SDR: 20–40 mEq per day
   Order: 30 mEq per day
   b. Safe to give
   c. Give less than dose per volume supplied of 15 mL (about 12 mL)
   d. 11.3 mL

$$? \frac{\text{mL}}{\text{dose}} = \frac{15 \text{ mL}}{\underset{4}{\cancel{40 \text{ mEq}}}} \times \frac{\overset{3}{\cancel{30 \text{ mEq}}}}{\text{dose}} = \frac{45}{4}$$

$$= 11.25, \text{ rounded to } \frac{11.3 \text{ mL}}{\text{dose}}$$

e. Equation is balanced. Estimate supports answer.

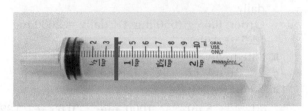

4 **a.** 1 mg per 7.5 mL
   b. Yes. Order is within SDR.
   c. Give two times dose per volume supplied: 15 mL
   d. 15 mL per dose

$$? \frac{\text{mL}}{\text{dose}} = \frac{7.5 \text{ mL}}{1 \text{ mg}} \times \frac{2 \text{ mg}}{\text{dose}} = \frac{15 \text{ mL}}{\text{dose}}$$

e. Equation is balanced. Estimate supports answer.

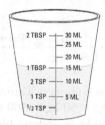

5 Estimated weight in kg: 25 kg; actual weight in kg: 24 kg
   a. 75 mg per 5 mL
   b. Yes. Order is within SDR. Patient is receiving 120 mg q8h, which equals 360 mg per day which is 15 mg per kg and within the safe dosage range.

$$? \frac{\text{mg}}{\text{day}} = \frac{10 \text{ mg}}{\text{kg} \times \text{day}} \times \frac{24 \text{ kg}}{1} = \frac{240 \text{ mg}}{\text{day}}$$
$$= 240 \text{ mg per day low safe dose}$$

$$? \frac{\text{mg}}{\text{day}} = \frac{25 \text{ mg}}{\text{kg} \times \text{day}} \times \frac{24 \text{ kg}}{1} = \frac{600 \text{ mg}}{\text{day}}$$
$$= 600 \text{ mg per day high safe dose}$$

   c. 8 mL
   d. 8 mL
   e. This is a safe dose to give.

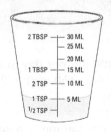

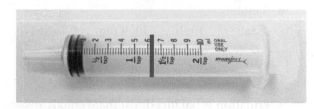

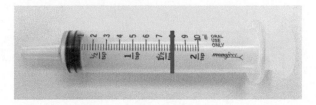

3 **a.** SDR 325–650 mg q4h up to 12 tablets per day or 2–3 tablets (325–975 mg) q6h up to 12 tablets in 24 hr. Order: 0.65 g (625 mg) six times a day (12 tablets)

b. Safe to give

c. 2; more

d. Will give 2 tabs (325 mg mEq $\times$ 2 = 650 mg)

$$?\frac{\text{tab}}{\text{dose}} = \frac{1\text{ tab}}{325\text{ mg}} \times \frac{1000\text{ mg}}{1\text{ g}} \times \frac{0.65\text{ g}}{\text{dose}}$$
$$= \frac{2\text{ tablets}}{\text{dose}}$$

e. Equation is balanced. Answer equals estimate.

4 **a.** SDR: 8–16 mg sol 1 hr preoperatively
Order: 14 mg 1 hr preoperatively

b. Safe to give

c. 4 $\times$ 5 mL= 20 mL

d. 17.5 mL

$$?\frac{\text{mL}}{\text{dose}} = \frac{5\text{ mL}}{\underset{2}{4\text{ mg}}} \times \frac{\overset{7}{14\text{ mg}}}{\text{dose}} = \frac{35}{2} = \frac{17.5\text{ mL}}{\text{dose}}$$

e. Equation is balanced. Estimate supports answer.

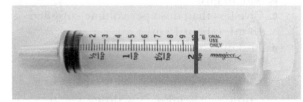

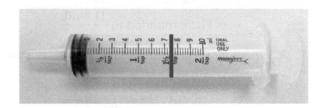

5 **a.** SDR: 50-400 mg per day in divided doses
Order: 0.15 g (150 mg) $\times$ 2 doses = 300 mg

b. Safe to give

c. 0.15 g ordered = (150 mg);
50 mg $\times$ 3 = 150 mg = 3 tablets

d. 3 tablets

$$?\frac{\text{tab}}{\text{dose}} = \frac{1\text{ tab}}{50\text{ mg}} \times \frac{1000\text{ mg}}{1\text{ g}} \times \frac{0.15\text{ g}}{\text{dose}}$$
$$= \frac{150}{50} = \frac{3\text{ tablets}}{\text{per dose}}$$

e. Equation is balanced. Estimate equals answer.
Note: Recheck orders for doses exceeding 1 or 2 tablets. In this case the patient diagnosis and the current drug literature support the administration of up to 150 mg per dose twice daily.

6 **a.** SDR: 60 mg daily
Order: 0.06 g (60 mg) $\times$ 2 = 120 mg ordered daily

b. Unsafe. Order exceeds SDR. Hold medication. Call prescriber promptly.

c. N/A

d. N/A

e. N/A

7 **a.** SDR: 325–650 mg q4–6h up to 4 g (4000 mg) daily
Order: 0.65 g (650 mg 4$\times$ daily = 2600 mg [2.6 g] daily)

b. Safe to give

c. 2 $\times$ 10 mL (2 $\times$ 325) (about 20 mL)

d. 20 mL

$$?\frac{\text{mL}}{\text{dose}} = \frac{5\text{ mL}}{160\text{ mg}} \times \frac{1000\text{ mg}}{1\text{ g}} \times \frac{0.65\text{ g}}{\text{dose}} \times \frac{325\theta}{16\theta}$$
$$= 20.31\text{ mL} = 20.3\text{ mL}$$

e. Equation is balanced. Answer equals estimate.

8 **a.** SDR maintenance: 75–125 mcg daily
Order: 0.1 mg = 100 mcg daily

b. Safe to give

c. 2 tablets (0.05 $\times$ 2 = 0.1)

d. 2 tablets

$$?\frac{\text{tab}}{\text{dose}} = \frac{1\text{ tab}}{\underset{1}{0.05\text{ mg}}} \times \frac{\overset{2}{0.1\text{ mg}}}{1} = \frac{2\text{ tabs}}{\text{dose}}$$

e. Equation is balanced. Estimate equals answer.

9 **a.** SDR: 10 mg $\times$ 50 kg = 500 mg low safe daily dose.
15 mg $\times$ 50 kg = 750 mg high safe daily dose.
Order: 300 mg bid (600 mg per day)

b. Safe to give

c. Estimate: slightly more than 5 mL unit dose

d. 6 mL (need two packages)

$$?\frac{\text{mL}}{\text{dose}} = \frac{5\text{ mL}}{\underset{5}{250\text{ mg}}} \times \frac{\overset{6}{300\text{ mg}}}{\text{dose}} = \frac{30}{5} = \frac{6\text{ mL}}{\text{dose}}$$

e. Need two packages

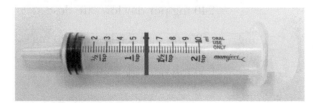

f. Equation is balanced. Estimate equals answer.

10 a. SDR: 125-250 mg q6-8h
Order: 0.25 g (250 mg) q8h
b. Safe to give
c. 1 tablet (0.25 g = 250 mg)
d. 1 tablet

$$? \frac{\text{tab}}{\text{dose}} = \frac{1 \text{ tab}}{\underset{1}{\cancel{250 \text{ mg}}}} \times \frac{\overset{4}{\cancel{1000 \text{ mg}}}}{1 \cancel{\text{ g}}} \times \frac{0.25 \cancel{\text{ g}}}{\text{dose}}$$

$$= \frac{1 \text{ tab}}{\text{dose}}$$

e. Equation is balanced. Estimate equals answer.

Suggestions for Further Reading

Clayton BD, Willihnganz M: *Basic pharmacology for nurses,* 18 ed, St. Louis, 2020, Elsevier.

Skidmore-Roth L: *Mosby's 2021 nursing drug reference,* 34ed., St. Louis, 2021, Mosby.

http://www.cwladis.com/math104/lecture3.php

http://quizlct.com/18124377/chapter-12-oral-medication-labels-and-dosage-calculations-flash-cards/

Ⓔvolve   For additional practice problems, refer to the Oral Dosages section of the Elsevier's Interactive Drug Calculation Application, Version 1 on Evolve.

Chapter 6 covers syringe measurements in preparation for measuring injectable medication doses.

6 Syringes for Injection

OBJECTIVES

- State the total volume capacity for various syringes.
- Differentiate the calibrations (quantity values) for various syringe sizes per milliliter.
- State the lowest and nearest measurable dose for syringes.
- Select the appropriate syringe size for stated volumes.
- Draw a vertical line through an accurate dose on a syringe.
- Select the appropriate syringe for selected purposes.
- Identify safety principles related to syringes and needles.
- Define needle gauge and three criteria for needle selection.

ESTIMATED TIME TO COMPLETE CHAPTER: 30 minutes to 1 hour

The measurement and use of oral syringes were covered in Chapter 5. This chapter focuses on the parts of the syringe, measurement calibrations, syringe selection, safety precautions, and disposal methods. Additional practice will be offered in this chapter so that volume measurements for syringes of multiple sizes can be identified for providing the nearest measurable dose.

Examining and handling a variety of syringes and needles in the laboratory will be necessary to obtain a more comprehensive view and competence in the use of the equipment.

VOCABULARY

Hypodermic	General term used to describe injectables under the skin.
Insulin Syringe	Small syringe, with a 0.3- to 1-mL capacity, calibrated for specific insulin mixtures in standardized units.
Intradermal (ID)	Shallow injection to be given just under the skin between the dermis and the epidermis. Used mainly for skin tests. Not used to deliver medications. *0.1 mL* is the usual volume for skin test injections. A 1-mL tuberculin syringe is used.
Intramuscular (IM)	Into the muscle. The muscle is able to accept more irritating substances than other injectable routes.
Intravenous (IV)	Into the vein. These injections provide *instant* drug access to the circulation.
Needle Gauge	Diameter (thickness) of the needle shaft. The lower the gauge number, the larger the diameter of the needle. An 18-gauge needle is much larger than a 27-gauge needle.
Parenteral Medications	Injectable medications. Excludes oral, nasogastric, gastric, topical, and intestinal routes.
Prefilled Syringe	Syringe prefilled by manufacturer or pharmacy with specific frequently ordered doses of medication. This method is thought to reduce dose measurement errors.

Continued

Safety Syringe	Syringe designed with a variety of locking sheath covers to protect needle sterility and prevent accidental injury during and after disposal.
Subcutaneous	Under the skin into the fatty layer. Used for less irritating substances than are intramuscular injections. Insulin and heparin are given subcutaneously.
Syringe Holder	Specially designed device to be used only with an inserted prefilled medication cartridge.
Tuberculin Syringe	Small-volume syringe, with a 1-mL capacity, used for intradermal skin tests and small-volume injections in frail at-risk populations.
Viscosity	Ability to flow; thickness of a solution. A highly viscous solution may have directions for dilution. High viscosity solutions such as blood products and some reconstituted. Medications may require the use of a larger-gauge needle.

Syringe Sizes

20-mL, 10-mL, 5-mL, 3-mL, and 1-mL syringes

Syringes are available in many sizes, ranging from *0.3-mL* insulin syringe to *60-mL* or greater capacity. The decision to use a specific syringe is based on the volume of medication to be administered and the route of administration.

The 3-mL and 5-mL syringes were introduced in Chapter 5 for oral liquid medications.

Intravenous medications should be given with large-volume syringes to avoid excessive pressure in the line (Figures 6-1 and 6-2). Check agency policy for additional clarification.

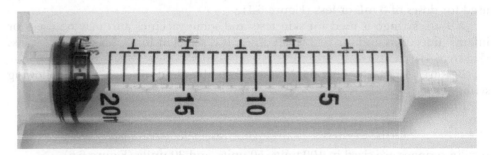

FIGURE 6-1 20-mL syringe with 1-mL calibrations.

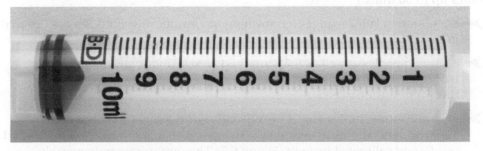

FIGURE 6-2 10-mL syringe with 0.2-mL calibrations.

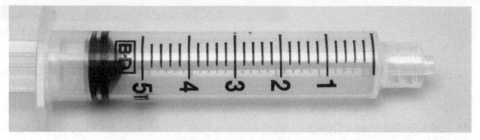

FIGURE 6-3 5-mL syringe with 0.2-mL calibrations.

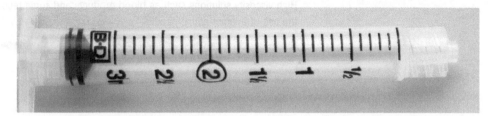

FIGURE 6-4 3-mL syringe with 0.1-mL calibrations.

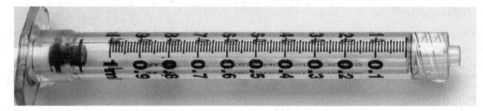

FIGURE 6-5 1-mL tuberculin syringe with 0.01-mL calibrations.

Intramuscular injections may be given with either a 3-mL or a 5-mL syringe (Figures 6-3 and 6-4).

Many subcutaneous and intramuscular injections are given with a 3-mL syringe, used for doses of 3 mL or less (Figure 6-4).

A 1-mL syringe is used for skin tests and some vaccines and may be used for infants' injections and for very small doses. It is selected for doses of 1 mL or less (Figure 6-5).

Be sure you can identify the lowest measurable dose on each of the following syringes.

Insulin syringes

Insulin syringes are sized in 100 units, 50 units, and 30 units (Figure 6-6).

A 100-unit insulin syringe is selected for insulin doses up to 100 units.

A 50-unit insulin syringe is selected for better visualization of insulin doses up to 50 units. A 30-unit insulin syringe is selected for better visualization of insulin doses up to 30 units.

➤ Do not use insulin syringes for anything but insulin. Insulin doses are ordered in units. Avoid confusing insulin syringes with tuberculin syringes.

➤ All used needles as well as their attached used syringes must be placed in hazardous waste sharps containers immediately after use. They may not be thrown in trash baskets.

➤ Do not confuse 1-mL syringes or tuberculin syringes marked in milliliters (or cubic centimeters) with 1-mL *insulin* syringes, which are marked with the word *insulin* and calibrated in *units* (Figure 6-7).They are not interchangeable.

➤ Do not substitute a tuberculin syringe for insulin.

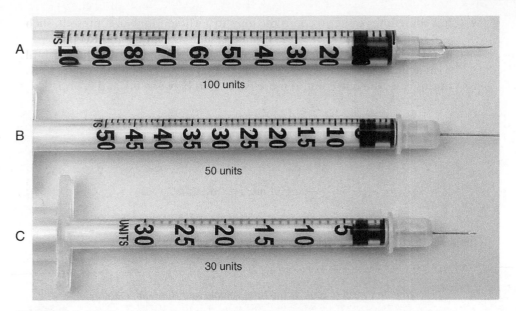

FIGURE 6-6 Insulin syringes. **A,** 100 units (1 mL). **B,** 50 units (0.5 mL). **C,** 30 units (0.3 mL).

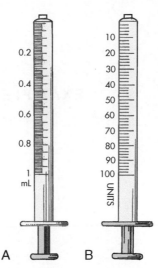

FIGURE 6-7 **A,** 1-mL tuberculin syringe. **B,** 100-unit 1-mL insulin syringe. (From Potter PA, Perry AG, Stockert PA, Hall AM: *Fundamentals of nursing,* ed 10, St Louis, 2021, Elsevier.)

Parts of the Syringe

Figure 6-8 shows the parts of a syringe. Syringes are supplied without needles or with attached needles. Supervised clinical practice is required to learn safe handling of syringes and needles.

The 3-mL syringe is the most commonly used syringe for intramuscular injections. The arrows illustrate the location of the 1- and 0.5-mL markings (Figure 6-9). The lowest measurable dose is 0.1 mL.

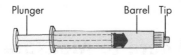

FIGURE 6-8 Parts of a syringe. (From Potter PA, Perry AG, Stockert PA, Hall AM: *Fundamentals of nursing,* ed 10, St Louis, 2021, Elsevier.)

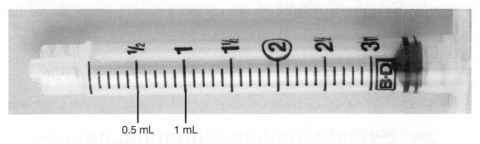

FIGURE 6-9 3-mL syringe showing 0.5-mL and 1-mL calibrations.

Total Capacity and Lowest Measurable Dose

Finding the total capacity and the lowest measurable dose involves the same process for all syringes. Syringe size selection is based on the medication dose ordered, the total volume of the syringe, and nearest *measurable* dose on the syringe. Examine the empty 3-mL syringe shown in Figure 6-9 for a review:
- The total capacity is 3 mL.
- The lowest measurable dose is 0.1 mL.
- Medications for this syringe can be given to the *nearest tenth of a milliliter* (2.2 mL, 2.3 mL, etc.) because that is the *lowest measurable dose.*
- The calibrations are slightly more prominent for the *whole*-milliliter marks.

- It is sometimes easier to count the lines to a whole number, if present, such as 0 to 1 mL, or between whole numbers, such as 1 and 2 mL. Keep in mind that smaller syringes may not have whole numbers. Examine the 1-mL syringe illustrated in Figure 6-5. It has 100 calibrations between 0 and 1 mL. In this case, the line count is more easily read between 0.1 and 0.2 mL.

EXAMPLES

$$\frac{1 \text{ mL}}{100 \text{ calibrations}} = 0.01 \text{ mL lowest measurable dose}$$

$$\frac{1 \text{ mL}}{10 \text{ calibrations}} = 0.1 \text{ mL lowest measurable dose}$$

$$\frac{1 \text{ mL}}{5 \text{ calibrations}} = 0.2 \text{ mL lowest measurable dose}$$

FAQ *Why do I need to look at the total volume and the 1-mL markings?*

ANSWER To avoid medication dose errors, you need to know the precise measurements. After the dose is calculated, select a syringe that will contain the total number of milliliters that you need to give. You would not select a 3-mL syringe if you had to give 4.5 mL, unless you planned to give two separate injections. The best way to avoid making a syringe measurement error is to locate the 1-, 0.5-, or other major mL mark if available and then to observe the value of each calibration. Larger syringes will not have all the smaller calibrations. Misreading *1.5 mL* for *0.5 mL* is a major error. Nevertheless, it has occurred.

Where to Measure the Dose on Syringes

The dose in syringes is measured at the upper flat ring of the plunger, the ring closest to the needle end. For practice measurements, the plunger will not be shown.

RAPID PRACTICE 6-1 Measuring Syringe Capacities

ESTIMATED COMPLETION TIME: 10 to 15 minutes   **ANSWERS ON:** page 230

DIRECTIONS: *Examine the numbers and calibrations on the syringe, and provide the answer in the space provided.*

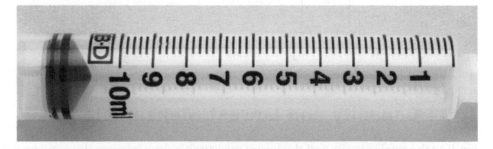

1 Draw a vertical line through the syringe at 5.6 mL.

2 Draw a second vertical line through the syringe at 8.8 mL.

3 What is the total capacity of the syringe in milliliters? _____

4 How many calibrations are there between 0 and 5 mL? _____

5 How many calibrations are there between 0 and 1 mL? _____

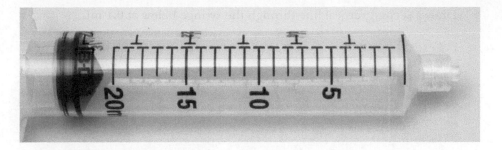

6 What is the smallest measurable dose (the first space up to the first line) on the syringe? _____

7 Draw a vertical line through the syringe above at 1 mL.

8 Draw a second vertical line through the syringe above at 14 mL.

9 What is the total capacity of this syringe in milliliters? _____

---

1 How do the lowest measurable doses on the 10- and 20-mL syringe shown in the text differ from the lowest measurable doses on the 3- and 5-mL syringes?

ASK YOURSELF **Q & A**

_____

MY ANSWER

RAPID PRACTICE 6-2   Measuring Syringe Capacities

ESTIMATED COMPLETION TIME: 10 minutes   **ANSWERS ON:** page 230

DIRECTIONS: *Examine the numbers and calibrations on the syringe and provide the answers in the space provided.*

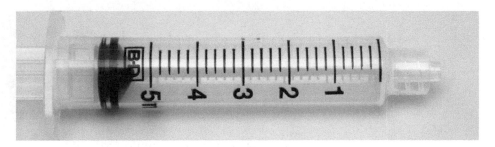

1 Draw a vertical line through the syringe above at 0.6 mL. (Note: There are also 5-mL syringes that have 10 calibrations per milliliter.)

2 Draw a second vertical line through the syringe above at 3.4 mL.

3 Draw a vertical line through the syringe below at 0.05 mL.

4   Draw a second vertical line through the syringe below at 0.1 mL.

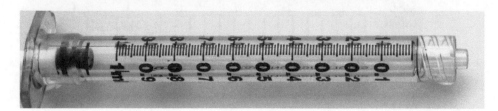

5   How many calibrations are there between 0 and 0.1 mL? _____

6   How many calibrations are there between 0 and 1 mL? _____

7   What is the total capacity of the syringe above in milliliters? _____

8   What is the smallest measurable dose on the syringe? _____

➤ Pay special attention to the decimal place in the doses for the 1-mL syringe.

Q & A ASK YOURSELF	**1**	What are the two most commonly used sizes of syringes?
MY ANSWER		_____

RAPID PRACTICE 6-3   ## Measuring Syringe Capacities

ESTIMATED COMPLETION TIME: 5 minutes   **ANSWERS ON:** page 230

DIRECTIONS: *Examine the numbers and calibrations on the syringe and provide the answers in the space provided or by putting a line on the syringe drawing.*

1   Draw a vertical line through the syringe below at 1.6 mL.

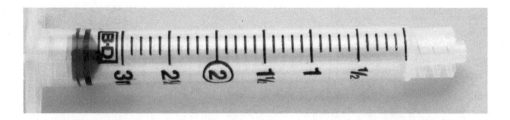

2   What is the total capacity of the syringe below in milliliters? _____

3   What is the smallest measurable dose on this syringe? _____

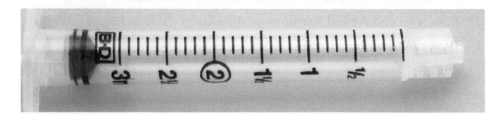

4 Draw a vertical line through the syringe below at 0.9 mL.

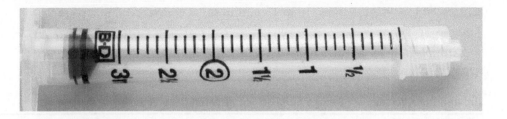

5 Draw a vertical line through the syringe below at 2.7 mL.

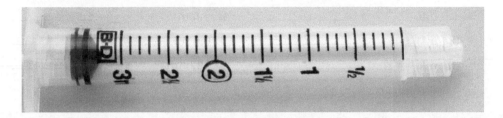

The 3- and 5-mL syringes are the most commonly used. However, nurses must know how to distinguish the differences in calibrations in the other sizes to avoid a dose measurement error.

ASK YOURSELF **Q & A**

1 What is the difference in the lowest measurable dose between the 3-mL and the 5-mL syringe shown in this text?

MY ANSWER

_____

2 Of the 3-mL and the 5-mL syringe shown in this text, which one can accommodate a 2.7-mL ordered dose?

_____

Examining the Calculated Doses for Correct Syringe Selection

- If the amount ordered is a whole number (e.g., 3 mL) or in tenths of a milliliter (e.g., 2.8 or 1.8 mL), the 3-mL syringe would be appropriate.
- If the amount ordered was 0.8 mL, then a 1-mL syringe would be appropriate. A 3-mL *could* also be used, but for amounts less than 1 mL, a 1-mL syringe would be the best choice.
- If the amount to be given is 0.08 mL, the 3-mL syringe would not be used because it is not calibrated in hundredths of a milliliter. A 1-mL (tuberculin) syringe would be selected.
- If the amount to be given is 3.6 mL, the 3-mL syringe would not be used because the patient would have to receive two injections. A 5-mL syringe would be selected.

| RAPID PRACTICE 6-4 | Identifying the Syringe for the Dose Ordered |

ESTIMATED COMPLETION TIME: 10 to 15 minutes　　**ANSWERS ON:** page 230

DIRECTIONS: *State the preferred syringe size in mL that provides the nearest measurable dose for the dose ordered. Note that a tuberculin syringe is a 1-mL syringe.*

Ordered Dose Volume	Syringe Size	Ordered Dose Volume	Syringe Size
1　1.7 mL	_____	6　2.8 mL	_____
2　3.2 mL	_____	7　0.08 mL	_____
3　1.5 mL	_____	8　9.6 mL	_____
4　6.4 mL	_____	9　0.6 mL	_____
5　0.1 mL	_____	10　12.6 mL	_____

| RAPID PRACTICE 6-5 | Syringe Selections and Disposal |

ESTIMATED COMPLETION TIME: 5 minutes　　**ANSWERS ON:** page 230

DIRECTIONS: *Refer to the preceding text and syringe photographs that follow to answer the following questions.*

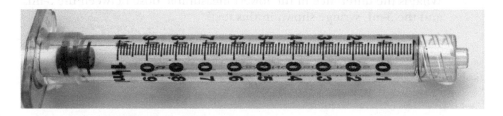

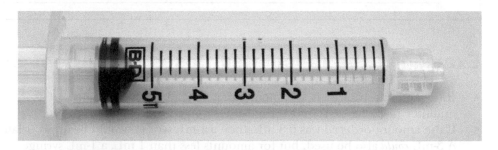

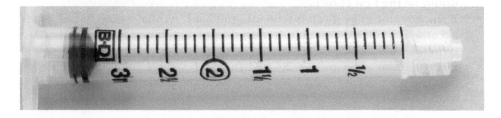

1　What is the main criterion for selection of syringe size? _____

2　Can used syringes without needles be placed in ordinary trash containers? ____

3　If a nurse prepares 0.06 mL of a medication, which size syringe should the nurse select? _____

4 If a nurse calculates a dose of 2.9 mL of a medication, which size syringe should the nurse select? _____ How much medication will be drawn up in the syringe for the nearest measurable dose? _____

5 If a nurse calculates a dose of 3.19 mL of a medication, which size syringe should the nurse select? _____ What will be the nearest measurable dose on the syringe? _____

Prefilled Injectable Syringes

Prefilled injectable syringes contain a single-dose of medication. They have a needle attached and are disposable (Figure 6-10). If the order calls for less than the supplied amount, the nurse adjusts the dose by discarding unneeded amounts before administration.

➤ Doses for prefilled syringes must be calculated before administration. There *may* be extra medication and air in the syringe that need to be expelled before administration. Check the package and/or label directions.

➤ Check agency protocols for discard of controlled substances.

➤ Many prefilled syringe medications look similar. The nurse must check all the information on the syringe to avoid giving the wrong medicine or dose.

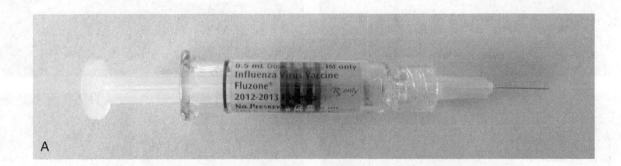

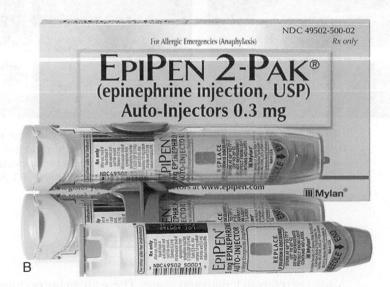

FIGURE 6-10 A, Prefilled flu vaccine. **B,** Prefilled epinephrine auto-injectors for anaphylaxis treatment. (From Mylan Specialty L.P., Morgantown, WV.)

Prefilled Medication Cartridges for Injection

Injectables may be supplied in a cartridge with an attached needle. The cartridge containing the medicine is to be locked in the plastic holder for injection of the medication.

Dexterity with this equipment requires *intermittent* practice sessions for insertion, locking, unlocking, and needle safety techniques (Figure 6-11). The cartridges usually have 0.1 or 0.2 mL extra medication in case of loss. The label and calibrations must be read and compared with the order *before* the cartridge is inserted. The cartridge can be rotated so that the calibrations are in view for adjusting the dose.

➤ Be especially careful to examine prefilled syringe labels and cartridge calibrations before administering them. Rotate the cartridge after placement in the holder so that the amounts and calibrations can be clearly seen.

➤ **Because of concern about transmission of infection, some facilities may no longer allow the use of the reusable cartridge holder. Follow your agency policy regarding this issue.**

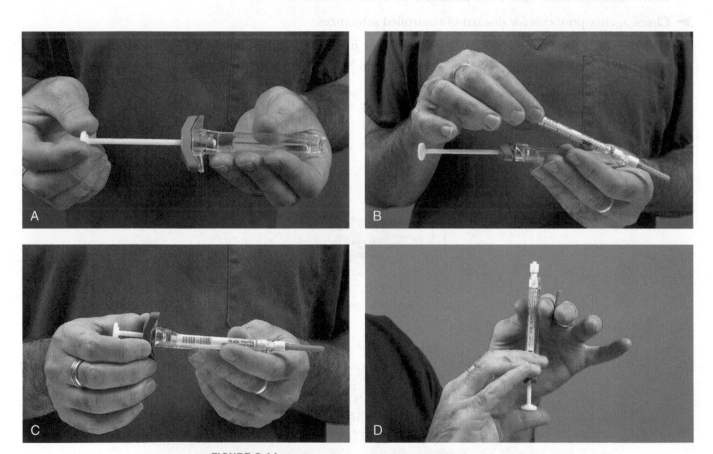

FIGURE 6-11 **A,** Carpuject syringe and prefilled sterile cartridge with needle. **B,** Assembling the Carpuject. **C,** The cartridge slides into the syringe barrel, turns, and locks at the needle end. The plunger then screws into the cartridge end. **D,** Expel excess medication to obtain accurate dose. (From Potter PA, Perry AG, Stockert PA, Hall A: *Essentials of nursing practice,* ed. 9, St. Louis, 2019, Elsevier.)

Needle Sizes

Needle size refers to length and gauge. There are many options available (Figure 6-12). Supervised laboratory and clinical experience is needed to master needle size selection, dexterity, and safe handling.

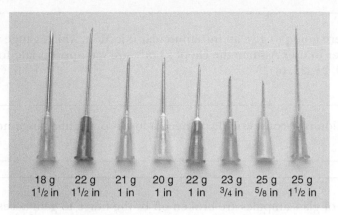

18 g 22 g 21 g 20 g 22 g 23 g 25 g 25 g
1½ in 1½ in 1 in 1 in 1 in ¾ in ⅝ in 1½ in

FIGURE 6-12 Needles of various gauges and lengths. (From Lilley LL, Rainforth Collins S, Snyder JS: *Pharmacology and nursing process,* ed. 9, St. Louis, 2020, Mosby.)

Needle lengths are as follows:
- Intramuscular: 1 to 2 inches
- Subcutaneous: ⅜ to ⅝ inch
- Intradermal: ⅜ to ½ inch

Basics of needle selection

Needle selection, length, and gauge depend on three criteria:

1 Purpose and route of the injection

2 Size and skin integrity of the patient

3 Viscosity of the solution

Intramuscular (IM) injections are inserted into the striated muscle fibers that are under the subcutaneous layers of the skin. The onset of action is longer than with intravenous administration but usually shorter than with oral administration.

Intramuscular injections require longer needles than do intradermal and subcutaneous injections. Irritating substances are not injected into *subcutaneous* tissue because they are not absorbed as quickly into the circulation. The muscle would be a better alternative for such a substance because it has a better blood supply. Larger adults require a longer needle than a frail adult or a child. The shortest needles are reserved for intradermal use. See Table 6-1 for usual needle sizes and their purposes. In addition to altering needle size, the angle of injection is altered for different-sized patients. This is learned in supervised clinical practice.

 Mnemonic

LL: **L**ower gauge number, **L**arger needle.

TABLE 6-1	Usual Needle Sizes and Purposes
Usual Needle Size (Gauge)*	**Purpose**
31	Subcutaneous insulin administration
27–30	Intradermal skin tests, subcutaneous insulin administration
25–27	Subcutaneous injections, heparin administration
22	Spinal canal insertion
20–23	Intramuscular injections
16–20	Intravenous injections
18	Preferred for blood administration because blood is viscous

*Check your agency supply and protocols. There are other sizes available.

Q & A   **ASK YOURSELF**   **1**   If you were going to give an intramuscular injection, which gauge would you prefer to use? Assume the client's body size was appropriate for any of them: 20, 21, 22, or 23?

MY ANSWER   _____

2   If a solution is viscous, would you need a lower- or higher-gauge needle?

_____

➤ The tips of glass ampules are broken off by the nurse to gain access to the contents.

➤ Special filter needles *must* be used when withdrawing medications from glass ampules so that small particles of glass cannot enter the syringe (Figure 6-13).

➤ The filter needle must be removed and discarded. A new needle is put on the syringe to give the injection.

CLINICAL RELEVANCE   Failure to remove the filter needle prior to giving the injection risks the patient receiving glass particles along with the medication.

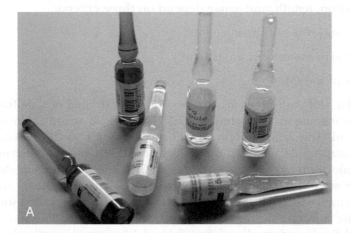

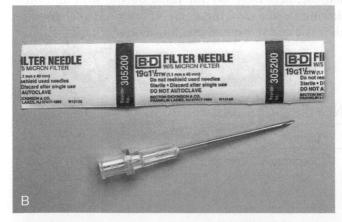

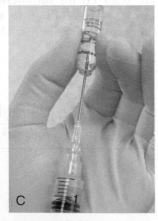

FIGURE 6-13 A, Ampules containing medications come in various sizes. The ampules must be broken carefully to withdraw the medication with the use of a filter needle. **B,** BD Filter needle. Some agencies require that filter needles be used for vials as well as ampules. **C,** Using a filter needle to withdraw medication from an ampule. (**C,** From Lilley LL, Rainforth Collins S, Snyder JS: *Pharmacology and nursing process,* ed. 9, St. Louis, 2020, Mosby.)

1 Why must the filter needles be replaced before injection?

_____

Safety Syringes

> The greatest risks for needle-stick injury are during the handling and disposal of used needles *after* injection. Needles should never be recapped after giving an injection. Risks of needle-stick injury include transmission of blood-borne pathogens such as hepatitis B and C and HIV.

Prepared medicines and needles have safety features to prevent needle stick injuries. Many syringes are supplied with a variety of sheaths and sliding or retracting devices to cover the needle as soon as it is withdrawn from the patient to prevent needle stick injuries (Figures 6-14 and 6-15).

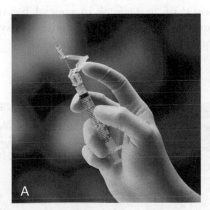 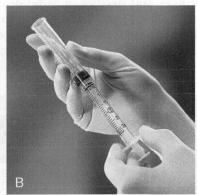

FIGURE 6-14 A, BD Safety Glide™. **B,** BD Safety-Lok™ Syringe. (**A,** From Becton, Dickinson, and Company, Franklin Lakes, NJ. **B,** From Becton, Dickinson, and Company, Franklin Lakes, NJ.)

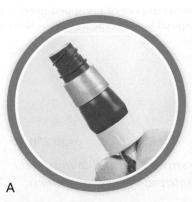 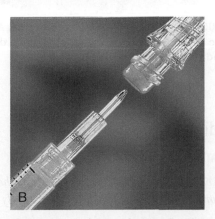

FIGURE 6-15 A, Clave Needlefree Antimicrobial IV Access Connection. **B,** BD Interlink Vial Access Cannula with syringe. Nurse can access vials without the use of a sharp needle. Blue vial access tip stays in vial. Needleless syringe is then ready for use. (**A,** ICU Medical, Inc. San Clemente, CA. **D,** From Becton, Dickinson, and Company, Franklin Lakes, NJ.)

CLINICAL RELEVANCE

➤ Do not recap used needles.

Beware of needles projecting from overfilled containers.

Beware of human traffic when crossing a room or exiting a curtained area with an exposed contaminated needle. The needle needs to be pointed away from the carrier and toward the floor (not angled toward the ceiling).

Sharps containers need to be replaced when they are ⅔ full.

Do not attempt to push a syringe into a filled sharps container. Your hand may be stuck by an upright needle in the container.

Be very careful if a bedside treatment that included an injection (e.g., a spinal tap) has been performed. A used needle inadvertently dropped in the bedding poses a needle stick risk.

➤ During orientation to any new clinical agency, nurses need to familiarize themselves with the types and uses of syringes and needles, the needleless equipment available, and the location of sharps disposal containers. Agency policies pertaining to handling of the equipment must also be checked.

Safety Issues and Disposal of Sharps

Used syringes and needles must be disposed of *immediately* in special hazardous waste containers (Figure 6-16). Check your agency policies for needle and syringe disposal. The trend is to use needleless equipment and safety syringes.

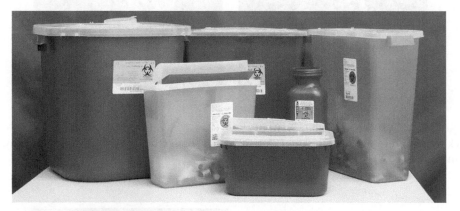

FIGURE 6-16 Never recap a used needle! Always dispose of uncapped needles in the appropriate sharps container. Needle disposal boxes come in various shapes and sizes to meet the needs of users.

RAPID PRACTICE 6-6   Reading Syringe Volumes

ESTIMATED COMPLETION TIME: 10 minutes   **ANSWERS ON:** page 230

DIRECTIONS: *Examine the calibrations of the syringes pictured to answer the questions. Follow these three steps to rapidly interpret syringe calibrations:*

- Identify the total capacity.
- Note the volume and number of calibrations between two adjacent dark lines.
- Calculate the smallest measurable dose (specific volume ÷ number of calibrations).

1

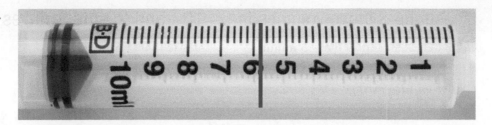

   a. Total volume of this syringe: _____
   b. Number of calibrations between 0 and 1 mL: _____
   c. The value of each calibration (smallest measurable dose): _____
   d. What is the amount marked on the syringe? _____

2

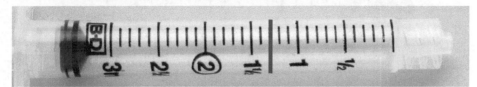

   a. Total volume of this syringe: _____
   b. Number of calibrations between 0 and 1 mL: _____
   c. The value of each calibration (smallest measurable dose): _____
   d. What is the amount marked on the syringe? _____

3

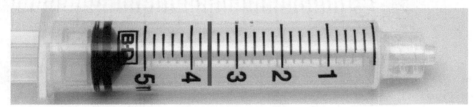

   a. Total volume of this syringe: _____
   b. Number of calibrations between 0 and 1 mL: _____
   c. Value of each calibration (smallest measurable dose): _____
   d. What is the amount marked on the syringe? _____

4

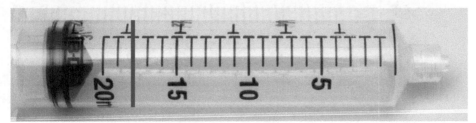

   a. Total volume of this syringe. _____
   b. Number of calibrations between 0 and 1 mL. _____
   c. The value of each calibration (smallest measurable dose) _____
   d. What is the amount marked on the syringe? _____

5

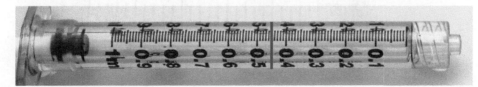

   a. Total volume of this syringe: _____
   b. Number of calibrations between 0 and 0.1 mL: _____
   c. The value of each calibration (smallest measurable dose): _____
   d. What is the amount marked on the syringe? _____

RAPID PRACTICE 6-7 | Measuring Syringe Volumes in 5-, 10-, and 20-mL Syringes

ESTIMATED COMPLETION TIME: 5 minutes   **ANSWERS ON:** page 231

DIRECTIONS: *Draw a vertical line through the calibrated line for the requested volume on each syringe.*

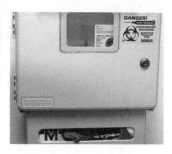

Needle sharps disposal for individual patient room.

1 14 mL

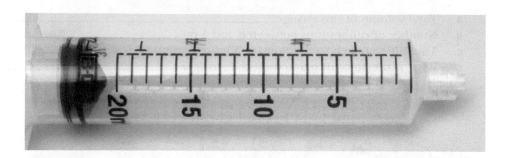

2 7.2 mL

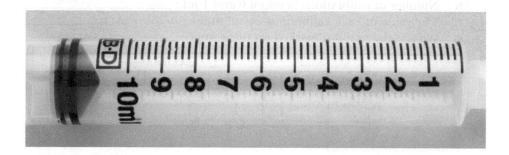

3 8.2 mL

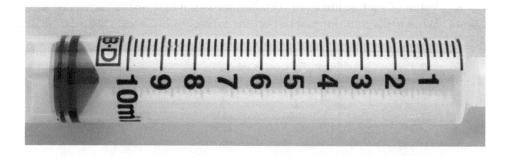

4 4.2 mL

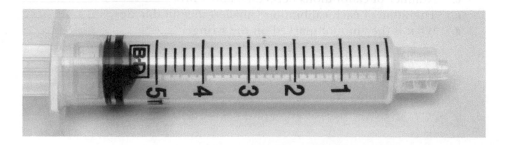

5   3.8 mL

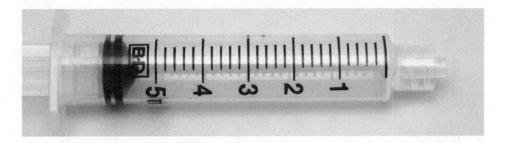

| RAPID PRACTICE 6-8 | 1-mL Syringe Measurements |

ESTIMATED COMPLETION TIME: 5 to 10 minutes   **ANSWERS ON:** page 231

DIRECTIONS: *Draw a vertical line through the calibrated line of each syringe for the dose to be given. The top ring of the plunger,* closest to the needle, *must rest on that calibrated line of the dose in milliliters when the medication is drawn into the syringe.*

1   0.86 mL

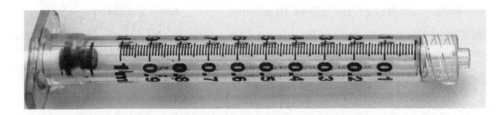

2   Draw an arrow pointing to 0.1 mL, the volume used for most skin tests (e.g., tuberculosis).

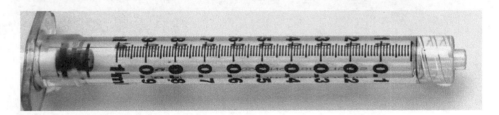

3   0.24 mL

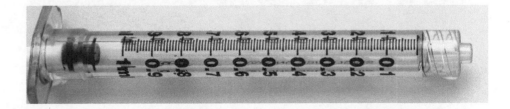

4 0.3 mL

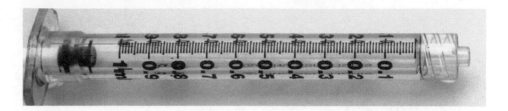

5 0.55 mL

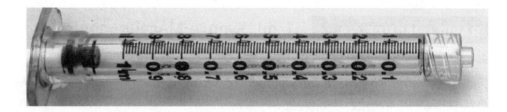

| RAPID PRACTICE 6-9 | 3-mL Syringe Measurements |

ESTIMATED COMPLETION TIME: 5 to 10 minutes   **ANSWERS ON:** page 231

DIRECTIONS: *Draw a vertical line through the calibrated line of each syringe for the dose requested.*

1 1.4 mL

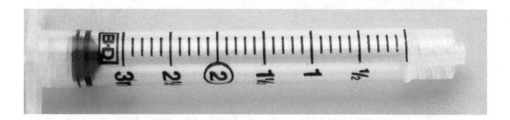

2 0.6 mL

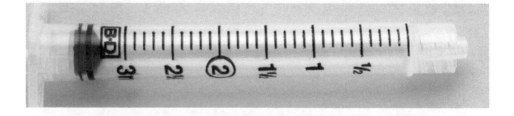

3 0.7 mL

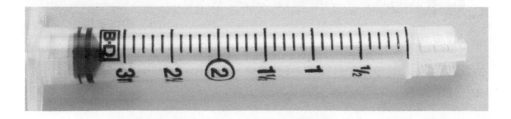

4   2.8 mL

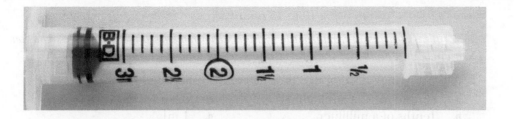

5   1.8 mL

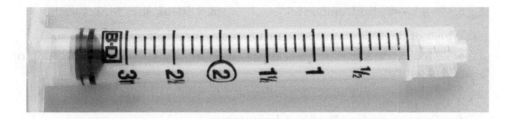

1	When you read and check volumes on a syringe, why is it advisable to have the calibrations at eye level and eyeglasses on hand, if needed?	**ASK YOURSELF**
		MY ANSWER

Recommended Fluid Volume for Selected Sites

An excess of injected fluid volume into tissue is not absorbed within a reasonable amount of time, and it causes discomfort for the patient. The recommended fluid volumes for selected sites are as follows:

- 0.1 mL for intradermal skin tests
- 0.5–1 mL for subcutaneous injections at a single site
- Up to 3 mL for intramuscular injections at a single site
- 1–60 mL for intravenous injections

➤ Assuming the correct syringe is selected, the nurse rounds the number of milliliters of medication to the *nearest measurable dose* on the syringe. If the syringe is calibrated in *tenths* of a milliliter, the medication is prepared to the *nearest tenth*. If the syringe is calibrated in *hundredths* of a milliliter, the medication is prepared to the *nearest hundredth*.

➤ Do *not* round up to whole numbers, such as from 0.8 to 1 mL or from 0.5 to 1 mL on a syringe. For a review of rounding instructions, see p. 21.

CHAPTER 6   MULTIPLE-CHOICE REVIEW

ESTIMATED COMPLETION TIME: 10 to 15 minutes   **ANSWERS ON:** page 231

DIRECTIONS: *If necessary, review the syringe measurements presented in this chapter. Then circle the number of the correct response, as shown in problem 1.*

1 A 1-mL syringe is calibrated in which of the following increments?
   - **a.** Hundredths of a milliliter
   - **b.** Tenths of a milliliter
   - **c.** 0.2 mL
   - **d.** 1 mL

2 The *syringe* size and amount used for skin tests is
   - **a.** 1-mL size, 0.1-mL amount
   - **b.** 3-mL size, 1-mL amount
   - **c.** 5-mL size, 0.2-mL amount
   - **d.** 10-mL size, 1-mL amount

3 Which of the following are the main criteria for selection of needle size?
   - **a.** Medication viscosity, medication route, size of patient, and skin condition of patient
   - **b.** Volume of fluid to be administered and number of milligrams of medication to be administered
   - **c.** Frequency of medication administration
   - **d.** Gauge and length of needle

4 If the dose ordered is 0.88 mL, to be administered with a 1-mL syringe, how many milliliters should the nurse administer?
   - **a.** 0.8 mL
   - **b.** 0.85 mL
   - **c.** 0.88 mL
   - **d.** 0.9 mL

5 Which of the following statements pertaining to needle gauge is true?
   - **a.** The highest-gauge needles have the smallest diameters.
   - **b.** An 18-gauge needle is narrower than a 23-gauge needle.
   - **c.** The needles with the smallest gauges are used for intradermal skin tests.
   - **d.** The needles with the largest gauges are used for intramuscular tests.

6 A 3-mL syringe is calibrated in which of the following increments?
   - **a.** Hundredths of a milliliter
   - **b.** Tenths of a milliliter
   - **c.** 0.2 mL
   - **d.** 1 mL

7 When do most needle stick injuries occur?
   - **a.** During medication preparation
   - **b.** During medication administration
   - **c.** After medication administration
   - **d.** When the patient self-administers

8 The most commonly used size of syringe for adult intramuscular injections is
   - **a.** 1 mL
   - **b.** 3 mL
   - **c.** 5 mL
   - **d.** 10 mL

9 If the dose ordered is 2.54 mL, to be administered with a 3-mL syringe, how many milliliters should the nurse administer?
   - **a.** 2.5 mL
   - **b.** 2.54 mL
   - **c.** 2.6 mL
   - **d.** 3 mL

10 Which of the following is the major criterion in *syringe* selection?
   - **a.** Volume of medication to be given
   - **b.** Route of administration specified by prescriber
   - **c.** Trade and generic names of the drug
   - **d.** Size of the patient in lb or kg

ESTIMATED COMPLETION TIME: 1 hour   **ANSWERS ON:** page 231

DIRECTIONS: *Estimate and calculate the dose using mental arithmetic and DA verification when requested. Evaluate the answer. Does the estimate support the answer? Draw a vertical line through the calibrated line of each syringe to indicate the dose to be given.*

1 **Ordered:** 120 mg of Drug Y. Available: 10 mg per mL.

   a. Examine the ordered dose and the dose available. Estimate your dose calculation. Will you need to give *more* or *less* than the unit mL dose available? (Circle one.)

   b. How many mL will you give?

   DA equation:

   c. Evaluation: _____

Draw a vertical line through the nearest measurable amount on the 20-mL syringe shown.

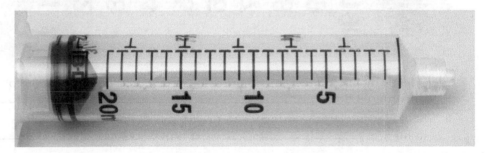

2 **Ordered:** 200 mg of Drug Y. Available: 100 mg per mL.

   a. Estimated dose: Will you need to give *more* or *less* than the unit mL dose available? (Circle one.)

   b. How many mL will you give? (Use mental arithmetic.) _____

   c. Evaluation: _____

Draw a vertical line through the nearest measurable amount on the 3-mL syringe shown.

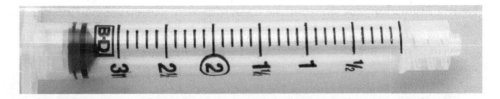

3 **Ordered:** 15 mg of Drug Y. Available: 30 mg per mL.

   a. Estimated dose: Will you need to give *more* or *less* than the unit mL dose available? (Circle one.)

   b. How many mL will you give? (Use mental arithmetic.) _____

   c. Evaluation: _____

Draw a vertical line through the nearest measurable amount on the 3-mL syringe shown.

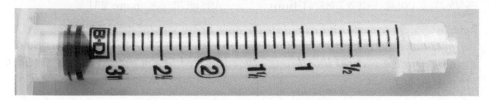

4 Ordered: 80 mg of Drug Y. Available: 10 mg per mL.

a. Estimated dose: Will you need to give *more* or *less* than the unit mL dose available? (Circle one.)

b. How many mL will you give? (Use mental arithmetic.) _____

c. Evaluation: _____

Draw a vertical line through the nearest measurable amount on the 5-mL syringe shown.

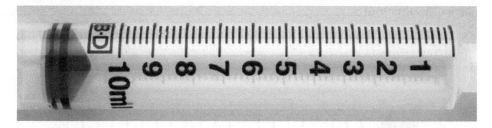

5 a. What is the most important criterion for syringe selection in relation to the ordered dose? _____

b. Should you select the syringe *before* or *after* calculating the dose volume in mL? _____

6 Ordered: 15 mg of Drug Y. Available: 100 mg per mL.

a. Examine the ordered dose and the dose available. Estimate your dose calculation. Will you need to give *more* or *less* than the unit mL dose available? (Circle one.)

b. How many mL will you give for the nearest measurable dose on the syringe provided?

DA equation:

c. Evaluation: _____

Draw an arrow pointing to the nearest measurable amount on the 1-mL syringe provided.

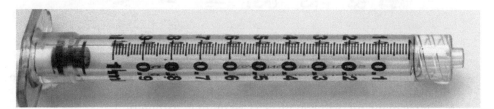

7 a. List two special precautions that must be taken when disposing of used and/or contaminated needles? _____

_____

b. Name two diseases mentioned in the chapter that can be acquired through needle stick injuries. _____

8 **Ordered:** 320 mg of Drug Y. Available: 50 mg per mL.

    a. Estimated dose: Will you need to give *more* or *less* than the unit mL dose available? (Circle one.)

    b. How many mL will you give?

      DA equation:

    c. Evaluation: _____

Draw a vertical line through the nearest measurable amount on the 10-mL syringe shown.

9 **Ordered:** 40 mg of Drug Y. Available 50 mg per mL.

    a. Examine the ordered dose and the dose available. Estimate your dose calculation. Will you need to give *more* or *less* than the unit mL dose available? (Circle one.)

    b. How many mL will you give?

      DA equation:

    c. Evaluation: _____

Draw a vertical line through the nearest measurable amount on the 3-mL syringe shown.

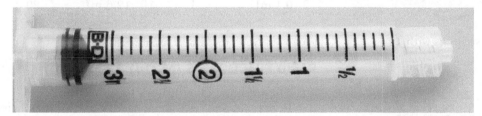

10 **Ordered:** 80 mg of Drug Y. Available: 75 mg per mL.

    a. Estimated dose: Will you need to give *more* or *less* than the unit mL dose available? (Circle one.)

    b. How many mL will you give?

      DA equation:

    c. Evaluation: _____

Draw a vertical line through the nearest measurable amount on the 3-mL syringe shown.

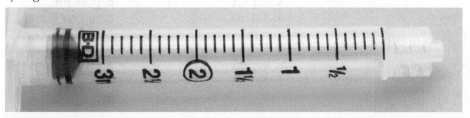

CHAPTER 6 ANSWER KEY

RAPID PRACTICE 6-1 (p. 210)

1-2

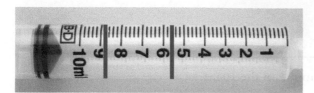

3 10 mL
4 25
5 5
6 1 mL

7-8

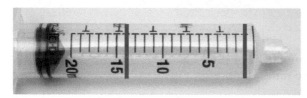

9 20 mL

RAPID PRACTICE 6-2 (p. 211)

1-2

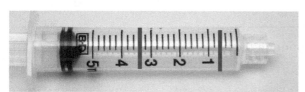

Note: There are also 5-mL syringes with 10 calibrations per mL.

3-4

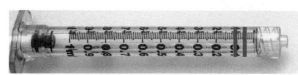

Note: Pay special attention to the decimal place when preparing small doses.

5 10
6 100 calibrations
7 1 mL
8 0.01 mL

RAPID PRACTICE 6-3 (p. 212)

1

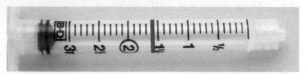

2 3 mL
3 0.1 mL
4

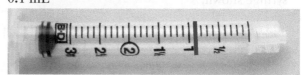

5

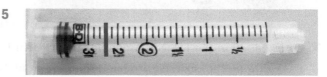

RAPID PRACTICE 6-4 (p. 214)

Ordered Dose	Syringe Size (in mL)	Ordered Dose	Syringe Size (in mL)
1 1.7 mL	3	6 2.8 mL	3
2 3.2 mL	5	7 0.08 mL	1
3 1.5 mL	3	8 9.6 mL	10
4 6.4 mL	10	9 0.6 mL	1
5 0.1 mL	1	10 12.6 mL	20

In some clinical situations a larger syringe may be selected.

RAPID PRACTICE 6-5 (p. 214)

1 The volume of medication to be administered
2 In many cases, yes. Check agency and state policies.
3 1 mL
4 3 mL; 2.9 mL
5 5 mL; 3.2 mL

RAPID PRACTICE 6-6 (p. 220)

1 a. 10 mL
   b. 5
   c. 0.2 mL
   d. 5.8 mL
2 a. 3 mL
   b. 10
   c. 0.1 mL
   d. 1.3 mL
3 a. 5 mL
   b. 5
   c. 0.2 mL
   d. 3.6 mL
4 a. 20 mL
   b. 1
   c. 1 mL
   d. 18 mL
5 a. 1 mL
   b. 10
   c. 0.01 mL
   d. 0.45 mL

RAPID PRACTICE 6-7 (p. 222)

1

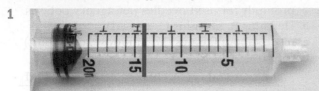

2

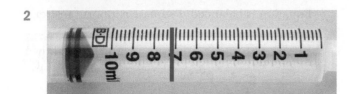

3

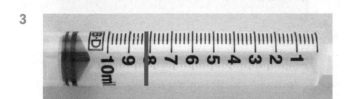

4

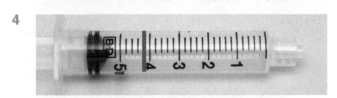

5

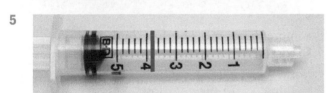

RAPID PRACTICE 6-8 (p. 223)

1

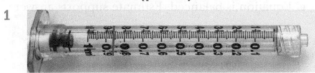

2

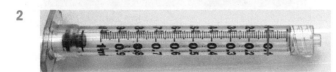

3

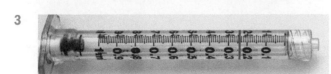

4

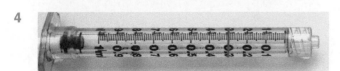

5

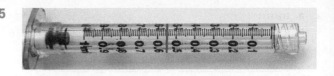

RAPID PRACTICE 6-9 (p. 224)

1

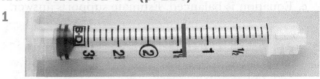

2

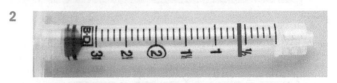

3

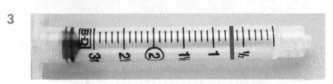

4

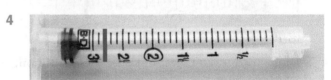

5

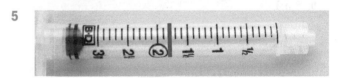

CHAPTER 6 MULTIPLE-CHOICE REVIEW (p. 226)

2 a   **7** c
3 a   **8** b
4 c   **9** a
5 a   **10** a
6 b

CHAPTER 6 FINAL PRACTICE (p. 227)

1 **a.** more (about 12 mL)
   b. 12 mL per dose

$$? \frac{mL}{dose} = \frac{mL}{\underset{1}{\cancel{10\ mg}}} \times \frac{\overset{12}{\cancel{120\ mg}}}{dose} = \frac{12\ mL}{dose}$$

   c. Equation is balanced. Estimate supports answer.

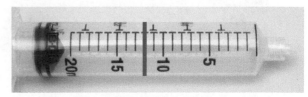

2 **a.** more
  b. give twice unit dose (2 mL)

$$? \frac{mL}{dose} = \frac{mL}{\overset{}{\underset{1}{100\ mg}}} \times \frac{\overset{2}{200\ mg}}{dose} = \frac{2\ mL}{dose}$$

  c. Equation is balanced. Estimate supports answer.

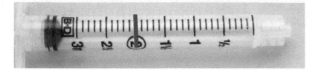

3 **a.** less
  b. give half of unit dose. (0.5 mL)

$$? \frac{mL}{dose} = \frac{mL}{\underset{2}{30\ mg}} \times \frac{\overset{1}{15\ mg}}{dose} = \frac{0.5\ mL}{dose}$$

  c. Equation is balanced. Estimate supports answer.

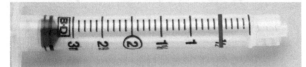

4 **a.** more (order is 8 times unit dose concentration, or about 8 mL)
  b. 8 mL

$$? \frac{mL}{dose} = \frac{mL}{\underset{1}{10\ mg}} \times \frac{\overset{8}{80\ mg}}{dose} = \frac{8\ mL}{dose}$$

  c. Equation is balanced. Estimate supports answer.

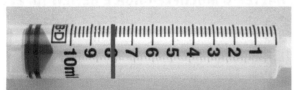

5 **a.** Total mL volume of the order
  b. After calculating dose
6 **a.** less (about 0.1 mL)
  b. 0.15 mL

$$? \frac{mL}{dose} = \frac{mL}{100\ mg} \times \frac{15\ mg}{dose} = \frac{0.15\ mL}{dose}$$

  c. Equation is balanced. Estimate supports answer.

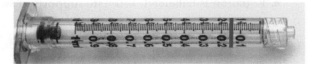

7 **a.** Never recap used needles. Use sharps container promptly for used needles per agency policies.
  b. Hepatitis B, hepatitis C, and HIV.
8 **a.** more (about 6 times the unit dose, or 6-7 mL)
  b. 6.4 mL

$$? \frac{mL}{dose} = \frac{mL}{50\ mg} \times \frac{320\ mg}{dose} = \frac{32}{5} = \frac{6.4\ mL}{dose}$$

  c. Equation is balanced. Estimate supports answer.

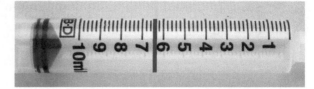

9 **a.** less than 1 mL
  b. 0.8 mL

$$? \frac{mL}{dose} = \frac{1\ mL}{\underset{5}{50\ mg}} \times \frac{\overset{4}{40\ mg}}{dose} = \frac{0.8\ mL}{dose}$$

  c. Equation is balanced. Estimate supports answer.

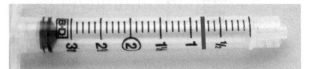

10 **a.** more than 1 mL, less than 2 mL
  b. 1.1 mL

$$? \frac{mL}{dose} = \frac{mL}{75\ mg} \times \frac{80\ mg}{dose}$$
$$= 1.066, \text{ rounded to } \frac{1.1\ mL}{dose}$$

  c. Equation is balanced. Estimate supports answer

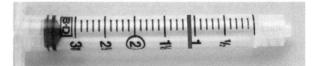

Suggestions for Further Reading

Perry AG, Potter PA, Ostendorf W: *Clinical nursing skills and techniques,* ed. 9,
    St. Louis, 2018, Mosby.
www.bd.com
http://www.fda.gov/drugs/drugsafety/medicationerrors
http://www.cdc.gov/niosh/topics/bbp/#prevent
http://www.ismp.org

Chapter 7 covers the calculations for reconstitution of powder and liquid medications. Syringes are often used to reconstitute medications. DA equations will be needed to calculate a variety of doses.

7 Reconstitution of Medications

OBJECTIVES

- Distinguish routes of drugs for reconstitution.
- Interpret directions for dilution of reconstituted medications.
- Select the appropriate concentration to prepare for the ordered dose.
- Calculate doses for reconstituted medications using DA equations.
- Measure the appropriate dose using a medicine cup and a syringe.
- Identify appropriate notation on reconstituted multidose medication labels.
- Interpret directions for safe storage of reconstituted medications.
- Calculate ratio dilutions for partial-strength solutions.

ESTIMATED TIME TO COMPLETE CHAPTER: 1 to 2 hours

Campers who have reconstituted dried food and caregivers who have mixed powdered baby formula with water to prepare a bottle have applied the technique of reconstitution of dry products. Some medications are supplied in the form of powders or crystals to which a liquid must be added for reconstitution shortly before use.

The medications are supplied in dry form because the product can be stored for a long time in dry form but becomes unstable and deteriorates in solution within a relatively short time. Such solutions are said to have a "short shelf life." The equipment used to reconstitute medications must be calibrated for the medicines being dispensed. The capacity of syringes, medicine droppers, and calibrated medication spoons is precise, whereas that of household equipment varies greatly from spoon to spoon and cup to cup.

VOCABULARY

Diluent	Fluid that makes a mixture less concentrated or viscous. The fluid dilutes the mixture. It is also used to convert a dry form of a substance to a liquid form. For example, water is used to liquefy a dry form of baby formula. When reconstituting medications, read the directions to find out which diluent needs to be used. Water or normal saline (NS) solution is often used to dilute medicines and to liquefy dry, powdered forms of medicines.
Dilution	Extent to which the concentration of a mixture is reduced.
Dilution Ratio	Special ratio indicating the number of parts of an active ingredient to the number of parts of inactive ingredients in a solution. For example, a 1:4 dilution ratio means that, out of 5 total parts, 1 part is active and 4 parts are inactive. Adding 4 parts water to 1 part powdered milk would provide a dilution ratio of 1:4.
Displacement	Volume occupied by a powder when a diluent is added during reconstitution.
Reconstitution	Process of combining the dry form of a mixture with a fluid to achieve a usable state. Process of diluting a liquid concentrate to achieve a usable state.
Solution Concentration (Strength)	Amount of drug in a quantity of solution expressed as a ratio (e.g., 100 mg per 100 mL, or 1:1) or as a fraction or a percentage (e.g., half strength, or 50% solution).

Suspension	Liquid in which fine particles are dispersed throughout a fluid, where they are supported by the buoyancy of shaking or stirring. If a suspension is left standing, the solid particles settle. Antibiotics are often supplied as oral suspensions.
SW	Sterile water.
Bacteriostatic SW	Sterile water with an antimicrobial agent, such as benzyl alcohol.
	➤ Sterile water and bacteriostatic sterile water cannot be used interchangeably with each other or with tap water. The product label specifies the diluent.
Unit	Standardized laboratory measure of the therapeutic strength, as opposed to the weight or volume, of a drug. Often used for insulin, heparin, and some antibiotics.
Unstable	Easily broken down to a state of diminished effectiveness. Breakdown can occur rapidly with reconstituted solutions. Foods, solutions, and certain medications that are unstable, such as reconstituted medications, have a short shelf life. Refrigeration may extend shelf life. Consult the label.

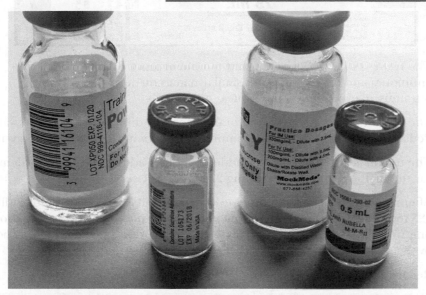

Powdered medication can be reconstituted to a liquid form by adding a specified amount of diluent.

Reconstituted Medications

Some medicines are very unstable in liquid form. Therefore, they are supplied in a dry form to which an inactive diluent is added just before use. The information about the specific type and amount of diluent to be added to achieve specific concentrations is provided on the label. The nurse selects the amount of diluent that will provide the concentration closest to the dose ordered.

Interpreting orders and reading labels for reconstituted medications

Examine the following order: Augmentin suspension 125 mg PO tid × 5 days. The order includes the form, oral *suspension*, but does *not* mention that the drug requires reconstitution or describe how to prepare it. The nurse must read the medication label and insert to determine how to prepare the medication.

➤ Pharmacists usually reconstitute large-volume oral suspensions and relabel with the quantity per dose to be given. Most times the pharmacist will premeasure each dose so that the nurse will administer the medication as if it were a unit dose medication.

Reading Labels Directions on the label state the precise amount and type of liquid diluent to add in order to achieve specific dilutions or concentrations of the drug per milliliter. The directions always state conditions and time limits for storage after reconstitution to liquid form. Some products must be discarded immediately, whereas others may be refrigerated for several hours or days so that they can be used for additional doses.

There is a lot of information on the label, but most of it is self-explanatory once you have read one or two types of labels. Examine the directions on the following label for an oral suspension to be reconstituted:

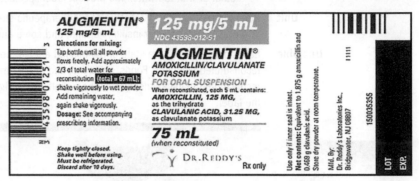

➤ The route is oral. This is important to note because there are injectable antibiotics and other drugs with similar names made specifically for intramuscular or intravenous routes.

➤ The type of *diluent* is water. Most oral suspension diluents use purified water. Pediatric patients and immunocompromised patients may need sterile water.

➤ The total *amount of diluent* to be added is 67 mL, added in two parts: 45 mL for the first mix and the remaining 22 mL for the second.

➤ After reconstitution, the unit drug *concentration* (unit dose concentration) will be 125 mg per 5 mL water. The total amount of medication will be 75 mL, although only 67 mL of water was added. This discrepancy is due to displacement of liquid by the powder. Both ingredients occupy space. Discard after 10 days.

➤ Reconstitution of an injectable is illustrated on p. 242.

CLINICAL RELEVANCE

It is critical to communicate the date and time of preparation and the specific concentration of reconstituted solutions to nursing staff on subsequent shifts with a *clearly marked label* that specifies all of the required components. Many facilities do not permit nurses to pass on a medication from one shift to the next.

Marking the label for reconstituted medications

The label is marked by the nurse only under the following conditions:

1   The drug label states that the medication may be used more than once after reconstitution.

2   The patient is eligible to receive another dose before the drug must be discarded.

➤ The label for reconstituted medications must contain the patient's name, the date and time of preparation, the diluent type and amount added, the concentration per milliliter after dilution, and the nurse's initials or name, according to agency policy. Discard date and time are added according to agency policy. Refer to the Augmentin label above and the reconstituted label on following page.

RECONSTITUTED AUGMENTIN ORAL SUSPENSION BOTTLE
Patient: John B. Doe
01/05/18 1800: 67 mL SW added; 125 mg per 5 mL, JM, RN
Discard date and time:*
_____

*Check institutional policies for their specific labeling, storage, and discard requirements.

EXAMPLES

Expired Reconstituted Drugs

Single-dose preparations cannot be stored. The remainder must be discarded. Only multidose preparations may be stored and reused according to label directions and hospital policy.

Because of the cost and short shelf life of reconstituted medications, it is appropriate that the nurse review the patient's records and recent orders to be sure that the medication order has not expired before preparing the medication.

CLINICAL RELEVANCE

RAPID PRACTICE 7-1 | ## Interpreting Labels for Reconstituted Medications

ESTIMATED COMPLETION TIME: 25 minutes   **ANSWERS ON:** page 260

DIRECTIONS: *Read the labels for the medications and supply the required information. Use brief phrases.*

1

NDC 0093-4170-64
DOXYCYCLINE
for Oral Suspension USP
25 mg/5 mL*

When reconstituted as directed,
each teaspoonful (5 mL) contains doxycycline
monohydrate equivalent to 25 mg of doxycycline.
RASPBERRY FLAVORED
℞ only

60 mL (when reconstituted)

TEVA

FOR ORAL USE ONLY
*Each bottle contains: doxycycline monohydrate equivalent to 300 mg of doxycycline.
Usual Dosage: See package insert for full prescribing information.
Store dry powder at 20° to 25°C (68° to 77°F) [See USP Controlled Room Temperature].
SHAKE WELL BEFORE EACH USE.
MIXING DIRECTIONS:
Tap bottle lightly to loosen powder. Add 47.6 mL of water to the bottle to make a total volume of 60 mL. Shake well. This prescription, when in suspension, will maintain its potency for two weeks when kept at room temperature.
DISCARD UNUSED PORTION AFTER TWO WEEKS
KEEP THIS AND ALL MEDICATIONS OUT OF THE REACH OF CHILDREN.
TEVA PHARMACEUTICALS USA
Sellersville, PA 18960
Iss. 5/2008

N 3 0093-4170-64

LOT:
EXP:

a. Form and route of medication: _____
b. Generic name: _____
c. Unit dose concentration after reconstitution (mg per mL):* _____
d. Unit dose or multidose container: _____
e. Total volume in container after reconstitution: _____
f. Storage directions: _____
g. Trade name: _____

---

*Milligram(s) per milliliter(s); the unit dose (drug) concentration is a multiple of the usual doses ordered. Note that mL is both the singular and plural abbreviation. Do not write mLs.

2

Directions for mixing: Tap bottle until all powder flows freely. Add approximately 1/3 total amount of water for reconstitution (total = 35 mL); shake vigorously to wet powder. Add remaining water, again shake vigorously.

Each 5 mL (1 teaspoonful) will contain amoxicillin trihydrate equivalent to 200 mg anhydrous amoxicillin.

Dosage: Administer every 12 hours. See accompanying prescribing information.

Keep tightly closed.

Shake well before using.

Refrigeration preferable but not required.

Discard suspension after 14 days.

M.L.No.: 57/RR/AP/2003/F/R

P1408309

NDC 65862-070-50

Amoxicillin

for Oral Suspension, USP

200 mg/5 mL

50 mL when reconstituted

Rx only

Net contents: Equivalent to 2 grams anhydrous amoxicillin.

Store dry powder at 20° to 25°C (68° to 77°F); excursions permitted to 15° to 30°C (59° to 86°F) [see USP Controlled Room Temperature].

Manufactured for:
Aurobindo Pharma USA, Inc.
2400 Route 130 North
Dayton, NJ 08810

Manufactured by:
Aurobindo Pharma Limited
Hyderabad-500 072, India

Batch :

Expiry :

AUROBINDO

a. Form and route of medication: _____
b. Type and amount of diluent to be used: _____
c. Total volume in container after reconstitution: _____
d. Unit dose concentration after reconstitution: _____
e. Storage directions: _____
f. Mixing directions after reconstitution: _____
g. Discard directions: _____

3

Net Contents: Contains 1 g cefixime as the trihydrate

Prior to reconstitution:
Store drug powder at 20 - 25°C (68 - 77°F) [See USP Controlled Room Temperature].

After reconstitution:
Store at room temperature or under refrigeration.
Keep tightly closed.

Usual dosage:
See package insert.

Manufactured for:
Lupin Pharmaceuticals, Inc.
111 South Calvert Street
Baltimore, Maryland 21202
United States

Manufactured by:
Lupin Limited
Mumbai 400 098 INDIA
Code No.MP/DRUGS/28/18/83

Lot No.
Exp. Date
Date of reconstitution:

NDC 68180-202-03

Suprax®

Cefixime for Oral Suspension, USP

100 mg/5 mL

When reconstituted, each teaspoonful (5 mL) contains 100 mg of cefixime as the trihydrate.

FOR ORAL USE ONLY

SHAKE WELL BEFORE USING

Discard any unused portion after 14 days

Rx only

50 mL (when reconstituted)

Lupin Pharmaceuticals, Inc.

TO THE PHARMACIST:
IMPORTANT
Use this bottle for dispensing.
Use only if inner seal is intact.

Directions for mixing:
To reconstitute, suspend with 34 mL water.

Method: Tap the bottle several times to loosen powder contents prior to reconstitution. Add approximately half the total amount of water for reconstitution and shake well. Add the remainder of water and shake well.

204041

a. Form and route of medication: _____
b. Type of diluent to be used: _____
c. Total amount of diluent to add to bottle: _____
d. Mixing directions: _____
e. Unit dose concentration after reconstitution: _____
f. Trade name: _____
g. Generic name: _____
h. Unit dose or multidose container: _____
i. Expiration, or discard time, after reconstitution: _____
j. Storage directions: _____

4

IMPORTANT - READ INSERT FOR PRECAUTIONS AND DIRECTIONS BEFORE USE.

*Each vial contains:
Vancomycin hydrochloride equivalent to 1 g vancomycin.

Inactive: May contain hydrochloric acid and/or sodium hydroxide for pH adjustment.

Usual Adult Dosage: 2 g daily in divided doses. See package insert. Dilute contents with 20 mL Sterile Water for Injection.

NDC 23360-152-50

STERILE VANCOMYCIN HYDROCHLORIDE, USP

1 g*/vial

For Intravenous Use

AFTER RECONSTITUTION MUST BE FURTHER DILUTED. SEE PACKAGE INSERT.

Rx only

LOT: EXP.:

Prior to reconstitution, store at 20° to 25°C (68° to 77°F) [see USP Controlled Room Temperature].
After dilution - Refrigerate

Lyophilized

Manufactured for:
Akorn - Strides, LLC
Lake Forest, IL 60045

Made in India

Code No.: KR/DRUGS/KTK/28/280/95
Revision: 11/08

a. Generic name: _____
b. Route: _____
c. Total amount in vial: _____
d. Type of diluent required: _____

5 **Ordered:** nystatin oral suspension 400,000 units, swish and swallow four times daily while awake for an adult with an oral candidiasis (yeast) infection secondary to antibiotic administration.*

Directions: Administer half of dose each side of the mouth and have patient swish thoroughly and swallow.

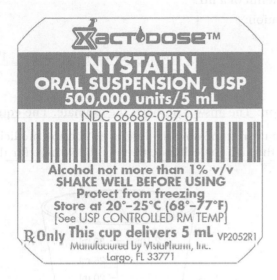

a. How many mL will you prepare? _____

b. How many mL will you administer each side of the mouth? _____

c. Where should the product be stored? _____

➤ If a slash (/) is used on a drug label or in a drug order, be careful to avoid reading it as the number 1. For example, 5 mg/5 mL could be misread as 5 mg per 15 mL.

_____

*Problem 1 is an example of a prepared suspension that does not need further dilution.

RAPID PRACTICE 7-2	Reconstituting, Calculating, and Measuring Oral Doses

ESTIMATED COMPLETION TIME: 30 minutes   **ANSWERS ON:** page 260

DIRECTIONS: *Read the order and the label, then estimate and calculate the dose using a DA equation. Shade in the medicine cup to the nearest multiple of 5 mL. Indicate the balance of the dose that will be added with the syringe, as shown in problem 1.*

1 **Ordered:** cephalexin oral suspension 0.3 g PO q6h for a patient with a respiratory tract infection.

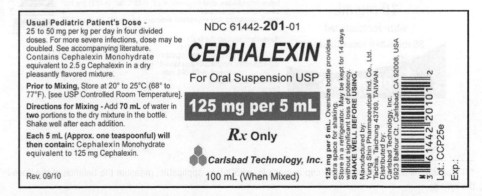

a. Total amount and type of diluent to be added: _____<u>70 mL</u>_____
   (*all at once* or ⟨*divided*⟩?)

b. Estimate: ⟨*more*⟩ or *less* than the dose per 5 mL after reconstitution
   (circle one)

c. How many mL will you prepare (per dose)? _____<u>12 mL</u>_____ to the
   nearest tenth of a mL?

   DA equation:

$$\frac{mL}{dose} = \frac{5\ mL}{\underset{1}{\cancel{125\ mg}}} \times \frac{\overset{8}{\cancel{1000\ mg}}}{1\ \cancel{g}} \times \frac{0.3\ \cancel{g}}{dose} = \frac{12\ mL}{dose}$$

d. Evaluation: <u>The answer supports the estimate. The equation is balanced.</u>

Shade in the nearest measurable dose in mL on the medicine cup and draw a
vertical line through the calibrated line of the syringe for the remaining mL
as applicable.*

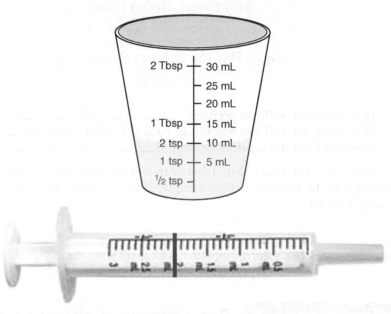

2 **Ordered:** fluconazole oral susp 0.03 g PO daily for a patient with oral
candidiasis.

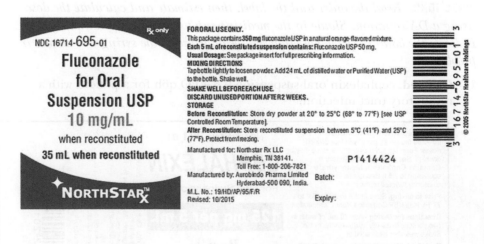

---

*Throughout, shade in the medicine cup in multiples of 5 mL as applicable; measure the balance of the dose in
the syringe.

a. Amount and type of diluent to be added: _____
b. Estimate: *more* or *less* than unit dose after reconstitution? (Circle one.)
c. How many milliliters will you prepare for each dose? _____

DA equation:

d. Evaluation: _____

Draw a vertical line through the calibrated line of the syringe as applicable.

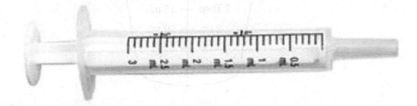

3 **Ordered:** cefaclor oral susp 0.25 g PO tid for a patient with an infection.

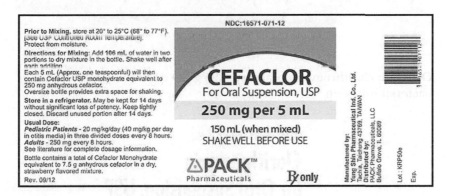

Prior to Mixing, store at 20° to 25°C (68° to 77°F).
(See USP Controlled Room Temperature).
Protect from moisture.
Directions for Mixing: Add 106 mL of water in two
portions to dry mixture in the bottle. Shake well after
each addition.
Each 5 mL (Approx. one teaspoonful) will then
contain Cefaclor USP monohydrate equivalent to
250 mg anhydrous cefaclor.
Oversize bottle provides extra space for shaking.
Store in a refrigerator. May be kept for 14 days
without significant loss of potency. Keep tightly
closed. Discard unused portion after 14 days.
Usual Dose:
Pediatric Patients - 20 mg/kg/day (40 mg/kg per day
in otitis media) in three divided doses every 8 hours.
Adults - 250 mg every 8 hours.
See literature for complete dosage information.
Bottle contains a total of Cefaclor Monohydrate
equivalent to 7.5 g anhydrous cefaclor in a dry,
strawberry flavored mixture.
Rev. 09/12

NDC:16571-071-12

CEFACLOR
For Oral Suspension, USP
250 mg per 5 mL
150 mL (when mixed)
SHAKE WELL BEFORE USE

△**PACK**™
Pharmaceuticals   Ɍonly

Manufactured by:
Yung Shin Pharmaceutical Ind. Co., Ltd.
Tacha, Taichung 43769, TAIWAN
Distributed by:
PACK Pharmaceuticals, LLC
Buffalo Grove, IL 60089

Lot.: KRP50e
Exp.

a. Amount and type of diluent to be added: _____
b. Estimate: *more* or *less* than dose after reconstitution? (Circle one.)
c. How many milliliters will you prepare to the nearest tenth of a mL? _____

DA equation:

d. Evaluation: _____

Shade in the dose in mL on the medicine cup and draw a vertical line
through the calibrated line of the syringe as applicable.

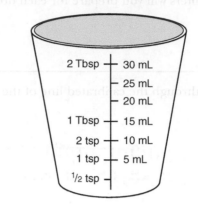

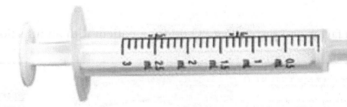

4   **Ordered:** clarithromycin oral susp 0.25 g PO q12h for a patient with a
bacterial infection.

NDC 0781-**6022**-52

Clarithromycin
for Oral Suspension, USP

125 mg* per 5 mL

when reconstituted

*When mixed as directed, each teaspoonful
(5 mL) contains 125 mg of clarithromycin in
a fruit-punch flavored, aqueous vehicle.

R̠ₓ only

50 mL (when mixed)

⚠ **SANDOZ**

a.   Reconstitute with 50 mL sterile water to make 50 mL of clarithromycin
suspension. Amount and type of diluent to be added: _____

b.   Estimate: *more* or *less* than unit dose after reconstitution?
(Circle one.)

c.   How many milliliters will you prepare? _____
DA equation:

d.   Evaluation: _____

Shade in the dose in mL on the medicine cup and draw a vertical line
through the calibrated line of the syringe as applicable.

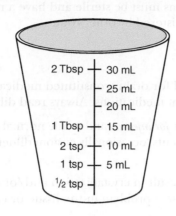

2 Tbsp — 30 mL
25 mL
20 mL
1 Tbsp — 15 mL
2 tsp — 10 mL
1 tsp — 5 mL
½ tsp —

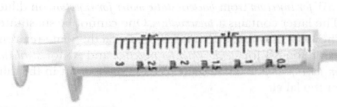

5   **Ordered:** cefprozil oral susp 0.2 g PO q12h for a patient with an infection.

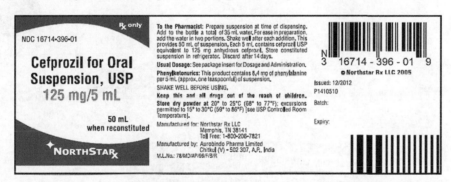

NDC 16714-396-01

**Cefprozil for Oral
Suspension, USP**
125 mg/5 mL

50 mL
when reconstituted

NORTHSTAR

R_x only

To the Pharmacist: Prepare suspension at time of dispensing. Add to the bottle a total of 35 mL water. For ease in preparation, add the water in two portions. Shake well after each addition. This provides 50 mL of suspension. Each 5 mL contains cefprozil USP equivalent to 125 mg anhydrous cefprozil. Store constituted suspension in refrigerator. Discard after 14 days.

Usual Dosage: See package insert for Dosage and Administration.

Phenylketonurics: This product contains 8.4 mg of phenylalanine per 5 mL (approx. one teaspoonful) of suspension.

SHAKE WELL BEFORE USING.

Keep this and all drugs out of the reach of children.

Store dry powder at 20° to 25°C (68° to 77°F); excursions permitted to 15° to 30°C (59° to 86°F) [see USP Controlled Room Temperature].

Manufactured for: Northstar Rx LLC
Memphis, TN 38141
Toll Free: 1-800-206-7821

Manufactured by: Aurobindo Pharma Limited
Chitkul (V) - 502 307, A.P., India

M.L.No.: 78/MD/AP/96/F/S/R

N 3   16714 - 396 - 01   9
© Northstar Rx LLC 2005

Issued: 12/2012
P1410510

Batch:

Expiry:

a.   Estimate: *more* or *less* than unit dose after reconstitution?
(Circle one.)

b.   How many milliliters will you prepare for each dose? _____
DA equation:

c.   Evaluation: _____

Draw a vertical line through the calibrated line of the syringe as applicable.

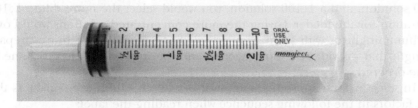

Reconstituted Parenteral Drugs

> Parenteral medications must be sterile and have a much shorter shelf life than do drugs administered by other routes.

Diluents

> Purified water is used for oral reconstituted medications; sterile diluents must be used for parenteral medications. Always read dilution directions.

Although sterile water *for injection* and sterile normal saline (NS) solution are the most commonly used diluents, occasionally custom diluents or dextrose solutions are required.

> Incompatibility can result in crystallization and/or clumping of the drug in solution and can cause a problem in the tissue or circulation of the patient.

> Distinguish *SW for injection* from *bacteriostatic water for injection* on diluent directions. The latter contains a *preservative*. One cannot be substituted for the other. The label must be read and followed exactly. Some references use the abbreviation *SW* for *sterile water for injection* and *NS* for *sterile normal saline solution for injection*. Bacteriostatic water is spelled out in the dilution directions on the label.

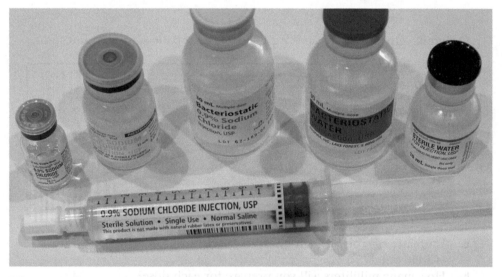

Diluents used to reconstitute medications. *Syringe:* 0.9% sodium chloride (normal saline). *Three bottles on left:* bacteriostatic 0.9% sodium chloride. *Second bottle from right:* bacteriostatic water. *Bottle on right:* preservative-free sterile water 0.9% sodium chloride.

Selecting the Appropriate Unit Dose Concentration Based on Dilution Directions When More Than One Dilution Is Offered If a 1:100 concentration of sugar water was needed for your hummingbird feeder and you had on hand a 1:30 solution, a 1:50 solution, and a 1:100 solution, you would select the more dilute 1:100 concentration for the feeder. Giving the more concentrated solutions would overdose the hummingbirds with sugar. Similarly, with medications the nurse prepares the strength that provides the dose needed and the most convenient volume for the route ordered.

In selecting the appropriate amount of diluent, the nurse considers the relevant factors in the following sequence when reading the label:
- Route ordered
- Dose ordered and amount needed
- Drug concentrations and volumes available that are close in amount to the ordered dose for that route

Based on the ordered amount, the nurse examines the label to make critical decisions. For example, consider an order of Drug A 200 mg IM. The label dilution directions state:

For IM injection:
Add 1.8 mL SW for injection to obtain 200 mg per mL.
Add 3.6 mL SW for injection to obtain 100 mg per mL.
Add 5.2 mL SW for injection to obtain 75 mg per mL.

For IV injection:
Add 8.4 mL SW for injection to obtain 50 mg per mL.

According to the label, three concentrations are safe to inject into the muscle. The nurse chooses a concentration based on the order. In this example, the first intramuscular option allows the patient to receive a smaller injected *volume*.

ASK YOURSELF **Q & A**

1 Which is the more concentrated solution after reconstitution according to the reconstitution directions cited above for Drug A?

MY ANSWER

_____

2 Can SW, NS, and bacteriostatic water be used interchangeably to dilute medicines?

_____

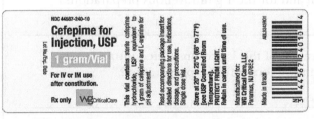

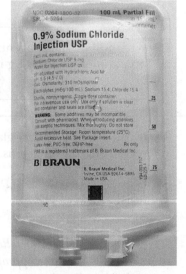

PREPARATION OF CLAFORAN STERILE

Claforan for IM or IV administration should be reconstituted as follows:

Strength	Diluent (mL)	Withdrawable Volume (mL)	Approximate Concentration (mg/mL)
1g vial (IM)*	3	3.4	300
2g vial (IM)*	5	6.0	330
1g vial (IV)*	10	10.4	95
2g vial (IV)*	10	11.0	180
1g infusion	50-100	50-100	20-10
2g infusion	50-100	50-100	40-20
10g bottle	47	52.0	200
10g bottle	97	102.0	100
*in conventional vials			

Shake to dissolve; inspect for particulate matter and discoloration prior to use. Solutions of Claforan range from very pale yellow to light amber, depending on concentration, diluent used, and length and condition of storage.

IV drugs that are not stable for long periods when mixed can be reconstituted immediately before administration by breaking a flexible piece of plastic separating the medication powder and then mixing the attached IV solution with the powder.

These labels are included to illustrate medications that need to be reconstituted for routes other than oral and that offer *multiple options for dilution*. If the label permits several choices of dilution to obtain different unit dose strengths, the nurse must take special care to focus on the appropriate dilution. Several choices of dilution are more likely to be found with reconstituted parenteral drugs.

Diluting oxacillin sodium in sterile water for injection. (From Brown M, Mulholland J: *Drug calculations: ratio and proportion problems for clinical practice,* ed. 9, St. Louis, 2012, Mosby.)

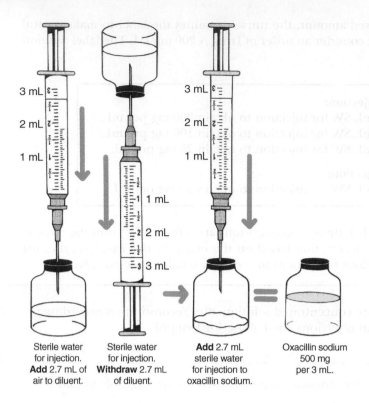

Sterile water for injection.
Add 2.7 mL of air to diluent.

Sterile water for injection.
Withdraw 2.7 mL of diluent.

Add 2.7 mL sterile water for injection to oxacillin sodium.

Oxacillin sodium 500 mg per 3 mL.

Q & A **ASK YOURSELF**

1 What are the amounts of diluent recommended for the 1 g reconstituted intramuscular preparation and for the 1 g intravenous preparation?

MY ANSWER _____

2 What will be the concentration of the 1 g reconstituted intramuscular preparation and the 1 g intravenous infusion preparation?

_____

➤ If you require reading glasses, keep them handy for reading the reconstitution directions.

RAPID PRACTICE 7-3 ## Selecting Diluents to Calculate Doses

ESTIMATED COMPLETION TIME: 20 to 30 minutes **ANSWERS ON:** page 261

DIRECTIONS: *Examine the following reconstitution directions and the example in problem 1. Select the appropriate dilution for problems 2 to 5 using the reconstitution directions provided. Evaluate your equations for problems 4 to 5.*

Reconstitution directions for Drug Y for IM administration

Diluent SW	Total Volume	Solution Concentration
1 mL	1.4 mL	480 mg per mL
2 mL	3 mL	250 mg per mL
4 mL	5.8 mL	100 mg per mL
For IV administration		
12 mL	15.8 mL	50 mg per mL

> The more diluent added, the weaker the concentration of the solution.

> Keep in mind that the average-sized adult should receive no more than 3 mL in one intramuscular site.

> The nurse should select a dilution that permits a minimum of 0.5 mL for an intramuscular injection.

CLINICAL RELEVANCE

Select the dilution from the list above that is closest to the unit dose you need and that meets the foregoing criteria. Calculate doses to the *nearest tenth of a milliliter.* Examine the routes first. Then compare the order to the concentrations to find a reasonable low-volume dose. Verify the answer with a DA equation where requested.

1   **Ordered:** Drug Y, 50 mg IM.
   a.   How much diluent will you add? <u>4 mL</u>
   b.   What will be the unit dose concentration? <u>100 mg per mL</u>
   c.   How many milliliters will you give? <u>0.5 mL</u>

2   **Ordered:** Drug Y, 0.5 g IV.
   a.   How much diluent will you add? _____
   b.   What will be the unit dose concentration? _____
   c.   How many milliliters will you give? _____
      DA equation:

   d.   Evaluation: _____

3   **Ordered:** Drug Y, 0.1 g IM.
   a.   How much diluent will you add? _____
   b.   What will be the unit dose concentration? _____
   c.   How many milliliters will you give? _____

4   **Ordered:** Drug Y, 0.3 g IM.
   a.   How much diluent will you add? _____
   b.   What will be the unit dose concentration? _____
   c.   How many milliliters will you give? _____
      DA equation:

   d.   Evaluation: _____

5   **Ordered:** Drug Y, 0.25 g IM.
   a.   How much diluent will you add? _____
   b.   What will be the unit dose concentration? _____
   c.   How many milliliters will you give? _____

---

1   If you were to receive 150 mg of an intramuscular injection and the directions for reconstitution of the medicine specified (a) add 20 mL to obtain 50 mg per mL or (b) add 10 mL to obtain 100 mg per mL, which concentration would you select for reconstitution?

ASK YOURSELF **Q & A**

_____   **MY ANSWER**

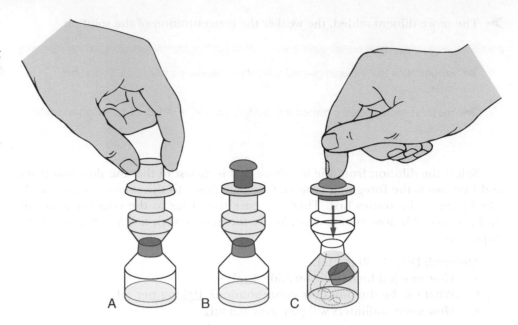

Reconstituted Drug Prefilled Containers

Some parenteral medications for reconstitution are supplied with diluents that are in prefilled syringe cartridges, ampules, or vials. Others are attached to the vial (Figure 7-1) and can be mixed by depressing the stopper without opening the vials. There is less chance for contamination of the contents when the ingredients are not exposed to air.

| **RAPID PRACTICE 7-4** | Interpreting Directions and Calculating Reconstituted Injectables |

ESTIMATED COMPLETION TIME: 30 minutes   **ANSWERS ON:** page 262

DIRECTIONS: *Examine the worked-out problem 1. Read the labels to answer the questions for problems 2 to 5. Calculate doses to the nearest measurable dose on the syringe provided.*

1 **Ordered:** ceftazidime 0.5 g IM, an antibiotic, for a patient with *Klebsiella* pneumonia.

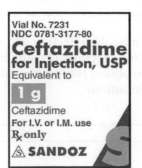

Vial No. 7231
NDC 0781-3177-80
Ceftazidime for Injection, USP
Equivalent to
1 g
Ceftazidime
For I.V. or I.M. use
℞ only
⚠ SANDOZ

RECONSTITUTION

Single Dose Vials:
For I.M. injection, I.V. direct (bolus) injection, or I.V. infusion, reconstitute with Sterile Water for injection according to the following table. The vacuum may assist entry of the diluent. SHAKE WELL.

Table 5

Vial Size	Diluent to Be Added	Approx. Avail. Volume	Approx. Avg. Concentration
Intramuscular or Intravenous Direct (bolus) Injection			
1 gram	3.0 ml.	3.6 ml.	280 mg./ml.
Intravenous Infusion			
1 gram	10 ml.	10.6 ml.	95 mg./ml.
2 gram	10 ml.	11.2 ml.	180 mg./ml.

Withdraw the total volume of solution into the syringe (the pressure in the vial may aid withdrawal). The withdrawn solution may contain some bubbles of carbon dioxide.
NOTE: As with the administration of all parenteral products, accumulated gases should be expressed from the syringe immediately before injection of 'Tazicef'.
These solutions of 'Tazicef' are stable for 18 hours at room temperature or seven days if refrigerated (5°C.). Slight yellowing does not affect potency.

For I.V. infusion, dilute reconstituted solution in 50 to 100 ml. of one of the parenteral fluids listed under COMPATIBILITY AND STABILITY.

a. What kind of diluent is specified? <u>SW for injection</u>
b. How much diluent will you add? <u>3 mL</u>
c. What will the total volume in milliliters be after the diluent is added? <u>3.6 mL</u>
d. Unit dose concentration IM per mL after dilution: <u>280 mg per mL</u>
e. Is the dose ordered (after you move decimal places) [more] or *less* than the unit dose after dilution? <u>0.5 g = 500 mg, which is more than the unit dose of 280 mg</u>
f. Estimated dose in milliliters: <u>A little less than 2 mL</u>
g. Actual dose in milliliters calculated with a DA equation to the nearest measurable dose on a 3-mL syringe:

$$\frac{mL}{dose} = \frac{mL}{\underset{14}{\cancel{280\ mg}}} \times \frac{\overset{25}{\cancel{500\ mg}}}{dose} = \frac{25}{14} = 1.78, \text{ rounded to } 1.8\ mL \text{ per dose for the 3-mL syringe}$$

h. Evaluation: <u>Estimate supports answer. Equation is balanced</u>. If satisfactory, draw a vertical line through the calibrated line of the exact dose on the syringe.

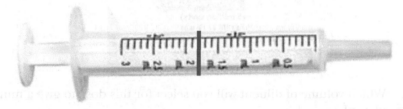

i. How will you mark label? Patient: <u>John Doe, 2/01/18 1800, 3 mL sterile H₂O added, 280 mg per mL, jm reeze, RN</u>
j. Storage and/or discard directions: <u>Stable 18 hours at room temperature or 7 days if refrigerated (5° C)</u>

2 **Ordered:** streptomycin 0.5 g IM q12h for a patient with *Klebsiella* pneumonia.

Directions: Dilute vial with 1.8 mL SW for injection.

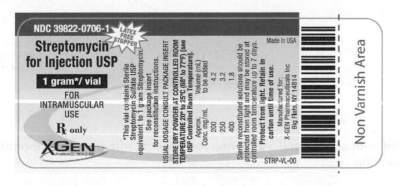

a. Which type of diluent will you use: tap water or sterile water? _____
b. Will you give more or less than the unit dose per mL after reconstitution?

_____
c. How many mL will you administer per dose? _____
DA equation:

d. Evaluation: _____

e. Draw a vertical line through the calibrated line of the nearest measurable dose on the syringe.

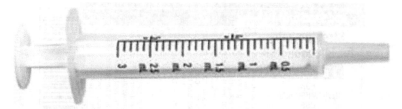

3 **Ordered:** penicillin G potassium 400,000 units IM q8h for 10 days for a patient with a streptococcal infection. Add 18.2 mL sterile water to make a concentration of 250,000 units per milliliter.

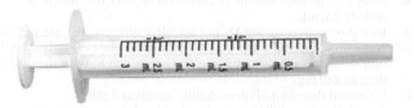

a. Which volume of diluent will you select for this dose to give a minimum of 1 mL? _____

b. How many mL will you administer per dose?

DA equation:

c. Evaluation: _____

If satisfactory, draw a vertical line through the calibrated line of the nearest measurable dose on the syringe.

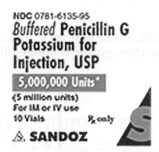

4 **Ordered:** ampicillin 0.5 g IM q6h for a patient with an upper respiratory infection (URI).

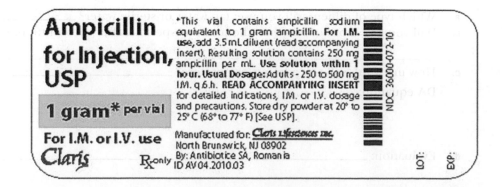

a. How much diluent should be added for IM use? _____
b. What is the concentration after the reconstitution? _____
c. How soon should the reconstituted solution be used? _____
d. Estimated dose in mL: _____
e. How many mL will you administer (per dose)? _____

   DA equation:

f. Evaluation: _____

If satisfactory, draw a vertical line through the calibrated line of the exact dose on the syringe.

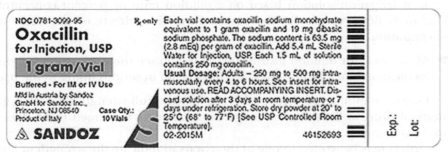

5   **Ordered:** oxacillin 400 mg IM, an antibiotic, for a patient with an infection.

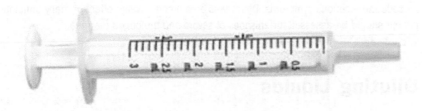

NDC 0781-3099-95
Oxacillin
for Injection, USP

1 gram/Vial

Buffered · For IM or IV Use
Mfd in Austria by Sandoz
GmbH for Sandoz Inc.,
Princeton, NJ 08540   Case Qty.:
Product of Italy   10 Vials

⚠ **SANDOZ**

℞ only Each vial contains oxacillin sodium monohydrate equivalent to 1 gram oxacillin and 19 mg dibasic sodium phosphate. The sodium content is 63.5 mg (2.8 mEq) per gram of oxacillin. Add 5.4 mL Sterile Water for Injection, USP. Each 1.5 mL of solution contains 250 mg oxacillin.
Usual Dosage: Adults – 250 mg to 500 mg intramuscularly every 4 to 6 hours. See insert for intravenous use. READ ACCOMPANYING INSERT. Discard solution after 3 days at room temperature or 7 days under refrigeration. Store dry powder at 20° to 25°C (68° to 77°F) [See USP Controlled Room Temperature].
02-2015M   46152693

Exp.:
Lot:

a. What kind of diluent or diluents are specified? _____
b. How much diluent will you add? _____
c. Drug concentration after dilution: _____
d. Estimated dose: Is the dose ordered (after you move decimal places) *more* or *less* than the unit dose after dilution? (Circle one.)
e. Actual dose in milliliters calculated with a DA equation.

   DA equation:

f. Evaluation: _____

CLINICAL RELEVANCE

Many of the medications for reconstitution are antibiotics. They may be supplied in several forms and a variety of concentrations for oral, topical, intramuscular, or intravenous routes. Some have similar-sounding generic and trade names. Compare the order to the label carefully.

➤ Each antibiotic is targeted for specific kinds of infections.

Generic Name	Trade Name
cefaclor	Ceclor
cefprozil	Cefzil
cefuroxime	Ceftin
cephalexin	Keflex
cephazolin	Kefzol
ciprofloxacin	Cipro, Cipro XR

CLINICAL RELEVANCE

Some patients are allergic to certain antibiotics. Assess the patient's lung sounds for wheezes and the skin for rashes, and ask the patient if there have been any severe bowel changes (e.g., severe diarrhea). These are the most common symptoms of allergic reactions. A skin rash may precede more serious symptoms. Diarrhea is a common adverse effect of many antibiotics. The patient should be assessed for episodes of severe and prolonged diarrhea.

Liquid Concentrates: Diluting Liquids

The pharmacy usually dilutes medication solutions to the ordered strength. Occasionally, the nurse will need to dilute a medication, nutritional beverage supplement, or irrigation solution based on a dilution ratio or percent concentration. Dilution is done to protect the patient from side effects of an overly strong concentration.

➤ Always look for dilution instructions when you see the word *concentrate* on a medication label. Failure to do so could result in serious injury to the patient.

Liquids administered through feeding tubes at full strength may cause gastrointestinal distress. Solutions for irrigation treatments may need to be diluted to avoid tissue injury.

Orders may be written in one of three ways to indicate the strength or concentration of a solution:

Order	Meaning
Percentage	*Percent* means "per 100." For example, *50% strength* denotes a solution that contains 50% active ingredient (the drug) plus 50% inactive ingredient (the diluent).
Fraction	For example, $\frac{1}{2}$ or "half strength" indicates that 1 part out of a total of 2 parts is the active ingredient and the other part is the inactive ingredient. The *denominator* of the fraction denotes the total number of parts.
Ratio	For example, $1:1$ denotes 2 total parts: 1 part active ingredient *added to* 1 part inactive ingredient. The *left* number is the *active* ingredient, or the drug. The *right* number is the inactive ingredient, or the diluent.

Inactive Ingredients Used for Dilutions

Water or normal saline (NS) is often the *inactive* ingredient used for dilution. Check the order and label for the diluent. Sterile solutions may be indicated for wound irrigations, pediatric formulas, or medications for immunocompromised patients. Normal saline solution is supplied as a sterile solution. Read the label and check agency protocols. Order the supplies from the pharmacy or central supply, according to agency guidelines.

Percent or fractional strengths are written more frequently for dilution than are ratios.

➤ The two sides of a ratio need to be added to obtain the total number of parts (e.g., 1:3 = 4 total parts).

Converting Dilution Ratios to Fractions and Percentages

➤ To convert a ratio to a fraction, add the *total number of parts* to create a *denominator.* Place the number of active-ingredient parts in the numerator.

➤ To convert a fraction to a percentage, multiply the fraction by 100 and add a percent sign.

➤ To convert a percentage to a fraction, divide the percentage by 100, remove the percent sign, and reduce the fraction.

➤ The nurse must be able to interpret dilution orders.

EXAMPLES

1. **Ordered:** 120 mL q2h Ensure formula 50%. Preparation: 60 mL Ensure plus 60 mL water to make a 1:1 ratio, $\frac{1}{2}$ strength, or 50% solution. 1:1 = 1 part active ingredient "per", "to", or "plus" 1 part inactive ingredient (ratio of Ensure to water). Total parts = 2 = $\frac{1}{2}$ strength = 50% solution ($\frac{1}{2} \times 100$).

2. **Ordered:** Isomil baby formula 10 mL 1:4 solution q3h. 1:4. 1:4 = 1 part active ingredient (Isomil) "per", "to", or "plus" 4 parts inactive ingredient (water). Total parts = 5, $\frac{1}{5}$, or 20% solution. Use 1 part active ingredient, and add 4 parts diluent.

➤ Note that the dilution ratio 1:4 does not convert to the fraction $\frac{1}{4}$.

➤ Think of the dilution ratio 1:4 as 1 part added to 4 parts (1 + 4 = 5 total parts).

➤ Read the fraction as 1 part out of 5 total parts, or $\frac{1}{5}$.

➤ Read 20% strength as 20 parts per 100 parts, or $\frac{1}{5}$.

Recall from Chapter 1, "Essential Math Review," that the denominator of a fraction indicates the *number of total parts* and that *percent* means "per 100." Read $\frac{1}{5}$-strength concentration as 20%.

Using a DA Equation to Calculate the Amount of Concentrate

Most dilution orders can be solved with mental arithmetic or simple arithmetic. The nurse needs to know the concentration and the total amount to be given in order to calculate the amount of active ingredients per the amount of inactive ingredients in milliliters.

➤ Simple DA-style equations are solved using fraction forms. Change the percentage in the order to a fraction.

EXAMPLES

Ordered: 120 mL of 25% formula per feeding tube q2h for 12 hours per day.

$25\% = \dfrac{25}{100} = \dfrac{1}{4}$. The desired answer is the amount in milliliters of the *active ingredient*:

mL active ingredient:	Total mL	×	fraction	=	answer
(formula)	120 mL	×	$\dfrac{1}{4}$	=	30 mL *active ingredient*
		120 mL total − 30 mL active ingredient = 90 mL *diluent* (water)			

Evaluation: 30 is 25%, or $\dfrac{1}{4}$, of 120. 30 + 90 = 120 = 1:3 ratio. Both sides of the equation balance mathematically.

➤ When in doubt about dilutions, consult the agency pharmacist.

RAPID PRACTICE 7-5

Interpreting Dilution Orders

ESTIMATED COMPLETION TIME: 25 minutes   **ANSWERS ON:** page 262

DIRECTIONS: *Fill in the dilution tables from left to right with the correct equivalent terms and solution amounts, as shown in the first row of the table that follows.*

	Fractional Strength	Ratio of Active to Inactive Ingredients	Percent	Order	Amount of Active Ingredient	Amount of Diluent (Inactive Ingredient)
1	$\dfrac{1}{4}$	1:3	25%	100 mL q1h	25 mL	75 mL
2			20%	240 mL four times daily		
3			10%	50 mL once a day		
4			50%	60 mL tid		
5			75%	1000 mL q8h		

Q & A   **ASK YOURSELF**   **1**   What is the difference between a dilution ratio and a fraction? How will I remember? Which one is easier (one less step) to convert to a percentage: the ratio or the fractional strength?

MY ANSWER _____

ESTIMATED COMPLETION TIME: 20 to 30 minutes   **ANSWERS ON:** page 262

DIRECTIONS: *Circle the correct answer for the following.*

1 Which of the following statements can lead to medication calculation errors?

  a. Suspensions must be combined with a precise amount of diluent and thoroughly mixed.
  b. Elixirs are solutions that contain alcohol.
  c. Extracts are solutions that are concentrated.
  d. It is acceptable to use household teaspoons and tablespoons to measure liquids.

2 One way to detect major errors in the dose calculations is to:

  a. Estimate the answer.
  b. Pour oral medications to the nearest tenth of a milliliter.
  c. Move decimal places to obtain equivalent measurements.
  d. Rely on the calculations from another nurse.

3 Which of the following statements defines *displacement*?

  a. Liquid oral medications are prepared using clean technique and nonsterile equipment.
  b. The diluent for oral liquid medications is usually water.
  c. The volume after reconstitution exceeds the amount of liquid diluent added.
  d. Oral liquid medications are usually prepared to the nearest tenth of a milliliter for adults.

4 The usual adult dose for oral liquid medications is measured to the:

  a. Nearest tenth of a milliliter   **c.** Nearest 0.5 mL
  b. Nearest hundredth of a milliliter   **d.** Nearest whole milliliter

5 If a liquid oral medication order calls for 13 mL, how will the nurse prepare it?

  a. Pour at eye level to just below the 15 mL line.
  b. Pour to 10 mL at eye level and add 3 mL with a needleless syringe.
  c. Pour to 15 mL, remove 2 mL, and return the 2 mL to the medication bottle.
  d. Draw 20 mL in a 20-mL syringe and discard 7 mL.

6 Which conversion is most commonly used in medication problems?

  a. 2.54 cm = 1 inch   **c.** 1,000,000 mcg = 1 g
  b. 1000 mg = 1 g   **d.** 1000 mL = 1 L

7 Most plastic medication cups have the following milliliter calibrations:

  a. Multiples of 5   **c.** Multiples of 15
  b. Multiples of 10   **d.** Multiples of 30

8 If a liquid oral medication order calls for 7.5 mL, how will the nurse prepare it?

  a. Pour at eye level to 5 mL and add 2.5 mL with a needleless syringe.
  b. Pour to 10 mL, remove 2.5 mL, and return the 2.5 mL to the medication bottle.
  c. Withdraw 7.5 mL in a 10-mL syringe and place it in the medication cup.
  d. Give $1\frac{1}{2}$ medication teaspoonful.

9 If a drug label states 250 mg per 5 mL, which of the following statements would be correct?

a. There are 5 mL of active drug concentrated in the solution.

b. The medicine has a concentration of 250 mg of drug in each 5 mL of solution.

c. There is 250 mg of diluent in each 5 mL of solution.

d. A ratio of 125 mg per 5 mL of the same drug would be more concentrated.

10 An order calls for a wound irrigation with 120 mL of a mixture of hydrogen peroxide solution and sterile normal saline at a 1:1 ratio, followed by a normal saline rinse. How many mL of hydrogen peroxide solution will be used?

a. 240   b. 120   c. 60   d. 30

CHAPTER 7   FINAL PRACTICE

ESTIMATED COMPLETION TIME: 1 hour   **ANSWERS ON:** page 263

DIRECTIONS: *Examine the labels, change the units to equivalents by moving decimal places, estimate the answer, calculate the dose to the nearest tenth of a milliliter, and evaluate your answer. Then shade in the dose on the medicine cup and draw a vertical line through the calibrated line of each syringe for the dose to be given.*

1 **Ordered:** ceftriaxone 0.45 g IM bid for a child with a skin infection.

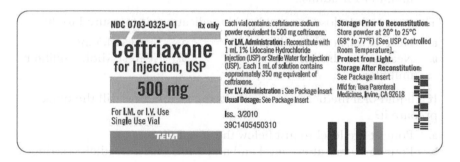

NDC 0703-0325-01   Rx only

Ceftriaxone
for Injection, USP

500 mg

For I.M. or I.V. Use
Single Use Vial

TEVA

Each vial contains: ceftriaxone sodium powder equivalent to 500 mg ceftriaxone.
For I.M. Administration : Reconstitute with 1 mL 1% Lidocaine Hydrochloride Injection (USP) or Sterile Water for Injection (USP). Each 1 mL of solution contains approximately 350 mg equivalent of ceftriaxone.
For I.V. Administration : See Package Insert
Usual Dosage: See Package Insert

Iss. 3/2010
39C1405450310

Storage Prior to Reconstitution: Store powder at 20° to 25°C (68° to 77°F) [See USP Controlled Room Temperature].
Protect from Light.
Storage After Reconstitution: See Package Insert
Mfd for: Teva Parenteral Medicines, Irvine, CA 92618

a. What is the unit dose concentration once it is reconstituted? _____

b. Estimate: more or less than unit dose?

     DA equation:

c. How many milliliters of medication will you give with each dose?

d. Evaluation: _____

Draw a line through the nearest measurable dose on the syringe provided.

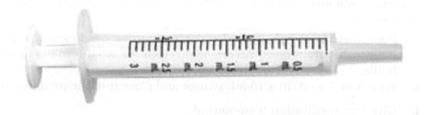

2 A wound irrigation order calls for 50 mL $\frac{1}{2}$ strength NS irrigations tid. The nurse needs to prepare the irrigation from full-strength NS by adding SW.

   a. What will be the ratio of NS solution to SW? _____

   b. How much NS solution will the nurse pour? _____

   c. How much SW will the nurse add? _____

3 **Ordered:** cefadroxil oral suspension 0.2 g PO twice daily for a patient with cystitis.

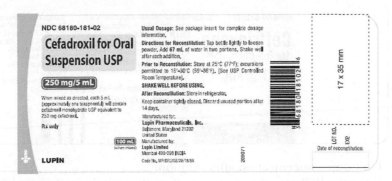

   a. Estimated dose: _____

   b. Calculated dose with equation to nearest tenth of a milliliter:

      DA equation:

   c. Evaluation: _____

Shade in the dose in mL on the medicine cup and draw a vertical line through the calibrated line of the syringe as applicable.

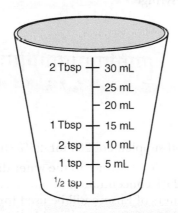

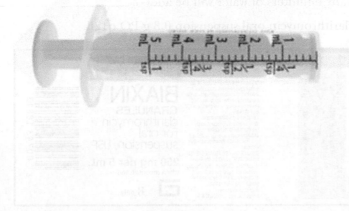

4 An NS solution has a concentration of sodium chloride (NaCl) 0.9%. NaCl is supplied in grams. The diluent is SW.

   a. Is the NS concentration more or less than a 1% solution? _____

   b. How many grams of solute (0.9 g solute NaCl concentrate) are contained in 100 mL of NS? _____

   c. How many grams of solute are contained in 1000 mL (1 L) of NS? _____

5 **Ordered:** ceftriaxone 750 mg IM q12h for a patient with a genitourinary infection.

<table>
<tr><td>NDC 0703-0335-01   Rx only</td><td>Each vial contains: ceftriaxone sodium powder equivalent to 1 gram ceftriaxone.
For I.M. Administration : Reconstitute with 2.1 mL 1% Lidocaine Hydrochloride Injection (USP) or Sterile Water for Injection (USP). Each 1 mL of solution contains approximately 350 mg equivalent of ceftriaxone.
For I.V. Administration : See Package Insert
Usual Dosage: See Package Insert
Iss. 9/2009
39C1701450909</td><td>**Storage Prior to Reconstitution:** Store powder at 20° to 25°C (68° to 77°F) [See USP Controlled Room Temperature].
Protect from Light.
Storage After Reconstitution: See Package Insert
Mfd for: Teva Parenteral Medicines Irvine, CA 92618</td></tr>
<tr><td>**Ceftriaxone**
for Injection, USP
1 gram
For I.M. or I.V. Use
Single Use Vial
TEVA</td><td></td><td></td></tr>
</table>

   a. Unit dose concentration after dilution: _____

   b. Estimate: Will you give *more* or *less* than the unit dose concentration? (circle one)

   c. Estimated round dose in milliliters: _____

   d. Actual dose: _____

   DA equation:

   e. Evaluation: _____

   If satisfactory to give, draw a vertical line through the calibrated line of the dose on this syringe.

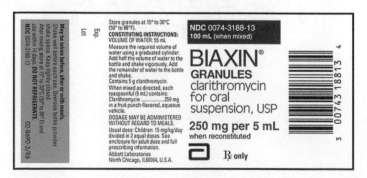

6 **Ordered:** Ensure food supplement 200 mL 25% strength q8h for 3 days.

   a. What will be the ratio of Ensure to the water diluent? _____

   b. How would the 25% concentration be expressed as a fraction? _____

   c. How many milliliters of Ensure will be used for the dose? _____

   d. How many milliliters of water will be added? _____

7 **Ordered:** clarithromycin oral suspension 0.3 g PO q12h.

<table>
<tr><td>Store granules at 15° to 30°C (59° to 86°F).
CONSTITUTING INSTRUCTIONS:
VOLUME OF WATER: 55 mL
Measure the required volume of water using a graduated cylinder. Add half the volume of water to the bottle and shake vigorously. Add the remainder of water to the bottle and shake.
Contains 5 g clarithromycin.
When mixed as directed, each teaspoonful (5 mL) contains:
Clarithromycin ....250 mg
in a fruit punch-flavored, aqueous vehicle.
DOSAGE MAY BE ADMINISTERED WITHOUT REGARD TO MEALS.
Usual dose: Children: 15 mg/kg/day divided in 2 equal doses. See enclosure for adult dose and full prescribing information.
Abbott Laboratories
North Chicago, IL60064, U.S.A.</td><td>NDC 0074-3188-13
100 mL (when mixed)

BIAXIN®
GRANULES
clarithromycin for oral suspension, USP
250 mg per 5 mL
when reconstituted
℞ only</td></tr>
</table>

   a. Estimated dose: _____

   b. Calculated dose with equation to nearest tenth of a milliliter:

     DA equation:

   c. Evaluation: _____

Shade in the dose in mL on the medicine cup and draw a vertical line
through the calibrated line of the syringe as applicable.

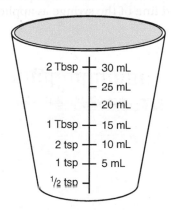

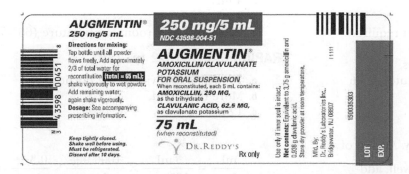

8 Ordered: Baby formula $\frac{1}{3}$ strength, 30 mL/hr to be diluted with SW.

   a. What is the equivalent percent concentration to the nearest whole
number? _____

   b. What is the equivalent ratio of active to inactive ingredients? _____

   c. How much formula will the nurse pour per hr? _____

   d. How much diluent will the nurse add per hr? _____

9 Ordered: amoxicillin clavulanate potassium oral suspension 0.6 g PO q12h.

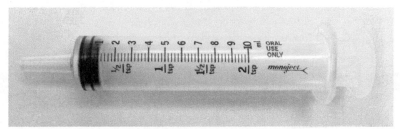

This drug is a combination drug.

a. Estimated dose: _____

b. Calculated dose with equation to the nearest tenth of a milliliter:

DA equation:

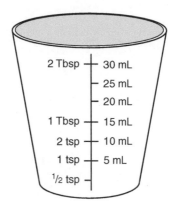

c. Evaluation: _____

Shade in the dose in mL on the medicine cup and draw a vertical line through the calibrated line of the syringe as applicable.

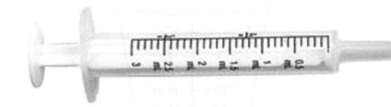

CHAPTER 7 ANSWER KEY

RAPID PRACTICE 7-1 (p. 237)

1
a. Oral suspension
b. Doxycyline
c. 25 mg per 5 mL
d. Multidose
e. 60 mL
f. Room temperature
g. None

2
a. Oral suspension when reconstituted from powder
b. 35 mL of water
c. 50 mL
d. 200 mg per 5 mL
e. Refrigeration preferable but not required.
f. Shake well before using.
g. Discard suspension after 14 days.

3
a. Oral suspension when reconstituted from powder
b. Water
c. 34 mL of water
d. Tap until all powder flows freely. Add $\frac{1}{2}$ of 34 mL (17 mL). After shaking well, add remaining $\frac{1}{2}$ (17 mL) and shake well.
e. 100 mg per 5 mL

f. Suprax
g. Cefixime
h. Multidose
i. Discard suspension after 14 days.
j. Store at room temperature or under refrigeration. Keep tightly closed.

4
a. Vancomycin hydrochloride
b. IV
c. 1 g
d. Sterile water

5
a. 4 mL
b. 2 mL
c. In a location at room temperature (68°–77° F)

RAPID PRACTICE 7-2 (p. 239)

1
a. 70 mL water divided in 2 portions
b. More than 5 mL
c. 12 mL

$$\frac{mL}{dose} = \frac{5\ mL}{\underset{1}{\cancel{125\ mg}}} \times \frac{\overset{8}{\cancel{1000\ mg}}}{1\ \cancel{g}} \times \frac{0.3\ \cancel{g}}{dose} = \frac{12\ mL}{dose}$$

d. The estimate supports the answer. Only mL remain. The equation is balanced.

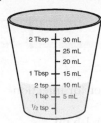

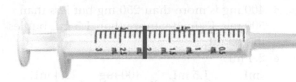

2 **a.** 24 mL distilled or purified water
b. More than 1 mL or 3 times more ($10 \times 3 = 30$)
c. 3 mL

$$\frac{mL}{dose} = \frac{1\ mL}{\underset{1}{\cancel{10\ mg}}} \times \frac{\overset{100}{\cancel{1000\ mg}}}{1\ \cancel{g}} \times \frac{0.03\ \cancel{g}}{dose} = \frac{3\ mL}{dose}$$

d. Equation is balanced. Estimate supports answer.

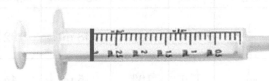

3 **a.** 106 mL of water in two portions
b. same ($0.25\ g = 250\ mg$)
c. 5 mL

$$\frac{mL}{dose} = \frac{5\ mL}{\underset{1}{\cancel{250\ mg}}} \times \frac{\overset{4}{\cancel{1000\ mg}}}{1\ \cancel{g}} \times \frac{0.25\ \cancel{g}}{dose}$$
$$= \frac{5\ mL}{dose}$$

d. Equation is balanced. Estimate supports answer.

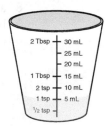

4 **a.** Add 14 mL water followed by 13 mL of water for a total of 27 mL.
b. Estimate will give more than 2 times unit dose of 5 mL ($0.25\ g = 250\ mg$).
c. 10 mL

$$\frac{mL}{dose} = \frac{5\ mL}{\underset{1}{\cancel{125\ mg}}} \times \frac{\overset{8}{\cancel{1000\ mg}}}{1\ \cancel{g}} \times \frac{0.25\ \cancel{g}}{dose}$$
$$= \frac{10\ mL}{dose}$$

d. Equation is balanced. Estimate supports answer.

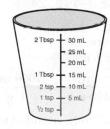

A syringe is not needed.

5 **a.** More than 5 mL ($0.2\ g = 200\ mg$)
b. 8 mL

$$\frac{mL}{dose} = \frac{5\ mL}{\underset{1}{\cancel{125\ mg}}} \times \frac{\overset{8}{\cancel{1000\ mg}}}{1\ \cancel{g}} \times \frac{0.2\ \cancel{g}}{dose} = \frac{8\ mL}{dose}$$

c. Equation in balanced. Estimate supports answer.

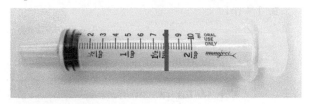

RAPID PRACTICE 7-3 (p. 246)

2 **a.** 12 mL
b. 50 mg per mL
c. 10 mL

$$\frac{mL}{dose} = \frac{1\ mL}{\underset{1}{\cancel{50\ mg}}} \times \frac{\overset{20}{\cancel{1000\ mg}}}{1\ \cancel{g}} \times \frac{0.5\ \cancel{g}}{dose} = \frac{10\ mL}{dose}$$

d. Equation is balanced. Estimate supports answer.
3 **a.** 4 mL ($0.1\ g = 100\ mg$) (know your metric equivalents)
b. 100 mg per mL
c. 1 mL ($100\ mg = 0.1\ g$)
4 **a.** 2 mL ($0.3\ g = 300\ mg$)
b. 250 mg per mL

c. 1.2 mL (300 mg is more than 250 mg)

$$\frac{mL}{dose} = \frac{1\ mL}{\underset{1}{\cancel{250\ mg}}} \times \frac{\overset{4}{\cancel{1000\ mg}}}{1\ \cancel{g}} \times \frac{0.3\ \cancel{g}}{dose}$$

$$= 4 \times 0.3 = \frac{1.2\ mL}{dose}$$

d. Equation is balanced. Estimate supports answer.

5 a. 2 mL (0.25 g = 250 mg)
   b. 250 mg per mL
   c. 1 mL (250 mg = 0.25 g)

RAPID PRACTICE 7-4 (p. 248)

2 a. Sterile water
   b. Slightly more
   c. More than 1 mL

$$\frac{mL}{dose} = \frac{mL}{\cancel{400\ mg}} \times \frac{1000\ \cancel{mg}}{1\ \cancel{g}} \times \frac{0.5\ \cancel{g}}{dose} = \frac{5}{4}$$

$$= 1.25\ mL,\ rounded\ to\ \frac{1.3\ mL}{dose}$$

d. Equation is balanced. Estimate supports answer.

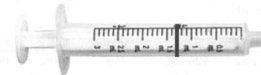

3 a. 18.2 mL
   B. 1.4 mL

$$\frac{mL}{dose} = \frac{1\ mL}{\underset{5}{\cancel{250,000\ units}}} \times \frac{\overset{8}{\cancel{400,000\ units}}}{dose}$$

$$= 1.6\ mL\ per\ dose$$

C. Equation is balanced. Estimate supports answer.

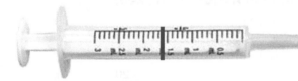

4 a. 3.5 mL
   b. 250 mg per mL
   c. Within 1 hour
   d. About twice as many mL as unit dose
   e. 2 mL per dose

$$\frac{mL}{dose} = \frac{1\ mL}{\underset{1}{\cancel{250\ mg}}} \times \frac{\overset{4}{\cancel{1000\ mg}}}{1\ \cancel{g}} \times \frac{0.5\ \cancel{g}}{dose} = \frac{2\ mL}{dose}$$

f. Estimate supports answer. Equation is balanced.

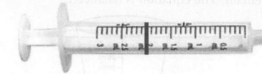

5 a. Sterile water for injection
   b. 5.4 mL
   c. 250 mg per 1.5 mL
   d. 400 mg is more than 250 mg but less than 500 mg. Estimate: more than 1.5 mL but less than 3 mL.
   e. 2.4 mL

$$\frac{mL}{dose} = \frac{1.5\ mL}{\cancel{250\ mg}} \times \frac{\cancel{400\ mg}}{dose} = \frac{2.4\ mL}{dose}$$

f. Equation is balanced. Estimate supports answer.

RAPID PRACTICE 7-5 (p. 254)

	Fractional Strength	Ratio	Percent	Amount Active Ingredient	Amount Diluent Inactive Ingredient
2	$\frac{1}{5}$	1:4	20%	48 mL	192 mL
3	$\frac{1}{10}$	1:9	10%	5 mL	45 mL
4	$\frac{1}{2}$	1:1	50%	30 mL	30 mL
5	$\frac{3}{4}$	3:1	75%	750 mL	250 mL

CHAPTER 7 MULTIPLE-CHOICE REVIEW (p. 255)

1	d	6	b
2	a	7	a
3	c	8	a
4	a	9	b
5	b	10	c

CHAPTER 7 FINAL PRACTICE (p. 256)

1 **a.** 350 mg per mL

b. Estimate: more than unit dose

$$DA \frac{mL}{dose} = \frac{1\ mL}{\underset{7}{\cancel{350\ mg}}} \times \frac{\overset{20}{\cancel{1000\ mg}}}{1\ \cancel{g}} \times \frac{0.45\ \cancel{g}}{dose}$$

$$= \frac{1.28\ mL}{dose} = \frac{1.3\ mL}{dose}$$

c. 1.3 mL per dose

d. Estimate supports answer. The equation is balanced.

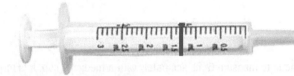

2 **a.** 1 : 1

b. 25 mL

c. 25 mL (25 + 25 = 50 mL)

3 **a.** Less than 5 mL (0.2 g = 200 mg)

b. 4 mL

$$\frac{mL}{dose} = \frac{5\ mL}{\underset{1}{\cancel{250\ mg}}} \times \frac{\overset{4}{\cancel{1000\ mg}}}{1\ \cancel{g}} \times \frac{0.2\ \cancel{g}}{dose} = \frac{4\ mL}{dose}$$

c. Equation is balanced. Estimate supports answer.

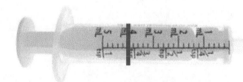

Note: A medicine cup is not appropriate for an amount less than 5 mL.

4 **a.** Less ($1\% \times \frac{1}{100}$) ($0.9\% = \frac{0.9}{100}$)

b. 0.9 g solute

c. 9 g

$$\frac{g}{solute} = \frac{0.9\ g\ solute}{\underset{1}{\cancel{100\ mL}}} \times \frac{\overset{10}{\cancel{1000\ mL}}}{1} = 9\ g\ solute$$

5 **a.** 350 mg per mL

b. More

c. Near 2 mL

d. 2.14, rounded to 2.1 mL per dose

$$\frac{mL}{dose} = \frac{1\ mL}{\underset{7}{\cancel{350\ mg}}} \times \frac{\overset{15}{\cancel{750\ mg}}}{dose} = \frac{15}{7}$$

$$= 2.14 = 2.1\ mL\ per\ dose$$

e. Estimate supports answer. Equation is balanced.

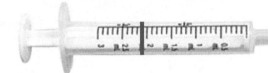

6 **a.** 1 : 3

b. $\frac{25}{100} = \frac{1}{4}$

c. mL : 200 mL × 0.25 = 50 mL

(or 200 mL × $\frac{1}{4}$ = 50 mL Ensure)

d. 200 mL − 50 mL = 150 mL water

7 **a.** slightly more than 5 mL

b. 6 mL

$$\frac{mL}{dose} = \frac{5\ mL}{\underset{1}{\cancel{250\ mg}}} \times \frac{\overset{4}{\cancel{1000\ mg}}}{1\ \cancel{g}} \times \frac{0.3\ \cancel{g}}{1} = \frac{6\ mL}{dose}$$

c. Equation is balanced. Estimate supports answer.

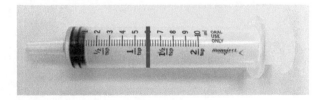

8 **a.** 33%

b. 1 : 2

c. mL : 30 mL × 0.33 = 9.9 mL (or 30 × $\frac{1}{3}$ = 10 mL formula)

d. 30 mL − 10 mL = 20 mL diluent of SW

9 **a.** Slightly more than 10 mL

b. 12 mL

$$\frac{mL}{dose} = \frac{5\ mL}{\underset{1}{\cancel{250\ mg}}} \times \frac{\overset{4}{\cancel{1000\ mg}}}{1\ \cancel{g}} \times \frac{0.6\ \cancel{g}}{dose}$$

$$= \frac{12\ mL}{dose}$$

c. Equation is balanced. Estimate supports answer.

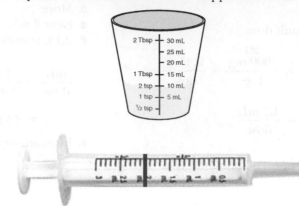

CLINICAL RELEVANCE	It is difficult to measure 6 mL accurately with a medicine cup. It is more accurate to use a calibrated syringe.

Suggestions for Further Reading

http://www.cwladis.com/math104/lecture4.php

web.cerritos.edu/rsantiago/SitePages/Reconstitution%20of%20Powdered%20Meds.htm

Chapter 8 builds on early chapters to provide a variety of practice problems for subcutaneous and intramuscular dose calculations, with labels of commonly used medications. Injection sites are illustrated.

PART IV

Parenteral Medications

8

Injectable Medications

OBJECTIVES

- Calculate and prepare intradermal, subcutaneous, and intramuscular doses.

- Calculate and combine doses for two medications to be mixed in one syringe.
- Identify safety hazards of injectable medications.

ESTIMATED TIME TO COMPLETE CHAPTER: 1 to 2 hours

This chapter offers a variety of practice problems involving subcutaneous and intramuscular dose calculations. This practice will improve your calculations in the clinical setting so that you can focus on injection technique. Some injectable drugs are mixed in one syringe to avoid giving the patient two separate injections.

VOCABULARY

Drug Incompatibilities	Consider all drugs incompatible unless compatibility is stated. Compatibility is affected by several factors, including pH, temperature, strength, and composition. Compatibility data are listed in drug package inserts and current drug references. This information includes the choice of diluents, such as SW or sterile NS solution. One may be compatible with a drug and the other may not.
	➤ When in doubt, check with the pharmacist and document the finding.
Hypodermic	General term used for injections "under the skin."
Intradermal (ID) Injection	Injection into the dermal layer, just under the epidermis, as for many skin tests.
Intramuscular (IM) Injection	Injection into a muscle.
Parenteral	Medications given outside the gastrointestinal (GI) tract. Includes medications delivered via IV, IM, subcutaneous, and intradermal injections.
Parenteral Mix	Two or more compatible liquid medications combined in one syringe for injection. Medication combinations may include a narcotic and an anticholinergic agent to reduce nausea or dry secretions. Mixing relieves the patient from having to receive two separate IM injections.
Subcutaneous (Subcut) Injection	Injection into loose connective tissue, or fatty layer, underlying the dermis.

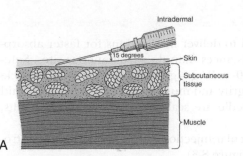

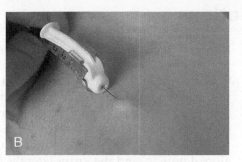

FIGURE 8-1 A, Intradermal needle tip inserted into dermis. **B,** Intradermal injection creates a small bleb. (From Potter PA, Perry AG, Stockert PA, Hall AM: *Fundamentals of nursing,* ed 10, St Louis, 2021, Elsevier.)

✳ **Communication**

Many patients are afraid of "needles." When giving vaccines and administering skin tests, the nurse can reassure patients about INTRADERMAL injections by showing them how little medicine will be given and how small and fine the needle is, if the patient is willing to take a look. Do not give false reassurances, such as, "Oh, you won't feel a thing." Prepare the patient for some discomfort even though there usually is minimal pain with these types of injections: "Mrs. Brown, most people dislike injections. This is just a drop or two of medicine. This will just feel like a little mosquito bite."

Intradermal Injections

Small-volume injections usually administered as skin tests are injected intradermally just under the epidermis at a very shallow angle. A small fluid-filled wheal or bleb like a mosquito bite forms. The area is examined daily for a few days to see if there is an antibody reaction to the antigen injected. The observations are measured and documented.

Medications are not delivered via the ID route because this route offers poor absorption capability.

The usual dose for a skin test is 0.1 mL. Skin tests are administered with a 1-mL syringe and a 26- to 29-gauge needle (Figure 8-1).

Subcutaneous Injections

Nonirritating substances up to 1 mL may be injected into subcutaneous fatty tissue sites, usually with a 25- to 31-gauge needle. Insulin and anticoagulants, such as heparin, and enoxaparin and dalteparin, are medications that are delivered through the subcutaneous route. The fluid volume needle gauge, needle length (average $\frac{1}{2}$ inch), and angle of injection depend on the patient's size, skin thickness, and condition.

The most common sites for subcutaneous injection are the subcutaneous fatty areas of the upper posterior arm, the abdomen, and the anterior thigh (Figure 8-2).

➤ A 2-inch zone around the umbilicus is to be avoided. As with all injections, the sites must be rotated systematically to avoid tissue injury.

➤ It is best to write out *subcutaneous* or *subcut* on medical records to avoid misinterpretation; *subq, subc,* and *SQ* can be misinterpreted. Printed materials do use abbreviations such as *subc* or *subQ* but are less likely to be misinterpreted than is handwriting.

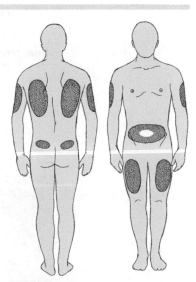

FIGURE 8-2 Sites recommended for subcutaneous injections. (From Potter PA, Perry AG, Stockert PA, Hall AM: *Fundamentals of nursing,* ed 10, St Louis, 2021, Elsevier.)

Intramuscular Injections

Intramuscular injection sites are selected to deliver medications for faster absorption and tolerate more concentrated substances than do subcutaneous sites. Solutions up to 3 mL may be injected with a 20- to 23-gauge needle into a single muscle site, depending on the patient's skin integrity and muscle size. The volume of fluid and the length, gauge, and angle of needle are scaled down for smaller adults, children, and infants.

The most common sites for intramuscular injection are the deltoid, the ventrogluteal muscle, and the vastus lateralis (Figure 8-3).

➤ The dorsogluteal site is considered to be the most dangerous site for giving an IM injection, and it is generally avoided. The sciatic nerve is located

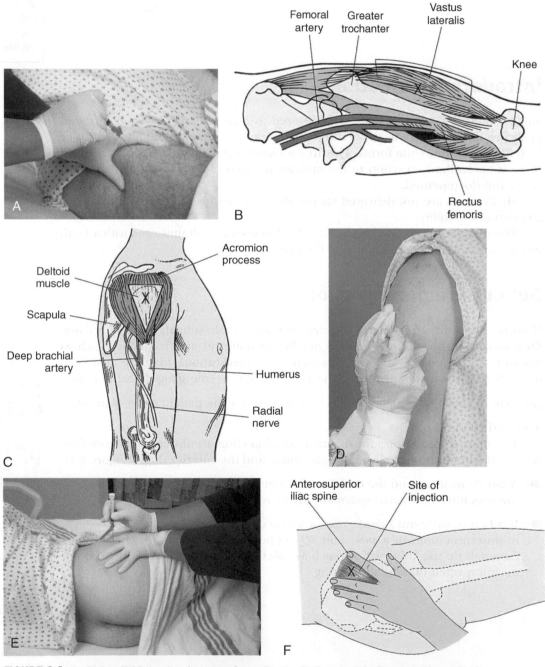

FIGURE 8-3 A, Giving IM injection in vastus lateralis site. **B,** Landmarks for vastus lateralis site. **C,** Landmarks for deltoid site. **D,** Giving IM injection in deltoid site. **E,** Ventrogluteal site avoids major nerves and blood vessels. **F,** Hand placement for selecting correct ventrogluteal site for injection. (From Perry AG, Potter PA, Ostendorf WR: *Clinical nursing skills and techniques,* ed. 9, St. Louis, 2021, Mosby.)

only a few centimeters away and, if damaged, can be a painful complication (immediate and long term) if struck. The superior gluteal artery is also near this region, and if the injected medication enters this artery, the medication becomes an unplanned intravenous push injection.

➤ Check workplace policies and procedures for acceptable injection sites. Assess integrity of skin sites prior to injection.

Administering Injections

Mastery of the technique of delivering injections to the correct layer of tissue requires supervised laboratory and clinical practice with anatomical models and a variety of different-sized patients.

Medications for subcutaneous and intramuscular injections are administered with a variety of equipment, including vials, ampules, prefilled syringes, and syringe cartridges, as illustrated in Figure 8-4. Ampules are single-dose glass containers containing liquid medications and solutions. Vials are supplied as single-dose or multidose glass containers and may contain liquid or dry medication forms.

➤ Remember that a filter needle must be used to withdraw medicines from glass ampules.
➤ Replace the filter needle with a regular needle *BEFORE* administering the injection to avoid injecting glass or rubber particles into the patient.

Prefilled syringes reduce the chance of contamination during preparation of the medication.

➤ However, they do not entirely eliminate that risk because dose adjustments may be required with prefilled syringes. They may contain 0.1 to 0.2 mL of extra medication in case of loss during preparation.

FAQ *What is the quickest way to learn selection of syringe and needle sizes?*

ANSWER There is no substitute for supervised and, later, independent experience, but learning can be greatly expedited. Assuming that you have learned to identify syringe capacities and calibration amounts (covered in Chapter 6), focus on a commonly used syringe size for each route and an approximate needle size and typical amount. Try to learn syringe and needle size selection in sequential order from the intradermal to intramuscular or vice versa (Table 8-1). Then, in the clinical setting, modifications and the selection of needles and the appropriate angle of injection for specific-sized patients can be added to the body of knowledge.

➤ There are many variations on the sizes and amounts shown in Figure 8-5. These figures are just averages.

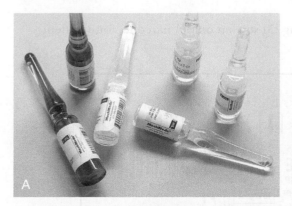
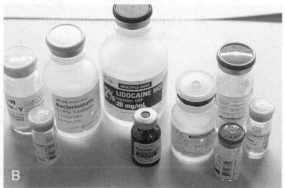

FIGURE 8-4 A, Medication in ampules. **B,** Medication in vials.

TABLE 8-1	Usual Syringe Size, Needle Size, and Doses			
Route	**Usual Syringe Size**	**Needle Size**	**Average/Usual Amount**	**Maximum Amount per Site**
Intradermal*	1-mL syringe	$\frac{1}{2}$ inch or less	0.1-mL injection	0.5 mL*
Subcutaneous	1- to 3-mL syringe	$\frac{1}{2}$ to 1 inch	0.5 mL	1 mL
Intramuscular	3-mL syringe	1 to 2 inches	2 mL	3 mL

*The intradermal route is not used for medication administration. Skin test amounts are usually 0.1 mL.

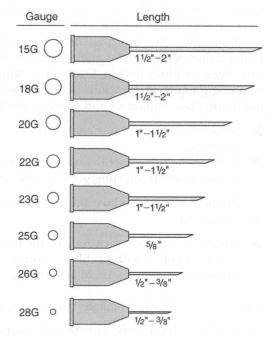

FIGURE 8-5 Needle gauge and length. (From Willihnganz M, Gurevitz S, Clayton B: *Clayton's Basic pharmacology for nurses,* ed 18, St Louis, 2020, Elsevier.)

➤ Note that the 3-mL syringe for intramuscular injections corresponds to the maximum 3-mL amount for intramuscular injections to be used in one site.

➤ Remember: Never recap a used needle.

RAPID PRACTICE 8-1 | Parenteral Dose Calculations

ESTIMATED COMPLETION TIME: 20 to 30 minutes   **ANSWERS ON:** page 292

DIRECTIONS: *Estimate the dose, verify it with a DA-style equation to the nearest tenth of a mL, and evaluate. Draw a vertical line through the calibrated line of each syringe for the dose to be given.*

1   **Ordered:** morphine sulfate 9 mg IM stat, an opioid narcotic, for a patient with pain.

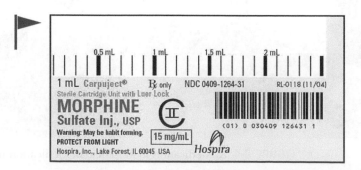

a. Drug concentration: _____

b. Estimated dose: _____

c. How many mL will you prepare?

➤ Write out morphine sulfate. Do not abbreviate.

DA equation:

d. Evaluation: _____

Draw a vertical line through the nearest measurable dose on the syringe provided.

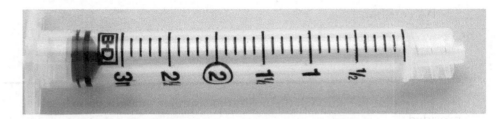

➤ Note the *C II* on the morphine label. This means that the drug is a federally controlled substance, Schedule II, a category of drugs with strong potential for abuse as well as its useful medical purposes. Morphine is an opium-derived narcotic. There are strict record-keeping requirements for controlled drugs.

➤ Assess the patient for respiratory depression before giving an opioid medication and periodically thereafter until the drug effect has diminished. There are several visual scales available for assessing current pain levels. The patient identifies the current level on a range from "no pain" to "worst pain" or "severest pain" subjective rating. This practice may reduce the risk of overmedication.

CLINICAL RELEVANCE

2 **Ordered:** digoxin 0.125 mg deep IM daily for 3 days, for a patient with heart failure.

a. Drug concentration: _____

b. Estimated dose: _____

c. How many mL will you prepare?

DA equation:

d. Evaluation: _____

Draw a vertical line through the nearest measurable dose on the syringe provided.

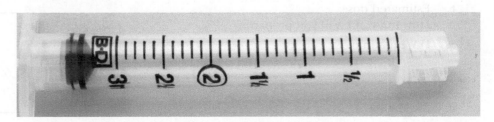

Non-varnish area

NDC 0641-1410-31   2 mL Ampul

Digoxin Injection, USP

500 mcg/2 mL   Rx only

0.5 mg/2 mL (250 mcg/mL)

FOR SLOW IV OR DEEP IM USE

Distr. by: ✺ WEST-WARD

(01)00306411410316

PLB669-WES/1

Lot:

Exp: Non-varnish area

3   **Ordered:** diazepam 6 mg IM stat for a patient with anxiety.

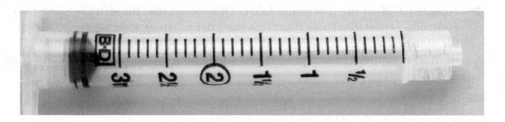

10 mL Multiple-dose   ℞ only   NDC 0409-3213-02
DIAZEPAM
Injection, USP
5 mg/mL
HOSPIRA, INC., LAKE FOREST, IL 60045 USA

Each mL contains 5 mg diazepam; 40% propylene glycol; 10% alcohol; 5% sodium benzoate and benzoic acid added as buffers and 1.5% benzyl alcohol added as a preservative. pH 6.6 (6.2 to 6.9). Store at 20 to 25°C (68 to 77°F). For I.V. or I.M. use. Usual dosage: See insert. NOTE: Solution may appear colorless to light yellow.   RL-0644 (10/04)

Hospira

a.   Drug concentration: _____

b.   Estimated dose: _____

c.   How many mL will you prepare?

DA equation:

d.   Evaluation: _____

Draw a vertical line through the nearest measurable amount on the syringe provided.

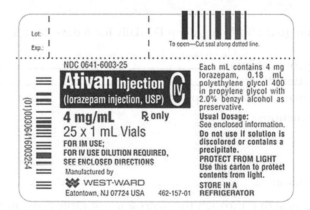

4   **Ordered:** lorazepam 2 mg deep IM stat, a sedative and anti-anxiety agent, for an agitated elderly patient. Note: Ativan (lorazepam) is a very irritating substance and should be given undiluted deep IM.

Lot:
Exp.:
To open—Cut seal along dotted line.

NDC 0641-6003-25
Ativan Injection ℞ only
(lorazepam injection, USP)
4 mg/mL   ℞ only
25 x 1 mL Vials
FOR IM USE;
FOR IV USE DILUTION REQUIRED,
SEE ENCLOSED DIRECTIONS
Manufactured by
✖ WEST-WARD
Eatontown, NJ 07724 USA   462-157-01

(01)00306416003254

Each mL contains 4 mg lorazepam, 0.18 mL polyethylene glycol 400 in propylene glycol with 2.0% benzyl alcohol as preservative.
Usual Dosage:
See enclosed information.
Do not use if solution is discolored or contains a precipitate.
PROTECT FROM LIGHT
Use this carton to protect contents from light.
STORE IN A REFRIGERATOR

a.   Drug concentration: _____

b.   Estimated dose: _____

c.   How many mL will you prepare?

DA equation:

d.   Evaluation: _____

Draw a vertical line through the nearest measurable dose on the syringe provided.

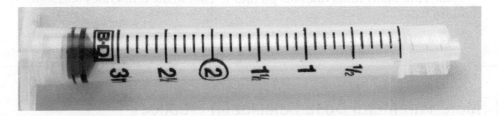

Note that Ativan (lorazepam) is labeled *C IV* (i.e., controlled substance Schedule IV). Drugs in this category have *less* potential for abuse or addiction than do Schedule II, or III drugs. Schedule IV drugs include phenobarbital and certain other anti-anxiety agents.

➤ Focus intently on decimals when they appear in medication orders or drug labels. Dose calculation errors are large if a decimal point is misplaced. Write neatly and make decimal points prominent. If there is no whole number preceding the decimal then use a "leading zero" to avoid an error. Never use a "trailing zero" at the end of a decimal.

CLINICAL RELEVANCE

5 **Ordered:** nafcillin 0.45 g IM q4h, an antibiotic, for a patient with infection.

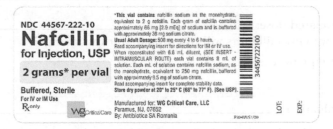

a. Drug concentration after reconstitution: _____
b. Estimated dose: _____
c. How many mL will you prepare for the syringe provided below?

DA equation:

d. Evaluation: _____

Draw a vertical line through the nearest measurable amount on the syringe provided.

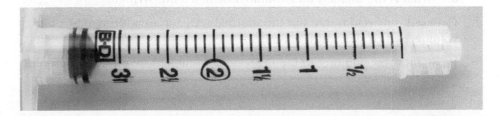

Q & A **ASK YOURSELF** **1** How many times does 0.05 go into 0.1? How many times does 0.25 go into 0.5? How many times does 0.5 go into 1? How many times does 0.025 go into 0.05?

MY ANSWER _____

RAPID PRACTICE 8-2 | **More Parenteral Dose Calculation Practice**

ESTIMATED COMPLETION TIME: 20 to 30 minutes   **ANSWERS ON:** page 293

DIRECTIONS: *Examine the order and calculate the dose. Recalculate if the estimate does not support the answer.*

1 **Ordered:** Furosemide 35 mg IM, a diuretic, for a patient with edema.

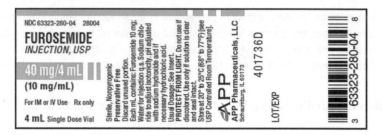

NDC 63323-280-04 28004
FUROSEMIDE
INJECTION, USP
40 mg/4 mL
(10 mg/mL)
For IM or IV Use   Rx only
4 mL Single Dose Vial

Sterile, Nonpyrogenic
Preservative Free
Discard unused portion.
Each mL contains: Furosemide 10 mg;
Water for Injection q.s. Sodium chlo-
ride to adjust isotonicity, pH adjusted
with sodium hydroxide and if
necessary hydrochloric acid.
Usual Dosage: See Insert.
PROTECT FROM LIGHT. Do not use if
discolored. Use only if solution is clear
and seal intact.
Store at 20° to 25°C (68° to 77°F) [see
USP Controlled Room Temperature].

APP Pharmaceuticals, LLC
Schaumburg, IL 60173
401736D
LOT/EXP

a. Estimated dose: _____

b. How many milliliters will you prepare for this syringe?

DA equation:

c. Evaluation: _____

Draw a vertical line through the nearest measurable amount on the syringe provided.

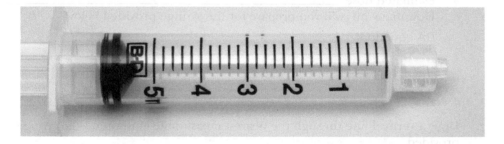

d. What is the smallest measurable dose in a 5-mL syringe?

2 **Ordered:** tuberculin skin test intradermal (ID) for an adult patient. The volume for this skin test is 0.1 mL.

Draw an arrow pointing to the nearest measurable dose on the tuberculin syringe provided.

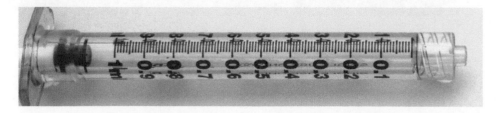

3   **Ordered:** Solu-Cortef 0.3 g IM, an anti-inflammatory steroid, for a patient
     with severe inflammatory response.

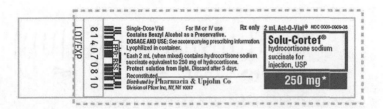

   a.   Estimated dose: _____
   b.   How many milliliters will you prepare for this syringe?

        DA equation:

   c.   Evaluation: _____

Draw a vertical line through the nearest measurable amount on the syringe
provided.

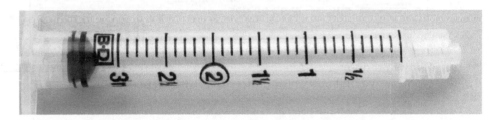

4   **Ordered:** oxymorphone 0.0015 g IM q3–4h prn for pain, a narcotic analgesic,
     for a patient with pain.

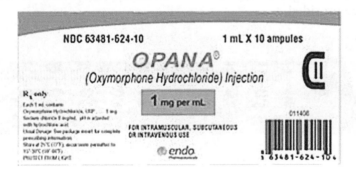

   a.   Estimated dose: _____
   b.   How many milliliters will you prepare for this syringe to the nearest tenth
        of a mL?

        DA equation:

   c.   Evaluation: _____

Draw a vertical line through the nearest measurable amount on the syringe provided.

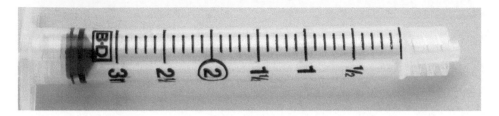

5   **Ordered:** atropine 0.3 mg IM on call to OR, an anticholinergic, for a preoperative patient.

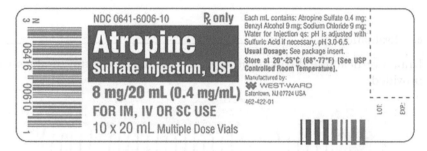

a.   Estimated dose: _____

b.   How many milliliters will you prepare for the 1-mL syringe?

DA equation:

c.   Evaluation: _____

Draw an arrow pointing to the nearest measurable amount on the syringe provided.

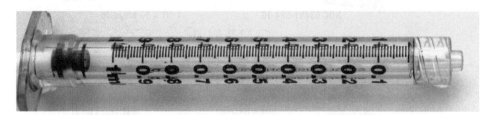

Q & A   **ASK YOURSELF**   1   Why is it important to make a habit of evaluating the equations and comparing the answers to the estimates? What are the risks if this step is skipped?

MY ANSWER   _____

Parenteral Mixes

When two medications are administered together in one syringe, the order is bracketed:

$$\left.\begin{array}{l}\text{morphine 5 mg IM}\\ \text{atropine 0.2 mg IM}\end{array}\right\}\text{on call to OR}$$

The use of preoperative sedation via the parenteral route is much less common than it used to be. Now, most patients receive preoperative sedation via IV push injection in the holding room of the operating room suite.

On a few rare occasions a preoperative injection that requires the mixing of two medications may be ordered. The use of parenteral mixes spares the patient the discomfort of two separate intramuscular injections. Even though they are now very rarely ordered, if used, they usually consist of a narcotic and either an anticholinergic or an antihistamine-type medication that extends the action of the narcotic, decreases nausea, or dries respiratory secretions for patients who are to receive general anesthesia.

It is essential for the nurse to check the compatibility of the two medications that are to be mixed. The nurse may either consult a current drug reference or call the pharmacy.

➤ Consider all drugs incompatible unless otherwise documented

Example of Parenteral Mix Order

Ordered:

$$\left.\begin{array}{l}\text{hydromorphone 2 mg}\\ \text{hydroxyzine 25 mg}\end{array}\right\}\text{IM q4h prn pain}$$

Note the brackets, which indicate the medications should be mixed together.

CLINICAL RELEVANCE

There is an automatic expiration date (called a "stop order") on narcotics and medications that have the potential for dependence or abuse or that are ineffective if given beyond a specified period. It is usually 48 to 72 hours for controlled substances. In order to continue the medications, the order must be renewed in a timely manner so that the medication schedule proceeds without interruption. Check agency policy.

➤ The nurse cannot legally continue to administer any drug after the "stop order" date, be it automatic or written out. The prescriber must be contacted promptly if the medication is still perceived to be needed. By giving a drug where the order is expired, the nurse then becomes a prescriber without the license to prescribe—an illegal practice.

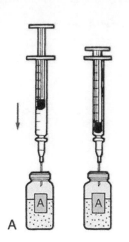
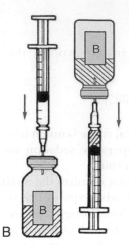
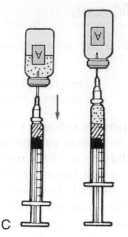
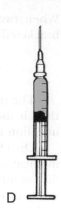

FIGURE 8-6 **A,** Injecting air into vial A. **B,** Injecting air into vial Band withdrawing dose. **C,** Withdrawing medication from vial A. **D,** Medications are now mixed. (Modified from Perry AG, Potter PA, Stockert PA, Hall A: *Essentials of nursing practice,* ed. 9, St. Louis, 2019, Mosby.)

Mixing two medications in one syringe

Mixtures may be combinations of vial, ampule, prefilled syringe, and/or prefilled cartridge medications. This technique requires supervised clinical practice (Figure 8-6).

Calculating the dose for a parenteral mix

Calculate each dose separately to the nearest tenth of a milliliter. Add them together. Round the dose to the nearest tenth of a milliliter. For example,

morphine sulfate	0.4 mL
atropine sulfate	+0.2 mL
	0.6 mL total volume for syringe

RAPID PRACTICE 8-3   Calculating Parenteral Mix Doses

ESTIMATED COMPLETION TIME: 10 to 15 minutes   **ANSWERS ON:** page 293

DIRECTIONS: *Examine the order and the labels. Estimate the ordered doses. Calculate the two individual doses to the nearest tenth of a milliliter using DA-style equations. Evaluate the equation. Is the equation balanced? Does the estimate support the answer? Draw a vertical line through the* total *desired amount to the nearest measurable dose on the available 3-mL syringe. Follow the example given in problem 1. The order of the questions for each problem suggests the order to follow to solve these problems.*

➤ Although preoperative sedation is given less frequently today than in the past, nurses need to know how to mix a narcotic with another medication in case it is ordered. Postoperative IM injections have become less common as well, but nurses need to be prepared to give IM pain medication, which can be a single drug or a combination of two drugs to potentiate the narcotic effects.

1 **Ordered:** meperidine hydrochloride 75 mg ⎫ IM q4–6h prn pain for a
hydroxyzine hydrochloride 25 mg ⎭ patient allergic to morphine
and hydromorphone

Rx only   NDC 76045-008-10

Morphine ℂ

Sulfate Injection, USP **10** mg/mL

For Intramuscular or Intravenous use.
Do **NOT** place syringe on a Sterile Field.

24 x **1** mL Prefilled single-use syringes
Discard unused portion.

Simplist™   PRESENIUS KABI

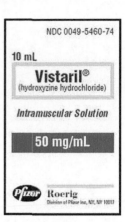

NDC 0049-5460-74

10 mL

Vistaril®
(hydroxyzine hydrochloride)

Intramuscular Solution

50 mg/mL

Pfizer Roerig
Division of Pfizer Inc, NY, NY 10017

Morphine

a. Estimate: Does the order call for *more* or ⟨*less*⟩ than the unit dose available?
Less. Estimated dose: about $\dfrac{4}{5}$ mL.

b. How many mL will you prepare?
DA equation:

$$\frac{mL}{dose} = \frac{mL}{\cancel{10\ mg}} \times \frac{\cancel{8\ mg}}{dose} = \frac{4}{5} = \frac{0.8\ mL}{dose}$$

c. Evaluation: Is the equation balanced? <u>Yes.</u> Does the estimate support the answer? <u>Yes.</u>

Hydroxyzine HCl

d. Estimate: Does the order call for *more* or ⟨*less*⟩ than the dose available?
Less. Estimated dose: about $\dfrac{1}{2}$ of 1 mL.

e. How many mL will you prepare?
DA equation:

$$\frac{mL}{dose} = \frac{1\ mL}{\underset{2}{\cancel{50\ mg}}} \times \frac{\overset{1}{\cancel{25\ mg}}}{dose} = \frac{0.5\ mL\ hydroxyzine}{dose}$$

f. Evaluation: Is the equation balanced? <u>Yes.</u> Does the estimate support the answer? <u>Yes.</u>

Total Dose

g. *Total combined volume* in milliliters *to nearest tenth:* <u>0.8 + 0.5 mL = 1.3 mL</u>

Draw a vertical line through *the nearest measurable amount* for the total dose on the syringe.

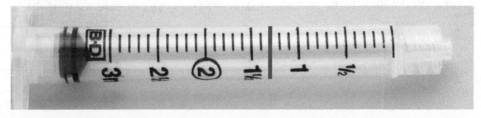

The only difference between this calculation and other calculations of liquid doses learned earlier is the addition of the two doses together.

2 **Ordered:** hydromorphone HCl 3 mg
Promethazine 10 mg } IM stat

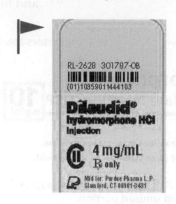

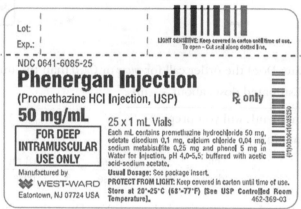

Hydromorphone

a. Estimated dose: _____

b. How many mL will be prepared?

DA equation:

c. Evaluation: Is the equation balanced? Does the estimate support the
answer? _____

Promethazine

d. Estimated dose: _____

e. How many mL will you prepare?

DA equation:

f. Evaluation: Is the equation balanced? Does the estimate support the
answer? _____

Total Dose

g. Total combined volume: _____

Draw a vertical line through the nearest measurable amount for the total dose on the syringe provided.

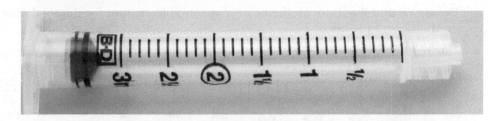

3 **Ordered:** hydromorphone HCl 1.5 mg ⎫ IM at 0800
atropine 0.4 mg ⎭

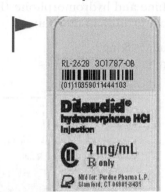

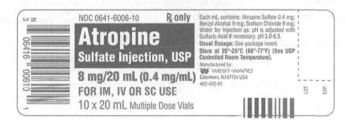

Hydromorphone

a. Estimated dose: _____

b. How many mL will you prepare?

DA equation:

c. Evaluation: Is the equation balanced? Does the estimate support the answer? _____

Atropine

d. Estimated dose: _____

e. How many mL will you prepare?

DA equation:

f. Evaluation: Is the equation balanced? Does the estimate support the answer? _____

Total Dose

g. Total combined volume: _____

Draw a vertical line through the nearest measurable amount for the total dose on the syringe provided.

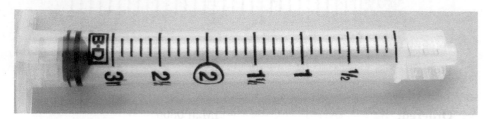

➤ Do not confuse morphine and hydromorphone (Dilaudid). Hydromorphone is considerably more powerful than morphine.

4 **Ordered:** $\left.\begin{array}{l}\text{Morphine sulfate 8 mg}\\\text{Glycopyrrolate 0.4 mg}\end{array}\right\}$ IM now

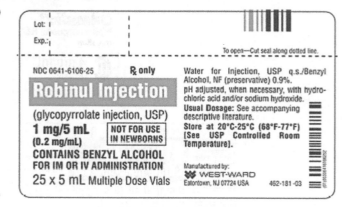

Morphine

a. Estimated dose: _____

b. How many mL will you prepare?

DA equation:

c. Evaluation: Is the equation balanced? Does the estimate support the answer? _____

Glycopyrrolate

d. Estimated dose: _____

e. How many mL will you prepare?

DA equation:

f. Evaluation: Is the equation balanced? Does the estimate support the answer? _____

Total Dose

g. Total combined volume: _____

Draw a vertical line through the nearest measurable amount for the total dose on the syringe provided.

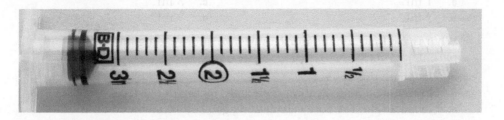

Medicines Supplied in Units

Medicines that are supplied in units and also may be administered via the subcutaneous route are covered in Chapters 11 and 12.

CHAPTER 8   MULTIPLE-CHOICE REVIEW

ESTIMATED COMPLETION TIME. 30 minutes to 1 hour   ANSWERS ON: page 294

DIRECTIONS: *Place a circle around the letter of the correct answer. Select reconstituted drugs for an IM injection with a 3-mL syringe.*

1 Ordered: morphine sulfate 6 mg. Available: morphine sulfate 10 mg/mL. What is the estimated dose?

  a. 0.06 mL   **c.** 1.2 mL

  b. 0.6 mL   **d.** 6 mL

2 Identify the difference between SW and bacteriostatic water, if any.

  a. Bacteriostatic water contains a preservative and may be used as a diluent only if the medication label so states.

  b. Both solutions are sterile and may be used interchangeably.

  c. SW may be used in place of bacteriostatic water.

  d. Both are bacteriostatic.

3 Examine the following dose concentrations. Which dilution would be most appropriate for a 10-mg IM dose? (Consider the volume to be administered.)

  a. Add 20 mL to make 1 mg per mL

  b. Add 10 mL to make 2 mg per mL

  c. Add 5 mL to make 5 mg per mL

  d. Add 1 mL to make 40 mg per mL

4 Parenteral mixes most often include which types of medications?

  a. A narcotic and another medication, for example, to control nausea

  b. Potassium and bacteriostatic sterile water for injection

  c. Two different kinds of antibiotics

  d. An intravenous medication and an intramuscular medication

5 Skin tests are administered via which route?

  a. Subcutaneous   **c.** Intramuscular

  b. Intradermal   **d.** Intravenous

6 The maximum amount of fluid that is recommended for one site for adult intramuscular injections is:

a. 1 mL

b. 2 mL

c. 3 mL

d. 5 mL

7 What is the first step the nurse must take after reading an order for a parenteral mix?

a. Estimate the doses.

b. Prepare each medication separately, maintaining sterile technique.

c. Evaluate the DA dose calculation against the estimated dose.

d. Check current drug literature for drug compatibility.

8 Examine the following dose concentrations. Which dilution would be appropriate for a 50-mg IM dose? (Consider the volume of the prepared dose.)

a. Add 10 mL to make 5 mg per mL

b. Add 8 mL to make 10 mg per mL

c. Add 5.6 mL to make 12 mg per mL

d. Add 3 mL to make 25 mg per mL

9 The most commonly used syringe size for intramuscular injections is:

a. 1 mL

b. 2 mL

c. 3 mL

d. 5 mL

10 Ordered: Butorphanol tartrate 1 mg ⎱ IM stat for a patient with a severe
Promethazine 10 mg ⎰ migraine headache

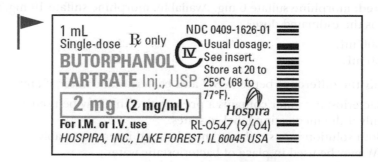

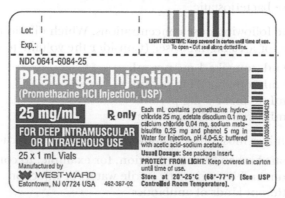

How many total milliliters will you administer?

a. 0.8 mL

b. 1.2 mL

c. 1.4 mL

d. 0.9 mL

ESTIMATED COMPLETION TIME: 1 hour   **ANSWERS ON:** page 294

DIRECTIONS: *Analyze the problems. Estimate and calculate the requested doses to the nearest tenth of a mL. Use a calculator for long division and multiplication. Evaluate your equations and answers on your own.*

1 Ordered: Olanzapine 6 mg ⎱ IM now for a patient exhibiting
               diphenhydramine 30 mg ⎰ combative behavior

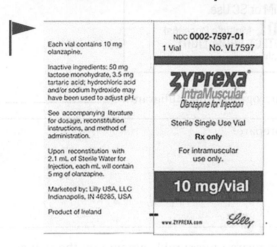

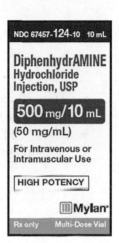

Olanzapine

a. Estimated dose: _____

b. How many mL will be prepared?

DA equation:

Evaluation: _____

Diphenhydramine

c. Estimated dose: _____

d. How many mL will be prepared?

DA equation:

Evaluation: _____

Total Combined Dose

e. Total dose in mL to nearest tenth: _____

Draw a vertical line through the nearest measurable amount on the syringe provided.

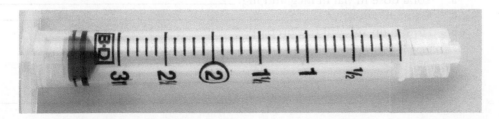

2 Ordered: cyanocobalamin 0.75 mg IM weekly × 1 month.

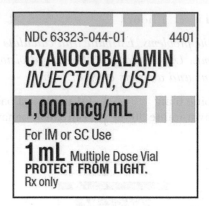

NDC 63323-044-01   4401

CYANOCOBALAMIN
INJECTION, USP

1,000 mcg/mL

For IM or SC Use
1 mL Multiple Dose Vial
PROTECT FROM LIGHT.
Rx only

a. Dose concentration in micrograms and milligrams: _____
b. Estimated dose: _____
c. How many mL will you prepare?

    DA equation:

Evaluation: _____

Draw an arrow pointing to the nearest measurable amount on the syringe provided.

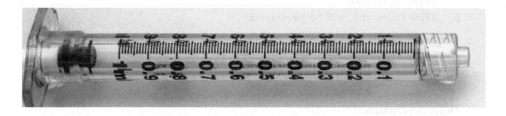

3 Ordered: Buprenex 250 mcg IM q6h for a patient with postoperative pain.

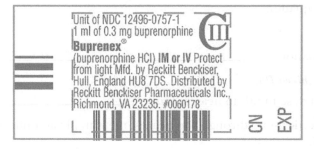

Unit of NDC 12496-0757-1
1 ml of 0.3 mg buprenorphine

Buprenex®
(buprenorphine HCl) **IM or IV** Protect
from light Mfd. by Reckitt Benckiser,
Hull, England HU8 7DS. Distributed by
Reckitt Benckiser Pharmaceuticals Inc.,
Richmond, VA 23235. #0060178

CN   EXP

a. Total dose in vial in mcg and mg: _____
b. Estimated dose: _____
c. How many mL will you prepare?

    DA equation:

Evaluation: _____

Draw a vertical line through the nearest measurable amount on the syringe provided.

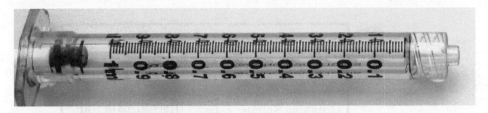

4 **Ordered:** streptomycin 0.3 g IM bid, an antibiotic, for a patient with an infection.

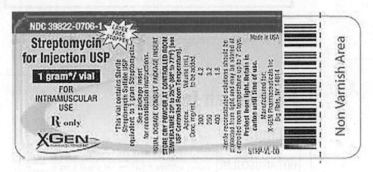

a. Total dose in vial: _____

b. Dose concentration after reconstitution: _____

c. Estimated dose: _____

d. How many mL will you prepare?

DA equation:

Evaluation: _____

Draw a vertical line through the nearest measurable amount on the syringe provided.

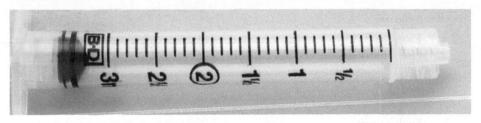

5 **Ordered:** morphine sulfate 7 mg ⎤
              promethazine 20 mg ⎦ IM for a patient with postoperative discomfort

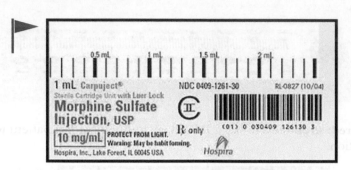

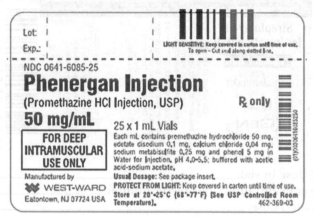

Morphine

a. Estimated dose: _____

b. How many mL will be prepared?

DA equation:

Evaluation: _____

Promethazine

c. Estimated dose: _____

d. How many mL will be prepared?

DA equation:

Evaluation: _____

Total Combined Dose

e. Total dose in mL to nearest tenth: _____

Draw a vertical line through the nearest measurable amount on the syringe
provided.

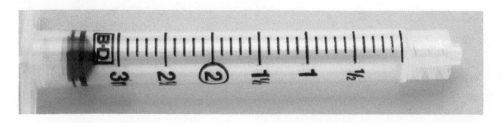

6 Ordered: metoclopramide 4 mg IM q4h to suppress chemotherapy-related nausea.

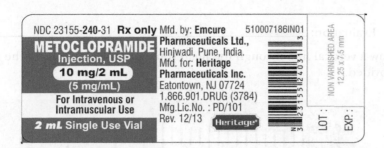

a. Estimated dose: _____

b. How many mL will be prepared?

   DA equation:

   Evaluation: _____

If estimated dose is confirmed, draw a vertical line through the nearest measurable amount on the syringe provided.

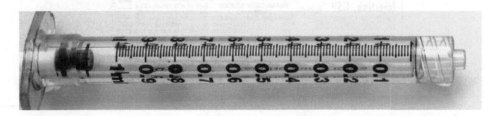

7 Ordered: phenobarbital sodium 0.1 g IM, a barbiturate, for a patient who needs sedation.

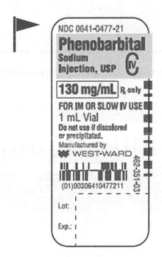

a. Total dose in vial: _____

b. Dose concentration: _____

c. Estimated dose: _____

d. How many mL will you prepare?

DA equation:

Evaluation: _____

Draw a vertical line through the nearest measurable amount on the syringe provided.

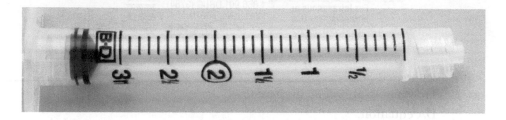

8 **Ordered:** penicillin G potassium 400,000 units IM q6h, an antibiotic, for a patient with an infection. Directions: Add 18 mL SW to make 250,000 units per mL.

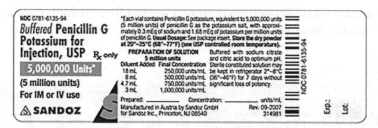

a. Total number of units in vial: _____
b. Dose concentration after reconstitution: _____
c. Estimated dose: _____
d. How many mL will you prepare?

DA equation:

Evaluation: _____

Draw a vertical line through the nearest measurable amount on the syringe provided.

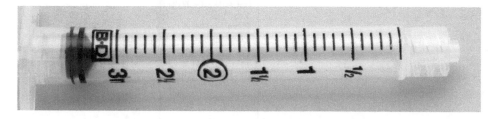

9 Ordered: haloperidol 35 mg
chlorpromazine 20 mg } IM stat for a patient with severe agitation

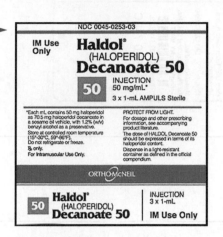

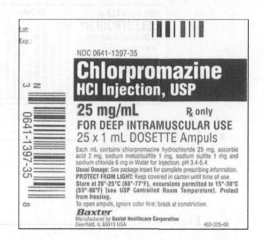

Haloperidol

a. Estimated dose: _____

b. How many mL will be prepared?

DA equation:

Evaluation: _____

Chlorpromazine

c. Estimated dose: _____

d. How many mL will be prepared?

DA equation:

Evaluation: _____

Total Combined Dose

e. Total dose in milliliters to nearest tenth: _____

Draw a vertical line through the nearest measurable amount on the syringe provided.

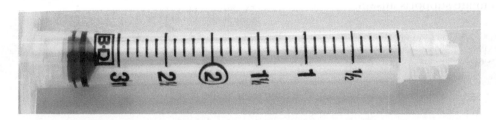

10 **Ordered:** estradiol valerate 25 mg IM × 1.

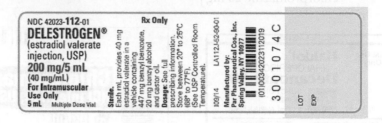

a. Estimated dose: _____

b. How many mL will you prepare?

DA equation:

Evaluation: _____

Draw a vertical line through the nearest measurable amount on the syringe provided.

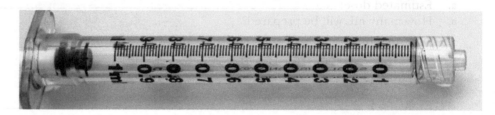

CHAPTER 8	ANSWER KEY

RAPID PRACTICE 8-1 (p. 270)

1 **a.** 15 mg per mL
b. give slightly more than 0.5 mL
c. 0.6 mL

$$\frac{mL}{dose} = \frac{1\ mL}{\underset{5}{\cancel{15\ mg}}} \times \frac{\overset{3}{\cancel{9\ mg}}}{dose} = \frac{3}{5} = \frac{0.6\ mL}{dose}$$

d. Equation is balanced. Estimate supports answer.

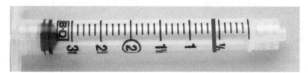

2 **a.** 0.5 mg per 2 mL

b. 0.125 mg is $\frac{1}{4}$ of 0.5 mg.
Give $\frac{1}{4}$ of 2 mL, or 0.5 mL.

c. 0.5 mL

$$\frac{mL}{dose} = \frac{\overset{4}{\cancel{2}}\ mL}{\underset{1}{\cancel{0.5\ mg}}} \times \frac{0.125\ \cancel{mg}}{dose} = \frac{0.5\ mL}{dose}$$

d. Equation is balanced. Estimate supports answer.

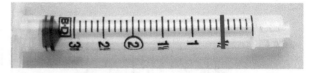

3 **a.** 5 mg per 1 mL
b. between 1 and 2 mL
c. 1.2 mL

$$\frac{mL}{dose} = \frac{1\ mL}{5\ \cancel{mg}} \times \frac{6\ \cancel{mg}}{dose} = \frac{1.2\ mL}{dose}$$

d. Equation is balanced. Estimate supports answer.

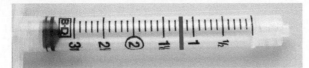

4   **a.** 4 mg per mL
   b. give one half or 0.5 mL
   c. 0.5 mL

$$\frac{mL}{dose} = \frac{1\ mL}{\underset{2}{\cancel{4\ mg}}} \times \frac{\overset{1}{\cancel{2\ mg}}}{dose} = \frac{1}{2} = \frac{0.5\ mL}{dose}$$

d. Equation is balanced. Estimate supports answer.

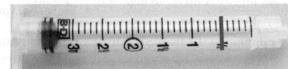

5   **a.** 250 mg per mL
   b. 0.15 g = 450 mg. Give almost 2 mL.
   c. 1.8 mL

$$\frac{mL}{dose} = \frac{1\ mL}{\underset{1}{\cancel{250\ mg}}} \times \frac{\overset{4}{\cancel{1000\ mg}}}{1\ \cancel{g}} \times \frac{0.45\ \cancel{g}}{dose}$$

$$= \frac{1.8\ mL}{dose}$$

d. Equation is balanced. Estimate supports answer.

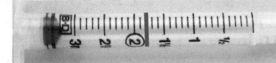

RAPID PRACTICE 8-2 (p. 274)

1   **a.** give between 3 mL and 4 mL
   b. 3.5 mL

$$\frac{mL}{dose} = \frac{\overset{1}{\cancel{4}}\ mL}{\underset{10}{\cancel{40\ mg}}} \times \frac{35\ \cancel{mg}}{dose} = \frac{35}{10} = \frac{3.5\ mL}{dose}$$

c. Equation is balanced. Estimate supports answer.

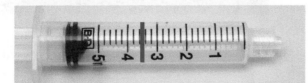

d. 0.2 mL

2

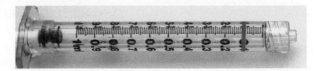

3   **a.** Give more than 2 mL. Two vials will be needed.
   b. 2.4 mL

$$\frac{mL}{dose} = \frac{2\ mL}{\underset{1}{\cancel{250\ mg}}} \times \frac{\overset{4}{\cancel{1000\ mg}}}{1\ \cancel{g}} \times \frac{0.3\ \cancel{g}}{dose}$$

$$= \frac{2.4\ mL}{dose}$$

c. Equation is balanced. Estimate supports answer.

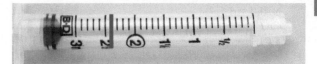

4   **a.** about 1.5 mL (will need two ampules)

   b. 1.5 mL

$$\frac{mL}{dose} = \frac{1\ mL}{1\ \cancel{mg}} \times \frac{1000\ \cancel{mg}}{1\ \cancel{g}} \times \frac{0.0015\ \cancel{g}}{dose} = \frac{1.5\ mL}{dose}$$

   c. Equation is balanced. Estimate supports answer.

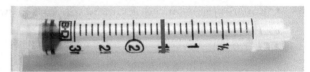

5   **a.** give less than 1 mL
   b. 0.75 mL

$$\frac{mL}{dose} = \frac{1\ mL}{0.4\ \cancel{mg}} \times \frac{0.3\ \cancel{mg}}{dose} = \frac{0.75\ mL}{dose}$$

c. Equation is balanced. Estimate supports answer.

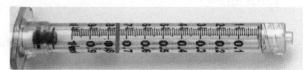

RAPID PRACTICE 8-3 (p. 278)

2   **a.** Prepare less than 1 mL.
   b. $\dfrac{mL}{dose} = \dfrac{1\ mL}{4\ \cancel{mg}} \times \dfrac{3\ \cancel{mg}}{dose}$

   $= 0.75$, rounded to $\dfrac{0.8\ mL}{dose}$ Dilaudid

   c. Equation is balanced. Estimate supports answer.
   d. Prepare less than 1 mL.

   e. $\dfrac{mL}{dose} = \dfrac{1\ mL}{\underset{5}{\cancel{50}}\ mg} \times \dfrac{\overset{1}{\cancel{10}}\ mg}{dose} = \dfrac{1}{5} = \dfrac{0.2\ mL}{dose}$

   f. Equation is balanced. Estimate supports answer.

g. 0.8 mL Dilaudid
<u>+ 0.2 mL Promethazine</u>
1.0 mL Total Volume

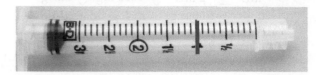

3 **a.** Give less than half of 1 mL.
b. 0.4 mL

$$\frac{mL}{dose} = \frac{1\ mL}{4\ mg} \times \frac{1.5\ mg}{dose}$$

$$= 0.37, \text{rounded to } \frac{0.4\ mL}{dose}\ \text{Dilaudid}$$

c. Equation is balanced. Estimate supports answer.
d. 1 mL
e. 1 mL

$$\frac{mL}{dose} = \frac{1\ mL}{0.4\ mg} \times \frac{0.4\ mg}{dose} = \frac{1\ mL}{dose}\ \text{Atropine}$$

f. Equation is balanced. Estimate supports answer.

g. 0.4 mL Dilaudid
<u>+ 1.0 mL Atropine</u>
1.4 mL Total Volume

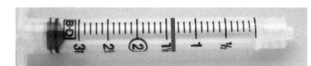

4 **a.** Prepare slightly less than 1 mL.
b. 0.8 mL

$$\frac{mL}{dose} = \frac{1\ mL}{\underset{5}{10\ mg}} \times \frac{\overset{4}{8\ mg}}{dose} = \frac{0.8\ mL}{dose}\ \text{Morphine}$$

c. Equation is balanced. Estimate supports DA equation.
d. Prepare about 2 mL.
e. 2 mL

$$\frac{mL}{dose} = \frac{5\ mL}{1\ mg} \times \frac{0.4\ mg}{dose} = \frac{2\ mL}{dose}\ \text{Glycopyrrolate}$$

f. Equation is balanced. Estimate supports DA equation.

g. 0.8 mL Morphine
<u>+ 2.0 mL Glycopyrrolate</u>
2.8 mL Total Volume

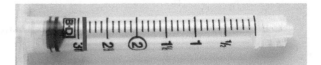

CHAPTER 8 MULTIPLE-CHOICE REVIEW (p. 283)

1	b	**8**	d
2	a	**9**	c
3	c	**10**	d (0.5 mL
4	a		Butorphanol
5	b		tartrate + 0.4 mL
6	c		Promethazine)
7	d (**Note:** This applies		= 0.9 mL

to IV fluids and
medications also.)

CHAPTER 8 FINAL PRACTICE (p. 285)

1 **a.** A little more than 1 mL
b. 1.2 mL

$$\frac{mL}{dose} = \frac{1\ mL}{5\ mg} \times \frac{6\ mg}{dose} = \frac{6}{5} = \frac{1.2\ mL}{dose}\ \text{Zyprexa}$$

Equation is balanced. Estimate supports answer.

c. A little more than $\frac{1}{2}$ mL

d. $\frac{mL}{dose} = \frac{10\ mL}{500\ mg} \times \frac{30\ mg}{dose} = \frac{300}{500} = \frac{0.6\ mL}{dose}$
$= 0.6$ mL diphenhydramine

Equation is balanced. Estimate supports answer.

e. 1.2 mL Zyprexa
<u>+ 0.6 mL diphenhydramine</u>
1.8 mL Total Volume

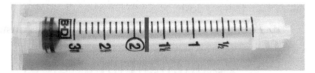

2 **a.** 1000 mcg per mL = 1 mg per mL
b. 0.75 mL (0.75 mg = 750 mcg)
c. 0.75 mL

$$\frac{mL}{dose} = \frac{1\ mL}{1000\ mcg} \times \frac{1000\ mcg}{1\ mg} \times \frac{0.75\ mg}{dose}$$
$$= \frac{0.75\ mL}{dose} = 0.75\ mL$$

Equation is balanced. Estimate supports answer.

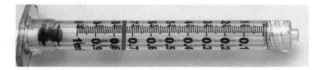

3 **a.** 0.3 mg = 300 mcg

b. A little more than $\frac{3}{4}$ of a mL.

$$\frac{mL}{dose} = \frac{1\ mL}{0.3\ \cancel{mg}} \times \frac{1\ \cancel{mg}}{\underset{4}{1000\ \cancel{mcg}}} \times \frac{\overset{1}{250\ \cancel{mcg}}}{dose} = \frac{1}{1.2}$$

$$= \frac{0.8333\ mL}{dose} = \text{rounded to } 0.83\ mL$$

Equation is balanced. Estimate supports answer.

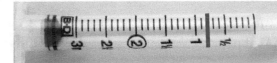

4 **a.** 1 g

b. 400 mg per mL

c. $\frac{3}{4}$ of a mL

d. 0.8 mL

$$\frac{mL}{dose} - \frac{1\ mL}{\underset{4}{400\ \cancel{mg}}} \times \frac{\overset{10}{1000\ \cancel{mg}}}{1\ \cancel{g}} \times \frac{0.3\ \cancel{g}}{dose}$$

$$= 0.75\ mL, \text{ rounded to } \frac{0.8\ mL}{dose}$$

Equation is balanced. Estimate supports answer.

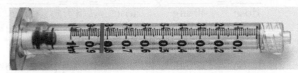

5 **a.** less than 1 mL

b. 0.7 mL

$$\frac{mL}{dose} = \frac{1\ mL}{10\ \cancel{mg}} \times \frac{7\ \cancel{mg}}{dose} = \frac{0.7\ mL}{dose}\ \text{Morphine}$$

Equation is balanced. Estimate supports answer.

c. less than $\frac{1}{2}$ mL

d. 0.4 mL

$$\frac{mL}{dose} = \frac{1\ mL}{\underset{5}{50\ \cancel{mg}}} \times \frac{\overset{2}{20\ \cancel{mg}}}{dose}$$

$$= \frac{0.4\ mL}{dose}\ \text{Promethazine}$$

Equation is balanced. Estimate supports answer.

e. 0.7 mL Morphine
+ 0.4 mL Promethazine
‾‾‾‾‾‾‾‾‾‾‾‾‾‾‾‾
   1.1 mL Total Volume

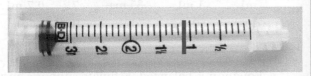

6 **a.** 0.8 mL

b. 0.8 mL

$$\frac{mL}{dose} = \frac{2\ mL}{\underset{5}{10\ \cancel{mg}}} \times \frac{\overset{2}{4\ \cancel{mg}}}{dose} = \frac{4}{5} = \frac{0.8\ mL}{dose}$$

$$= 0.8\ mL$$

Equation is balanced. Estimate supports answer.

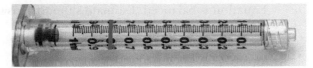

7 **a.** 130 mg

b. 130 mg per mL

c. Slightly less than 1 mL (0.1 g = 100 mg)

d. 0.8 mL

$$\frac{mL}{dose} = \frac{1\ mL}{\underset{13}{130\ \cancel{mg}}} \times \frac{\overset{100}{1000\ \cancel{mg}}}{1\ \cancel{g}} \times \frac{0.1\ \cancel{g}}{dose} = \frac{10}{13}$$

$$= 0.76\ mL, \text{ rounded to } \frac{0.8\ mL}{dose}$$

Equation is balanced. Estimate supports answer.

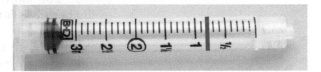

8 **a.** 5,000,000 units

b. 250,000 units per mL unit dose concentration

c. about 1.5 mL

d. 2 mL

$$\frac{mL}{dose} = \frac{1\ mL}{\underset{5}{250,000\ \cancel{units}}} \times \frac{\overset{8}{400,000\ \cancel{units}}}{dose}$$

$$= \frac{1.6\ mL}{dose}$$

Equation is balanced. Estimate supports answer.

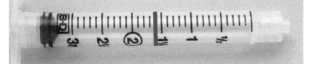

9 a. Slightly less than 1 mL

b. 0.7 mL

$$\frac{mL}{dose} = \frac{1\ mL}{\underset{10}{\cancel{50\ mg}}} \times \frac{\overset{7}{\cancel{35\ mg}}}{dose} = \frac{7}{10} = \frac{0.7\ mL}{dose}$$

$$= 0.7\ mL$$

Equation is balanced. Estimate supports answer.

c. Slightly less than 1 mL

d. 0.8 mL

$$\frac{mL}{dose} = \frac{1\ mL}{\underset{5}{\cancel{25\ mg}}} \times \frac{\overset{4}{\cancel{20\ mg}}}{dose} = \frac{4}{5} = \frac{0.8\ mL}{dose}$$

$$= 0.8\ mL$$

Equation is balanced. Estimate supports answer.

e. 0.7 + 0.8 mL = 1.5 mL Total Volume

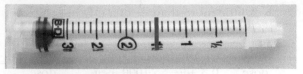

10 a. A little more than $\frac{1}{2}$ of an mL.

b. 0.63 mL

$$\frac{mL}{dose} = \frac{1\ mL}{\underset{8}{\cancel{40\ mg}}} \times \frac{\overset{5}{\cancel{25\ mg}}}{dose} = \frac{5}{8} = \frac{0.625\ mL}{dose}$$

$$= 0.625\ mL\ rounded\ to\ 0.63\ mL$$

Equation is balanced. Estimate supports answer.

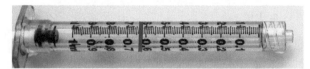

Suggestions for Further Reading

Clayton BD, Willihnganz M: *Basic pharmacology for nurses,* ed. 18, St. Louis, 2021, Mosby.

Lilley LL, Collins SR, Harrington S, Snyder JS: *Pharmacology and the nursing process,* ed. 9, St. Louis, 2021, Mosby.

Perry AG, Potter PA: *Clinical nursing skills and techniques,* ed. 10, St. Louis, 2021, Mosby.

www.cdc.gov/medicationsafety/program_focus_activities.html#3

www.drugs.com/drug_interactions.php

⊖volve For additional practice problems, refer to the Parenteral Dosages section of the Elsevier's Interactive Drug Calculation Application, Version 1 on Evolve.

Chapter 9 introduces basic intravenous flow rate calculations and the equipment used to deliver intravenous medications. These calculations are used daily in most clinical agencies. Much of the math needed to solve intravenous dose and rate problems has been covered in earlier chapters and can be applied to the intravenous route with some modifications.

9 Basic Intravenous Calculations

OBJECTIVES

- Interpret basic intravenous (IV) solution orders for peripheral infusion.
- Identify contents of commonly ordered IV fluids.
- Identify average flow rates for adults who are NPO and the general rationale for variations.
- Estimate, calculate, and verify flow rates for intermittent and continuous IV solutions with gravity and electronic devices.

- Calculate grams of dextrose and sodium chloride in IV fluids.
- Estimate and calculate the duration of flow for IV solutions in hours and minutes.
- Identify patient safety assessments related to IV solution therapy.

ESTIMATED TIME TO COMPLETE CHAPTER: 3 hours

Most patients receive at least one source of IV solution during a hospitalization. Monitoring the site and flow rate is a basic skill. Reporting concerns to the primary nurse is appropriate to protect the patient. Complications that a patient can incur are fluid overload or underdose, and tissue damage at the IV insertion site.

Basic IV calculations require only the simplest arithmetic. Examining each piece of IV equipment encountered in the laboratory and clinical agency and noting the key features, functions, similarities, and differences will expedite understanding.

➤ Be aware that IV equipment varies with facility purchase agreements.

➤ Patients may have some ability to monitor their therapy with oral medications because they may have knowledge and experience with them at home. However, patients are generally dependent on the nurse for safe IV administration. Life-threatening hazards from improper IV administration can occur more rapidly than from other, slower routes of absorption and may not be reversible.

VOCABULARY

Bolus	Fluids or concentrated medication solution given by IV route over a relatively brief period of time. Equipment used to deliver varies, depending on existing IV lines, volume, and time to be infused.
Continuous IV Infusion	IV solution that flows continuously (until further notice) as the name implies (e.g., dextrose 5% in water at 75 mL per hr). Patients who are NPO and surgical patients are two of the many types of patients who receive continuous infusions.

continued

VOCABULARY—cont'd

Drop Factor (DF)	Number of drops per milliliter (mL) delivered through various sizes of IV tubing. The tubing diameter affects the size of the drop. The DF is used to calculate flow rates on gravity administration sets. The abbreviation *gt(t)* was used for *gutta* (plural, guttae), the Latin word for *drop(s)*. It is an outdated apothecary term, but it may be seen on some prescriber's orders. It is recommended that the word *drops* be written out.
Electronic Infusion Pump	Electronic positive pressure pump that delivers fluid and/or medication at a preselected rate. Pumps have a variety of safety features that protect the patient from an unwanted bolus, running dry, or running at an infusion rate inconsistent with the usual administration of the medication or fluid.
Flow Rate	Rate at which fluid is delivered by IV infusion devices, in milliliters per hour (mL/hr).
Administration Set	This is another term for IV tubing; it may be used by gravity or with an electronic infusion pump.
Infusion Line, Primary	Main IV line or lines connected to the patient. Also called primary tubing on the IV administration set label. A patient may have more than one primary line. The first one is usually "dedicated" to fluid delivery and maintenance. Additional primary and secondary lines are usually reserved for medications or medicated solutions that are incompatible with other fluids.
Infusion Line, Secondary	Tubing that connects to ports on the primary line and permits an additional medication or fluid to be added without disruption of the primary line. Labels on the administration set indicate "secondary." ➤ Compatibility must be carefully checked before "mixing" a secondary medication into the primary line.
IV Injection Ports	An accessible port located on the IV line or IV solution container that permits access for injection of additional fluids or medications. A port adapter may also be attached directly to a cannula that is in a vein (also known as an IV lock, heparin lock, or saline lock).
Intermittent Infusions	Usually small-volume infusions (up to 250 mL) of IV solutions with medication added delivered at intervals. A variety of devices and methods are available, the most common being IV piggyback equipment, syringe pumps, and calibrated volume-control burette chambers.
IV Piggyback (IVPB)	Small-volume infusions, usually 50 to 250 mL, infused through a short secondary tubing line that is "piggybacked" to a port on a primary line. Intermittent infusions are delivered over 20 to 90 minutes, as specified by the pharmacy or pharmaceutical manufacturer.
IV Push	IV medication intermittent bolus dose of 1 to 50 mL, usually administered by manual direct injection with a syringe, sometimes via an infusion pump. ➤ It is occasionally written incorrectly as "IVP," which can be confused with the common abbreviation for the intravenous pyelogram (IVP) test. Also, do not confuse with IVPB (IV piggyback).
KVO, TKO	"Keep vein open" or "To keep open"; a flow rate order that may be given for a minimum rate that will keep the IV line patent and prevent coagulation. Some institutions specify a TKO rate in their standardized procedures.
Macrodrip	Gravity IV infusion tubing set that has a wide diameter to deliver large drops (most common is 10 drops per mL).
Microdrip	Gravity IV infusion tubing set that has a narrow diameter to deliver small drops and slower flow rates. Also known as pediatric tubing (most common is 60 drops per mL).
Osmolarity, Tonicity	Solute concentration in solution. The unit of measurement is the osmol. The milliosmol (mOs) is the unit of measurement in *plasma* and is used as a basis for comparison with the contents of IV solutions. *Isotonic* solutions, such as normal saline solution, 5% dextrose in water, and lactated Ringer's solution, approximate plasma osmolality. *Hyper*tonic solutions contain a higher number of milliosmols per liter and have higher tonicity. *Hypo*tonic solutions contain a lower number of milliosmols per liter and have lower tonicity.
Parenteral Fluids	Fluids administered outside of the digestive tract (e.g., IM, IV, subcutaneous).

Patency	State of being open and unblocked, such as a "patent IV site" or "patent airway." Sites are checked for patency during every visit to the bedside to ensure that the ordered fluids and medications are flowing into the vein and not into tissue.
PCA Pump	Patient-controlled analgesia pump. An electronic IV pump with a syringe or IV bag programmed to dispense prescribed amounts of analgesic narcotics at prescribed intermittent intervals with lockout intervals. Patients self-administer boluses of medication to control pain by remote push-button control.
Saline Lock	Resealable *access* device that permits additional IV lines or medications to be added into or on primary (main) IV tubing without initiating another injection site or disrupting the main IV line. Ports may also be indwelling venous cannulas that can be capped and kept patent with a saline or heparin (lock) flush solution and accessed when needed. The latter type of port frees the patient of the need to have IV solutions and tubing connected continuously.
Volume-Control Burette Device	Transparent, calibrated small-volume container, with a capacity of 100 to 150 mL, that is manually connected to an IV line just below the main IV solution container. It is filled with only 1 or 2 hours' worth of IV fluid and/or smaller amounts of medicated solution at a time. As the name implies, it protects at-risk patients from fluid or medication overload by limiting the total amount of solution available in case of equipment or a rate failure incident.

Overview of Intravenous Therapy

Oral medications and IV solutions that have medications added are the two most common routes of medication administration. The nursing responsibilities related to the patient's safety during oral and IV medication therapy are paramount.

Purpose of intravenous solutions

Intravenous solutions are ordered to:
- Provide daily maintenance fluid and electrolyte therapy.
- Replace prior fluid and electrolyte deficits.
- Administer medications and nutrients.

The fluids may contain dextrose solutions, electrolytes, medications, nutrients, or blood products as needed. They may be *isotonic, hypotonic,* or *hypertonic,* based on the prescriber's assessment of current laboratory test results and the patient's clinical needs.

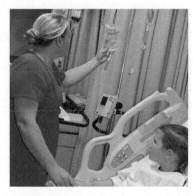

Nurse checking a primary maintenance IV solution.

Intravenous solutions are ordered to be either *continuous* or *intermittent,* depending on the patient's fluid and medication needs and fluid intake status. They are administered through peripheral or larger-diameter central veins. They are supplied in *nonvented plastic* or *vented* and nonvented glass containers.

Continuous IV lines are placed on *primary infusion administration lines. Intermittent* infusions are administered in a variety of ways but are frequently connected (piggybacked) to a port on a primary line via a *secondary* tubing set.

1	What are three purposes for ordering IV solutions? (Use one- or two-word answers.)	**ASK YOURSELF** **Q & A**
	_____	**MY ANSWER**

Maintenance intravenous flow rates

The average-sized adult patient who is to be NPO for a short period of time but is otherwise well hydrated, with good heart, lung, and renal function, may have a *maintenance isotonic* continuous IV solution ordered at about *75 to 125 mL per hr*. When an order calls for much less or more than this flow rate, the nurse needs to research the need for the variation. It is easier to keep in mind an average of about 1 L q8h or 2 to 3 L q24h for the hypothetical hydrated adult who is NPO for a limited period of time. Often, the reason for variation is obvious: fever, bleeding, diarrhea, etc.

CLINICAL RELEVANCE

A dehydrated patient will receive a higher-than-average volume and flow rate, depending on their clinical tolerance. A patient with compromised heart, lung, or renal function or a baby will receive a lower-than-average flow rate. The more the patient is able to drink, the less the need for a high flow rate or a continuous IV infusion. Even if the patient is able to take 2 to 3 L of fluid a day by mouth, an IV access line is frequently established and "saline locked" in order to provide prompt access for IV medications or fluids if needed.

Q & A **ASK YOURSELF**

1 What are examples of the patient-related criteria that the prescriber uses to make an informed decision about the flow rate for an IV order? (Give a brief answer.)

MY ANSWER _____

2 What are the main purposes of a primary line, a secondary line, and a port?

_____

_____

3 What is an average range of isotonic maintenance solution flow rates that might be ordered for a maintenance IV for an adult patient who is NPO and has good heart, lung, and renal function?

_____

Basic Intravenous Equipment

The essential elements of infusion equipment are:
- A prescribed solution with or without medication added
- A pole or stand to hold the solution and delivery devices
- Infusion pump(s)
- Infusion tubing of various sizes and types to connect the solution to the access device, needle, or needleless port
- Dressings and tape to protect and secure the injection site

CLINICAL RELEVANCE

Safety trends pertaining to IV equipment include increasing use of premixed medicated IV solutions supplied by the pharmacy or the manufacturer; needleless equipment; and sophisticated electronic IV pump(s) that are capable of extensive programming of medication libraries, alarms, drug doses, and flow rates. Many times patients will have multiple infusion pumps to handle their many IV fluid and medication needs. A patient in the ICU may have five or more infusion pumps at one time.

Types of Intravenous Solutions

There are many types of IV solutions. The contents depend on the purpose of the IV order, the condition of the patient, the laboratory test results, the hydration and fluid and electrolyte status of the patient, and compatible parenteral medications that need to be added to the solution.

The following are some of the most frequently ordered solutions to which medications can be added if necessary. Their names and abbreviations must be learned. Dextrose (D), normal saline (NS) solution, water (W), and lactated Ringer's (L/R) solution may contain varying percentages of dextrose or electrolytes. The nurse needs to focus on the percentage of contents ordered and match that with the label.

➤ A number indicates the percent of grams of solute per 100 mL; for example, D5 = 5% dextrose or 5 grams of dextrose per 100 mL of solution.

Tonicity of Intravenous Solutions

➤ Examine and learn the names and contents of the isotonic solutions *first*. Then contrast the isotonic solution with the selected hypotonic and hypertonic solutions.

Hypotonic	Isotonic (290 mOs)	Hypertonic
	5% dextrose in water (D5W)	10% dextrose in water or (D10W)
0.45% NaCl (sodium chloride) solution (0.45NS, $\frac{1}{2}$ NS)	Normal saline (NS) solution (0.9% NaCl solution)	D5W in 0.45% NaCl solution or D5W in $\frac{1}{2}$ NS
	Lactated Ringer's solution (RL, or LR)	D5LR
		D5NS or D5W in 0.9% NaCl solution

Additives such as vitamins, minerals, potassium chloride (KCl), and many other medications may be ordered for inclusion in these solutions. Figure 9-1 shows labels of selected isotonic solutions.

ASK YOURSELF

1 Which type of solution most closely approximates the tonicity of plasma: hypotonic, isotonic, or hypertonic? Refer to "Osmolarity" in the Essential Vocabulary.

_____

MY ANSWER

2 How does the percentage of solute in hypotonic and hypertonic solutions differ from that in isotonic solutions? (Give a brief answer and refer to Essential Vocabulary if necessary.)

_____

FAQ   *Why is $\frac{1}{2}$ NS labeled 0.45% rather than 0.5% NaCl?*

ANSWER   Because it contains half the NaCl content of NS solution. NS solution contains 0.9%, not 1%, NaCl.

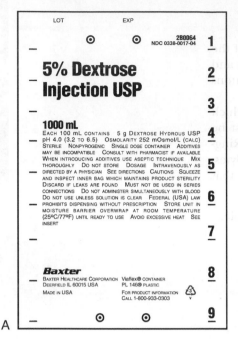

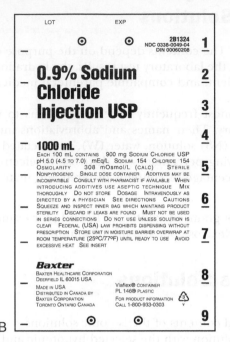

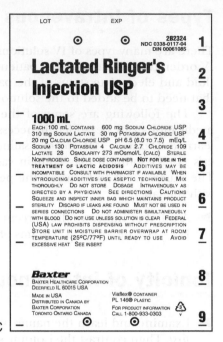

FIGURE 9-1 Labels of isotonic solutions. **A,** 5% dextrose. **B,** 0.9% sodium chloride. **C,** Lactated Ringer's solution.

➤ All IV solutions and medications must be checked for compatibility using a current drug reference before being administered. When in doubt, the nurse should consult the pharmacy.

Q & A	**ASK YOURSELF**	1	What are five types of equipment needed for all IV infusions?
	MY ANSWER		_____
			_____

Intravenous Solution Volume

Volumes of solution per IV container are usually 500 or 1000 mL for maintenance and continuous solutions. Some solutions that have medications added are provided in 50-, 100-, and 250-mL containers.

If the order calls for a liter, the nurse selects a 1000-mL container. Often, the order for a continuous IV infusion states only the name of the solution and the flow rate per hour. The nurse selects the volume for the infusion that will last a reasonable amount of time.

Intravenous Solution Orders for Milliliters per Hour

➤ One calculation needed for *all* infusions so that flow rate can be monitored is a determination of the number of milliliters per hour (mL per hr).

The following are two typical orders for a *continuous* IV infusion:

Order	Meaning
1000 mL D5W at 125 mL per hr	1 Liter of 5% dextrose in water to flow at a rate of 125 mL per hour until further notice
1 liter L/R solution q8h	1000 mL of lactated Ringer's solution every 8 hours

- Identify the ordered flow rate in mL per hr and any special instructions.
- Determine how long the IV solution will last.
  The calculations are usually very basic.
- If the prescriber orders D5W at 125 mL per hr, the nurse administers a *continuous* flow rate of *125 mL per hr* until the order is discontinued or changed. The equipment may vary and require further calculations, but the essential rate in mL per hr must be known.
- If the prescriber orders 1 L D5W q8h, the flow rate is derived with a simple calculation:

$$\frac{mL}{hr} = \frac{1000 \text{ mL}}{8 \text{ hr}} = 125 \text{ mL per hr}$$

- Milliliters and hours are both desired in the answer. This distinguishes hours from minutes or other time frames that may be ordered. The *initial* entry in the equation setup is the matched units in the numerator (milliliters). Hours (hr) must be entered in a denominator.
- Flow rates are rounded to the nearest whole number unless medications have been added. When medications have been added frequently, the rate will be rounded to the nearest tenth or hundredth, depending on the facility's policy.

---

1 What is the one calculation that is needed for all infusion rates?   **ASK YOURSELF**

_____   **MY ANSWER**

Determining Infusion Durations

- If the order states *1 L q8h,* it is obvious that the IV infusion will require replacement in 8 hours. If the order states only the mL per hour, a simple calculation is required.

If the order states mL per hr such as *120 mL per hr,* and a liter (1000 mL) will be supplied: **EXAMPLES**
  1. Determine the hours of duration first (total mL ÷ mL per hr)
  2. Convert any remainder of hours to minutes using a conversion factor:
     60 minutes = 1 hr (60 × hr = minutes).

$$hr = \frac{1 \text{ hr}}{120 \text{ mL}} \times \frac{1000 \text{ mL}}{1} = 8.3 \text{ hr}$$

$$minutes = \frac{60 \text{ minutes}}{1 \text{ hr}} \times \frac{0.3 \text{ hr}}{1} = 18 \text{ min}$$

Total expected duration of 1000 mL flowing at 120 mL per hr = 8 hr and 18 min.

CLINICAL RELEVANCE

Calculating the duration of an infusion helps the nurse to know when to prepare the next infusion (i.e., *before* the current one runs dry) or when to discontinue the infusion. If an infusion runs dry, the site can occlude, requiring the patient to have a new site established.

✳ *Communication*

After patient identification, patient education should occur regarding the general purpose of the IV fluid or medication. "Mr. Smith, your doctor has ordered some fluids and (name) medications in your vein to help your (state the condition)." It is better to say "help" than "prevent." Accentuate the positive. "Have you had an IV before? How did it go?" or "How did you do with it?" "Do you have any allergies to these medications or any other medications? What kind of reaction did you have?" *Listen carefully* to the patient's responses to these questions.

Calculating milliliter per hour (mL per hr) orders

Experienced nurses calculate simple orders, such as 1 L q8h, by converting 1 L to 1000 mL and performing simple division, 1000 mL ÷ 8 (total volume of the container divided by hours) yields a flow rate of 125 mL per hr.

➤ When the question is: "How many mL per hr?" Think of *per* as a *division line:*

$$\text{total milliliters} \div \text{total hours} = \frac{\text{mL}}{\text{hr}}.$$

➤ Always double-check your answers.

Check agency policy pertaining to IV solution, tubing, and IV catheter replacement. Some solutions need to be changed every 24 hours, others every 48 hours. The Joint Commission requires facilities to have replacement guidelines. The product label may indicate an expiration date, but the facility policy may be far more stringent once the IV solution has been opened for use.

Q & A ASK YOURSELF	1	What are the abbreviations for three commonly ordered isotonic IV solutions?
MY ANSWER		_____

 RAPID PRACTICE 9-1 | Flow Rates and Infusion Times for Intravenous Solutions

ESTIMATED COMPLETION TIME: 15 to 20 minutes   **ANSWERS ON:** page 342

DIRECTIONS: *Using the flow rate supplied, fill in the abbreviations for the* solution *ordered, the flow rate in mL per hr, the nearest whole number, and the infusion time in hours and minutes, if applicable.*

Order	Abbreviation(s) for Solution	Flow Rate (mL per hr)	Infusion Time, Hours (and Minutes, If Applicable)
1	250 mL half-strength normal saline q4h	_____	_____	_____
2	Infuse 500 mL normal saline over 6 hr	_____	_____	_____
3	1 L lactated Ringer's q10h	_____	_____	_____
4	500 mL 5% dextrose in lactated Ringer's at 40 mL per hr	_____	_____	_____
5	1000 mL 5% dextrose in water at 125 mL per hr	_____	_____	_____

FAQ *How do I know which size, in milliliters, of IV bag to select?*

ANSWER There are three criteria:

- Infusion time
- Flow rate ordered
- Solutions available or supplied

The commonly available solutions are packaged in amounts of 250, 500, and 1000 mL. Smaller amounts, including medicated solutions, are also supplied by the pharmacy. If the infusion is to last 8 hours and the flow rate is 100 mL per hr, 800 mL would be the minimum needed. The closest amount that can be selected would be a 1000-mL bag. If the solution is to infuse at 50 mL per hr continuously, most nurses will select a bag that contains at least enough to last for an 8- or 12-hour shift: 50 mL × 8 = 400 mL, or 50 mL × 12 = 600 mL. The nurse would probably select a 500- or 1000-mL bag even for the 50 mL per 8 hr order, assuming that the IV infusion would be reordered.

Electronic Infusion Pumps

Electronic infusion pumps are used for most IV infusions, particularly solutions that contain medications and nutrients. Technological advances to reduce intravenous infusion errors have resulted in the development of increasingly sophisticated infusion equipment known as "smart pumps" (Figure 9-2). In addition to programmable flow rates, electronic infusion pumps contain software with drug libraries, data logs, and customized safe medication dose, rate, and concentration limit alarms that are customized for the patient. They are also programmed to sound an alarm to prevent free flow accidents resulting in fluid overloads.

CLINICAL RELEVANCE

It is essential for the nurse to verify that the infusion pump is programmed for the right dosage, at the right rate and volume to be infused. This is especially important at a change of shift, when any change is made to the infusion pump settings, a new bag of medication/fluid is hung, or new infusion tubing is primed.

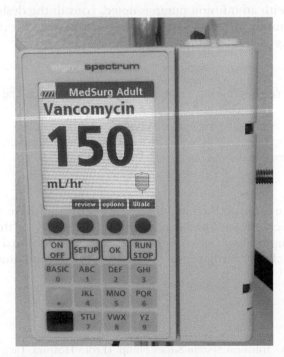

FIGURE 9-2 Sigma Spectrum Infusion System Smart Pump.

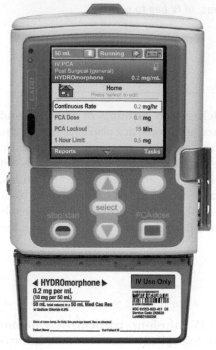

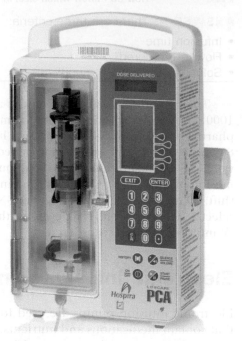

FIGURE 9-3 CADD Solis PCA Ambulatory Infusion Pump. (From Smiths Medical, Dublin, OH.)

FIGURE 9-4 Life Care PCA. (From Hospira, Inc., Lake Forest, IL.)

➤ With smart pump equipment, there can still be failures leading to adverse drug events, including mechanical failure, programming errors, data entry errors, and failure to double-check the prescriber's orders. Lack of knowledge about the contents of the IV, reason for the specific order, or about operation of the equipment can cause an error. Nurses need to be very familiar with the safe operation of the infusion equipment as well as agency infusion policies and procedures (Figures 9-3 and 9-4).

➤ If a problem with an infusion pump is noted, consult the designated agency resources promptly for assistance. Follow agency policies for defective equipment, e.g., tagging and prompt removal.

CLINICAL RELEVANCE

Obtain an independent double-check of infusion pump settings by a second nurse (per facility policy) when infusing high-risk medications such as insulin, heparin, total parenteral nutrition (TPN), morphine, and dilaudid (Figure 9-5). An independent double-check involves two nurses separately checking (alone and apart from each other, then comparing results) the infusion settings in accordance with the physician's order.

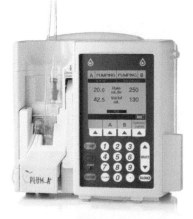

➤ Nurses need to monitor the patient for signs of over-infusion or under-infusion, particularly with high-risk medications. Observing the patient and monitoring vital signs are essential. The use of additional monitoring equipment such as a cardiac monitor, pulse oximetry, and glucose meter can be helpful.

FIGURE 9-5 Plum A+ Infusion System Smart Pump. (From Hospira, Inc., Lake Forest, IL.)

Gravity Infusions

Gravity infusions are used far less frequently than in the past. Outpatient centers, emergency vehicles, outpatient recovery units, home-care settings, rehabilitation units, and long-term care units are examples of places where gravity infusions may be encountered.

Gravity infusions are hung on a pole approximately 36 inches above the heart level of the patient. The flow rate is dependent on the flow rate control clamp adjustment, positioning of the solution, tubing patency, and the patient's position.

Intravenous Administration Sets

Intravenous tubing provides the connection between the IV solution and the patient. The nurse selects the tubing needed based on the order and the infusion equipment provided by the agency.

➤ The physician does not specify the equipment. Some tubing administration sets may be used interchangeably on infusion pumps and gravity devices. The tubing is supplied in various internal diameters to accommodate various flow rates and solution viscosities.

There are several types of specialized IV tubing. The main types include:
- Primary (main) tubing for "main" and "maintenance" IV lines, electronic infusion pumps, and gravity infusions (see Figure 9-6, *A*)
- Secondary, *shorter* tubing that connects to the primary tubing at a port to permit additional intermittent solutions to be added (piggybacked)

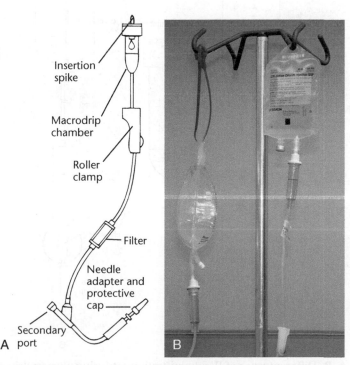

FIGURE 9-6 A, Gravity flow intravenous infusion equipment. (From Willihnganz M, Gurevitz S, Clayton B: *Clayton's Basic pharmacology for nurses,* ed 18, St Louis, 2020, Elsevier.)

without having to create an additional IV site on the patient (see Figure 9-6, *B*)

- Blood administration sets with special filters and a Y connector for NS solution to prime the lines before and flush after the blood transfusion or to use if the blood needs to be stopped or removed for any reason
- Extension tubings that are used when more length is needed (e.g., for ambulation)

A needle adapter with a cap, tubing, a clamp to stop and start the flow, a drip chamber, and an insertion spike are included in the administration sets.

Infusion Administration Sets for Gravity Infusions

For gravity infusions, the nurse selects the calibration of tubing needed based on the equipment available, the flow rate ordered, and the contents of the IV solution. The drop factor (DF) is listed on the tubing administration set. Figure 9-7 illustrates a DF of 60 (60 drops per mL).

Macrodrip (large-diameter) tubing usually has a drop factor (DF) of 10 and is selected for plain solutions, solutions requiring faster flow rates, solutions that have less powerful medications added, and solutions that are used on an infusion pump. A few manufacturers still make tubing with a DF of 15 and 20, but they are rarely used.

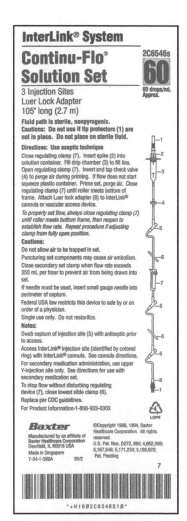

FIGURE 9-7 Packaging showing a drop factor of 60.

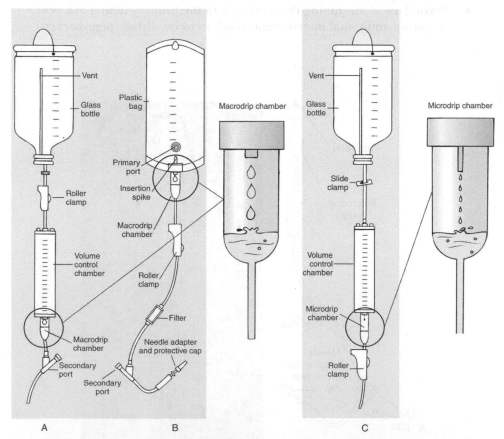

FIGURE 9-8 **A, B,** Different types of IV administration sets using a macrodrip chamber. **C,** An administration set using a microdrop chamber. (From Willihnganz M, Gurevitz S, Clayton B: *Clayton's Basic pharmacology for nurses,* ed 18, St Louis, 2020, Elsevier.)

Microdrip tubing (also known as pediatric tubing) has a DF of 60 and narrow tubing that delivers tiny drops from a *needle-like* projection to achieve 60 drops per mL. Because of the projection, microdrip sets can be recognized at a glance without having to go to a supply room to check the DF (Figure 9-8, *C*).

➤ Agency policies must be checked for regulations pertaining to choice of IV equipment. If a solution has medication added, it may be required to be on an electronic infusion pump.

Calculating Flow Rates for Gravity Infusions

The flow rate for simple gravity devices that consist of only an IV solution and tubing is derived from the number of mL per hr ordered and is delivered in *drops per minute*. The drop-per-minute rate is calculated by the nurse. The nurse adjusts the flow rate with a hand-operated slide pinch or roller clamp (Figure 9-9).

To convert mL per hr to drops per minute, identify the following factors:

1 Number of mL per hr ordered

2 Calibration (DF, or drops per milliliter) of the selected tubing administration set, stated on the administration set package: 10, 15, 20, or 60.

When the drop-per-minute count is correct, the flow rate will deliver an *approximate equivalent* of the number of mL per hr ordered.

The nurse needs to assess IV sites and flow rates during each visit to the bedside and/or every hour or more often. Check agency policies.

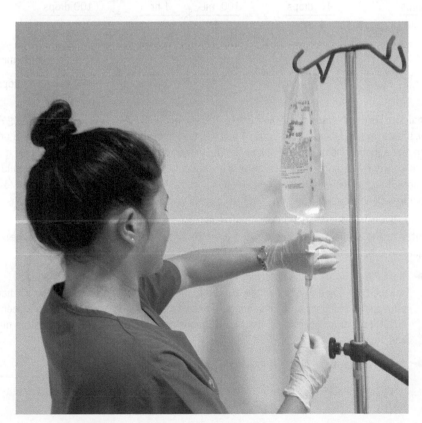

FIGURE 9-9 Nurse adjusting flow of IV gravity infusion.

Calculation of Gravity Infusion Rates

EXAMPLES

Ordered: IV D5W 1000 mL at 100 mL per hr or 1 L D5W q10h. How many drops per minute will the nurse set on the gravity infusion set?
- Identify the *mL per hour* to be infused: 100 mL per hr
- DF from the IV administration set: 10 drops per mL.

➤ Note that 10 drops per mL × 100 mL per hr ordered = 1000 drops per hr. The nurse cannot count the drops for an hour to see if the rate is correct. The nurse wants to know the count for 1 minute that would result in the desired number of drops per hour.

- Enter the data in a DA equation along with an hr-to-minute conversion.

All the data can be entered in *one* equation (when the number of mL per hr is known) to obtain the number of drops per minute. Examine the example that follows.

EXAMPLES

Ordered: IV D5W 1000 mL at 100 mL per hr
Drop factor (DF): 10 (10 drops per mL)
(The DF is found on the tubing administration set.)
The nurse will set the flow rate for how many drops per minute (min)?

Step 1	=	Step 2	×	Step 3	=	Answer
Desired Answer Units	=	Starting Factor	×	Given Quantity and Conversion Factor(s)	=	Estimate, Multiply, Evaluate
$\dfrac{\text{drops}}{\text{min}}$	=	$\dfrac{\overset{1}{\cancel{10}}\ \text{drops}}{1\ \cancel{\text{mL}}}$	×	$\dfrac{100\ \cancel{\text{mL}}}{1\ \cancel{\text{hr}}} \times \dfrac{1\ \text{hr}}{\underset{6}{\cancel{60}}\ \text{min}}$	=	$\dfrac{100\ \text{drops}}{6\ \text{min}}$
					=	$16\dfrac{2}{3}$ drops per min, rounded to 17 drops per min

Analysis: We need a *rate, drops,* and *time* in the answer. Once again, the selected Starting Factor, the conversion factor of 10 drops in 1 mL, was the factor containing the desired answer units. The rate and time factor was 100 mL per hr. The only time available was *hour,* so we used it and then converted hours to minutes. The rest of the factors were entered so that they could be canceled sequentially starting with mL. Drops has to be in a numerator and minutes has to appear in a denominator.

Evaluation: Only the desired answer units remain. Our estimate of about 1/6 of 100 is supported by the answer (Math check: 100 ÷ 6 = 16 2/3, rounded to 17 drops per minute). The equation is balanced. Note that once again, cancellation makes the math simple.

➤ Note the 1000 mL in the order was not needed. Rate, drops, and time were already selected. If we had also added the 1000 mL somewhere in the equation, mL would have appeared three times and could not have been canceled. The answer would have been 17,000 mL drops per minute; however, 60 drops per minute is about as fast as the nurse can count.

➤ Be aware that some orders still use the outdated abbreviation "gtt" for drops.

RAPID PRACTICE 9-2	Flow Rates for Gravity Infusions

ESTIMATED COMPLETION TIME: 15 minutes   **ANSWERS ON:** page 342

DIRECTIONS: *Examine the example on p. 306 and the example in problem 1. For problems 2 to 5, identify the number of mL per hr and the drop factor. Calculate the flow rates to the nearest whole drop per minute for the ordered solutions. Evaluate the equation.*

➤ Remember that the DF is in drops per 1 mL. The DF and the number of mL per hr ordered must be entered in the equation.

1   **Ordered:** IV 500 mL to infuse over 4 hours on a gravity infusion. Administration set DF: 15.

   a. How many mL per hr are ordered? mL per hr = 500 ÷ 4 = 125 mL/hr

   b. How many drops per minute will be set?

   DA equation:

$$\frac{\text{drops}}{\text{minute}} = \frac{\overset{1}{\cancel{15}} \text{ drops}}{1 \text{ }\cancel{mL}} \times \frac{125 \text{ }\cancel{mL}}{1 \text{ }\cancel{hour}} \times \frac{1 \text{ }\cancel{hour}}{\underset{4}{\cancel{60}} \text{ minute}} = 31.25, \text{ rounded to 31 drops/minute}$$

   c. Evaluation: The equation is balanced. The desired answer units are the only ones remaining. (Milliliters and hours had to be entered twice in order to be canceled.) All drops per minute equations use an hour-to-minutes conversion formula.

   ➤ Note that 500 mL total volume was not needed in the equation because the mL per hr was known. You can enter $\dfrac{500 \text{ mL}}{4 \text{ hr}}$ for the same result.

2   **Ordered:** IV 100 mL to infuse at 10 mL per hr. The drop factor is 60.

   a. How many hours will it last? _____

   b. How many drops per minute will be set? _____

   DA equation:

   c. Evaluation: _____

3   **Ordered:** IV 500 mL to infuse over 6 hours. Administration set DF: 20.

   a. How many mL per hr are ordered? _____

   b. How many drops per minute will be set? _____

   DA equation:

   c. Evaluation: _____

4   **Ordered:** IV 250 mL to infuse at 75 mL per hr. Administration set DF: 10.

   a. How many mL per hr are ordered? _____

   b. How many drops per minute will be set? _____

   DA equation:

   c. Evaluation: _____

5   **Ordered:** IV 1000 mL q12h on a gravity infusion device. Administration set DF: 20.

    a.   How many mL per hr are ordered? _____

    b.   How many drops per minute will be set? _____

    DA equation:

    c.   Evaluation: _____

Estimating drops per minute for a drop factor of 60

Equations must be set up for DFs of 10, 15, and 20 and can be set up for DF 60.

➤ Drop factors of 60, for microdrip pediatric administration sets, do *not* require equations *when the number of mL per hr is known.* Because a DF of 60 divided by 60 minutes provides a factor of 1, the number of mL per hr = the number of drops per minute. Study the example that follows.

EXAMPLES

Ordered: IV 50 mL to infuse over 1 hour, with a DF of 60.

$$\frac{\text{drops}}{\text{minute}} = \frac{\cancel{60}\text{ drops}}{1\ \cancel{mL}} \times \frac{50\ \cancel{mL}}{1\ \cancel{hr}} \times \frac{1\ hr}{\cancel{60}\text{ minutes}} = 50\text{ drops per minute}$$

Note how the quantity 60 in the *numerator* and the quantity 60 in the *denominator* are canceled, leaving only the 50 mL per hr. Thus, 50 mL per hr = 50 drops per min.

Microdrip (60 DF) flow rate in drops per minute = mL/hr.

➤ 60 DF = mL per hr applies only to *continuous infusions* or those that are to infuse for *60 minutes* or more.

Q & A   **ASK YOURSELF**

1   How many drops per minute would I estimate if the infusion was ordered for 30 mL per hr and the DF was 60?

MY ANSWER   _____

2   If the DF on the tubing administration is known to be 60 and the order is for 20 mL per hr, how many drops per minute would I estimate for the gravity device?

_____

➤ Microdrip tubing is used for low flow rates up to and including 60 drops per min (60 mL per hr). It is too difficult to count a faster drop flow than 1 drop per sec, or 60 drops per min.

➤ You will encounter the abbreviation gtt for the word *drops* in some written orders and printed literature.

RAPID PRACTICE 9-3	Calculating Flow Rates

ESTIMATED COMPLETION TIME: 20 to 25 minutes   **ANSWERS ON:** page 343

DIRECTIONS: *Calculate the flow rate in mL per hr or drops per minute depending on the equipment. Round all mL per hr and drops per minute to the nearest whole number. Label all answers in mL per hr or drops per minute, as appropriate for the equipment available.*

1   **Ordered:** 250 mL 0.45 NS at 25 mL per hr. Equipment: gravity infusion set with macrodrip tubing, DF 15.

   a.   Calculated flow rate:

      DA equation:

   b.   Evaluation: _____

   c.   Is the flow rate reasonable for counting drops per minute?
      Yes or No? _____

2   **Ordered:** 1000 mL D5LR at 100 mL per hr. Equipment: gravity infusion set with macrodrip tubing, DF 20.

   a.   Calculated flow rate:

      DA equation:

   b.   Evaluation: _____

   c.   Is the flow rate reasonable for counting drops per minute?
      Yes or No? _____

3   **Ordered:** 600 mL NS q8h to be infused continuously on an EID.
   What flow rate will the nurse set? (Use simple arithmetic.) _____

4   **Ordered:** 1000 mL LR at 80 mL per hr. Equipment: gravity infusion device with a DF 10.

   a.   Calculated flow rate:

      DA equation:

   b.   Evaluation: _____

   c.   Is the flow rate reasonable for counting drops per minute?
      Yes or No? _____

5   **Ordered:** 500 mL D5W at 25 mL per hr. Equipment: pediatric microdrip administration set for gravity infusion with a DF 60 (60 drops per mL).

   a.   What is the estimated flow rate? (Use mental calculation.) Label the answer. _____

   b.   Calculated flow rate:

      DA equation:

   c.   Evaluation: _____

➤ Remember that calculations of IV flow rates begin with examination of the prescriber's order to be able to determine milliliters for mL per hr. IV calculations require this value, not just for further calculations, but also to evaluate flow rate at the bedside.

ASK YOURSELF 1 If a flow rate is 50 mL per hr using a microdrip (pediatric) set, how many drops per minute will I set? (Use mental arithmetic.)

MY ANSWER _____

2 Noting that the DF denotes the number of drops per milliliter, which of three *macrodrip* sets—10, 15, and 20—would deliver the largest drop and therefore be suitable for a fastest rate of flow of more viscous fluids, such as blood products?

_____

➤ Remember that the microdrip set is selected for flow rates up to 60 drops per min.

Counting drops per minute

The nurse counts the drops at eye level for 15 or 30 seconds or 1 minute to ensure that the IV solution is flowing at the appropriate rate (Figure 9-10). The slower the rate, the longer the needed counting period. Multiply the 15-second count by 4 and the 30-second count by 2 to obtain the drops per minute.

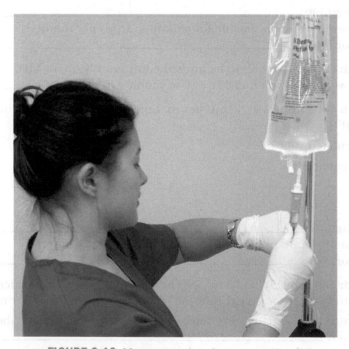

FIGURE 9-10 Nurse counting drops at eye level.

RAPID PRACTICE 9-4 | Gravity Infusion Rates

ESTIMATED COMPLETION TIME: 20 to 25 minutes   **ANSWERS ON:** page 343

DIRECTIONS: *Use DA equations to calculate the flow rates. Remember that gravity infusion calculations include an "hour-to-minute" conversion. Use mental calculations for continuous microdrip calculations.*

1 **Ordered:** IV D5NS at 100 mL per hr, DF 10 administration set selected.

   a. Flow rate will be set at _____

      DA equation:

   b. Evaluation: _____

2 **Ordered:** IV 0.45% NaCl sol at 120 mL per hr, DF 10 administration set selected.

   a. Flow rate will be set at _____

      DA equation:

   b. Evaluation: _____

3 **Ordered:** IV LR at 125 mL per hr, DF 15 administration set selected.

   a. Flow rate will be set at _____

      DA equation:

   b. Evaluation: _____

4 **Ordered:** IV D5W (continuous) at 10 mL per hr, DF 60.

   a. What flow rate will the nurse set? (Use mental calculation.) _____

   b. Is this a macrodrip or microdrip tubing factor? _____

   c. How can the nurse tell at a glance if a tubing factor is macrodrip or microdrip when it is infusing? _____

5 **Ordered:** IV D10W at 75 mL per hr, DF 20 administration set selected.

   a. Flow rate will be set at _____

      DA equation:

   b. Evaluation: _____

---

1 What does the DF on the gravity tubing mean exactly in terms of a milliliter?

ASK YOURSELF **Q & A**

MY ANSWER

2 Which is the DF of the narrowest tubing that delivers the smallest drops and therefore delivers the greatest number of drops per milliliter?

_____

| **RAPID PRACTICE 9-5** | Gravity Infusion Flow Rates |

ESTIMATED COMPLETION TIME: 15 minutes   **ANSWERS ON:** page 344

DIRECTIONS: *Use the hourly flow rate to calculate the IV flow rates. Use the simplified method for pediatric (microdrip) tubing if minutes equal 60. Verify with a DA equation.*

1 Ordered: D10W 500 mL at 75 mL per hr, DF 10.

    a.   Flow rate: _____

        DA equation:

    b.   Evaluation: _____

2 Ordered: 1000 mL D5W at 125 mL per hr, DF 10.

    a.   Flow rate: _____

        DA equation:

    b.   Evaluation: _____

3 Ordered: 500 mL NS at 50 mL per hr, DF 15.

    a.   Flow rate: _____

        DA equation:

    b.   Evaluation: _____

4 Ordered: D5LR 500 mL at 50 mL per hr, DF 20.

    a.   Flow rate: _____

        DA equation:

    b.   Evaluation: _____

5 Ordered: D5LR 250 mL at 40 mL per hr, DF 60.

    a.   Flow rate: _____

        DA equation:

    b.   Evaluation: _____

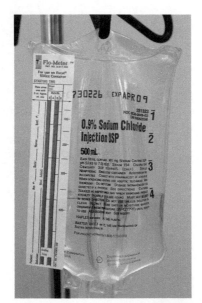

FIGURE 9-11 Time tape attached to Normal Saline IV bag to help monitor whether fluid is being administered as scheduled.

Intravenous Piggyback Solutions

For intermittent use, IV solutions with medication added are often prepared in the pharmacy and supplied in small volumes such as 50 or 100 mL to be administered through a secondary line for 30, 60, or 90 minutes (Figure 9-11). These solutions frequently contain antibiotics that may be infused intermittently (e.g., q4h or q6h) to maintain therapeutic blood levels of the medication.

They are connected (piggybacked) to a primary line port through a shorter secondary tubing set. Most intermittent infusions will be administered over 30, 60, or 90 minutes.

Flow rates for IVPB infusions

EXAMPLES

Ordered: IVPB antibiotic 50 mL in 30 minutes. How many mL per hr will be set on the electronic infusion pump? The equation will require a conversion formula from minutes to hours.

DA equation:

$$\frac{mL}{hr} = \frac{50 \text{ mL}}{\frac{30 \text{ min}}{1}} \times \frac{\overset{2}{\cancel{60} \text{ min}}}{1 \text{ hr}} = 100 \text{ mL per hr}$$

Evaluation: The equation is balanced. It is logical that, to infuse 50 mL in 30 minutes, the rate would have to be set at 100 mL per hr (60 min). The 60 min = 1 hr conversion is needed to convert the 30-min order to an hourly rate. ($\frac{mL}{hr}$ = mL per hour)

The flow rate for piggyback solutions is always set in *mL per hr* for electronic infusion pumps.

ASK YOURSELF

1   If I drink 60 mL in 60 minutes, how much fluid will I have consumed in
   30 minutes if I had been sipping at the same rate for the entire time?

   MY ANSWER

   _____

2   If an IV antibiotic label states, "Infuse at 60 mL per hr for 30 minutes,"
   what volume will have been completed in an hour if the infusion
   "continued" for the hour?

   _____

3   If an IV is to infuse at 20 mL per *hr* for 30 minutes, how much fluid should
   infuse in *30 minutes?*

   _____

Simplified piggyback calculations for milliliter-per-hour settings

Because many small-volume IVPB infusions are usually administered over 30 or 60 minutes on a secondary IV line, the nurse can perform mental calculations to obtain the flow rate in mL per hr. A simple DA equation can be employed for verification. No arithmetic is required for a 60-minute infusion.

➤ For 60-minute infusions, volume = milliliter-per-hour rate.

➤ For 30-minute infusions, *double* the amount of milliliters ordered for
   30 minutes to obtain the 60-mL (hourly) rate.

   Do not forget to check the infusion to be sure that the main IV line restarts after the 30- or 60-minute period is completed. On some electronic infusion pumps, each line is programmed separately. The nurse needs to confirm that the programming is accurate for both the primary and secondary solutions.

   The IV infusion will be completed in the ordered time period. The nurse then ensures that the primary IV line resumes at its ordered rate.

➤ The flow rate for the IVPB line is set at what would have been the volume for
   1 hour. That rate is often different from and may be faster than the primary
   IV infusion rate.

EXAMPLES

Primary rate: D5W continuous IV at 75 mL per hr.

Piggyback rate: 50 mL over 20 minutes, or 150 mL per hr.

Adjust the rate from 150 down to 75 mL per hr when the piggybacked solution is finished. The trend is to use electronic infusion pump equipment that has separate control devices for flow rates for primary and secondary lines.

FAQ   *Why are IVPB solutions given at different rates than the primary IV infusion?*

ANSWER   Effective treatment of acute infections or tumors requires heavily concentrated infusions of drugs at periodic intervals to maintain therapeutic blood levels of the medication. These infusions must be given on time and are ordered at a specific rate to deliver the amount of drug for maximum effectiveness. It is important to change the flow rate for the medication if the order so indicates and to change the rate back to the primary rate when the intermittent infusion is completed.

RAPID PRACTICE 9-6   IV Piggyback Flow Rates (mL per Hour)

ESTIMATED COMPLETION TIME: 30 minutes   **ANSWERS ON:** page 344

DIRECTIONS: *For problems 2 to 5, use mental calculations to calculate the milliliters-per-hour setting on an electronic infusion pump for the piggybacked solution. Verify the calculation with a DA equation.*

1   **Ordered:** 100 mL (IVPB) antibiotic over 30 minutes.

    a.   Estimated flow rate in mL/hr: <u>100 mL × 2, or 200 mL per hr for</u> <u>30 minutes</u>
DA verification:

$$\frac{mL}{hr} = \frac{100 \text{ mL}}{\overset{}{\underset{1}{\cancel{30 \text{ min}}}}} \times \frac{\overset{2}{\cancel{60 \text{ min}}}}{1 \text{ hour}} = 200 \text{ mL per hr*}$$

    b.   Evaluation: <u>The equation is balanced. The estimate supports the answer.</u>

➤ *Recheck calculations for high-volume flow rates such as this.

2   **Ordered:** 30 mL antibiotic (IVPB) over 20 minutes.

    a.   Estimated flow rate in mL per hr: _____
DA verification:

    b.   Evaluation: _____

3   **Ordered:** 50 mL antibiotic (IVPB) over 20 minutes.

    a.   Estimated flow rate in mL per hr: _____
DA verification:

    b.   Evaluation: _____

4 **Ordered:** 80 mL anti-cancer drug (IVPB) over 30 minutes.

  a. Estimated flow rate in mL per hr: _____
    DA verification:

  b. Evaluation: _____

5 **Ordered:** 25 mL anti-cancer drug (IVPB) over 30 minutes.

  a. Estimated flow rate in mL per hr: _____
    DA verification:

  b. Evaluation: _____

FAQ *Why is the DA verification needed if we can mentally calculate the flow rate for the IVPB solution?*

ANSWER As with all other calculations, the nurse must be proficient in setting up the DA equation as a back-up method in case an odd number of minutes is ordered, which would make a mental calculation difficult. Applying the DA setup to a variety of problems now and reviewing it periodically is necessary to *maintain* proficiency. Verify pharmacy calculations as well.

IVPB flow rates (drops per minute)

Equations used to calculate IVPB infusions on *gravity* devices are very simple and *different* from other infusion equations: They do not use a milliliter-per-hour calculation.

If an IVPB order is for 50 mL over 30 minutes with a DF administration set of 10, the question to be solved by a DA equation is: *How many drops per minute will be set?*

EXAMPLES

$$\frac{\text{drops}}{\text{minute}} = \frac{\overset{1}{10} \text{ drops}}{1 \text{ mL}} \times \frac{50 \text{ mL}}{\underset{3}{30} \text{ minute}} = 16.6, \text{ rounded to 17 drops per minute}$$

Analysis: The desired answer units are drops per minute. Enter the drop factor with its accompanying milliliter unit first to match the desired answer numerator. The order to be converted is 50 mL over 30 minutes.

➤ There is *no need to enter hours* in the equation. The answer will *not* be in mL per hr. Entry of the minutes unit is postponed until the entry of the denominator of the second fraction. Seventeen drops per minute will deliver 50 mL in 30 minutes.

IVPB Flow Rates for Gravity Devices

ESTIMATED COMPLETION TIME: 15 to 25 minutes   **ANSWERS ON:** page 344

DIRECTIONS: *Estimate the flow rate in mL per hour. Calculate the flow rate in drops/minute to the nearest whole number for gravity infusions. Label answers.*

1 **Ordered:** IVPB antibiotic 50 mL over 20 minutes, DF 10.

   a. Estimated flow rate in mL per hr: _____

   b. Flow rate in drops per minute: _____

   DA equation:

   c. Evaluation: _____

2 **Ordered:** IVPB cortisone product 50 mL over 20 minutes, DF 10.

   a. Estimated flow rate in mL per hr: _____

   b. Flow rate in drops per minute: _____

   DA equation:

   c. Evaluation: _____

3 **Ordered:** IVPB anti-cancer drug 75 mL over 60 minutes, DF 20.

   a. Estimated flow rate in mL per hr: _____

   b. Flow rate in drops per minute: _____

   DA equation:

   c. Evaluation: _____

4 **Ordered:** IVPB antibiotic 100 mL over 30 minutes, DF 15.

   a. Estimated flow rate in mL per hr: _____

   b. Flow rate in drops per minute: _____

   DA equation:

   c. Evaluation: _____

5 **Ordered:** IVPB anti-infective drug 30 mL over 30 minutes, DF 60.

   a. Estimated flow rate in mL per hr: _____

   b. Flow rate in drops per minute: _____

   DA equation:

   c. Evaluation: _____

Regulating and Positioning Gravity Infusion Devices

Note the positioning of the primary and secondary IVPB solutions in Figure 9-12. The higher IV solution is currently infusing. When it is empty, the lower solution will resume infusing. At this point, the nurse must change the flow rate back to the primary flow rate if the secondary rate is different.

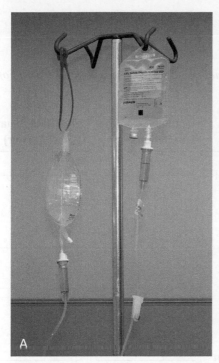
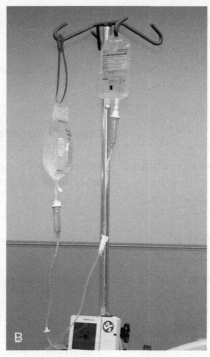

FIGURE 9-12 A, Gravity-flow intravenous piggyback (IVPB). The IVPB is elevated above the existing IV, allowing it to infuse by gravity. **B,** An electronic infusion pump may be used for both children and adults for intermittent infusions (IVPB).

Solutions for gravity flow devices need to be 3 feet above the patient's heart level. The solution that is on "hold" is lowered *below* the solution that is to flow. A simple hanger extender device is used to accomplish this.

RAPID PRACTICE 9-8	Calculating IVPB Flow Rates

ESTIMATED COMPLETION TIME: 15 minutes   **ANSWERS ON:** page 345

DIRECTIONS: *Fill in the following IVPB flow rate table with the needed flow rates in the spaces provided. Examine the example provided for the first entry. Label all answers in mL per hr or drops per minute.*

	IVPB Order and Equipment	Estimated Flow Rate (mL per hour)	Flow Rate Equation (in mL per hr or drops per min as needed)
1	50-mL antibiotic solution to infuse over 30 minutes on an electronic infusion pump	100 mL per hr	$\dfrac{50 \text{ mL}}{\cancel{30 \text{ minute}}_1} \times \dfrac{\cancel{60 \text{ minute}}^2}{1 \text{ hr}} = 100 \text{ mL per hr}$
2	20-mL antibiotic solution to infuse over 30 minutes by gravity, DF 60	_____	_____
3	25-mL antibiotic solution over 20 minutes by gravity infusion, DF 20	_____	_____
4	30-mL anti-cancer medication to infuse over 20 minutes on an electronic infusion pump	_____	_____
5	60-mL antibiotic solution to infuse over 40 minutes on an electronic infusion pump	_____	_____

RAPID PRACTICE 9-9	Intravenous Infusion Practice

ESTIMATED COMPLETION TIME: 15 minutes   **ANSWERS ON:** page 345

DIRECTIONS: *Read the IV order and equipment available, and supply the infusion information in the spaces provided.*

	Order	Equipment Available	Continuous or Intermittent	Flow Rate Equation (Label Answer)
1	30-mL antibiotic solution to infuse over 30 min	Pediatric microdrip administration set	_____	_____
2	1000 mL D5W q10h	IV administration set DF 10	_____	_____
3	50-mL antibiotic solution to infuse over 20 min	Volumetric pump	_____	_____
4	250 mL D5W over 4 hr	Electronic infusion pump	_____	_____
5	500 mL NS every 6 hr	IV administration set DF 15	_____	_____

The nurse always needs to know the ordered flow rate and must be able to verify that rate at the bedside, whether it is being administered on an electronic infusion pump or any other kind of equipment.

The prescriber orders mL per hr for maintenance solutions, not drops per minute.

Flow Rate Errors

Flow rates can get behind or ahead of schedule for many reasons:
- Positional dislodgement of the needle
- Movement of the patient
- Occlusion of the entry site
- Incorrect flow rate entry
- Administration of other fluids on a secondary line
- Incorrect positioning of the IV solutions
- Equipment failure
- Temporary discontinuance for travel to the x-ray or other department
- A change in flow rate orders by the prescriber since the nurse last checked for new orders

Monitoring the Flow Rate on Infusion Devices

The nurse verifies the *ordered flow rate* by
- Reading the entry on the infusion pump
- Counting the drops on a gravity infusion and converting to mL per hr
- Examining the timed tape, if present, on the solution container

➤ The flow rate and site must be monitored frequently.

The patient and family should have access to a call bell, should be advised that the nurse will be checking in on them, and should be advised to call the nurse if an alarm device becomes activated. "There will be an alarm to warn us when the solution gets low," "Here is the call light," or "Call me if the solution stops dripping." It is unnecessary discomfort to the patient when an IV must be restarted because of preventable occlusion from an IV running dry. The nurse has also not met the patient's needs when an IV that was supposed to infuse in 8 hours has infused in 2 hours. If the patient has orders to leave the bed for any reason, tell the patient to call for assistance before getting out of bed until there is assurance the patient can move independently with the equipment. Remember that IV fluids will increase the need to urinate. Do not forget to ask, "Do you have any questions?"

➤ Each hour and during visits to the bedside, the IV site is examined and the solution is examined to ensure that the site is patent, the appropriate volume has been infused to date, and the rate is correct. Previous caretakers may have set incorrect rates. The nurse also needs to be aware that orders may be changed frequently by the prescriber.

Timed tapes

Timed tapes can be placed on full IV solution containers by the nurse. The top calibration on the top of the tape is placed opposite the hanging fluid level, with the current time written next to it (Figure 9-13).

The nurse writes the anticipated time that the solution should reach the major volume calibrations based on the rate ordered.

➤ A timed tape can be placed on IV solution containers, both with electronic devices and with gravity devices, to further ensure that the volume infused matches the hourly ordered rate. The timed tape is very helpful but only if it is checked frequently as a rough gauge of fluid infused.

➤ Patients receiving intermittent infusions (piggybacks) in addition to their primary IV should not have timed tapes used because they will skew the primary IV times from the regular hourly IV rate marked on the timed tape.

CLINICAL RELEVANCE

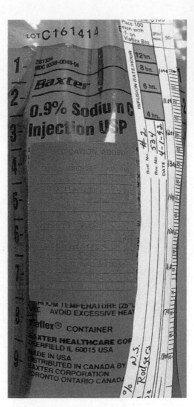

FIGURE 9-13 IV bag with timed tape. (From Potter PA, Perry AG, Stockert PA, Hall A: Basic nursing, ed 7, St. Louis, 2011, Mosby.)

CLINICAL RELEVANCE

➤ The nurse must be aware of the following *warnings about flow rate adjustments*. If the flow is deemed to be infusing too slowly or quickly, beware of "catching up." Flow rates affect major organ function. IV solutions with medications added are prescribed to deliver drugs at a therapeutic rate. It may seem safe to lower an IV rate, but if there is a medication included, slowing the infusion may cause the patient to suffer from abrupt withdrawal. Check with the prescriber about any adjustments and obtain changes in orders before adjusting the flow rate.

➤ The best way to keep IV flow rates on target is thorough knowledge of the current ordered IV infusion rate and frequent monitoring at every patient contact, and at least every hour.

➤ Never open up an IV line to full flow to catch up.

➤ Gravity flow rates have a high potential of inaccuracy as the tubing may become pinched; the clamp that regulates the flow may slip; or a positional change may cause a flow rate to increase, decrease, or halt. Educate the patient and family, if possible, to call for assistance if the flow rate stops or seems to be infusing too quickly.

➤ Infusion pumps are more reliable than gravity infusion devices but still must be monitored.

➤ Remember: The nurse cannot legally prescribe flow rates. Infusion times are recommended by the pharmaceutical company.

Question	Some Considerations
Is this an at-risk patient? De-hydrated, frail, poor heart, lung, or renal function?	Consult the prescriber.
When was the volume infused last monitored?	A significant change over an unknown time period requires consultation with the prescriber.
What was the purpose of the solution? Maintenance? Replacement?	These issues affect urgency of corrective actions (e.g., hydration status of the patient).
Have intake and output been adversely affected?	Assess and then consult with the prescriber.
Is the site patent?	The IV site may have to be changed before any decision is made about fluid rate changes.
Is there a positional problem with a gravity infusion?	This can be adjusted and calls attention to the need for more frequent monitoring in addition to patient or family teaching.
Is anyone tampering with the flow rate?	This is not a frequent occurrence but can happen and will need to be documented and reported.

Measures to prevent a flow rate error recurrence need to be put in place. The nurse cannot legally prescribe medications and flow rates unless the physician writes an order to titrate the drug.

➤ Above all, the nurse cannot "open up" the infusion line to try to catch up the flow rate. This is a totally unsafe practice that has potentially dire consequences for the patient.

An adult patient with good cardiac, lung, and renal function receiving an IV infusion of 75 to 125 mL per hr with no medications added can probably tolerate a small increase in rate without difficulty. If it is considered necessary by the prescriber to have the infusion complete on time, the calculation is very basic: Divide the remaining solution by the remaining number of hours as if it were a new IV infusion. Evaluate the difference in rate between the order and the new rate.

EXAMPLES

Ordered: 1000 mL D5W at 100 mL per hr. Total duration: 10 hr. Start time: 1200. Scheduled end time: 2200.

Evaluation: At 1800 hrs, there should be 400 mL remaining.

Remaining mL at 1800 Hours		Remaining Hours		New Flow Rate per Prescriber
600 mL	÷	4 hr	=	150 mL per hr

Do not forget to document the assessments and actions.

CLINICAL RELEVANCE

Obtaining an order to change from 100 to 150 mL per hr would be mandatory. Increases in rate need to be gradual to reduce physiological stress on the patient. Slowing down IV infusions that contain medications also often needs to be gradual. Remember the 75 to 125 mL per hr average figure for average healthy adults cited at the beginning of the chapter. During the infusion and on completion, assess the patient for signs of fluid overload—shortness of breath, bounding pulse, moist lung sounds, and complaints of discomfort—and document the findings.

What should I do if ordered IV fluids are delayed, are behind schedule, or have been infusing too fast?

ANSWER Consult with the healthcare provider to obtain new orders.

Question	Some Considerations
Is there medication in the solution?	Adjustments need to be made in consultation with the prescriber. There may be adverse consequences for underdose or sudden overdose and a need for a change in orders.
Has there been a significant drop or increase in percentage of IV infused? Over what time period? Was the ordered flow rate slow or rapid?	Consult with the prescriber. When the ordered flow rate is particularly slow or rapid, there is a medical reason that will make it necessary to consult with the prescriber for adjustment.

There have been incidents in which a patient or family member changed the setting on an electronic infusion pump. Also, staff on the previous shift may have entered the wrong setting or the order may have changed.

Drops per Minute to Milliliters per Hour

As mentioned before, the usual *ordered* flow rate for gravity infusions is in mL per hr, not drops per minute.

When caring for patients whose IV infusions have been initiated by someone else, the currently assigned nurse must verify during each visit that the flow rate is as ordered. For example, a nurse visits the bedside and notes that a gravity device has been used. They will count the current drop-per-minute flow rate. At that point, the nurse has two choices for verifying that *ordered flow rate* is infusing:

1 Calculate the derived flow rate in drops per minute from the mL per hr order and compare it to the current drops-per-minute flow rate.
2 Calculate the milliliters-per-hour flow rate from the current flow.

The nurse must be able to perform both calculations. A prescriber may ask at the bedside, "What is the current flow rate?," and will want the answer in mL per hr.

By counting the current flow rate in drops per minute, the nurse can verify the flow rate in mL per hr.

EXAMPLES

An IV is infusing at 30 drops per min. The DF is 20. How many mL per hr are being infused at this rate?

$$\frac{mL}{hr} = \frac{1\ mL}{\underset{2}{\cancel{20\ drops}}} \times \frac{\overset{3}{\cancel{30\ drops}}}{1\ \cancel{minute}} \times \frac{60\ \cancel{minute}}{1\ hr} = \frac{180}{2} = 90\ mL\ per\ hr$$

Analysis: The number of drops per minute and the DF are the known data. (Most agencies buy one brand of administration sets in bulk. The nurse learns the DFs for the main equipment used in the agency during orientation and initial observation of the tubing set labels.) The DF must be entered in the DA equation along with the number of drops per minute. If *hour* is needed in the answer, the conversion *60 minutes = 1 hour* is required in the equation to convert minutes to hours.

Evaluation: The equation is balanced. Only mL per hr remains.

RAPID PRACTICE 9-10 Milliliters per Hour for Gravity Infusions

ESTIMATED COMPLETION TIME: 20 to 30 minutes   **ANSWERS ON:** page 346

DIRECTIONS: *Calculate mL per hr from the drops per minute flowing on the gravity device. Use a calculator for long division and multiplication to solve the equations. Label all answers.*

Drops per 30 Sec Counted at Bedside	Drops per Min (Mental Calculation)	Administration Set DF	Flow Rate Equation
1 10 drops per 15 sec	40 (10 × 4)	20	$\dfrac{mL}{hr} : \dfrac{1\ mL}{\underset{1}{\cancel{20}}\ drops} \times \dfrac{40\ \cancel{drops}}{1\ \cancel{minute}} \times \dfrac{\overset{3}{\cancel{60}}\ minute}{1\ hr} = 120$ mL per hr
2 8 drops per 30 sec	_____	10	_____
3 6 drops per 15 sec	_____	60	_____
4 15 drops per 30 sec	_____	60	_____
5 12 drops per 30 sec	_____	15	_____

Electronic Infusion Pump Alarms

Electronic infusion pumps have a variety of safety alarm settings, depending on the sophistication of the device. In addition to setting the flow rate in mL per hr, the nurse programs the volume that will generate an alarm to give notice that the current infusion is almost finished. This warning serves several functions:

- The nurse has warning time to prepare a subsequent solution, if ordered.
- The IV line is prevented from running dry.
- The entry site will maintain patency and will not become coagulated.
- The patient will not have to be subjected to another venipuncture for a new site because of clot formation.
- Medications and fluids will be delivered at the scheduled time.

Maintaining patency means safety and comfort for the patient, on-time delivery of fluids and medications, and time saved for the nurse.

"Volume to Be Infused" Alarm

Setting the advance warning alarm time is simple. Usually, the nurse programs the alarm to sound based on three criteria:

- How many hours will the IV solution be infused and at what rate?
- How much notice does the nurse need or want in order to bring the next infusion solution and equipment, such as new tubing, that may be needed?
- How many milliliters will have been infused by the time the nurse wants the alarm to sound?

➤ The nurse does not enter the entire volume to be infused. That would not give advance warning time.

A rough guideline for determining the volume at which the alarm should sound is to subtract 50 mL from the total volume in the bag for faster infusion rates and 25 mL for slower flow rates. Experience, preference, and work load help the nurse to determine how much warning is needed.

✱ **Communication**

"Mr. and Mrs. Smith, I have set an alarm to let me know when the IV needs replacement. Please use the call bell to reach me if you have any concerns about the solution running out or if the flow stops or your arm hurts."

For a total IV infusion volume of 1000 mL:

Infusion Rate	Amount to Subtract from Total Volume	Volume to Be Infused for Alarm to Sound
150 mL per hr	50 mL	950 mL
75 mL per hr	25 mL	975 mL

➤ With or without an alarm, the nurse needs to develop a reminder for the anticipated time at which to prepare the next IV solution.

ASK YOURSELF   **Q & A**

1   If the flow rate was very rapid, would I want the alarm to sound earlier or later than average?

MY ANSWER

_____

EXAMPLES

➤ Disposal of IV tubing, needles, and dressings according to the guidelines and policies of the clinical agency and the federal Occupational Safety and Health Administration is a critical safety issue. Special hazardous waste containers must be used for sharps, and special care must be taken to avoid leaving any contaminated equipment at the bedside. Doing so could cause a needle-stick injury or bodily fluid exposure to a staff member at bedside or during transport for disposal.

RAPID PRACTICE 9-11   Intravenous Infusion Review

ESTIMATED COMPLETION TIME: 10 to 20 minutes   **ANSWERS ON:** page 346

DIRECTIONS: *Study the previous material and supply the requested information pertaining to basic IV infusions.*

1   How does the nurse determine the number of drops per milliliter for a gravity IV infusion line? _____
   a.   Refer to relevant IV pharmacology references.
   b.   Call the agency pharmacist or consult a wall chart on the unit.
   c.   Ask an experienced nurse on the unit.
   d.   Read the DF on the IV administration set container.

2   An IV device that permits the patient to control and administer an intermittent medicated (analgesic) solution for pain relief is called _____
   a.   IV push   c.   IV piggyback
   b.   PCA   d.   TKO

3   Basic intravenous flow rates are usually ordered in which of the following terms: _____
   a.   Drops per hour   c.   Liters per minute
   b.   mL per hr   d.   Liters per hour

4   A reasonable short-term IV maintenance rate for an NPO adult patient in good health would be _____
   a.   300 mL per hr   c.   75-125 mL per hr
   b.   150-200 mL per hr   d.   10-20 mL per hr

5   An example of an order indicating that a continuous IV infusion solution is to be started on a patient would be _____
   a.   Ampicillin 2 g IVPB q6h   c.   D5W 1 L q8h at 50 mL per hr
   b.   Pantoprazole 40 mg IV push daily d.   Lorazepam 1 mg IV push

| RAPID PRACTICE 9-12 | Gravity Device Flow Rate Practice |

ESTIMATED COMPLETION TIME: 20 to 25 minutes   **ANSWERS ON:** page 346

DIRECTIONS: *Assume that all the continuous IV infusions ordered in problems 1 to 5 are to be administered with gravity equipment. Calculate the flow rates as requested. Use a calculator for long division and multiplication.*

1   **Ordered:** IV D5W 1000 mL at 150 mL per hr
    DF: 15 drops per mL

   a.   Macrodrip or microdrip: _____

   b.   mL per hr flow rate: _____

   c.   Flow rate in drops per minute: _____

      DA equation:

   d.   Evaluation: _____

   e.   Infusion duration in hours (and minutes if applicable): _____

2   **Ordered:** IV D5LR 500 mL q10h

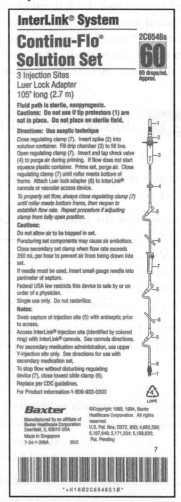

   a.   Macrodrip or microdrip: _____

   b.   Estimated flow rate in drops per minute: _____

      DA equation:

   c.   Evaluation: _____

3 **Ordered:** IV D5NS 1000 mL q8h
DF: 10 drops per mL

a. Macrodrip or microdrip: _____

b. Flow rate in drops per minute: _____

DA equation:

c. Evaluation: _____

4 **Ordered:** medicated IVPB of 40 mL to infuse in 1 hour (an intermittent IV)

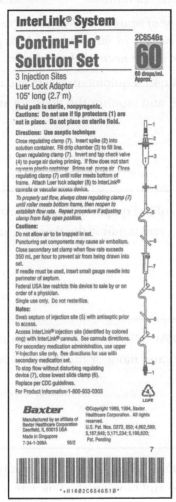

a. Macrodrip or microdrip: _____

b. Flow rate in drops per minute: _____

DA equation:

c. Evaluation: _____

5 **Ordered:** medicated IVPB of 100 mL to infuse in 1 hour (60 minutes)
DF: 10 drops per mL

a. Macrodrip or microdrip: _____

b. Flow rate in drops per minute: _____

DA equation:

c. Evaluation: _____

Q & A	ASK YOURSELF	1	Can I write the four drop factors for gravity infusions, starting with the microdrip?
	MY ANSWER		_____

RAPID PRACTICE 9-13   ## Determining Flow Rates

ESTIMATED COMPLETION TIME: 25 minutes   **ANSWERS ON:** page 347

DIRECTIONS: *Notice the type of equipment that will be used: pump or gravity infusion. Calculate the flow rate in mL per hr or drops per minute, whichever is needed. Round the answer to the nearest whole number. Label all answers.*

1   **Ordered:** 500 mL LR q4h. Equipment: electronic infusion pump.
   a.   The nurse will set and monitor the flow rate at _____
      DA equation:

   b.   Evaluation: _____

2   **Ordered:** 250 mL NS q6h. Equipment: gravity device with tubing DF 20.
   a.   The nurse will set and monitor the flow rate at _____
      DA equation:

   b.   Evaluation: _____

3   **Ordered:** 1000 mL D5W q8h. Equipment: electronic infusion pump.
   a.   The nurse will set and monitor the flow rate in mL per hr at _____
      DA equation:

   b.   Evaluation: _____

4   **Ordered:** 1000 mL D5LR q12h. Equipment: gravity device with tubing DF 10.
   a.   The nurse will set and monitor the flow rate at _____
      DA equation:

   b.   Evaluation: _____

5   **Ordered:** 1 L $\frac{1}{2}$ NS q24h. Equipment: gravity device with tubing DF 60.
   a.   The nurse will set and monitor the flow rate at _____
      DA equation:

   b.   Evaluation: _____

"To Keep Open" Flow Rates

The order "to keep open" (TKO) indicates the slowest rate that can be infused on the available equipment when the goal is to have a patent IV line available for potential future use. A TKO flow rate can be 10 to 20 mL per hr. Defer to facility policies. More frequently, prescribers order an indwelling injection port known as a "saline lock," or "IV lock." Infusions, syringes, and long, straight infusion lines can be connected to an indwelling capped cannula or needle only when needed. The lock is flushed with saline solution* to prevent clotting. It is accessed for IV solutions when needed. The IV lock provides convenience and more mobility for the patient.

Calculating Grams of Solute

➤ As stated in Chapter 1, % means "per 100."

Using D5W as an example, the percentage of dextrose in solution means 5 g dextrose per 100 mL.

Calculating total grams of solute in a solution

➤ To determine total grams of solute in a solution, given the percentage, change the percentage value to grams per 100 mL and multiply that fraction form by the total volume in milliliters.

Formula: g in solution = number of $\frac{g}{100\,mL}$ × total volume in mL = g in total volume.

Question: How many grams of dextrose are in the following solution: D5W in 1000 mL?

$$g\ dextrose = \frac{5\ g\ dextrose}{\cancel{100\ mL}\ 1} \times \frac{\overset{10}{\cancel{1000\ mL}}}{1} = 50\ g\ dextrose$$

Analysis: The starting factor matches the desired answer.
Evaluation: The equation is balanced. The equation eliminates milliliters so that only grams remain.

Question: How many grams of sodium chloride (NaCl) are in the following solution: 1000 mL NS solution (0.9% NaCl)?

$$g\ sodium\ chloride = \frac{0.9\ g\ NaCl}{\cancel{100\ mL}\ 1} \times \frac{\overset{10}{\cancel{1000\ mL}}}{1} = 0.9 \times 10 = 9\ g\ sodium\ chloride$$

Analysis: The starting factor matches the desired answer.
Evaluation: Equation is balanced. Only grams remain.

➤ Note that 0.9 is *less than* 1%. NaCl contains sodium *and* chloride. A liter of NS contains 9 g of NaCl and 3.6 g of sodium.

➤ Remember to make the decimal points prominent so they are not missed in calculations.

---

*Occasionally heparin is used for a flush.

Calculating Grams of Solute

ESTIMATED COMPLETION TIME: 10 minutes   **ANSWERS ON:** page 347

DIRECTIONS: *Calculate the total number of grams of solute in the IV solution supplied. Mentally change L to mL for the equation. Verify your answer using a calculator.*

1 **Solution:** 1 L of D10W

    a. What is the total number of grams of dextrose? <u>100 g dextrose</u>

      DA equation:

$$\text{g dextrose: } \frac{10 \text{ g}}{\overset{1}{\cancel{100 \text{ mL}}}} \times \frac{\overset{10}{\cancel{1000 \text{ mL}}}}{1} = 100 \text{ g dextrose}$$

    b. Evaluation: <u>Equation is balanced. Only grams remain.</u>

2 **Solution:** 2 L D10LR

    a. What is the total number of grams of dextrose? _____

      DA equation:

    b. Evaluation: _____

3 **Solution:** 0.5 L $\frac{1}{2}$ NS.

    a. What is the total number of grams of sodium chloride (NaCl)? _____

      DA equation:

    b. Evaluation: _____

4 **Solution:** 1.5 L of D5LR

    a. What is the total number of grams of dextrose? _____

      DA equation:

    b. Evaluation: _____

5 **Solution:** 1.5 L of NS.

    a. What is the total number of grams of sodium chloride (NaCl)? _____

      DA equation:

    b. Evaluation: _____

▶ A Word about Potassium Chloride

Potassium chloride (KCl) is ordered to be added to many primary IV solutions, particularly for patients who are NPO. It has been identified by the Institute for Safe Medication Practices (ISMP) as a high-risk medication, meaning that it has high potential to cause adverse effects. For safety reasons, KCl vials are not stocked on the nursing units. The pharmacy prepares the solution, or a premixed (diluted) solution is used. (Reminder: The red flag icon indicates a high-alert drug.)

➤ Consult agency and TJC guidelines regarding IV potassium administration. Following are some of the key considerations the nurse should keep in mind:
- The *amount* ordered
- The *concentration* ordered
- The *solids dilution rate* and *dilutions* recommended in the literature
- The *rate* ordered and the *rate* recommended in the literature
- Results of the patient's most recent *serum potassium* levels
- Results and implications of the patient's most recent *renal function* tests, including serum creatinine and blood urea nitrogen
- Results and implications of physical assessment for side effects of too little (hypokalemia) or too much potassium (hyperkalemia)

➤ Potassium is never administered undiluted in an IV. Even if it is to be added to a large-volume IV, measures must be taken to ensure that it is well mixed with the IV fluid before it gets into the tubing.

➤ On the rare occasion it is added by the nurse, it should be added to a full bag of the main IV solution.

➤ Never inject potassium directly into a currently hanging IV solution.

➤ If KCl is administered undiluted, it can cause tissue necrosis, vessel damage, and cardiac arrest. A rapid flow of diluted KCl can also cause cardiac arrest.

➤ Administering KCl preparations safely requires further study, supervision, and experience.

➤ You must be able to distinguish mEq from mg and mL on the label.

Intravenous Intermittent Solution Delivery Systems

Intermittent solutions, usually medicated, may be delivered in five ways: (1) IVPB solutions, (2) volume-control devices, (3) IV (direct) push with a syringe, (4) syringe pumps, or (5) PCA pumps.

There is a trend toward using more manufacturer-prepared IV medication systems. An example of a prepared IVPB solution container and medication is the Hospira ADD-Vantage® with a drug vial of vancomycin (Figure 9-14) and the Hospira ADD-Vantage® System (Figure 9-15).

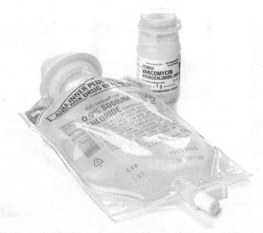

FIGURE 9-14 Hospira ADD-Vantage® with a drug vial of vancomycin. (From Hospira, Inc., Lake Forest, IL.)

Hospira

ADD–Vantage® System

As Easy as **1, 2, 3**

1 Assemble — Use Aseptic Technique

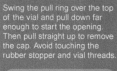

Swing the pull ring over the top of the vial and pull down far enough to start the opening. Then pull straight up to remove the cap. Avoid touching the rubber stopper and vial threads.

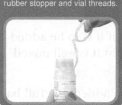

Hold diluent container and gently grasp the tab on the pull ring. Pull up to break the tie membrane. Pull back to remove the cover. Avoid touching the inside of the vial port.

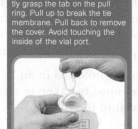

Screw the vial into the vial port until it will go no further. Recheck the vial to assure that it is tight. Label appropriately.

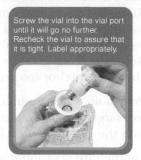

2 Activate — Pull Plug/Stopper to Mix Drug with Diluent

Hold the vial as shown. Push the drug vial down into container and grasp the inner cap of the vial through the walls of the container.

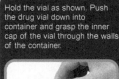
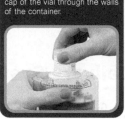

Pull the inner plug from the drug vial; allow drug to fall into diluent container for fast mixing. Do not force stopper by pushing on one side of inner cap at a time.

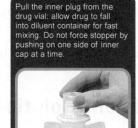

Verify that the plug and rubber stopper have been removed from the vial. The floating stopper is an indication that the system has been activated.

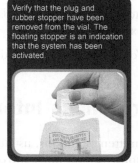

3 Mix and Administer — Within Specified Time

Mix container contents thoroughly to assure complete dissolution. Look through bottom of vial to verify complete mixing. Check for leaks by squeezing container firmly. If leaks are found, discard unit.

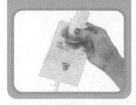

Pull up hanger on the vial.

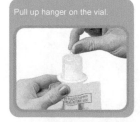

Remove the white administration port cover and spike (pierce) the container with the piercing pin. Administer within the specified time.

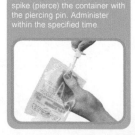

For more information on Advancing Wellness with ADD-Vantage® family of devices, contact your Hospira representative at **1-877-946-7747 (1-877-9Hospira)** or visit **www.Hospira.com**

©Hospira, Inc. - 275 North Field Drive, Lake Forest, IL 60045

6-131-1-Nov. 04

THE **ADD-Vantage®** SYSTEM

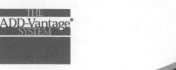

FIGURE 9-15 Hospira ADD-Vantage® System. (From Hospira, Inc., Lake Forest, IL.)

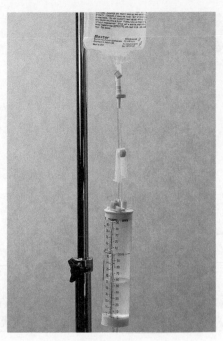

FIGURE 9-16 Volume control device. (From Potter PA, Perry AG, Stockert PA, Hall A: *Essentials of nursing practice,* ed 9, St. Louis, 2019, Elsevier.)

Volume-control device (calibrated burette chamber)

Now that electronic infusion pumps (smart pumps) are used, volume-control devises are less common; however, nurses must be familiar with them. When there is a need to protect the patient from a possible *fluid* or *medication overload,* a simple volume-control device may be placed between the main IV container and the drip chamber (Figure 9-16). If the volume-control device is being used for medication administration, the solutions in the primary bag and the medication must be checked for compatibility.

The calibrated chamber, which usually holds 100 to 150 mL, will be filled with a limited specific amount of the primary IV solution or with a medication. A *clamp above the chamber* to the main IV line *will be closed.* This system may be used for pediatric and other at-risk patients. Burettes have a DF of 60, so 1 mL = 1 drop.

➤ Agencies specify the *maximum amount* of fluid that may be placed in the burette at any one time: *1 to 2 hours' worth at the ordered flow rate.* Medications placed in the burette will need to be diluted according to the manufacturer's guidelines for IV infusion. Flushing procedures before and after administering medications with the device must be followed according to policy, and comprehensive labels stating date, time, medication contents, and flow rate need to be employed. The nurse opens the clamp to refill the calibrated chamber as needed.

➤ The nurse must have a system in place for the timing of the refill. If the chamber empties and the clamp to the primary bag is closed, the IV site will coagulate.

---

1 If the ordered flow rate is 15 mL per hr for a baby and the agency policy is a limit of 2 hours' worth of volume in the volume-control device, what is the maximum number of milliliters that may be placed in the device?

ASK YOURSELF

_____

MY ANSWER

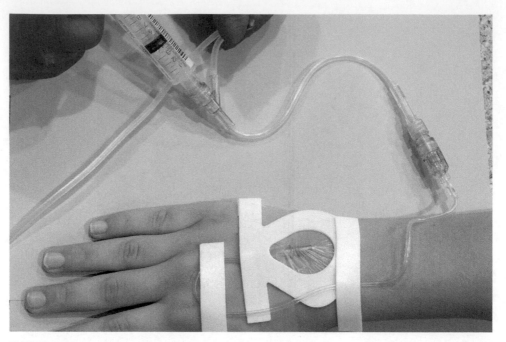

FIGURE 9-17 Slowly inject the intravenous push medication through the intravenous lock; use a watch to time the injection. When giving an intravenous push medication through an intravenous line, pinch the tubing just above the injection port.

Intravenous push medications (direct)

IV push medications are very-small-volume medications administered one time only or intermittently with a syringe directly into an infusion line or port closest to a vein (Figure 9-17). Most of these medications must be diluted in a small volume of a specific diluent, and all must be administered at a controlled rate. The pharmacy will generally specify these instructions, otherwise, an appropriate pharmacology reference must be used for dilution and rate instructions. IV push calculations are covered in more detail in Chapter 10.

➤ Do not abbreviate *IV push*. *IVP* refers to a kidney function test.

➤ IV push does not mean push hard or push fast.

Syringe pump

Syringe pumps are manual, electronic, or battery-operated devices that use positive pressure and a plunger to deliver a specific programmed amount of a smaller-volume medicated or unmedicated IV solution over a specific period of time. Tubing from the syringe is connected to an access device, such as a port on the patient's IV tubing.

Patient-Controlled Analgesia (PCA) Pump A PCA pump is an IV infusion syringe pump device connected to an indwelling line and programmed by the nurse to deliver pain medication in prescribed small increments at programmed intervals with lockout periods to prevent overdoses (Figure 9-18). These often deliver controlled drugs and require narcotic counts.

The patient pushes a button on a small remote control device that releases boluses of medication into the established IV line. A small basal (continuous) rate of the medication *may* be programmed to be administered continuously between boluses (Figure 9-19).

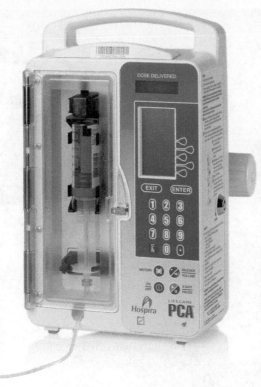

FIGURE 9-18 Lifecare® Patient-controlled analgesia 3 Infusion System. (From Hospira, Inc., Lake Forest, IL.)

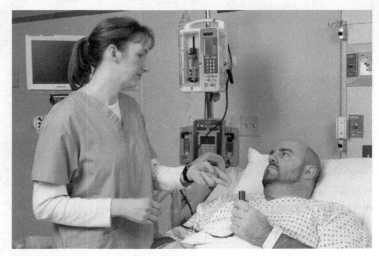

FIGURE 9-19 The nurse instructs the patient on the use of a PCA infusion pump for pain control. (From Potter PA, Perry AG, Stockert PA, Hall A: Essentials of nursing practice, ed 9, St. Louis, 2019, Elsevier.)

A sample order for a programmed dose regimen for a patient with pain would be:

> *Initial bolus: morphine 2 mg*
> *Incremental dose: morphine 1 mg*
> *Lockout (delay time) interval: 15 minutes*
> *Basal rate: 0 mg per hr*
> *One-hour limit: 4 to 6 mg (permits prn bolus)*
> *PRN bolus: 2 mg q4h*

The pharmacy provides a prefilled syringe with the analgesic. The nurse places the pump on an established continuous-flow IV line with a compatible solution, inserts the syringe in the pump, programs the orders, and monitors the use and effectiveness of the dose.

The PCA pump gives control of pain to the patient, relieves anxiety about having to wait for medication, provides a steadier degree of pain relief, and is thought to result in overall reduced total usage of analgesics. Assessments of the pump readouts of the number of attempts made, amounts used, and relief obtained are usually recorded hourly.

The nurse replaces the prefilled syringe cartridges as needed.

Blood Administration

- There are many steps in the protocols for blood administration. The agency procedures must be followed scrupulously by a registered nurse to avoid a potentially very serious adverse event (Figure 9-20).

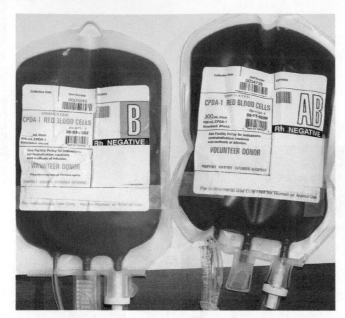

FIGURE 9-20 Blood products must be cross-checked by two nurses to ensure the patient receives the correct unit that has been crossmatched in the lab as compatible with the patient's blood.

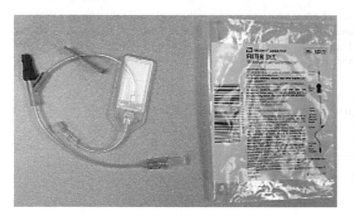

FIGURE 9-21 Filter used for blood administration.

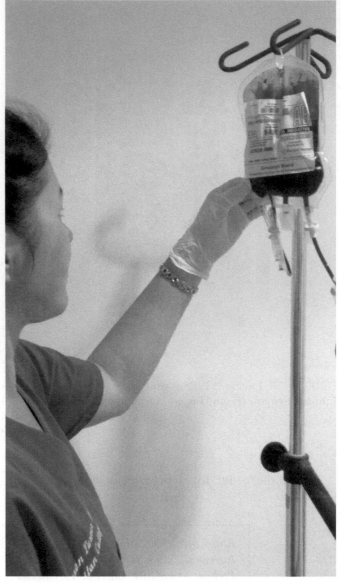

FIGURE 9-22 Blood administration with Y tubing and normal saline.

- Blood is administered only after a primary line is established with normal saline (NS) solution on Y tubing with a blood administration set for a pump or a gravity device (Figures 9-21 and 9-22).

➤ The usual initial flow rate for a unit of blood is 120 mL per hour for the first 15 to 30 minutes. Check agency policies. The nurse is required to be present for the initial part of the transfusion for a specified time period in case of adverse reaction.

A unit of whole blood is often administered without the plasma. Without plasma, the unit "packed cells" contains about 250 to 350 mL. With plasma, the amount will be closer to 500 mL.

➤ Agency protocols must be consulted for patient identification, patient care, blood storage and administration; disposal of used blood transfusion equipment; and actions to take should a suspected adverse event occur.

➤ Two nurses must verify accurate patient identification, blood and Rh factor compatibility of the donor unit of blood with the recipient patient, and the type and crossmatch done in the lab.

ESTIMATED COMPLETION TIME: 30 minutes   **ANSWERS ON:** page 347

DIRECTIONS: *Analyze the IV-related questions and select the best answer using the available equipment.*

1 **Ordered:** 30 mL antibiotic IVPB q4h infused over 30 minutes. Equipment available: infusion pump. The nurse will set the flow rate at _____.
   a. 25 mL per hr   c. 60 mL per hr
   b. 50 drops per min   d. 200 mL per hr

2 **Ordered:** 1000 mL D5NS 24h. Equipment available: Pediatric microdrip administration set. The nurse will set the flow rate at _____.
   a. 41 drops per min   c. 42 drops per min
   b. $41\frac{2}{3}$ mL per hr   d. 42 mL per hr

3 **Ordered:** 50 mL antibiotic IVPB q6h infused over 30 minutes. Equipment available: gravity device, DF 15. The nurse will set the flow rate at _____.
   a. 25 drops per min   c. 25 mL per hr
   b. 12.5 drops per min   d. 100 mL per hr

4 The average maintenance flow rate for a healthy adult who is NPO is _____.
   a. 10 to 15 mL per hr   c. 75 to 125 mL per hr
   b. 25 mL per hr   d. 150 to 250 mL per hr

5 **Ordered:** 1 unit of blood (250 mL) to be infused over 2 hours. Equipment available: an infusion pump. After initial slow flow, the nurse will set the flow rate at _____.
   a. 125 mL per hr   c. 12.5 mL per hr
   b. 125 drops per min   d. 12.5 drops per min

6 An isotonic electrolyte solution used for IV infusions is _____.
   a. 5DW   c. D5LR
   b. 10DW   d. 2.5% DW

7 **Ordered:** 500 mL D5W, an isotonic fluid maintenance solution to infuse over 12 hr. Equipment available: infusion pump. The nurse will set the flow rate at _____.
   a. 41 mL per hr   c. 43 mL per hr
   b. 41.7 mL per hr   d. 42.5 drops per min

8 D10W 1000 mL contains _____ grams of dextrose.
   a. 15   c. 50
   b. 25   d. 100

9 **Ordered:** LR 1000 mL q8h. Equipment available: gravity device, DF 20. The nurse will set the flow rate at _____.
   a. 20 mL per hr   c. 42 mL per hr
   b. 42 drops per min   d. 125 mL per hr

10 **Ordered:** NS 500 mL q4h. Equipment available: gravity device with rate controller. The nurse will set the flow rate at _____.
   a. 100 drops per min   c. 125 mL per hr
   b. 125 drops per min   d. 150 mL per hr

CHAPTER 9 FINAL PRACTICE

ESTIMATED COMPLETION TIME: 1 hour   **ANSWERS ON:** page 347

DIRECTIONS: *Show work, label answers. Calculate with a DA equation when requested. Use a calculator for long division and multiplication. All flow rates must be labeled drops per min or mL per hr.*

1 An IVPB of 20 mL is ordered to be infused over 20 minutes.

   a. Estimate the flow rate on a microdrip device. _____
         DA equation:

   b. Evaluation: _____

2 An IV of 1000 mL D5W at 100 mL per hr is ordered and started at 0800.

   a. Amount that should remain at 1200: _____
   b. Hour at which ordered IV should be completed: _____

3 **Ordered:** 50 mL 50% dextrose solution for a diabetic patient in insulin shock.

   a. How many grams of dextrose are contained in the solution? _____
         DA equation:

   b. Evaluation: _____

4 What type of IV solution is used when administering blood products such as a unit of packed red blood cells (RBCs)?

   _____

5 State the meaning of DF of 10 on a gravity infusion administration set.

   _____

6 **Ordered:** whole blood to be infused initially at 2 mL per minute for the first 15 minutes. Equipment available: infusion pump for blood and blood administration pump set.

   State the flow rate in mL per hr that the nurse would set on the pump for the first 15 minutes: _____

7 Select the type of administration set that would be selected for an IVPB solution: *primary* or *secondary*? (Circle one)

8 **Ordered:** 250 mL D5W at 50 mL per hr.

   a. How long will the IV infusion last? _____

   b. If an alarm is set for $\frac{1}{2}$ hour before the solution will be completely infused, how much volume to be infused would be entered for the alarm to sound? _____

9 Name the three purposes of IV therapy:

_____   _____

_____

10 What is a nursing responsibility pertaining to flow rate when a secondary infusion or IVPB has been completed and the primary IV resumes flow?

_____

11 **Ordered:** 500 mL LR q8h. Equipment available: electronic infusion pump

   a. State the flow rate that would be set to nearest 0.5 mL: _____

   b. If the IV infusion started at 1200, at what time (military time) would the nurse prepare the next solution to have it at the bedside $\frac{1}{2}$ hour before the container would be empty? _____

12 State the names of three isotonic IV solutions commonly ordered:

_____

_____

_____

13 State the most serious adverse effect of an error with overdose or over-concentration during KCl IV administration: _____

14 **Ordered:** 250 mL NS q4h. Equipment available: gravity device with DF 10.

   a. State the grams of sodium in the solution: _____

     DA equation:

   b. Evaluation: _____

   c. State the flow rate that would be set: _____

     DA equation:

   d. Evaluation: _____

15 **Ordered:** 250 mL whole blood to be infused over 2 hours. Equipment available: gravity blood administration set with DF 10.

   a. Calculate the flow rate with a DA equation:

   b. Evaluation: _____

16 **a.** State the DF for a microdrip, or pediatric, infusion administration step.

     _____

   b. State the flow rate limit for infusions using microdrip sets. _____

17 **Ordered:** 500 mL D5W q8h. Equipment available: gravity infusion device with DF 20.

   a. Calculate the flow rate with a DA equation:

   b. Evaluation: _____

18 **a.** What type of device would the nurse connect between an IV solution and tubing to protect a patient from a fluid or medication overload?

_____

b. What are the usual guidelines or criteria for the amount of fluid placed in this device? _____

19 An IVPB of 50 mL is ordered to be infused over 30 minutes. Estimate the flow rate on an infusion pump: _____

20 **Ordered:** 3 L D5LR q24h. Equipment available: gravity administration set with DF 15.

a. Calculate the flow rate with a DA equation:

b. Evaluation: _____

CHAPTER 9   ANSWER KEY

RAPID PRACTICE 9-1 (p. 304)

Order		Abbreviation(s) for Solution	Flow Rate (mL per hr)	Time to Infuse (hr and min if applicable)
1	250 mL half-strength normal saline q4h	0.45% NaCl Sol $\frac{1}{2}$ NS $\frac{1}{2}$ strength NS	63	4 hr
2	Infuse 500 mL normal saline over 6 hr	NS	83	6 hr
3	1 L lactated Ringer's q10h	LR RL	100	10 hr
4	500 mL 5% dextrose in lactated Ringer's at 40 mL per hr	D5 L/R D5 R/L D5RL or D5LR	40	12 hr, 30 min
5	1000 mL 5% dextrose in water at 125 mL per hr	D5W 5DW	125	8 hr

RAPID PRACTICE 9-2 (p. 311)

2 **a.** 10 hours; $100 \div 10 = 10$-hr duration

b. 10 drops per min

$$\frac{\text{drops}}{\text{min}} = \frac{60 \text{ drops}}{1 \text{ mL}} \times \frac{10 \text{ mL}}{1 \text{ hr}} \times \frac{1 \text{ hr}}{60 \text{ min}}$$

$$= 10 \text{ drops per min}$$

c. Equation is balanced. Only drops per min remain.

Note: Note that the 60 DF and 60 min cancel each other so that mL per hr (10) = drops per min (10).

3 **a.** 83 mL per hr

$$\frac{\text{mL}}{\text{hr}} = \frac{500 \text{ mL}}{6 \text{ hr}} = \frac{83.3, \text{ rounded to}}{83 \text{ mL per hr}}$$

b. 28 drops per min

$$\frac{\text{drops}}{\text{min}} = \frac{\overset{1}{20} \text{ drops}}{1 \text{ mL}} \times \frac{\overset{250}{500 \text{ mL}}}{\underset{3}{6 \text{ hr}}} \times \frac{1 \text{ hr}}{\underset{3}{60 \text{ min}}} = \frac{250}{9}$$

$$= 27.7, \text{ rounded to } 28 \text{ drops per min}$$

c. Equation is balanced. Only drops per min remain.

Note: $\frac{83 \text{ mL}}{1 \text{ hr}}$ could have been substituted for $\frac{500 \text{ mL}}{6 \text{ hr}}$ in the equation.

4 **a.** 75 mL per hr
b. 13 drops per min

$$\frac{\text{drops}}{\text{min}} = \frac{\overset{1}{\cancel{10}} \text{ drops}}{1 \text{ } \cancel{mL}} \times \frac{75 \text{ } \cancel{mL}}{1 \text{ } \cancel{hr}} \times \frac{1 \text{ } \cancel{hr}}{\underset{6}{\cancel{60}} \text{ min}}$$

$$= \frac{75}{6} = \begin{matrix} 12.5, \text{ rounded to} \\ 13 \text{ drops per min} \end{matrix}$$

c. Equation is balanced. Only drops per min remain.

5 **a.** 83 mL per hr (1000 ÷ 12)
b. 28 drops per min

$$\frac{\text{drops}}{\text{min}} = \frac{\overset{1}{\cancel{20}} \text{ drops}}{1 \text{ } \cancel{mL}} \times \frac{1000 \text{ } \cancel{mL}}{12 \text{ } \cancel{hr}} \times \frac{1 \text{ } \cancel{hr}}{\underset{3}{\cancel{60}} \text{ min}}$$

$$= \frac{1000}{36} = \begin{matrix} 27.7, \text{ rounded to} \\ 28 \text{ drops per min} \end{matrix}$$

c. Equation is balanced. Only drops per min remain. Min had to be entered in a conversion formula in the denominator to match the desired answer.

Note: You have a choice of substituting the $\frac{83 \text{ mL}}{\text{hr}}$ for $\frac{1000 \text{ mL}}{12 \text{ hr}}$.

RAPID PRACTICE 9-3 (p. 313)

1 **a.** 6 drops per min

$$\frac{\text{drops}}{\text{min}} = \frac{\overset{1}{\cancel{15}} \text{ drops}}{1 \text{ } \cancel{mL}} \times \frac{25 \text{ } \cancel{mL}}{1 \text{ } \cancel{hr}} \times \frac{1 \text{ } \cancel{hr}}{\underset{4}{\cancel{60}} \text{ min}} = \frac{25}{4}$$

$$= 6.25, \text{ rounded to } 6 \text{ drops per min}$$

b. Equation is balanced. Only drops per min remain.
c. Yes. 6 drops per min can be counted.

Note: It is a very slow rate. The site may coagulate.

2 **a.** 33 drops per min

$$\frac{\text{drops}}{\text{min}} = \frac{\overset{1}{\cancel{20}} \text{ drops}}{1 \text{ } \cancel{mL}} \times \frac{100 \text{ } \cancel{mL}}{1 \text{ } \cancel{hr}} \times \frac{1 \text{ } \cancel{hr}}{\underset{3}{\cancel{60}} \text{ min}} = \frac{100}{3}$$

$$= 33.3, \text{ rounded to } 33 \text{ drops per min}$$

b. Equation is balanced. Only drops per min remain.
c. Yes. 33 drops per min can be counted.

3 75 mL per hr

$$\frac{\text{mL}}{\text{hr}} = \frac{600 \text{ mL}}{8 \text{ hr}} = 75 \text{ mL per hr}$$

4 **a.** 13 drops per min

$$\frac{\text{drops}}{\text{min}} = \frac{\overset{1}{\cancel{10}} \text{ drops}}{1 \text{ } \cancel{mL}} \times \frac{80 \text{ } \cancel{mL}}{1 \text{ } \cancel{hr}} \times \frac{1 \text{ } \cancel{hr}}{\underset{6}{\cancel{60}} \text{ min}} = \frac{80}{6}$$

$$= 13 \text{ drops per minute}$$

b. Equation is balanced. Only drops per minute remain.
c. Yes. 13 drops per minute can be counted.

5 **a.** 25 mL per hr will equal 25 drops per min because the DF is 60.
b. 25 drops per min

$$\frac{\text{drops}}{\text{min}} = \frac{\overset{}{\cancel{60}} \text{ drops}}{1 \text{ } \cancel{mL}} \times \frac{25 \text{ } \cancel{mL}}{1 \text{ } \cancel{hr}} \times \frac{1 \text{ } \cancel{hr}}{\cancel{60} \text{ min}}$$

$$= 25 \text{ drops per minute}$$

c. Equation is balanced. Estimate equals answer.

RAPID PRACTICE 9-4 (p. 315)

1 **a.** 17 drops per min

$$\frac{\text{drops}}{\text{min}} = \frac{\overset{1}{\cancel{10}} \text{ drops}}{1 \text{ } \cancel{mL}} \times \frac{\overset{50}{\cancel{100}} \text{ } \cancel{mL}}{1 \text{ } \cancel{hr}} \times \frac{1 \text{ } \cancel{hr}}{\underset{3}{\cancel{60}} \text{ min}} = \frac{50}{3}$$

$$= 16.6, \text{ rounded to } 17 \text{ drops per min}$$

b. Equation is balanced. Only drops per min remain. Note that 1 hr = 60 min is often the last entry in DF equations.

2 **a.** 20 drops per min

$$\frac{\text{drops}}{\text{min}} = \frac{\overset{1}{\cancel{10}} \text{ drops}}{1 \text{ } \cancel{mL}} \times \frac{120 \text{ } \cancel{mL}}{1 \text{ } \cancel{hr}} \times \frac{1 \text{ } \cancel{hr}}{\underset{6}{\cancel{60}} \text{ min}}$$

$$= \frac{120}{6} = 20 \text{ drops per min}$$

b. Equation is balanced. Only drops per min remain.

3 **a.** 31 drops per min

$$\frac{\text{drops}}{\text{min}} = \frac{\overset{1}{\cancel{15}} \text{ drops}}{1 \text{ } \cancel{mL}} \times \frac{125 \text{ } \cancel{mL}}{1 \text{ } \cancel{hr}} \times \frac{1 \text{ } \cancel{hr}}{\underset{4}{\cancel{60}} \text{ min}}$$

$$= \frac{125}{4} = 31 \text{ drops per min}$$

b. Equation is balanced. Only drops per min remain.

4 **a.** 10 drops per min because DF is 60.
b. Microdrip
c. A needle-like projection delivers the small drops for the microdrip (pediatric) tubing.

5 **a.** 25 drops per min

$$\frac{\text{drops}}{\text{min}} = \frac{\overset{1}{\cancel{20}} \text{ drops}}{1 \text{ } \cancel{mL}} \times \frac{75 \text{ } \cancel{mL}}{1 \text{ } \cancel{hr}} \times \frac{1 \text{ } \cancel{hr}}{\underset{3}{\cancel{60}} \text{ min}} = \frac{75}{3}$$

$$= 25 \text{ drops per min}$$

b. Equation is balanced. Only drops per min remain.

RAPID PRACTICE 9-5 (p. 316)

1 **a.** 13 drops per min

$$\frac{\text{drops}}{\text{min}} = \frac{\overset{1}{\cancel{10} \text{ drops}}}{1 \ \cancel{\text{mL}}} \times \frac{75 \ \cancel{\text{mL}}}{1 \ \cancel{\text{hr}}} \times \frac{1 \ \cancel{\text{hr}}}{\underset{6}{\cancel{60} \text{ min}}} = \frac{75}{6}$$

$$= 12.5, \text{ rounded to 13 drops per min}$$

b. Equation is balanced. Only drops per min remain.

2 **a.** 21 drops per min

$$\frac{\text{drops}}{\text{min}} = \frac{\overset{1}{\cancel{10} \text{ drops}}}{1 \ \cancel{\text{mL}}} \times \frac{125 \ \cancel{\text{mL}}}{1 \ \cancel{\text{hr}}} \times \frac{1 \ \cancel{\text{hr}}}{\underset{6}{\cancel{60} \text{ min}}}$$

$$= 20.8, \text{ rounded to 21 drops per min}$$

b. Equation is balanced. Only drops per min remain.

3 **a.** 13 drops per min

$$\frac{\text{drops}}{\text{min}} = \frac{\overset{1}{\cancel{15} \text{ drops}}}{1 \ \cancel{\text{mL}}} \times \frac{50 \ \cancel{\text{mL}}}{1 \ \cancel{\text{hr}}} \times \frac{1 \ \cancel{\text{hr}}}{\underset{4}{\cancel{60} \text{ min}}}$$

$$= \frac{25}{2} = 12.5, \text{ rounded to 13 drops per min}$$

b. Equation is balanced. Only drops per min remain.

4 **a.** 17 drops per min

$$\frac{\text{drops}}{\text{min}} = \frac{\overset{1}{\cancel{20} \text{ drops}}}{1 \ \cancel{\text{mL}}} \times \frac{50 \ \cancel{\text{mL}}}{1 \ \cancel{\text{hr}}} \times \frac{1 \ \cancel{\text{hr}}}{\underset{3}{\cancel{60} \text{ min}}} = \frac{50}{3}$$

$$= 16.6, \text{ rounded to 17 drops per min}$$

b. Equation is balanced. Only drops per min remain.

5 **a.** 40 drops per min

$$\frac{\text{drops}}{\text{min}} = \frac{\cancel{60} \text{ drops}}{1 \ \cancel{\text{mL}}} \times \frac{40 \ \cancel{\text{mL}}}{1 \ \cancel{\text{hr}}} = \frac{1 \ \cancel{\text{hr}}}{\cancel{60} \text{ min}}$$
$$= 40 \text{ drops per min}$$

b. Equation is balanced. Only drops per min remain.

RAPID PRACTICE 9-6 (p. 318)

2 **a.** $30 \times 3 = 90$ mL per hr

$$\frac{\text{mL}}{\text{hr}} = \frac{30 \text{ mL}}{\underset{1}{\cancel{20} \ \cancel{\text{min}}}} \times \frac{\overset{3}{\cancel{60} \ \cancel{\text{min}}}}{1 \text{ hr}} = 90 \text{ mL per hr}$$

b. Equation is balanced. Estimate equals answer.

3 **a.** $3 \times 50 = 150$ mL per hr

$$\frac{\text{mL}}{\text{hr}} = \frac{50 \text{ mL}}{\underset{1}{\cancel{20} \ \cancel{\text{min}}}} \times \frac{\overset{3}{\cancel{60} \ \cancel{\text{min}}}}{1 \text{ hr}} = 150 \text{ mL per hr}$$

b. Equation is balanced. Estimate equals answer.

4 **a.** 160 mL per hr (80×2)

$$\frac{\text{mL}}{\text{hr}} = \frac{80 \text{ mL}}{\underset{1}{\cancel{30} \ \cancel{\text{min}}}} \times \frac{\overset{2}{\cancel{60} \ \cancel{\text{min}}}}{1 \text{ hr}} = 160 \text{ mL per hr}$$

b. Equation is balanced. Estimate equals answer.

5 **a.** $25 \text{ mL} \times 2 = 50$ mL per hr

$$\frac{\text{mL}}{\text{hr}} = \frac{25 \text{ mL}}{\underset{1}{\cancel{30} \ \cancel{\text{min}}}} \times \frac{\overset{2}{\cancel{60} \ \cancel{\text{min}}}}{1 \text{ hr}} = 50 \text{ mL per hr}$$

b. Equation is balanced. Estimate equals answer.

RAPID PRACTICE 9-7 (p. 320)

1 **a.** 150 mL per hr (50×3) (20 min periods)
b. 25 drops per min

$$\frac{\text{drops}}{\text{min}} = \frac{\overset{1}{\cancel{10} \text{ drops}}}{1 \ \cancel{\text{mL}}} \times \frac{50 \ \cancel{\text{mL}}}{\underset{2}{\cancel{20} \text{ min}}}$$

$$= \frac{50}{2} = 25 \text{ drops per min}$$

c. Equation is balanced. Only drops per min remain.

2 **a.** 150 mL per hr (50×3) (three 20-min periods = 1 hr)
b. 25 drops per min

$$\frac{\text{drops}}{\text{min}} = \frac{\overset{1}{\cancel{10} \text{ drops}}}{1 \ \cancel{\text{mL}}} \times \frac{50 \ \cancel{\text{mL}}}{\underset{2}{\cancel{20} \text{ min}}}$$

$$= 25 \text{ drops per min}$$

c. Equation is balanced. Only drops per min remain.

3 **a.** 75 mL per hr
b. 25 drops per min

$$\frac{\text{drops}}{\text{min}} = \frac{\overset{1}{\cancel{20} \text{ drops}}}{1 \ \cancel{\text{mL}}} \times \frac{75 \ \cancel{\text{mL}}}{\underset{3}{\cancel{60} \text{ min}}} = \frac{75}{3}$$

$$= 25 \text{ drops per min}$$

c. Equation is balanced. Only drops per min remain.

4 **a.** 100×2 (30-min periods) $= 200$ mL per hr
b. 50 drops per min

$$\frac{\text{drops}}{\text{min}} = \frac{\overset{1}{\cancel{15} \text{ drops}}}{1 \ \cancel{\text{mL}}} \times \frac{100 \ \cancel{\text{mL}}}{\underset{2}{\cancel{30} \text{ min}}} = \frac{100}{2}$$

$$= 50 \text{ drops per min}$$

c. Equation is balanced. Only drops per min remain.

5 **a.** 60 mL per hr (30 min × 2) with microdrip mL
per hr = 60 drops per min

b. 60 drops per min

$$\frac{\text{drops}}{\text{min}} = \frac{\overset{2}{\cancel{60}} \text{ drops}}{1 \text{ } \cancel{mL}} \times \frac{30 \text{ } \cancel{mL}}{\underset{1}{\cancel{30}} \text{ min}}$$

$$= 60 \text{ drops per min}$$

c. Equation is balanced. Only drops per minute remain.

RAPID PRACTICE 9-8 (p. 321)

	IVPB Order and Equipment	Estimated Flow Rate	DA
2	20-mL antibiotic solution to infuse in 30 min on gravity infusion device with DF 60	40 mL per hr (20 mL × 2) (2 × 30 min = 60 min)	$\frac{\text{drops}}{\text{min}} = \frac{\overset{2}{\cancel{60}} \text{ drops}}{1 \text{ } \cancel{mL}} \times \frac{20 \text{ } \cancel{mL}}{\underset{1}{\cancel{30}} \text{ min}} = 40$ drops per min $\left(\text{DF } 60 \frac{\text{drops}}{\text{min}} = \frac{\text{mL}}{\text{hr}} \right)$
3	25-mL antibiotic solution in 20 min on gravity infusion device with DF 20	75 mL per hr (3- to 20-min periods in 60 min)	$\frac{\text{drops}}{\text{min}} = \frac{\cancel{20} \text{ drops}}{1 \text{ } \cancel{mL}} \times \frac{25 \text{ mL}}{\cancel{20} \text{ min}} = \frac{50}{2} = \frac{25 \text{ drops}}{\text{per min}}$
4	30-mL anti-cancer medication to infuse in 20 min on EID	90 mL per hr (three 20-min volumes in 60 min per 1 hr)	$\frac{\text{mL}}{\text{hr}} = \frac{30 \text{ mL}}{\underset{1}{\cancel{20 \text{ min}}}} \times \frac{\overset{3}{\cancel{60 \text{ min}}}}{1 \text{ hr}} = 90$ mL per hr
5	60-mL antibiotic solution to infuse in 40 min on EID	90 mL per hr (half the rate of a 20-min order) (180 ÷ 2)	$\frac{\text{mL}}{\text{hr}} = \frac{60 \text{ mL}}{\underset{2}{\cancel{40 \text{ min}}}} \times \frac{\overset{3}{\cancel{60 \text{ min}}}}{1 \text{ hr}} = \frac{180}{2} = 90$ mL per hr

RAPID PRACTICE 9-9 (p. 322)

	Order	Equipment Available	Continuous or Intermittent	Flow Rate Equation (Label Answer)
1	30-mL antibiotic solution to infuse over 30 min	Pediatric microdrip administration set	Intermittent	$\frac{\text{drops}}{\text{min}} = \frac{60 \text{ drops}}{1 \text{ } \cancel{mL}} \times \frac{\cancel{30 \text{ } mL}}{\cancel{30} \text{ min}} = 60$ drops per min
2	1000 mL D5W q10h	IV administration set DF 10	Continuous	$\frac{\text{drops}}{\text{min}} = \frac{\cancel{10} \text{ drops}}{1 \text{ } \cancel{mL}} \times \frac{1000 \text{ } \cancel{mL}}{\cancel{10} \text{ hr}} \times \frac{1 \text{ } \cancel{hr}}{60 \text{ min}} = \frac{1000}{60}$ $= 17$ drops per min
3	50-mL antibiotic solution to infuse over 20 min	Volumetric pump	Intermittent	$\frac{\text{mL}}{\text{hr}} = \frac{50 \text{ mL}}{\underset{1}{\cancel{20 \text{ min}}}} \times \frac{\overset{3}{\cancel{60 \text{ min}}}}{1 \text{ hr}} = 150$ mL per hr
4	250 mL D5W over 4 hr	Electronic infusion pump	Intermittent	$\frac{\text{mL}}{\text{hr}} = \frac{250 \text{ mL}}{4 \text{ hr}} = 62.5$, rounded to 63 mL per hr
5	500 mL NS q6h	IV administration set DF 15	Continuous	$\frac{\text{drops}}{\text{min}} = \frac{\cancel{15} \text{ drops}}{1 \text{ } \cancel{mL}} \times \frac{500 \text{ } \cancel{mL}}{6 \text{ } \cancel{hr}} \times \frac{1 \text{ } \cancel{hr}}{\underset{4}{\cancel{60} \text{ min}}} = \frac{500}{24}$ $= 20.8$, rounded to 21 drops per min

RAPID PRACTICE 9-10 (p. 326)

	Drops per 30 Sec Counted at Bedside	Drops per min (Mental Calculation)	Administration Set DF	Flow Rate Equation
2	8 drops per 30 sec	16	10	$\dfrac{mL}{hr} = \dfrac{1\ mL}{\underset{1}{\cancel{10}\ \cancel{drops}}} \times \dfrac{\overset{}{16}\ \cancel{drops}}{1\ \cancel{min}} \times \dfrac{\overset{6}{\cancel{60}\ \cancel{min}}}{1\ hr} = 96\ mL\ per\ hr$
3	6 drops per 15 sec	24	60	$\dfrac{mL}{hr} = \dfrac{1\ mL}{\cancel{60}\ \cancel{drops}} \times \dfrac{24\ \cancel{drops}}{1\ \cancel{min}} \times \dfrac{\cancel{60}\ \cancel{min}}{1\ hr} = 24\ mL\ per\ hr$
4	15 drops per 30 sec	30	60	$\dfrac{mL}{hr} = \dfrac{1\ mL}{\cancel{60}\ \cancel{drops}} \times \dfrac{30\ \cancel{drops}}{1\ \cancel{min}} \times \dfrac{\cancel{60}\ \cancel{min}}{1\ hr} = 30\ mL\ per\ hr$
5	12 drops per 30 sec	24	15	$\dfrac{mL}{hr} = \dfrac{1\ mL}{\underset{1}{\cancel{15}\ \cancel{drops}}} \times \dfrac{24\ \cancel{drops}}{1\ \cancel{min}} \times \dfrac{\overset{4}{\cancel{60}\ \cancel{min}}}{1\ hr} = 96\ mL\ per\ hr$

RAPID PRACTICE 9-11 (p. 327)

1 d   4 c
2 b   5 c
3 b

RAPID PRACTICE 9-12 (p. 328)

1 **a.** macrodrip
   b. 150 mL per hr
   c. 38 drops per min

$$\frac{drops}{min} = \frac{\overset{1}{\cancel{15}}\ drops}{1\ \cancel{mL}} \times \frac{150\ \cancel{mL}}{1\ \cancel{hr}} \times \frac{1\ \cancel{hr}}{\underset{4}{\cancel{60}}\ min}$$

$$= 37.5,\ rounded\ to\ 38\ drops\ per\ min$$

   d. Equation is balanced. Only drops per min remain.
   e. 6 hr 42 min infusion duration time

$$hr = \frac{1\ hr}{\underset{3}{\cancel{150}\ \cancel{mL}}} \times \overset{20}{\cancel{1000}\ \cancel{mL}}$$

$$= 6.66,\ rounded\ to\ 6.7\ hr$$

$$min = \frac{60\ min}{1\ \cancel{hr}} \times 0.7\ \cancel{hrs} = 42\ min$$

2 **a.** microdrip
   b. 50 drops per min

$$\frac{drops}{min} = \frac{\cancel{60}\ drops}{1\ \cancel{mL}} \times \frac{500\ \cancel{mL}}{10\ \cancel{hr}} \times \frac{1\ \cancel{hr}}{\cancel{60}\ min}$$

$$= \frac{500}{10} = 50\ drops\ per\ min$$

   c. Equation is balanced. Only drops per min remain.

3 **a.** macrodrip
   b. 21 drops per min

$$\frac{drops}{min} = \frac{\overset{1}{\cancel{10}}\ drops}{1\ \cancel{mL}} \times \frac{1000\ \cancel{mL}}{8\ \cancel{hr}} \times \frac{1\ \cancel{hr}}{\underset{6}{\cancel{60}}\ min} = \frac{1000}{48}$$

$$= 20.8,\ rounded\ to\ 21\ drops\ per\ min$$

   c. Equation is balanced. Only drops per min remain.

4 **a.** microdrip
   b. 40 drops per min

$$\frac{drops}{min} = \frac{\overset{1}{\cancel{60}}\ drops}{1\ \cancel{mL}} \times \frac{40\ \cancel{mL}}{\underset{1}{\cancel{60}}\ min}$$

$$= 40\ drops\ per\ min$$

   c. Equation is balanced. Only drops per min remain.

5 **a.** macrodrip
   b. 17 drops per min

$$\frac{drops}{min} = \frac{\overset{1}{\cancel{10}}\ drops}{1\ \cancel{mL}} \times \frac{100\ \cancel{mL}}{\underset{6}{\cancel{60}}\ min} = \frac{100}{6}$$

$$= 16.7,\ rounded\ to\ 17\ drops\ per\ min$$

   c. Equation is balanced. Only drops per min remain.

RAPID PRACTICE 9-13 (p. 330)

1 **a.** 125 mL per hr

$$\frac{mL}{hr} = \frac{500}{4} = 125 \text{ mL per hr}$$

b. Equation is balanced. Only mL per hr remain.

2 **a.** 14 drops per min

$$\frac{drops}{min} = \frac{\overset{1}{\cancel{20} \text{ drops}}}{1 \cancel{mL}} \times \frac{250 \cancel{mL}}{6 \cancel{hr}} \times \frac{1 \cancel{hr}}{\underset{3}{60} \text{ min}}$$

$$= \frac{250}{18} = \begin{matrix}13.9, \text{ rounded to} \\ 14 \text{ drops per min}\end{matrix}$$

b. Equation is balanced. Only drops per min remain.

3 **a.** 125 mL per hr

$$\frac{mL}{hr} = \frac{1000 \text{ mL}}{8 \text{ hr}} = 125 \text{ mL per hr}$$

b. Equation is balanced. Only mL per hr remain.

4 **a.** 14 drops per min

$$\frac{drops}{min} = \frac{10 \text{ drops}}{1 \cancel{mL}} \times \frac{1000 \cancel{mL}}{12 \cancel{hr}} \times \frac{1 \cancel{hr}}{60 \text{ min}}$$

$$= \frac{166.66}{12} = 13.88 = 14 \text{ drops per min}$$

b. Equation is balanced. Only drops per min remain.

5 **a.** 42 drops per min

$$\frac{drops}{min} = \frac{\overset{1}{\cancel{60} \text{ drops}}}{1 \cancel{mL}} \times \frac{1000 \cancel{mL}}{24 \cancel{hr}} \times \frac{1 \cancel{hr}}{\underset{1}{60} \text{ min}}$$

$$= \frac{1000}{24} = \begin{matrix}41.6, \text{ rounded to} \\ 42 \text{ drops per min}\end{matrix}$$

b. Equation is balanced. Only drops per min remain.

Note: With 60 DF and a continuous IV, mL per hr = drops per min.

RAPID PRACTICE 9-14 (p. 332)

2 **a.** 200 g dextrose

$$g \text{ dextrose} = \frac{10 \text{ g}}{100 \cancel{mL}} \times \frac{\overset{20}{\cancel{2000} \cancel{mL}}}{1}$$

$$= 200 \text{ g dextrose}$$

b. Equation is balanced. Only g remain.

3 **a.** 2.25 g NaCl

$$g \text{ NaCl} = \frac{0.45 \text{ g}}{\underset{1}{100 \cancel{mL}}} \times \frac{\overset{5}{\cancel{500} \cancel{mL}}}{1} = 2.25 \text{ g NaCl}$$

b. Equation is balanced. Only grams remain.

Remember: NS contains slightly less than 1% NaCl. Watch the decimal.

4 **a.** 75 g dextrose

$$g \text{ dextrose} = \frac{5 \text{ g}}{\underset{1}{100 \text{ mL}}} \times \frac{\overset{15}{\cancel{1500} \cancel{mL}}}{1}$$

$$= 75 \text{ g dextrose}$$

b. Equation is balanced. Only grams remain.

5 **a.** 13.5 g NaCl

$$g \text{ NaCl} = \frac{0.9 \text{ g}}{\underset{1}{100 \cancel{mL}}} \times \frac{\overset{15}{\cancel{1500} \cancel{mL}}}{1} = 13.5 \text{ g NaCl}$$

b. Equation is balanced. Only grams remain.

CHAPTER 9 MULTIPLE-CHOICE REVIEW (p. 339)

1	c	**6**	a
2	c	**7**	b
3	a	**8**	d (100 g per 1000 mL)
4	c	**9**	b
5	a	**10**	c

CHAPTER 9 FINAL PRACTICE (p. 340)

1 **a.** 60 drops per min (20×3)

$$\frac{mL}{hr} = \frac{\overset{3}{\cancel{60} \text{ drops}}}{1 \cancel{mL}} \times \frac{20 \cancel{mL}}{\underset{1}{\cancel{20} \text{ min}}}$$

$$= 60 \text{ drops per min}$$

b. Equation is balanced. Only drops per min remain.

2 **a.** 600 mL

b. 1800 hr

3 **a.** 25 g dextrose

$$g \text{ dextrose} = \frac{50 \text{ g}}{\underset{2}{100 \cancel{mL}}} \times \frac{\overset{1}{\cancel{50} \cancel{mL}}}{1}$$

$$= 25 \text{ g dextrose}$$

b. Equation is balanced. Only g remain.

4 Normal saline.

5 The tubing delivers a drop factor of 10 drops per mL.

6 120 mL per hr

$$\frac{mL}{hour} = \frac{2 \text{ mL}}{1 \cancel{min}} \times \frac{60 \cancel{min}}{1 \text{ hr}} = 120 \text{ mL per hr}$$

7 secondary

8 a. 5 hr

b. 225 mL

$$\frac{50 \text{ mL}}{1 \text{ hr}} \times 4.5 \text{ hr} = 225 \text{ mL}$$

9 Fluid and electrolyte maintenance, replacement of prior losses, and administration of medications and nutrients

10 Ensure that the primary IV is flowing at its ordered rate.

11 a. 63 mL per hr

$$\frac{\text{mL}}{\text{hr}} = \frac{500 \text{ mL}}{8 \text{ hr}} = 62.5 \text{ mL per hr}$$

b. 1200 + 7.5 hr = 1930 hr

12 0.9% NaCl, D5W, L/R (RL) (R/L)

13 Cardiac arrest (a sentinel event)

14 a. 2.25 g NaCl

$$g \text{ NaCl} = \frac{0.9 \text{ g}}{\overset{}{\underset{2}{100 \text{ mL}}}} \times \frac{\overset{5}{250 \text{ mL}}}{1} = \frac{4.5}{2}$$

$$= 2.25 \text{ g NaCl}$$

b. Equation is balanced.

c. 10 drops per min

$$\frac{\text{drops}}{\text{min}} = \frac{\overset{1}{10} \text{ drops}}{1 \text{ mL}} \times \frac{250 \text{ mL}}{4 \text{ hr}} \times \frac{1 \text{ hr}}{\underset{6}{60} \text{ min}}$$

$$= \frac{250}{24} = \begin{array}{l}10.4, \text{ rounded to} \\ 10 \text{ drops per min}\end{array}$$

d. Equation is balanced. Only drops per min remain.

15 a. $\dfrac{\text{drops}}{\text{min}} = \dfrac{\overset{1}{10} \text{ drops}}{1 \text{ mL}} \times \dfrac{\overset{125}{250 \text{ mL}}}{\underset{1}{2 \text{ hr}}} \times \dfrac{1 \text{ hr}}{\underset{6}{60} \text{ min}}$

$$= \frac{125}{6} = \begin{array}{l}20.8, \text{ rounded to} \\ 21 \text{ drops per min}\end{array}$$

b. Equation is balanced. Only drops per min remain.

Note: Equation can be simplified by substituting mL per hr for total mL per total hours.

16 a. 60 drops per mL

b. 60 drops per min (60 mL per hr)

17 a. $\dfrac{\text{drops}}{\text{min}} = \dfrac{\overset{1}{20} \text{ drops}}{1 \text{ mL}} \times \dfrac{500 \text{ mL}}{8 \text{ hr}} \times \dfrac{1 \text{ hr}}{\underset{3}{60} \text{ min}}$

$$= \begin{array}{l}20.8, \text{ rounded to} \\ 21 \text{ drops per min}\end{array}$$

b. Equation is balanced. Only drops per min remain.

18 a. Volume-control burette device

b. 1-2 hr worth of ordered fluid. Refer to agency policy.

19 100 mL per hr (50 × 2)

20 a. $\dfrac{\text{drops}}{\text{min}} = \dfrac{\overset{1}{15} \text{ drops}}{1 \text{ mL}} \times \dfrac{3000 \text{ mL}}{24 \text{ hr}} \times \dfrac{1 \text{ hr}}{\underset{4}{60} \text{ min}}$

$$= \begin{array}{l}31.25, \text{ rounded to} \\ 31 \text{ drops per min}\end{array}$$

b. Equation is balanced. Only drops per min remain.

Suggestions for Further Reading

Gahart BL, Nazareno AR: *2017 Intravenous medications: a handbook for nurses and health professionals,* ed. 33, St. Louis, 2021, Mosby.
www.baxter.com
www.cc.nih.gov/nursing
www.ismp.org
www.jointcommission.org
www.ccforpatientsafety.org
http://www.baxter.com/healthcare_professionals/products/infusion_systems_products.html

⊖volve   For additional practice problems, refer to the Intravenous Flow Rates section of the Elsevier's Interactive Drug Calculation Application, Version 1 on Evolve.

Chapter 10 covers advanced IV infusion calculations using this chapter as a foundation. Note the high-alert drugs.

10 Advanced Intravenous Calculations

OBJECTIVES

- Calculate infusion flow rates for the following units of measurement: mg per mL, mg per hr, mg per min, mcg per mL, mcg per hr, mcg per min, mcg per kg, mcg per kg per hr, mcg per kg per min, mg per kg, mg per kg per hr, mg per kg per min, and mEq per hr.
- Confirm IV medication orders with safe dosage range (SDR) criteria.
- Calculate rate of administration for direct IV push medications.

- Calculate the parameters of flow rates for titrated IV infusions.
- State the difference between central venous lines and peripheral venous lines.
- Calculate the calories in selected IV solutions.
- State the general purpose, contents, and types of hyperalimentation (PN) infusions.
- Identify patient safety issues for the administration of IV medications, and PN infusions.

ESTIMATED TIME TO COMPLETE CHAPTER: 3 hours

Chapter 9 focused on prepared IV solutions that required simple flow rate calculations. This chapter emphasizes more complex dose-based flow rate calculations for a variety of IV solutions containing medications. The principles of the equation setup are the same as in earlier chapters.

Although D5W, NS, and D5LR solutions are vehicles for many IV medications, certain medications require a specific solution. The trend for safety purposes is to have pharmacy-prepared IV mixtures.

➤ Always check for compatibilities *and incompatibilities* before mixing and/or administering medications and solutions. It must be assumed that IV solutions and medications, including diluents, are incompatible unless the literature states otherwise.

VOCABULARY

Central Venous Line	Central venous sites are large blood volume sites (such as the superior vena cava and right atrium) that can be accessed by catheter from large veins (such as the jugular) or surgically accessed chest veins. They can also be accessed from peripherally inserted central catheters (PICCs), which are less invasive and threaded to the superior vena cava–right atrial junction from a peripheral vein. The central venous sites provide rapid dilution of concentrated solutions such as PN and medications and are more suitable for longer term therapy and more concentrated solutions than smaller peripheral veins.
IV Filters	Used in some IV medication lines to prevent contaminants, particles, and clots from reaching patient circulation. Liquids can pass through the filter. Specific guidelines for use and filter size must be checked with agency and manufacturer guidelines prior to administration of medications. Blood administration sets are supplied with a clot filter, and other filters may be added for specific purposes, depending on the type of blood product. Filters are frequently used for infusions through central lines.
IV Flush (SAS) (SASH)	Technique that maintains patency of IV sites used before and after infusion of medications and for periodic maintenance. Saline solution or less frequently, low-dose heparin solution is injected through infusion ports in accordance with agency protocols for milliliter amounts for each type of flush solution and the equipment being flushed. The longer the line, the more solution must be used. Also used to clear lines of solutions before administering a potentially incompatible solution. *SAS* means "saline, administer drug, saline flush." *SASH* means "saline, administer drug, saline, heparin flush."
Kilocalorie (Kcal)	Metric measurement of a unit of energy, necessary to raise the temperature of 1 kg of water by 1° C. Commonly described as "calorie," even though there are 1000 calories in a *kilo*calorie, as the metric prefix indicates. The "Calories" on food labels are actually kilocalories.
⚑ **Parenteral Nutrition (PN) (also known as "Total Parenteral Nutrition (TPN),"** **"Hyperalimentation," "Hyperal")**	*Parenteral nutrition* (PN) refers to an IV caloric infusion of nutrients, vitamins, minerals, lipids, and electrolytes through a central or peripheral venous line. Contents and amounts are prescribed on an individual basis.
Peak and Trough Levels	Serum levels of drugs derived from blood samples drawn 30 minutes before the next dose is due (trough) and/or 30 minutes after administration (peak) for IV drugs and 1-2 hours after oral drugs (peak). Guides the prescriber for effective dosing and avoidance of toxicity or damage to renal function. The nurse must label specimen with peak or trough, exact time drawn, and time and dose of last medication infusion. Certain drugs, such as vancomycin, an antibiotic, have widely varying rates of individual absorption and necessitate peak and trough measurements to avoid severe toxic effects and are usually done after three doses are given and when there are dosage changes.
Peripherally Inserted Central Catheter (PICC)	A peripherally inserted central catheter (PICC line) is a form of intravenous access that can be used for a prolonged time (e.g., chemotherapy, extended antibiotic therapy, total parenteral nutrition) or to administer substances that should not be given peripherally because of vascular irritation. The catheter enters the body through the skin (percutaneously) at a peripheral site, and extends to the superior vena cava. It stays in place for days, weeks, and sometimes months. Blood for laboratory tests can also be withdrawn from a PICC. An ultrasound or a chest x-ray is obtained to confirm proper placement of the catheter tip.
Titrated Medication	Flexible drug order for dose adjustments to achieve desired therapeutic result, such as a specific urinary output, systolic or diastolic blood pressure, or glucose level (e.g., "dobutamine 2 to 8 mg per kg per min IV infusion. Increase or lower by 1 to 2 mg every 30 min to achieve/maintain systolic pressure between 90 and 110 mm Hg"). These are administered and adjusted by competency proven registered nurses.
Vascular Implanted Devices **Vascular Access Devices (VADs)**	Surgically implanted, subcutaneous, self-sealing injection ports that can tolerate repeated access with a special Huber needle. The port is attached to a catheter threaded most commonly through the subclavian vein into the right atrium. Saves the patient the discomfort of multiple needlesticks for blood draws and administration of IV medications.

Advanced Intravenous Calculations

Practice a few exercises to prepare for setting up and understanding medicated IV calculations.

RAPID PRACTICE 10-1	Intravenous Calculations

ESTIMATED COMPLETION TIME: 20 to 25 minutes   **ANSWERS ON:** page 383

DIRECTIONS: *Estimate and calculate the requested IV infusion as shown.*

1 **Ordered:** 2 mL per minute. Need to know: mL per hr.

   a. Estimated answer: $2 \times 60 = 120$ mL per hr.

   DA equation:

$$\frac{mL}{hr} = \frac{2 \text{ mL}}{1 \text{ min}} \times \frac{60 \text{ min}}{1 \text{ hr}} = 120 \text{ ml per hr}$$

   b. Evaluation: Equation is balanced. Only mL/hr remain.

2 **Ordered:** 60 mg per hr. Need to know: mg per min.

   a. Estimated mg per min: _____

   DA equation.

   b. Evaluation: _____

3 **Ordered:** 4 mg per min. Need to know: mg per hr.

   a. Estimated mg per hr:

   DA equation:

   b. Evaluation: _____

4 **Ordered:** 120 mL per hr. Need to know: mL per min to nearest tenth of a mL.

   a. Estimated mL per min: _____

   DA equation:

   b. Evaluation: _____

5 **Ordered:** 2 mg per kg per min. Weight: 10 kg.* Need to know: mg per min.

   a. Estimated mg per min: _____

   DA equation:

   b. Evaluation: _____

   c. Estimated mg per hr: _____

   DA equation:

   d. Evaluation: _____

---

*Kg weight-based dosing is recommended by many agencies.

Using Conversion Factors

One or more conversion factors may be required to complete IV infusion calculations. Refer back to these as you work through the chapter.

Conversion Factors	Purpose
60 minutes = 1 hour	Often needed to obtain milliliters or medication dose per hour, this formula also may be needed to verify how much drug per minute or volume per minute is being infused. For example: **Ordered:** Drug Y, 1 mg per min. Question: How many milligrams or milliliters per hour will be infused?
1000 mg = 1 g 1000 mcg = 1 mg	Needed for conversion when the drug units supplied do not match the drug units ordered. For example: **Ordered:** Drug Y, 2 mcg per min. Supplied: Drug Y, 500 mg.
1000 mL = 1 L	Needed to convert liters to milliliters for IV flow rate calculations. IV flow rates are delivered in milliliters. **Ordered:** 1 L q8h. 1 L = 1000 mL. 1000 mL ÷ 8 = 125 mL per hr.
2.2 lb = 1 kg	Occasionally needed to calculate the dose ordered when the dose is based on weight and the weight in pounds is known and in kilograms is not. For example: **Ordered:** Drug Y, 2 mg per kg per min. Weight: 50 lb.

 ASK YOURSELF 1 What are four conversion factors that may be needed for IV infusion calculations? (Give a brief answer.)

MY ANSWER _____

Calculating Flow Rates

Intravenous flow rates are usually calculated in milliliters per hour (mL per hr) but may be ordered in units of a drug to be infused per hour or per minute. Following are some examples of how the amount of a drug to be given per a unit of time may be expressed in medication orders:

2 mg per min	5 mcg per min	3 units per min
4 mg per hr	3 mcg per hr	10 mEq per hr
0.3 mg per kg per min	1 mcg per kg per min	0.5 milliUnits per min

Orders for powerful drugs may be written for a drug dose per minute or per hour. Following are some examples of drug concentrations supplied in IV solutions:

250 mg drug per 500 mL D5W	500 mg drug per 250 mL NS	100 mg drug per 250 mL D5W
250 mg drug per 1000 mL NS	100 mg drug per 50 mL NS	1 g drug per 1000 mL D5W

EXAMPLES

Ordered: Drug Y, 5 mg per min. Available: Drug Y, 400 mg per 200 mL. Question: The flow rate must be set at how many mL per hr to deliver 5 mg per min?

Three factors must be entered in the medication equation to determine mL per hour flow rates:
1. Ordered medication amount and time frame to be infused
2. Available drug concentration
3. Needed conversion factors

$$\frac{mL}{hr} = \frac{\overset{1}{\cancel{200}}\ mL}{\underset{\underset{1}{2}}{\cancel{400}\ \cancel{mg}}} \times \frac{5\ \cancel{mg}}{1\ \cancel{min}} \times \frac{\overset{30}{\cancel{60}\ \cancel{min}}}{1\ hr} = 150\ mL\ per\ hr$$

Analysis: The data with mL will be entered *in the first numerator.* Milligrams will need to be canceled. The order is in mg, and that quantity ordered is entered next to cancel the mg in the drug concentration. Hours are entered in the last *denominator* with the required min-to-hr conversion. Note the progression for canceling undesired units from one denominator to the next numerator—mg to mg and min to min—as in prior DA equations.

Evaluation: The equation is balanced. Only mL per hr remain.

➤ *One* conversion factor is needed. Because the drug ordered and the drug supplied are in the *same terms—milligrams—*a minutes-to-hours conversion is the *only* factor needed.

➤ The drug concentration is entered as one factor. Reduction and cancellation makes the math easy.

➤ If the drug ordered was ordered in mg, and the amount supplied in g, a conversion formula from mg to g would have to be entered.

ASK YOURSELF

1 What are three factors that need to be entered in the equation to calculate medicated IV infusion rates in mL per hr? (Use one- or two-word answers.)

MY ANSWER

_____

RAPID PRACTICE 10-2   Converting Milligrams per Minute to Milliliters per Hour

ESTIMATED COMPLETION TIME: 20 minutes   **ANSWERS ON:** page 383

DIRECTIONS: *For each problem, determine which conversion formula will be needed. Calculate the mL per hr flow rate as shown in the preceding example. Cancel units before doing the math. Label answers.*

TEST TIP   After cancellation of units in the equation, it often simplifies the math to reduce the available drug concentration fraction if it can be reduced.

---

1   **Ordered:** Drug Y, 0.4 mg per min. Available: 250 mg in 1 L D5W.

   a. mL per hr flow rate?

      DA equation:

   b. Evaluation: _____

2   **Ordered:** Drug Y, 1 mg per min. Available: 500 mg Drug Y in 1000 mL LRS.

    a. mL per hr flow rate?

        DA equation:

    b. Evaluation: _____

3   **Ordered:** Drug Y, 0.5 mg per min. Available: 500 mg per 250 mL 0.45 NS.

    a. mL per hr flow rate?

        DA equation:

    b. Evaluation: _____

4   **Ordered:** Drug Y, 0.2 mg per min. Available: 100 mg per 100 mL D5W.

    a. mL per hr flow rate?

        DA equation:

    b. Evaluation: _____

5   **Ordered:** Drug Y, 2 mg per min. Available: 1000 mg Drug Y in 1000 mL D5W.

    a. mL per hr flow rate?

        DA equation:

    b. Evaluation: _____

Flow Rates Requiring Two Conversion Factors

The nurse is liable for any medication administration errors regardless of whether they may be computer, prescriber, or pharmacy errors. It is essential for the nurse to know how to calculate flow rates no matter how they are ordered.

➤ The drug ordered and the drug supplied must be converted to the same terms.

➤ A time conversion, 60 minutes = 1 hour, is needed when the IV order is per minute.

Ordered: Drug Y, 100 mcg per min. Available: Drug Y, 400 mg per 250 mL.

Calculate flow rate in mL per hr.

EXAMPLES

Conversion factors available: 1000 mcg = 1 mg, 1000 mg = 1 g, 60 min = 1 hr, and 1000 mL = 1 L.

$$\frac{mL}{hr} = \frac{\overset{5}{\cancel{250}}\ mL}{\underset{8}{\cancel{400}\ mg}} \times \frac{1\ \cancel{mg}}{\underset{\underset{1}{10}}{\cancel{1000}\ \cancel{mcg}}} \times \frac{\overset{1}{\cancel{100}\ \cancel{mcg}}}{1\ \cancel{min}} \times \frac{\overset{6}{\cancel{60}\ \cancel{min}}}{1\ hr} = \frac{30}{8} = \begin{array}{l}3.75, \text{ rounded}\\ \text{to 4 mL per hr}\end{array} *$$

Analysis: Drug concentration was entered first because it contained mL for the desired answer. In addition to the drug order, two conversion formulas will be needed: mg to mcg to cancel mg in the first denominator and to cancel mcg in the drug order. Finally, the min-to-hr conversion formula was entered to provide hr for the desired answer. Stop before doing the math. Do only the desired answer units remain? Answer: Yes.

Evaluation: The equation is balanced. Only mL per hr remain.

➤ Note how sequential cancellation guides the setup.

_____

*Many IV pumps can deliver tenths of a mL such as 3.8 mL per hr (rounded from 3.75). The equipment determines the nearest measurable flow rate.

RAPID PRACTICE 10-3	Flow Rates Requiring Two Conversion Factors

ESTIMATED COMPLETION TIME: 20 to 25 minutes   **ANSWERS ON:** page 384

DIRECTIONS: *Analyze the preceding example and worked-out problem 1. Determine how many conversion factors are needed. Calculate using needed conversion factors. Conversion factors: 60 min = 1 hr, 1000 mcg = 1 mg, and 1000 mg = 1 g.*

1 Ordered: Drug Y, IV infusion 200 mcg per min. Available: Drug Y, 250 mg per 1000 mL D5W.

   a. What will the flow rate be in mL per hr?

   DA equation:

$$\frac{mL}{hr} = \frac{\overset{4}{\cancel{1000}}\ mL}{\underset{1}{\cancel{250}\ mg}} \times \frac{1\ \cancel{mg}}{\underset{\underset{1}{5}}{\cancel{1000}\ \cancel{mcg}}} \times \frac{\overset{1}{\cancel{200}\ \cancel{mcg}}}{1\ \cancel{min}} \times \frac{\overset{12}{\cancel{60}\ \cancel{min}}}{1\ hr} = 48\ \frac{mL}{hr}$$

   b. Evaluation: Equation is balanced. Only mL per hr remain.

2 Ordered: Drug Y, IV infusion 200 mcg per min. Available: Drug Y, 500 mg per 250 mL D5W.

   a. What will the flow rate be in mL per hr? _____

   DA equation:

   b. Evaluation: _____

3   **Ordered:** Drug Y, IV infusion 75 mcg per minute. Available: Drug Y, 10 mg per 100 mL NS.*

   a. What will the flow rate be in mL per hr?

       DA equation:

   b. Evaluation: _____

4   **Ordered:** Drug Y, IV infusion 5 mg per min. Available: Drug Y, 1 g per 200 mL LRS.

   a. What will the flow rate be in mL per hr? _____

       DA equation:

   b. Evaluation: _____

5   **Ordered:** Drug Y, IV infusion 1.5 mg per min. Available: Drug Y, 2 g per 200 mL NS.

   a. What will the flow rate be in mL per hr? _____

       DA equation:

   b. Evaluation: _____

| **Q & A** | **ASK YOURSELF** | 1 | Why are two conversion factors needed in problems 1 and 2? Which factors are they? |
| | **MY ANSWER** | | _____ |

Flow Rates for Weight-Based Doses

An order for a continuous IV infusion may read: dopamine 2 mcg per kg per min. The solution available may be: dopamine 200 mg per 250 mL D5W. How many mL per hr will be set? The patient weight today is 50 kg.

1   Identify the desired answer units.
2   Calculate the ordered dose based on the requested units of weight.
3   Enter the drug concentration available, the ordered dose, and any needed conversion formulas in a DA equation to obtain the desired answer.

As stated earlier, the dose ordered must always be entered in the medication equation along with the concentration available and the conversion factors.

➤ Step 2, calculating the ordered dose based on weight, is the only additional step compared with the problems in Rapid Practice 10-3.

➤ The desired answer is a mL-per-hr flow rate.

_____

*NS solution is 0.9% NaCl solution. Refer to Chapter 9. Any concentration other than 0.9% is stated, e.g., 0.45% NaCl ($\frac{1}{2}$NS).

Total dose for weight-based orders

Calculate the *total drug ordered* using the patient's body weight in kilograms.

Ordered: Dopamine 2 mcg per kg per min IV. Patient's weight: 50 kg.
How many total micrograms per minute are ordered?
Estimated dose in micrograms: (2 mcg $\times$ 50 kg) = 100 mcg total dose per min.

Step 1	=	Step 2	$\times$	Step 3	=	Answer
Desired Answer Units	=	Starting Factor	$\times$	Given Quantity and Conversion Factor(s)	=	Estimate, Multiply, Evaluate
$\dfrac{mcg}{min}$	=	$\dfrac{2\ mcg}{1\ \cancel{kg} \times min}$	$\times$	$\dfrac{50\ \cancel{kg}}{1}$	=	$\dfrac{100\ mcg}{min}$

Analysis:

➤ Note how the 2 mcg per kg per min will always set up with the kg per min(s) in the accompanying denominator in this kind of order that contains 3 units (e.g., 5 mg per kg per hr or 10 mcg per kg per hr).

If the patient's weight is 110 lb and the weight in kilograms is not known, just enter one more conversion factor for pounds to kilograms (1 kg = 2.2 lb).

$$\frac{mcg}{min} = \frac{2\ mcg}{1\ \cancel{kg}\ per\ min} \times \frac{1\ \cancel{kg}}{2.2\ \cancel{lb}} \times \frac{50\ \cancel{lb}}{1} = 100\ mcg\ per\ min$$

➤ $\dfrac{100\ mcg}{min}$ can be written as 100 mcg per min.

➤ Many IV medications are high-alert medications.

FAQ *Why are kilograms not retained in the answer for milligrams-per-kilogram problems?*

ANSWER The desired answer is in *micrograms per minute*. The dose is *based on the patient's weight: 2 mcg for each kilogram of weight*. After factoring in the kilogram weight by multiplying micrograms by kilograms, the kilogram units *are eliminated* from the answer.

If you were asked how many cups of water you drink during the day, you might respond, "I drink about 1 cup *per hour*, so I drink 8 cups a day." The desired units in the answer are *cups per day*. Hours were only factored in to get the total amount, just as kilograms of body weight are factored in only to get a total amount of milligrams. Hours would be eliminated from the final answer, as are kilograms.

Flow rate in milliliters per hour (mL per hr) for weight-based orders

The example that follows illustrates a one-step equation for IV weight-based orders.

EXAMPLES

Ordered: Dopamine 2 mcg per kg per min. On hand: An IV of dopamine 200 mg in 250 mL of D5W. Patient's weight: 60 kg.

What flow rate will be set on the IV pump to the nearest tenth of a mL?

Conversion factors: 60 minutes = 1 hr; 1000 mcg = 1 mg.

Step 1

Starting

Step 1 = Factor = Answer

$$\frac{mL}{hr} = \frac{\overset{1}{\underset{\underset{4}{\cancel{200}\;mg}}{\cancel{\underset{5}{\cancel{250}}}\;mL}}}{} \times \frac{1\;\cancel{mg}}{\underset{\underset{\underset{1}{100}}{200}}{\cancel{1000}\;\cancel{mcg}}} \times \frac{\overset{1}{\cancel{2}\;\cancel{mcg}}}{\cancel{kg} \times \cancel{min}} \times \frac{\cancel{60}\;\cancel{kg}}{1} \times \frac{\cancel{60}\;\cancel{min}}{1\;hr} = 9\frac{mL}{hr}$$

➤ 60 minutes = 1 hour provides a needed conversion for the answer.

➤ Remember to cancel units to verify the setup *before* doing the math cancellations.

Analysis: Each denominator leads to the placement of the next numerator for cancellation of unwanted units. Note how the math is greatly simplified with the reduction of the IV starting factor as well as cancellation of zeros. In these problems, the medicated IV concentration becomes the starting factor because it contains the needed mL. Concentrations can be inverted to be placed correctly to match the desired answer.

➤ Note that the trend is for the pharmacy to prepare and supply premixed IV medicated solutions. They also usually supply the ordered flow rate. Verify the rate.

FAQ　*Can the weight-based ordered dose calculation (2 mcg per kg per min = 60 mcg per minute or 3600 mcg per hr or 3.6 mg per hr) be calculated separately and then entered in the equation to shorten it?*

ANSWER　You have the option of entering all of the data in one equation or breaking it up into two steps. One step makes a very long equation as shown in the preceding example. There are two considerations: The more steps in the process, the greater the likelihood of error. But, as shown, the longer one-step equation can be greatly simplified with reduction and cancellation. The one-step equation also reveals that all the needed data are entered.

FAQ　*Why do medication infusion orders sometimes specify a range for drug dose or flow rate?*

ANSWER　A range allows the nurse to titrate the dose or rate, starting with the lowest dose, until the desired response is achieved (e.g., a pulse over 60, or to maintain a minimum urinary output). Based on intervals of time and dose specified in the order, the rate or dose is increased at a specified interval or gradually until the desired response is achieved and maintained. This may require many adjustments if the patient's condition is unstable.

The order may read: Drug Y at 10 to 20 mcg per min to maintain a systolic pressure of 90 to 100 mm Hg or a minimum urinary output of 30 mL per hr. May be increased by 2 mcg per min every hr. The calculations are performed separately for each amount in a range.

FAQ *If the pharmacy supplies IV solutions with medications, does the nurse still have to do the calculations?*

ANSWER Physicians as well as pharmacists are capable of making medication errors. The nurse must double-check the current order, the SDR references, the contents, and the flow rates in order to protect the patient.

RAPID PRACTICE 10-4 Flow Rates for Weight-Based Orders

ESTIMATED COMPLETION TIME: 25 minutes   **ANSWERS ON:** page 384

DIRECTIONS: *Study the preceding example and the following worked-out problem 1. Identify the desired answer units. Identify and calculate the dose ordered. Calculate the desired flow rate with a DA equation. Remember that reducing the drug concentration fraction after cancellation of units simplifies the math.*

1 **Ordered:** dobutamine hydrochloride IV infusion 0.5 mcg per kg per min for 24 hr for a patient with cardiac decompensation. Available: dobutamine 250 mg per 250 mL D5W. Patient's weight: 100 kg.

  a. DA equation to calculate mL per hr:

$$\frac{mL}{hr} = \frac{\overset{1}{\cancel{250}}\ mL}{\underset{1}{\cancel{250}\ mg}} \times \frac{1\ \cancel{mg}}{\underset{\underset{1}{10}}{\cancel{1000}\ \cancel{mcg}}} \times \frac{0.5\ \cancel{mcg}}{\cancel{kg} \times \cancel{minute}} \times \frac{\overset{1}{\cancel{100}\ \cancel{kg}}}{1} \times \frac{\overset{6}{\cancel{60}\ \cancel{minute}}}{1\ hr} = 3\ mL\ per\ hr$$

  b. Evaluation: <u>Equation is balanced. Only mL per hr remain.</u>

2 **Ordered:** aminophylline IV infusion 0.5 mg per kg per hr for a patient with asthma. Available: aminophylline 500 mg in 250 mL D5W. Patient's weight: 80 kg.

  a. DA equation to calculate mL per hr:

  b. Evaluation: _____

3 **Ordered:** isoproterenol hydrochloride IV infusion 0.1 mcg per kg per min for 8 hr for a patient with arrhythmia. Available: isoproterenol hydrochloride 1 mg in 250 mL D5W. Patient's weight: 40 kg (88 lb).

  a. DA equation to calculate mL per hr:

  b. Evaluation: _____

4 **Ordered:** bretylium tosylate IV infusion 2 mg per min for a patient with ventricular arrhythmia. Available: 1 g bretylium tosylate in 1 L NS.

  a. DA equation to calculate mL per hr to nearest tenth:

  b. Evaluation: _____

5 **Ordered:** dopamine hydrochloride IV infusion 3 mcg per kg per min for 24 hr to maintain a patient's blood pressure. Available: dopamine hydrochloride 400 mg in 500 mL D5W. Patient's weight: 70 kg.

  a. DA equation to calculate mL per hr to nearest tenth:

  b. Evaluation: _____

Equipment for Intravenous Solutions Containing Medications

The patient's safety is never more critical than when administering IV medications. The trend is to provide prepackaged IV medications in a variety of dosages and concentrations. Needleless medication systems and infusion pumps that calculate dose rates reflect the effort to reduce medication errors. Many of the electronic infusion pumps, unlike gravity devices, do not need secondary infusions to be hung at a higher level.

Remember that it is preferable to infuse IV solutions containing medications on electronic infusion pumps, and many facilities require this (Figure 10-1).

This infusion pump can be programmed by the nurse for the dose ordered, drug, concentration, and patient's weight. The pump then calculates the flow rate. The nurse then confirms all the data (Figure 10-2).

CLINICAL RELEVANCE

Although high-technology equipment offers greater flexibility, such as IV pumps that can be used for any medication dose on a patient of any age, there is also an increased risk for serious programming errors that can result in an adverse drug event, including fatalities, for example, if a decimal point is entered as a 0.

IV pumps, called *smart pumps,* use input from multiple sources for the designated clinical area, target patient population, and usual doses to provide alarms and alerts. For instance, they can sound an alarm if someone programs a dose for mg per kg per min *instead of* mcg per kg per min (an error of 1000 times the ordered dose). The alarm or alert would sound or occur if the nurse entered pound weight instead of kilogram weight (a 2.2 times overdose) because the pump is programmed for the usual dose parameters for that population.

➤ Remember that there is a 1000-fold difference between a microgram and a milligram. Be scrupulous about entering the correct units of measurement when programming doses. Sentinel events have occurred from confusing units of measurement, such as mcg and mg.

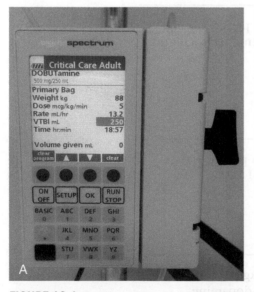

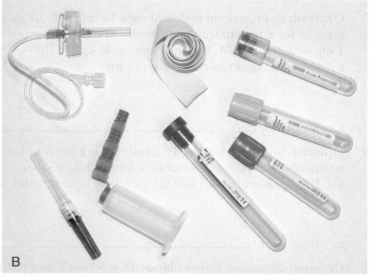

FIGURE 10-1 A, Sigma Spectrum Infusion Smart Pump has a master drug library that helps minimize the risk of pump-related programming medication errors. **B,** Some medications require drug levels to be drawn to ensure the patient is receiving the correct (therapeutic) dose.

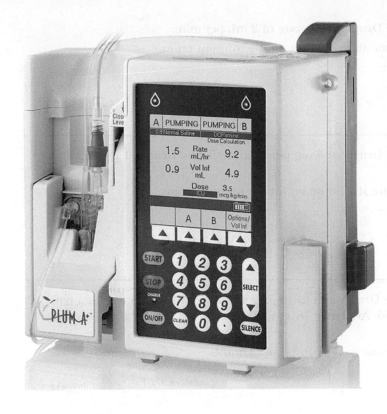

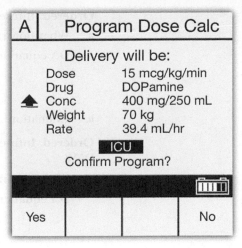

A	Program Dose Calc
	Delivery will be:

Delivery will be:

Dose	15 mcg/kg/min
Drug	DOPamine
Conc	400 mg/250 mL
Weight	70 kg
Rate	39.4 mL/hr

ICU

Confirm Program?

Yes   No

FIGURE 10-2 Plum A+® Drug Confirmation Screen.
(From Hospira, Inc., Lake Forest, IL.)

➤ Note that the flow rate in Figure 10-2 is in tenths of a mL. Some pumps deliver flow rates in hundredths of mL per hr.

If an infusion pump is unavailable and a gravity device must be used, a microdrip pediatric set may be used for some infusions. The flow rate would be in drops per min equal to the mL per hr calculated flow rate. Check agency policy.

➤ Powerful medications are often given at low flow rates. Careful attention must be given to dilution directions.

RAPID PRACTICE 10-5   Flow Rates for IV Infusions Containing Medications

ESTIMATED COMPLETION TIME: 15 to 20 minutes   **ANSWERS ON:** page 384

DIRECTIONS: *Identify the desired answer units and conversion factors needed. Calculate the ordered dose if it is weight based. Enter the critical factors and cancel unwanted units so that only the desired answer units of mL per hr remain. Calculate to the nearest tenth of a mL per hr. Label answers.*

1 **Ordered:** Infuse Drug Y at 0.1 mg per min. Available: Drug Y, 200 mg per 250 mL NS.

  a. What flow rate should be set on the infusion pump?

     DA equation:

  b. Evaluation: _____

2   **Ordered:** Infuse Drug Y at the rate of 2 mL per min.

   a.   What flow rate should be set on the infusion pump?

       DA equation:

   b.   Evaluation: _____

3   **Ordered:** Infuse Drug Y at 5 mg per min. Available: Drug Y, 1 g per 250 mL D5W.

   a.   What flow rate should be set on the infusion pump?

       DA equation:

   b.   Evaluation: _____

4   **Ordered:** Titrate Drug Y at 8 to 10 mcg per kg per min to maintain a patient's heart rate over 60. Available: Drug Y, 500 mg per 1 L LRS. Patient's weight: 44 kg.

   a.   Initial total dose to be infused per minute:

       DA equation:

   b.   What flow rate (to the nearest tenth of a mL) should be set on an infusion pump?

       DA equation:

   c.   Evaluation: _____

5   **Ordered:** Increase the drug dosage in problem 1 to 10 mcg per kg per min.

   a.   Total dose to be infused per minute:

       DA equation:

   b.   What flow rate (to the nearest tenth of a mL) should be set on the infusion pump?

       DA equation:

   c.   Evaluation: _____

Q & A   **ASK YOURSELF**   1   If the flow rate is 10 mL per hr on a pump for an infusion-containing medication, how would you set the rate on a pediatric microdrip set?

   MY ANSWER   _____

Calculating Milligrams per Milliliter (mg per mL)

The nurse needs to be able to calculate the number of mg per mL contained in any IV solution.

Some IV solutions offer multiple dilution directions. The concentration of mg per mL will have specified limits for various routes; for example:

"For IV infusion: do not exceed a concentration of 1 mg per mL."
"For IV push: do not exceed a concentration of 10 mg per mL."

The *greater the amount* of drug per milliliter, the more concentrated the solution. (Think of 1 teaspoon of lemon juice per glass of water versus 10 teaspoons of lemon juice.) This is a very basic calculation: think of *per* as a division line.

➤ To obtain mg per mL, divide the total number of milligrams of drug by the total number of mL of solution.

For example, if the available concentration is 500 mg of drug in a 250-mL solution, the number of mg per mL is obtained as follows:

$$\frac{mg}{mL} = \frac{\overset{2}{\cancel{500}}\ mg}{\underset{1}{\cancel{250}}\ mL} = \frac{2\ mg}{mL}$$

Evaluation: Equation is balanced. Only mg per mL remain.

---

1   Which is *less* concentrated: Drug Y, 100 mg per mL or Drug Y, 250 mg per mL?

ASK YOURSELF   **Q & A**

MY ANSWER

_____

Calculating the Dose of an Infusing Solution

The nurse may be asked how many milligrams or micrograms of a drug a patient is currently receiving per minute at the existing flow rate.

An IV solution labeled Drug Y, 500 mg per 250 mL, is infusing at 15 mL per hr. How many mg per min are being delivered? The equation setup begins with the same rule as for other equations: identify the desired answer units.

Two factors are known:
- Drug concentration ratio of the prepared solution: 500 mg per 250 mL
- Current flow rate: 15 mL per hr

$$\frac{mg}{min} = \frac{\overset{2}{\cancel{500}}\ mg}{\underset{1}{\cancel{250}}\ mL} \times \frac{\overset{1}{\cancel{15}}\ mL}{1\ \cancel{hr}} \times \frac{1\ \cancel{hr}}{\underset{4}{\cancel{60}}\ min} = \frac{2}{4} = \frac{0.5\ mg}{min}$$

Evaluation: Equation is balanced. Only mg per minute remain.

Analysis: The three primary factors in IV infusion calculations are the dose ordered, the drug concentration, and the flow rate. When *any two of the three* are known, the third can be obtained. Earlier equations calculated the flow rate from the drug concentration and dose ordered. Any relevant conversion factors, such as minutes to hours or hours to minutes, must also be entered in the equation.

EXAMPLES

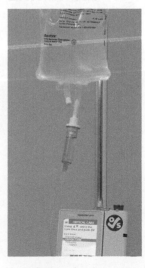

IV infusion (maintenance) on Sigma Spectrum Infusion Smart Pump.

RAPID PRACTICE 10-6   Calculating Infusion Rates

ESTIMATED COMPLETION TIME: 20 to 25 minutes   **ANSWERS ON:** page 385

DIRECTIONS: *Identify the desired answer units and conversion formulas. Calculate the number of milligrams per milliliter and milligrams per minute to the nearest hundredth as shown in the preceding examples and problem 1. Evaluate the equation. Label answers.*

TEST TIP   Take a moment to decide which of the conversion formulas will be needed for the equation: metric and minutes per hours.

1   Available: Drug Y, 500 mg per 1000 mL. Existing flow rate: 20 mL per hr.

    a.   mg per mL concentration: 0.5 mg per 1 mL $\left(\dfrac{500 \text{ mg}}{1000 \text{ mL}} \right)$
    b.   mg per min flow rate:

       DA equation:

$$\frac{\text{mg}}{\text{min}} = \frac{\overset{1}{\cancel{500}} \text{ mg}}{\underset{2}{\cancel{1000}} \text{ mL}} \times \frac{\overset{1}{\cancel{20}} \text{ mL}}{1 \text{ hr}} \times \frac{1 \text{ hr}}{\underset{3}{\cancel{60}} \text{ min}} = \frac{1}{6} = 0.166, \text{ rounded to } 0.17 \text{ mg per min}$$

    c.   Evaluation: Equation is balanced. Only mg per min remain.

2   Available: Drug Y, 500 mg per 500 mL. Existing flow rate: 12 mL per hr.
    a.   mg per mL concentration: _____
    b.   mg per min flow rate: _____
       DA equation:

    c.   Evaluation: _____

3   Available: Drug Y, 1 g per 250 mL. Existing flow rate: 10 mL per hr.
    a.   mg per mL concentration: _____
    b.   mg per min flow rate: _____
       DA equation:

    c.   Evaluation: _____

4   Available: Drug Y, 500 mg per 250 mL. Existing flow rate: 25 mL per hr.
    a.   mg per mL concentration: _____
    b.   mg per min flow rate: _____
       DA equation:

    c.   Evaluation: _____

5   Available: Drug Y, 250 mg per 1000 mL. Existing flow rate: 30 mL per hr.
    a.   mg per mL concentration: _____
    b.   mcg per min flow rate: _____
       DA equation:

    c.   Evaluation: _____

Intravenous Solution and Medications

Generally, the pharmacy prepares all IV solutions and medications that do not come premixed by the manufacturer. In some circumstances, the nurse may need to prepare a drug and add it to the appropriate IV infusion. For the initial drug dose ordered, preparation is exactly the same as for all injectables.

Medications for IV infusion often call for two dilutions:

- The first dilution is reconstitution of the drug with a specific diluent, such as SW or sterile saline solution for injection. A small amount of diluent is added according to manufacturer directions, usually just enough so that the ordered dose can be withdrawn. This preparation is often too *concentrated* to administer to the patient.
- The second dilution, if required, provides a safe concentration for IV administration.

EXAMPLES

Ordered: ampicillin 1.2 g over 30 min. Available: ampicillin 500 mg powder. Directions: Each 500-mg ampule is to be reconstituted with 5 mL of SW for injection. May be further diluted in 50 mL or more of NS, D5W, or LR and given as an infusion over not more than 4 hr. Final concentration should not exceed 30 mg per mL and may be added to the last 100 mL of a compatible IV solution.

1. Reconstitution (*First dilution*). Prepare the drug so that the precise dose ordered may be withdrawn from the total amount in the vial. This is the same preparation as for any injectable. Three ampules will have to be reconstituted to have enough for 1200 mg of ampicillin. Fifteen milliliters of SW for injection will be used to reconstitute the 1500 mg. From that amount, the nurse will calculate the number of mL needed for the 1200 mg ordered.

$$\frac{mL}{dose} = \frac{\overset{1}{\cancel{15}} \text{ mL}}{\underset{1}{\cancel{1500} \text{ mg}}} \times \frac{\cancel{1200} \text{ mg}}{dose} = \frac{12 \text{ mL}}{dose}$$

After reconstitution, there may be *more* than 12 mL because the powder will displace some of the solution. Read the label for that information.

Evaluation: Is the answer reasonable? Yes, because the answer has to be slightly less than 15 mL, which contained 1500 mg.

2. *Second dilution.* This dilution is for safe IV infusion. If 50 mL of IV solution is used, will the concentration be *less than* the 30 mg per mL safe maximum limit stated on the label?

$$50 \text{ mL plus } 12 \text{ mL} = 62 \text{ mL}$$

$$\frac{mg}{min} = \frac{1200 \text{ mg}}{62 \text{ mL}} = 19.35, \text{ or } \frac{19 \text{ mg}}{mL}$$

The 19 mg per mL is *less* concentrated than 30 mg per mL, so it is safe to use 50 mL of diluent. It also would be safe to dilute "to 50 mL" because the concentration would still be below 30 mg per mL (1200 per 50 = 24 mg per mL).

3. *Flow rate.* The order is to infuse 62 mL over 30 minutes. Calculate as for any infusion. Mental estimate: 62 mL over 30 min = 124 mL per hr.

$$\frac{mL}{hr} = \frac{62 \text{ mL}}{\underset{1}{\cancel{30} \text{ min}}} \times \frac{\overset{2}{\cancel{60} \text{ min}}}{1 \text{ hr}} = \frac{124 \text{ mL}}{hr}$$

Evaluation: The equation is balanced. Only mL per hr remain.

Set the flow rate at 124 mL per hr. The 62 mL will have infused in 30 min. The infusion pump is preferred for medicated solutions.

CLINICAL RELEVANCE

➤ More medications are being supplied in various concentrations, which requires increased responsibility for verification. Was a 10%, 20%, or 50% dextrose solution ordered? Was 100 mcg or 100 mg ordered? Was 1 mg given IV instead of 0.1 mg because a decimal was not seen? Was there a leading zero that indicated a decimal would follow? Was the medication supposed to be diluted once or twice?

➤ Always check the manufacturer's literature or a current IV drug reference for preparation including dilution directions and compatible solutions. Do not hesitate to call the pharmacy for assistance.

FAQ *What is the difference between "dilute in" 100 mL and "dilute to" 100 mL?*

ANSWER "Dilute in" means add the drug, whether it is powder or liquid, to the specified amount of diluent. This is often written for the *first* dilution of a drug so that the dose ordered may be withdrawn. "Dilute 25 mg in 5 mL of SW" means add the 25 mg to 5 mL water. This will result in more than 5 mL. The label will state the concentration after dilution. "Dilute to" means that the drug plus the diluent will add up to the specified amount. Dilute 25 mg of the drug to 5 mL (total) of SW or "further dilute" to 50 mL (total). This is often written when there is to be a second dilution of the medication in an IV infusion solution. The nurse can remove excess diluent before mixing the medication to obtain the desired total amount.

EXAMPLES

Ordered: Drug Y 100 mg in IV infusion. Available: Drug Y, 100 mg powder. Directions: Dilute each 100 mg in 3 mL of SW. Further dilute to 50 mL with IV solution. The nurse prepares the ordered amount first by reconstituting it with 3 mL SW. After that is gently and thoroughly mixed, it will be added to 47 mL of the IV solution.

Intravenous Push Medications

IV push medications are usually diluted in 1 to 50 mL. They may be administered over a minute to 30 minutes or more. A 5-mL minimum volume facilitates administration and titration rates.

The equipment selected depends on the amount of solution and duration of administration. If the injection is to be given through a distal port or an infusion line, agency flushing procedures must be followed. Current IV drug references must be consulted for safe dosage ranges, dilutions, rates, and compatibility with the infusing solution.

Small amounts of some drugs are usually to be given over a period of 1 to 5 minutes and may be administered manually and slowly by the nurse with a syringe directly into an infusion line or a port closest to the patient. Larger amounts of solutions to be administered over a longer period of time may be administered using an infusion pump.

CLINICAL RELEVANCE

➤ As with all IV medications—and this is even more urgent for patients receiving IV push medications—the patient must be assessed before, during, and after the medication is administered. The assessments include mental status, vital signs, and specific drug-related reactions and side effects.

Agencies are now required by OSHA to supply IV tubing with specially designed ports or adapters so that needles are not needed for IV push injections. This prevents needlestick injuries. Figure 10-3 shows an example of medication being administered by IV push into an infusion line.

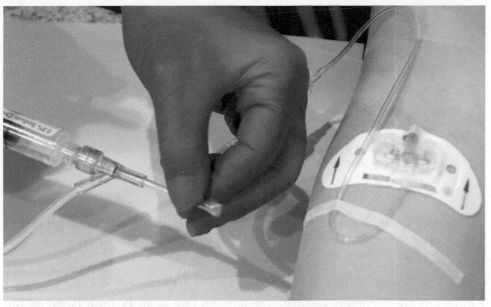

FIGURE 10-3 IV push (bolus) into existing infusion line; always use needleless equipment.

IV Push Administration

An IV push medication is given over a *specified* period of time. A reliable drug reference must be consulted for the administration time. It is important to focus, use a watch, and note the time started and the time it should be finished so that the patient does not receive the medication too quickly. There are many distractions in the workplace that may contribute to a rate error. Medications given IV push are very concentrated and if administered too quickly can cause severe harm to the patient.

The schedule is based on two factors:

1   Total number of mL in the *prepared* syringe after dilution
2   Total number of minutes and/or seconds to be injected

➤ A syringe with a wide diameter barrel (standard for a 10-mL syringe) needs to be used for all IV push medications.

➤ A narrow diameter syringe (such as a standard 1- or 3-mL syringe) can place excessive pressure on the vascular access device, whether it is peripheral or central.

➤ Some syringe manufacturers now make a 3-mL syringe with a wide barrel (like the barrel on a 10-mL syringe) that can be used safely for IV push medications.

➤ IV push (direct) is administered into an established line or port.

➤ Check agency policies for syringe sizes for IV push medications.

Method 1: milliliters per minute

The drug is *first prepared* according to directions and then diluted with a compatible solution according to current IV drug references for IV push medications and the manufacturer's guidelines. If the amount of mL per min to be injected is a whole number, this method works easily.

EXAMPLES

Prepare the drug dose ordered, and then dilute according to directions. Determine the number of mL per min (total mL in syringe ÷ total min to be given).

Treat "per" as a dividing line.

4 mL *prepared* to be given over 4 min: <u>1 mL per min</u>

4 mL *prepared* to be given over 2 min: <u>2 mL per min</u>

$$\frac{mL}{min} = \frac{\cancel{4}\ mL}{\cancel{4}\ min} = 1\ mL\ per\ min \qquad \frac{mL}{min} = \frac{\overset{2}{\cancel{4}}\ mL}{\underset{1}{\cancel{2}}\ min} = 2\ mL\ per\ min$$

Decide on a time to start and the exact stop time. Start when the second hand is on 12. Inject slowly and steadily. Avoid all distractions.

Method 2: seconds per calibration line on a syringe

Two factors are needed to calculate the infusion rate of an IV push based on the number of seconds needed to inject a solution per calibration mark on a syringe:

1 Number of calibrations occupied by the *prepared, diluted* drug in solution
2 Number of total seconds the drug is to be administered*

The syringe is examined for the number of calibrated lines the medication and diluent occupy. The total number of minutes for the injection is converted to seconds. How many seconds per calibration?

EXAMPLES

Ordered: morphine 4 mg direct IV push. Available: morphine sulfate 10 mg per mL. Literature: May be given undiluted, but it is appropriate to further *dilute to* 5 mL with SW, NS, or other compatible solutions. "Current drug reference": Administer over 5 minutes.

$$mL\ prepared\ dose = \frac{1\ mL}{\underset{5}{\cancel{10\ mg}}} \times \frac{\overset{2}{\cancel{4\ mg}}}{dose} = 0.4\ mL\ to\ be\ administered$$

Preparation: Withdraw ordered dose, 0.4 mL of morphine sulfate in a 10-mL syringe, and add 4.6 mL SW. This will make a total prepared volume of 5 mL.

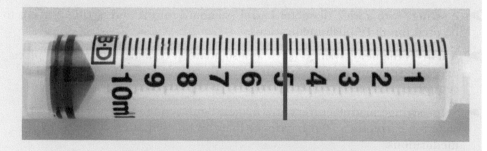

$$\frac{seconds}{calibration} = \frac{60\ second}{1\ \cancel{minute}} \times \frac{\overset{1}{\cancel{5\ minute}}}{\underset{5}{\cancel{25}\ calibrations}} = \frac{60}{5} = 12\ seconds\ per\ calibration$$

➤ Note that the calibrations replace the mL volume in this type of equation.

---

*Consult a current drug reference for the exact time limits for the push.

➤ Prepare the precise ordered dose before adding diluent. The total amount in the syringe is the prepared precise ordered dose plus the specified diluent. The total volume of the two solutions is used to calculate the schedule.

The nurse uses a watch to count 12 seconds while pushing each increment on the syringe. It is important *not to exceed* the prescribed rate of injection. The drugs may be powerful enough to cause severe adverse effects from too rapid injection.

---

1 When the seconds per calibration method is used to calculate rate of injection, why aren't the total mL needed in the equation? What data replace the total mL?

ASK YOURSELF **Q & A**

_____

MY ANSWER

Any site to be used for IV administration first needs to be checked for patency. If using an implanted IV port device to administer the medication, patency can be assessed by slight withdrawal of the syringe plunger to observe a blood return, followed by a flush injection of a 2- or 3-mL of sterile NS solution, with observation for swelling or discomfort. Neither method guarantees patency.

CLINICAL RELEVANCE

| **RAPID PRACTICE 10-7** | **IV Push Calculations** |

ESTIMATED COMPLETION TIME: 20 to 25 minutes   **ANSWERS ON:** page 386

DIRECTIONS: *Calculate the medication dose. Using the directions for administration rate, examine the syringe for the calibrations occupied by the medication volume. Calculate the number of mL per min and seconds per calibration. Label answers. Evaluate your own equations.*

1 **Ordered:** Cidofovir 60 mg IV push for cytomegalovirus retinitis in a patient with AIDS. Dilute to 5 mL of SW or NS. Give over 5 min. Available: Cidofovir, 75 mg per mL.

   a. Total amount of prepared medication in mL to the nearest hundredth:

   _____

   DA equation:

   _____

   b. Total amount of diluted medication in mL (if applicable): _____
   c. Total min to administer: _____
   d. mL per min to be administered: _____
   e. Total calibrations for the diluted medication: _____

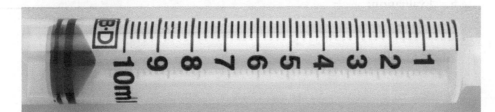

2 **Ordered:** phenobarbital 100 mg IV push, as a second-line drug for a patient with seizures. Follow directions on label for dilution and rate of injection. For IV use, dilute to 3 mL of NS for injection. Do not exceed injection rate of 1 mL per min. Do not use if solution is not clear.

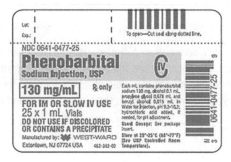

a. Total amount of prepared medication in mL to the nearest tenth: _____

DA equation:

b. Total amount of diluted medication in mL (if applicable): _____
c. Total min to administer: _____
d. mL per min to be administered: _____
e. Total calibrations for the diluted medication: _____

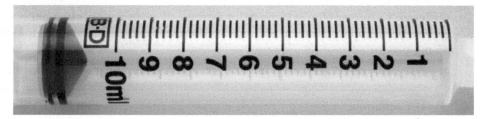

f. Total seconds to administer: _____
g. Seconds per calibration: _____

DA equation:

h. Evaluation: _____

3   **Ordered:** diazepam 10 mg IV push for sedation. Directions: Give undiluted.
Rate: Inject at rate of 5 mg per min prior to endoscopy procedure.

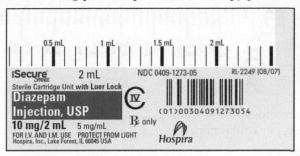

a.   Total amount of ordered medication in mL: _____

DA equation:

b.   Total amount of diluted medication in mL (if applicable): _____
c.   Total minutes to administer: _____
d.   mL per minute to be administered: _____
e.   Total calibrations for the diluted medication: _____

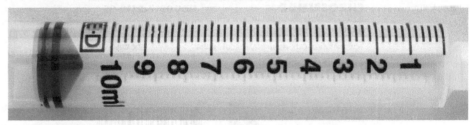

f.   Total seconds to administer: _____
g.   Seconds per calibration: _____

DA equation:

h.   Evaluation: _____

4   **Ordered:** Atropine 0.8 mg IV, for bradyarrhythmia. Directions: Dilute in up
to 10 mL of NS. The nurse adds enough NS to the prepared medication to
make 5 mL. Inject 1 mg or less over 1 minute.

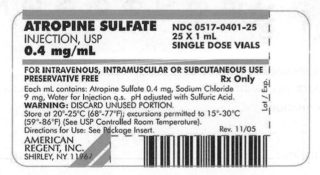

a.   Total amount of prepared medication in mL: _____

DA equation:

b.   Total amount of diluted medication in mL (if applicable): _____
c.   Total minutes to administer: _____
d.   mL per minute to be administered: _____

e.   Total calibrations for the diluted medication: _____

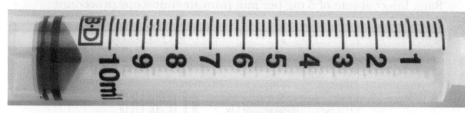

f.   Total seconds to administer: _____
g.   Seconds per calibration: _____
         DA equation:

h.   Evaluation: _____

5   Ordered: furosemide 40 mg IV push, for a patient with anuria. Directions:
Should be infused in anuric patients at a rate of 4 mg per minute. May be
given undiluted.

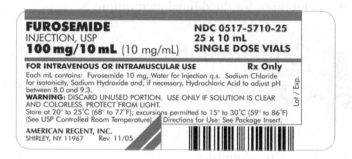

a.   Total amount of prepared medication in mL: _____
b.   Total amount of diluted medication in mL (if applicable): _____
c.   Total min to administer: _____
d.   mL per min to be administered: _____
e.   Total calibrations for the medication: _____

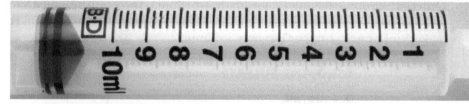

f.   Total seconds to administer: _____
g.   Seconds per calibration: _____
         DA equation:

h.   Evaluation: _____

CLINICAL RELEVANCE   ➤ Existing IV lines must be flushed before and after medication injection according
to agency policy. Such procedures are written for flushes of implanted IV ports and
IV infusion lines. Any existing site for IV administration needs to be checked for patency
and solution compatibility. IV medication injections can cause adverse reactions (e.g.,
sudden changes in mental status, blood pressure, and pulse). Assess the patient before,
during, and after the procedure.

1 Why is it suggested that the nurse start the push count with the second hand of the watch on the 12 o'clock mark?

_____

Hyperalimentation: Parenteral Nutrition

➤ All total parenteral solutions are on the ISMP list of high-alert medications (see Appendix B).

Hyperalimentation (*hyperal*, for short) provides high-calorie IV nutrition. Also known as parenteral nutrition (PN or TPN), it can provide up to 1 kcal per mL with amino acids, dextrose, electrolytes, vitamins, and minerals to meet total nutritional needs. About 10% or 20% lipid emulsions can also be delivered intravenously as part of the PN order. Lipids may be added intermittently to provide needed calories (Figure 10-4). Insulin, a high-alert medication, is ordered as an additive to normalize glucose levels based on the results of frequently drawn samples for glucose tests and prescriber's orders.

Ordinary IV fluids such as D5W only supply 5 g dextrose per 100 mL of solution, or 50 g dextrose (200 kcal) per 1000 mL. Three L per day would supply the patient with only 600 kcal per day, a starvation diet. Adults usually consume between 1500 and 2500 or more kcal per day of protein, carbohydrate, and fat to meet nutritional needs and maintain health and energy levels.

Solutions' contents are customized by the prescriber and prepared by the pharmacy based on frequent, current laboratory tests and the patient's condition.

1 How many calories do you consume on an average day?

_____

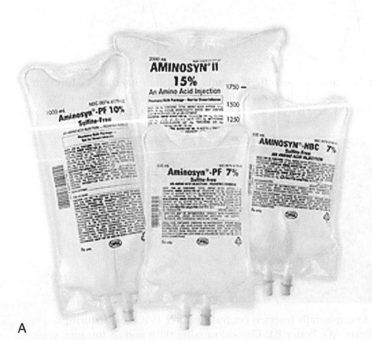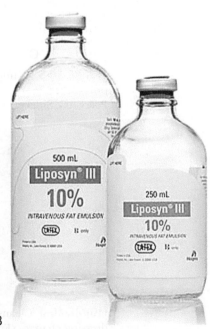

FIGURE 10-4 A, Amino acids. **B,** Lipids. (From Hospira, Inc., Lake Forest, IL.)

For long-term therapy and concentration solutions, a centrally inserted catheter into the superior vena cava is usually used. It may be an implantable port (Figure 10-5), a tunneled catheter, or an external catheter inserted into a large vein. A peripherally inserted central catheter (PICC) (Figure 10-6) may also be threaded into the vena cava from a large peripheral vein, usually for short or intermediate periods.

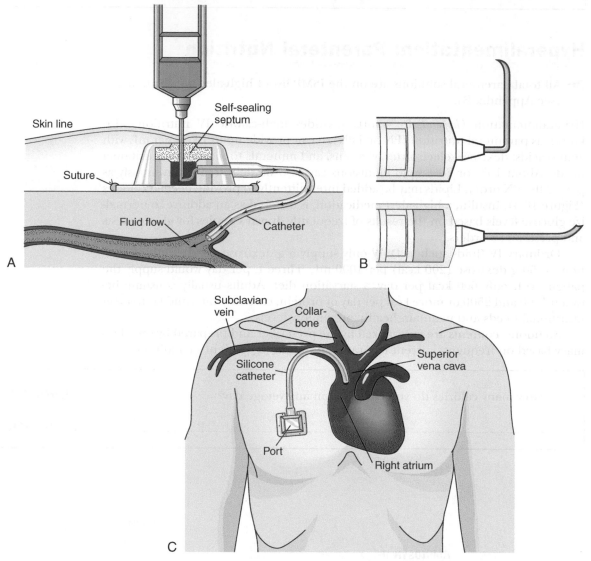

Skin line

Self-sealing septum

Suture

Fluid flow

Catheter

A

B

Subclavian vein

Collar-bone

Silicone catheter

Superior vena cava

Port

Right atrium

C

FIGURE 10-5 **A,** Implantable infusion port. **B,** Assortment of Huber needles. **C,** Infusion port placed in subcutaneous pocket with centrally inserted catheter. (From Potter PA, Perry AG, Stockert PA, Hall A: Essentials of nursing practice, ed 9, St. Louis, 2019, Elsevier.)

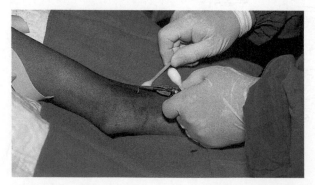

FIGURE 10-6 Cleansing a peripherally inserted central catheter (PICC) site during a dressing change. (From Perry AG, Potter PA: Clinical nursing skills and techniques, ed 5, St. Louis, 2004, Mosby.)

For short-term therapy, large peripheral veins can be used; this is known as *peripheral parenteral nutrition* (PPN). PPN uses more dilute solutions than total parenteral nutrition to protect the peripheral vein wall from irritation.

ASK YOURSELF **Q & A**

1   Is the PN solution for the home infusion order shown in Figure 10-7 isotonic, hypotonic, or hypertonic?

MY ANSWER

_____

2   What are two main differences between TPN and PPN?

_____

3   Which components provide (a) protein, (b) carbohydrate, and (c) fat (see Figure 10-7)?

_____

4   Which high-risk medication must be added just before infusion (see Figure 10-7)?

_____

➤ The nurse must compare the label contents and percentage of each PN solution with the prescriber's current order. Orders may be changed daily.

➤ The site used for PN cannot be used for the simultaneous administration of medications, blood, or other products.

➤ Central parenteral nutrition, more commonly known as total parenteral nutrition (TPN), is always administered through an electronic infusion pump.

➤ The solution decomposes quickly. Keep refrigerated and check expiration dates. Generally, once opened solutions expire in 24 hours. Check agency policy.

Amino acids provide protein.
Lipids provide fat and calories.
Dextrose provides carbohydrate.
MVI = multivitamins and gives it a yellow color.

Additives per Liter – in this prescription all of the additives are electrolytes.

Home Infusion Pharmacy
(408) 848-3400

| Smith, John | Rx# 763486 |
| m 48 | S. Chan MD |

Amino Acids 10% = 425 mL
Dextrose 10% = 125 mL
Sterile Water = 341 mL
Lipids 20% = 125 mL
MVI = 10 mL

Additives Per Liter
NaCl = 35 mEq
KCl = 25 mEq
Calcium = 5 mEq
Magnesium = 5 mEq

TPN 40–51 grams protein + Lipids

Infuse 8 PM to 8 AM through IV PICC line using infusion pump @ 104 mL per hour.

Total Volume = 1248 mL

Refrigerate Until Use

Expiration date 5/7/2018

FIGURE 10-7 Total parenteral nutrition bag label for home infusion therapy.

CLINICAL RELEVANCE

➤ To preserve the IV line, and avoid the risk of infection, air emboli, incompatibilities, precipitation, coagulation, hyperglycemia and hypoglycemia, familiarize yourself with the procedures, including changes of tubing, aseptic technique for site care, flushing protocols, and equipment permitted for approved compatible additives (e.g., Y tubing). Following the assessment protocols for weight, signs of infection, and laboratory tests permits early detection of complications.

CHAPTER 10 MULTIPLE-CHOICE REVIEW

ESTIMATED COMPLETION TIME: 30 minutes   **ANSWERS ON:** page 386

DIRECTIONS: *Select the correct IV-related response. Verify answers with a DA equation. Use a calculator for long division and multiplication.*

1 An order of 500 mg of a drug in 1000 mL is being infused at 10 mL per hr. The hourly amount of drug infused is:

  a. 2 mg per hr   **c.** 10 mg per hr
  b. 5 mg per hr   **d.** 15 mg per hr

2 How many kilocalories of dextrose are contained in a TPN solution of 1 L that contains 25% dextrose? (Conversion factor: 4 kcal = 1 g of dextrose.)

  a. 25   **c.** 250
  b. 100   **d.** 1000

3 **Ordered:** IV of 500 mL D5 NS with KCl 40 mEq, for a patient with hypokalemia, at 10 mEq per hr. Check serum potassium level when completed. Continue until serum potassium level greater than 4, then discontinue. The nurse will set the flow rate at:

  a. 10 mL per hr for 4 hours   **c.** 50 mL per hr for 4 hours
  b. 40 mL per hr for 10 hours   **d.** 125 mL per hr for 4 hours
Direct injection of concentrated KCl can cause cardiac arrest.

4 **Ordered:** IVPB antibiotic of 30 mL to infuse in 30 min. What flow rate will be set on a gravity device with a microdrip set? (Use mental arithmetic.)

  a. 30 mL per hr   **c.** 90 drops per min
  b. 60 drops per min   **d.** 100 drops per min

5 An available IV solution contains 1 g in 250 mL. How many milligrams per milliliter are contained in the solution? (Use mental arithmetic.)

  a. 4   **c.** 25
  b. 0.25   **d.** 100

6 **Ordered:** morphine sulfate 3 mg IV push, for a patient with pain. Drug reference directions for IV direct injection: Dilute to 5 mL with SW. Available: morphine sulfate 10 mg per mL. Directions: Administer over 5 min. How many mL per min will the medication deliver?

  a. 1   **c.** 10
  b. 5   **d.** 50

7 The recommendation for adjusting medicated IV infusions that are behind the ordered schedule for the amount infused is:

  a. Adjust up to 25% more than the ordered rate.
  b. Adjust up to 10% more than the ordered rate.
  c. Let the rate stay behind the ordered rate for the remainder of the infusion.
  d. Assess the patient condition and consult with the licensed prescriber.

8 Which of the following is the most concentrated IV solution?

a. 250 mg per 1000 mL

c. 100 mg per 100 mL

b. 250 mg per 500 mL

d. 50 mg per 100 mL

9 An existing unmedicated IV solution is flowing at 100 mL per hr when the nurse arrives to care for the patient. 500 of 1000 mL have been infused in 5 hours. The order reads: 1000 mL q8h. The patient is NPO 1 day postoperatively and has good heart, lung, and renal function. The urinary output appears concentrated. The nurse's assessment is that it would be safe to adjust the IV to complete it on time. The adjustment would be:

a. The flow rate needs adjustment to 125 mL per hr.

b. The flow rate needs adjustment to 167 mL per hr.

c. The flow rate needs to be opened up until it is on target for the current time and then adjusted to 125 mL per hr.

d. The flow rate should be adjusted to 155 mL per hr until completed.

10 An IV flow rate of 2 mL per min of D5LR would be set at which flow rate on an infusion pump?

a. 60 drops per min

c. 120 drops per min

b. 60 mL per hr

d. 120 mL per hr

CHAPTER 10 FINAL PRACTICE

ESTIMATED COMPLETION TIME: 1 to 2 hours   **ANSWERS ON:** page 387

DIRECTIONS: *Calculate the advanced intravenous problems. Verify your answers with a DA equation. Label answers. Evaluate your equations.*

1 Ordered: naloxone infusion, to wean a patient with narcotic depression, to be infused over 6 hr at 0.03 mg per hr. Directions: Dilute 2 mg in 500 mL NS or D5W.

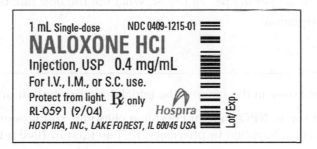

a. How many mL of naloxone will be added to the 500 mL? _____

DA equation:

Evaluation: _____

b. The nurse will set the flow rate on the infusion pump at (round to the nearest tenth of a mL): _____

DA equation:

Evaluation: _____

2 **Ordered:** KCl 10 mEq per hr, for a patient with hypokalemia. Available: KCl 40 mEq per 500 mL D5 $\frac{1}{2}$ NS. The nurse will set the flow rate on the infusion pump at: _____

DA equation:

Evaluation: _____

3 **Ordered:** aminophylline IV infusion for a patient with acute asthma. Titrate: 0.3 to 0.6 mg per kg per hr. Patient's weight: 75 kg. Directions: Dilute in 250 mL NS. Consult the label for drug amount placed in the IV. The nurse will withdraw 20 mL of NS before adding the aminophylline.

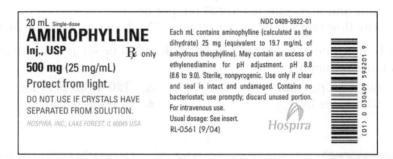

a. What flow rate, to the nearest tenth of a mL, will be set on the infusion pump for 0.3 mg per kg per hr? _____

DA equation:

Evaluation: _____

b. The patient's respiratory status does not improve. The theophylline serum levels are still within normal levels. The nurse increases the flow rate to 0.4 per mg per kg per hr. What will the flow rate be adjusted to?

DA equation:

Evaluation: _____

➤ The lowest dose in the range is the initial dose for titration orders.

4 **Ordered for an NPO patient:** Potassium chloride* continuous infusion of 5 mEq per hr. Supplied by pharmacy: KCl 40 mEq in 1000 mL of D5W.

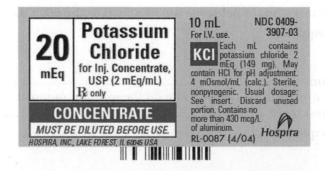

➤ *Potassium chloride is a common additive to IV solutions and should be prepared by the pharmacy. Concentrated KCl can cause arrhythmias and cardiac arrest if given undiluted. IV bags must be gently rotated several times before hanging to ensure that the potassium is dispersed *throughout* the bag. It *must be administered* via an infusion pump in concentrations greater than 20 mEq per 1000 mL. A timed tape is helpful for monitoring volume infused even when a pump is being used.

a. Is potassium chloride compatible with D5W (using a current drug reference)? _____

b. What flow rate will be set on the infusion pump? _____

DA equation:

Evaluation: _____

c. How long will the infusion last (using mental arithmetic)? _____

5 **Ordered:** atropine sulfate 1 mg bolus IV push, for a patient with bradyarrhythmia. Directions: Dilute to 10 mL NS for injection (total amount) and give over 1 min.

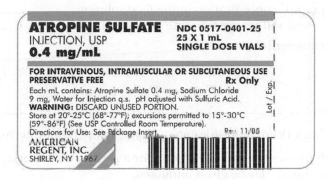

a. How many mL of atropine will the nurse prepare? _____

DA equation:

Evaluation: _____

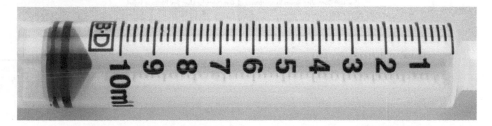

b. After dilution, how many seconds per mL will the atropine be injected?

_____

DA equation:

Evaluation: _____

6 **Ordered:** dobutamine 2.5 mcg per kg per min for a patient with heart failure. Directions: Dilute in 500 mL D5W. The nurse will withdraw 20 mL of the D5W, discard it, and use 480 mL of the D5W plus 20 mL of the dobutamine solution to make a 500-mL medicated solution. Patient weight: 64 kg.

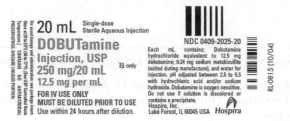

a. mg per mL concentration in the final solution: _____

b. The nurse will set the flow rate on the infusion pump at: _____

DA equation:

Evaluation: _____

➤ Always check IV solutions for compatibility before administering.

7 **Ordered:** furosemide 30 mg IV push, for a patient with anuria, at 4 mg per min. Directions: May be given undiluted.

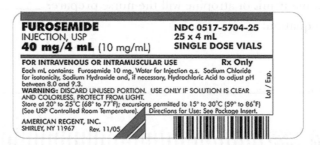

a. Total mL to inject: _____

DA equation:

Evaluation: _____

b. Calibrations occupied by the medication:

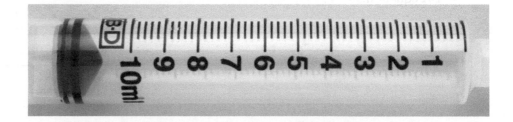

c. Total seconds for injection: _____

DA equation:

Evaluation: _____

d. Seconds per calibration for injection: _____

DA equation:

Evaluation: _____

8 **Ordered:** magnesium sulfate 2.5 mL per min IV infusion, for a patient with convulsions. Directions: Dilute 4 g in 250 mL of D5W. The label states 500 mg per mL. Prepare 4 g.

NDC 63323-064-02   96402
MAGNESIUM SULFATE
INJECTION, USP
50% (1 gram/2 ml)
For IM or IV Use
Must be diluted before IV use.
2 mL Single Dose Vial
4.06 mEq/mL   4.06 mOsmol/mL
APP Pharmaceuticals, LLC
Schaumburg, IL 30175

a. How many mL of magnesium sulfate will the nurse prepare for the infusion? _____

DA equation:

Evaluation: _____

The nurse will remove an amount of D5W equal to the amount of medication being added so that the IV solution remains 250 mL.

b. Following the ordered rate, what will be the flow rate on the infusion pump? _____

DA equation:

Evaluation: _____

c. How many mg per min will the patient receive? _____

DA equation:

Evaluation: _____

9 **Ordered:** dopamine HCl infusion 3 mcg per kg per min for a patient with shock syndrome. Patient's weight: 82 kg. Flow rate when the nurse begins the shift: dopamine HCl at 15 mL per hr.

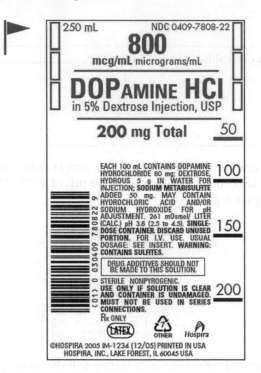

    a. How many mg per hr are ordered to the nearest whole number? _____
        DA equation:

    Evaluation: _____

    b. What is the ordered flow rate to the nearest tenth of a mL? _____
        DA equation:

    Evaluation: _____

10 **Ordered:** Nitropress IV infusion for a patient with hypertension. Start at 0.3 mcg per kg per min. Titrate to keep systolic blood pressure below 160 and diastolic pressure below 90 mm Hg. Directions: Dilute 50 mg in 250 mL D5W. The nurse will use 250 mL as the total amount of solution for calculation purposes. Patient weight: 60 kg.

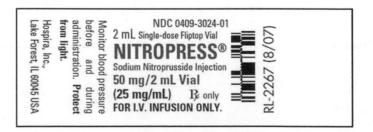

a. mg per mL concentration in the final solution: _____

DA equation:

Evaluation: _____

b. The nurse will set the flow rate on the infusion pump at (nearest tenth of a mL)_____.

DA equation:

Evaluation: _____

CHAPTER 10 ANSWER KEY

RAPID PRACTICE 10-1 (p. 351)

2 **a.** $60 \div 60 = 1$ mg per min

$$\frac{\text{mg}}{\text{min}} = \frac{\overset{1}{\cancel{60} \text{ mg}}}{1 \ \cancel{\text{hr}}} \times \frac{1 \ \cancel{\text{hr}}}{\underset{1}{\cancel{60} \text{ min}}}$$

$$= 1 \text{ mg per min}$$

b. Estimate equals answer.

3 **a.** $4 \text{ mg} \times 60 = 240$ mg per hr

$$\frac{\text{mg}}{\text{hr}} = \frac{4 \text{ mg}}{1 \ \cancel{\text{min}}} \times \frac{60 \ \cancel{\text{min}}}{1 \text{ hr}}$$
$$= 240 \text{ mg per hr}$$

b. Estimate equals answer.

4 **a.** $120 \div 60 = 2$ mL per min

$$\frac{\text{mL}}{\text{min}} = \frac{\overset{2}{\cancel{120} \text{ mL}}}{1 \ \cancel{\text{hr}}} \times \frac{1 \ \cancel{\text{hr}}}{\underset{1}{\cancel{60} \text{ min}}}$$

$$= 2 \text{ mL per minute}$$

b. Estimate equals answer.

5 **a.** $2 \text{ mg} \times 10 \text{ kg} = 20$ mg per min

$$\frac{\text{mg}}{\text{min}} = \frac{2 \text{ mg}}{1 \ \cancel{\text{kg}}} \times \frac{10 \ \cancel{\text{kg}}}{1 \text{ min}}$$
$$= 2 \text{ mg} \times 10 \text{ kg}$$
$$= 20 \text{ mg per min}$$

b. Estimate equals answer.

c. $20 \text{ mg} \times 60 \text{ min} = 1200$ mg per hr

$$\frac{\text{mg}}{\text{hr}} = \frac{2 \text{ mg}}{1 \ \cancel{\text{kg}} \times \cancel{\text{min}}} \times \frac{10 \ \cancel{\text{kg}}}{1} \times \frac{60 \ \cancel{\text{min}}}{1 \text{ hr}}$$
$$= \frac{1200 \text{ mg}}{\text{hr}}$$

d. Estimate equals answer.

Remember: Units following "per" need to be in the denominator of equations; e.g., mL per hr $\left(\dfrac{\text{mL}}{\text{hr}}\right)$ and mg per min $\left(\dfrac{\text{mg}}{\text{min}}\right)$.

The answer can be in fraction form $\left(\dfrac{\text{mg}}{\text{hr}}\right)$ or written out (mg per hr).

RAPID PRACTICE 10-2 (p. 353)

1 **a.** 96 mL per hr

$$\frac{\text{mL}}{\text{hr}} = \frac{\overset{4}{\cancel{1000} \text{ mL}}}{\underset{1}{\cancel{250} \text{ mg}}} \times \frac{0.4 \ \cancel{\text{mg}}}{1 \ \cancel{\text{min}}} \times \frac{60 \ \cancel{\text{min}}}{1 \text{ hr}}$$

$$= \frac{96 \text{ mL}}{\text{hr}}$$

Note: 1 L = 1000 mL.

b. Equation is balanced. Only mL per hr remain.

2 **a.** 120 mL per hr

$$\frac{\text{mL}}{\text{hr}} = \frac{\overset{2}{\cancel{1000} \text{ mL}}}{\underset{1}{\cancel{500} \text{ mg}}} \times \frac{1 \ \cancel{\text{mg}}}{1 \ \cancel{\text{min}}} \times \frac{60 \ \cancel{\text{min}}}{1 \text{ hr}}$$

$$= \frac{120 \text{ mL}}{\text{hr}}$$

b. Equation is balanced. Only mL per hr remain.

3 **a.** 15 mL per hr

$$\frac{\text{mL}}{\text{hr}} = \frac{\overset{1}{\cancel{250} \text{ mL}}}{\underset{\underset{1}{2}}{\cancel{500} \text{ mg}}} \times \frac{0.5 \ \cancel{\text{mg}}}{1 \ \cancel{\text{min}}} \times \frac{\overset{30}{\cancel{60} \ \cancel{\text{min}}}}{1 \text{ hr}}$$

$$= \frac{15 \text{ mL}}{\text{hr}}$$

b. Equation is balanced. Only mL per hr remain.

4 **a.** 12 mL per hr

$$\frac{\text{mL}}{\text{hr}} = \frac{\overset{1}{\cancel{100} \text{ mL}}}{\underset{1}{\cancel{100} \text{ mg}}} \times \frac{0.2 \ \cancel{\text{mg}}}{1 \ \cancel{\text{min}}} \times \frac{60 \ \cancel{\text{min}}}{1 \text{ hr}}$$

$$= \frac{12 \text{ mL}}{\text{hr}}$$

b. Equation is balanced. Only mL per hr remain.

5 **a.** 120 mL per hr

$$\frac{mL}{hr} = \frac{\cancel{1000}\ mL}{\cancel{1000}\ mg} \times \frac{2\ \cancel{mg}}{1\ \cancel{min}} \times \frac{60\ \cancel{min}}{1\ hr}$$

$$= \frac{120\ mL}{hr}$$

b. Equation is balanced. Only mL per hr remain. Note that mL must be entered in the first numerator, and hr must be entered in a denominator in the equation.

RAPID PRACTICE 10-3 (p. 355)

2 **a.** 6 mL per hr

$$\frac{mL}{hr} = \frac{\overset{1}{\cancel{250}}\ mL}{\underset{2}{\cancel{500}}\ \cancel{mg}} \times \frac{1\ \cancel{mg}}{\underset{5}{\cancel{1000}}\ \cancel{mcg}} \times \frac{1}{\cancel{200}\ \cancel{mcg}}{1\ min}$$

$$\times \frac{60\ \cancel{min}}{1\ hr} = \frac{60}{10} = \frac{6\ mL}{hr}$$

b. Equation is balanced. Only mL per hr remain.

3 **a.** 45 mL per hr

$$\frac{mL}{hr} = \frac{\overset{1}{\cancel{100}}\ mL}{10\ \cancel{mg}} \times \frac{1\ \cancel{mg}}{\underset{\underset{1}{10}}{\cancel{1000}}\ \cancel{mcg}} \times \frac{75\ \cancel{mcg}}{1\ min}$$

$$\times \frac{\overset{6}{\cancel{60}}\ \cancel{min}}{1\ hr} = \frac{450}{10} = \frac{45\ mL}{hr}$$

b. Equation is balanced. Only mL per hr remain.

4 **a.** 60 mL per hr

$$\frac{mL}{hr} = \frac{\overset{1}{\cancel{200}}\ mL}{1\ \cancel{g}} \times \frac{1\ \cancel{g}}{\underset{5}{\cancel{1000}}\ \cancel{mg}} \times \frac{5\ \cancel{mg}}{1\ \cancel{min}}$$

$$\times \frac{60\ \cancel{min}}{1\ hr} = \frac{300}{5} = \frac{60\ mL}{hr}$$

b. Equation is balanced. Only mL per hr remain.

5 **a.** 9 mL per hr

$$\frac{mL}{hr} = \frac{\overset{1}{\cancel{200}}\ mL}{2\ \cancel{g}} \times \frac{1\ \cancel{g}}{\underset{5}{\cancel{1000}}\ \cancel{mg}} \times \frac{1.5\ \cancel{mg}}{1\ \cancel{min}}$$

$$\times \frac{60\ \cancel{min}}{1\ hr} = \frac{90}{10} = \frac{9\ mL}{hr}$$

b. Equation is balanced. Only mL per hr remain.

RAPID PRACTICE 10-4 (p. 359)

2 20 mL per hr

a. $$\frac{mL}{hr} = \frac{\overset{1}{\cancel{250}}\ mL}{\underset{\underset{1}{2}}{\cancel{500}}\ \cancel{mg}} \times \frac{0.5\ \cancel{mg}}{1\ \cancel{kg} \times hr} \times \frac{\overset{40}{\cancel{80}\ \cancel{kg}}}{1}$$

$$= \frac{20\ mL}{hr}$$

b. Equation is balanced. Only mL per hr remain.

3 60 mL per hr

a. $$\frac{mL}{hr} = \frac{\overset{1}{\cancel{250}}\ mL}{1\ \cancel{mg}} \times \frac{1\ \cancel{mg}}{\underset{\underset{1}{4}}{\cancel{1000}}\ \cancel{mcg}} \times \frac{0.1\ \cancel{mcg}}{\cancel{kg} \times \cancel{min}}$$

$$\times \frac{\overset{10}{\cancel{40}\ \cancel{kg}}}{1} \times \frac{60\ \cancel{min}}{1\ hr} = \frac{60\ mL}{hr}$$

b. Equation is balanced. Only mL per hr remain.

4 **a.** $$\frac{mL}{hr} = \frac{\overset{1}{\cancel{1000}}\ mL}{1\ \cancel{g}} \times \frac{1\ \cancel{g}}{\underset{1}{\cancel{1000}}\ \cancel{mg}} \times \frac{2\ \cancel{mg}}{\cancel{minute}}$$

$$\times \frac{60\ \cancel{min}}{1\ hr} = \frac{120\ mL}{hr}$$

b. Equation is balanced. Only mL per hr remain.

5 15.8 mL per hr

a. $$\frac{mL}{hr} = \frac{\cancel{500}\ mL}{\cancel{400}\ mg} \times \frac{1\ \cancel{mg}}{1000\ mcg}$$

$$\times \frac{3\ mcg}{\cancel{kg} \times \cancel{min}} \times \frac{70\ \cancel{kg}}{1} \times \frac{60\ \cancel{min}}{1\ hr}$$

$$= 15.75, rounded\ to\ \frac{15.8\ mL}{hr}$$

b. Equation is balanced. Only mL per hr remain.

RAPID PRACTICE 10-5 (p. 361)

1 **a.** 7.5 mL per hr

$$\frac{mL}{hr} = \frac{\overset{5}{\cancel{250}}\ mL}{\underset{4}{\cancel{200}}\ \cancel{mg}} \times \frac{0.1\ \cancel{mg}}{1\ \cancel{min}} \times \frac{\overset{15}{\cancel{60}\ \cancel{min}}}{1\ hr}$$

$$= \frac{7.5\ mL}{hr}$$

b. Equation is balanced. Only mL per hr remain.

2 **a.** 120 mL per hr

$$\frac{mL}{hr} = \frac{2\ mL}{1\ \cancel{min}} \times \frac{60\ \cancel{min}}{1\ hr} = \frac{120\ mL}{hr}$$

b. Equation is balanced. Only mL per hr remain.

3 a. 75 mL per hr

$$\frac{\text{mL}}{\text{hr}} = \frac{\overset{1}{\cancel{250}}\ \text{mL}}{1\ \cancel{g}} \times \frac{1\ \cancel{g}}{\underset{\underset{1}{4}}{\cancel{1000}\ \cancel{mg}}} \times \frac{5\ \cancel{mg}}{1\ \cancel{min}}$$

$$\times \frac{\overset{15}{\cancel{60}\ \cancel{min}}}{1\ \text{hr}} = \frac{75\ \text{mL}}{\text{hr}}$$

b. Equation is balanced. Only mL per hr remain.

4 a. 352 mcg

$$\frac{\text{mcg}}{\text{min}} = \frac{8\ \text{mcg}}{1\ \cancel{kg}} \times \frac{44\ \cancel{kg}}{1\ \text{min}}$$

$$= \frac{352\ \text{mcg}}{\text{min}}\ \text{per initial dose}$$

b. 42.2 mL per hr

$$\frac{\text{mL}}{\text{hr}} = \frac{\overset{1}{\cancel{1000}\ \text{mL}}}{500\ \cancel{mg}} \times \frac{1\ \cancel{mg}}{\underset{1}{\cancel{1000}\ \cancel{mcg}}}$$

$$\times \frac{8\ \cancel{mcg}}{1\ \cancel{kg} \times \cancel{min}} \times \frac{44\ \cancel{kg}}{1} \times \frac{60\ \cancel{min}}{1\ \text{hr}}$$

$$= \frac{2112}{50} = \frac{42.2\ \text{mL}}{\text{hr}}\ \text{initial flow rate}$$

c. Equation is balanced. Only mL per hr remain.

Note: Remember to enter calculations twice for verification.

5 a. 440 mcg

$$\text{mcg} = \frac{10\ \text{mcg}}{1\ \cancel{kg}} \times \frac{44\ \cancel{kg}}{1\ \text{min}} = \frac{440\ \text{mcg}}{\text{min}}$$

b. 52.8 mL per hr

$$\frac{\text{mL}}{\text{hr}} = \frac{\overset{1}{\cancel{1000}\ \text{mL}}}{500\ \cancel{mg}} \times \frac{1\ \cancel{mg}}{\underset{1}{\cancel{1000}\ \cancel{mcg}}}$$

$$\times \frac{10\ \cancel{mcg}}{1\ \cancel{kg} \times \cancel{min}} \times \frac{44\ \cancel{kg}}{1} \times \frac{60\ \cancel{min}}{1\ \text{hr}}$$

$$= \frac{2640}{50} = \frac{52.8\ \text{mL}}{\text{hr}}$$

Note: Experienced nurses mentally convert 1 L to 1000 mL.

c. Equation is balanced. Only mL per hr remain.

RAPID PRACTICE 10-6 (p. 364)

2 a. 1 mg per mL (500 mg per 500 mL)
b. 0.2 mg per min

$$\frac{\text{mg}}{\text{min}} = \frac{\overset{1}{\cancel{500}\ \text{mg}}}{\underset{1}{\cancel{500}\ \text{mL}}} \times \frac{\overset{1}{\cancel{12}\ \text{mL}}}{1\ \cancel{hr}} \times \frac{1\ \cancel{hr}}{\underset{5}{\cancel{60}\ \text{min}}}$$

$$= \frac{1}{5} = \frac{0.2\ \text{mg}}{\text{min}}$$

c. Equation is balanced. Only mg per min remain.

3 a. 4 mg per mL (1000 mg per 250 mL)
b. 0.67 mg per min

$$\frac{\text{mg}}{\text{min}} = \frac{\overset{4}{\cancel{1000}\ \text{mg}}}{1\ \cancel{g}} \times \frac{1\ \cancel{g}}{\underset{1}{\cancel{250}\ \text{mL}}}$$

$$\times \frac{\overset{1}{\cancel{10}\ \text{mL}}}{\cancel{hr}} \times \frac{1\ \cancel{hr}}{\underset{6}{\cancel{60}\ \text{min}}} = \frac{4}{6}$$

$$= 0.666,\ \text{rounded to } 0.67\ \text{mg per min}$$

c. Equation is balanced. Only mg per min remain.

Note: The mg-to-g conversion formula was first because mg were needed in the first numerator.

4 a. 2 mg per mL (500 mg per 250 mL)
b. 0.83 mg per min

$$\frac{\text{mg}}{\text{min}} = \frac{\overset{2}{\cancel{500}\ \text{mg}}}{\underset{1}{\cancel{250}\ \text{mL}}} \times \frac{\overset{5}{\cancel{25}\ \text{mL}}}{1\ \cancel{hr}} \times \frac{1\ \cancel{hr}}{\underset{12}{\cancel{60}\ \text{min}}}$$

$$= 0.83\ \text{mg per min}$$

c. Equation is balanced. Only mg per min remain.

5 a. 0.25 mg per mL
b. 125 mcg per minute

$$\frac{\text{mcg}}{\text{min}} = \frac{\overset{1}{\cancel{1000}\ \text{mcg}}}{1\ \cancel{mg}} \times \frac{250\ \cancel{mg}}{\underset{1}{\cancel{1000}\ \text{mL}}} \times \frac{\overset{1}{\cancel{30}\ \text{mL}}}{1\ \cancel{hr}}$$

$$\times \frac{1\ \cancel{hr}}{\underset{2}{\cancel{60}\ \text{min}}} = \frac{250}{2} = \frac{125\ \text{mcg}}{\text{min}}$$

c. Equation is balanced. Only mcg per min remain.

Note: The mcg-to-mg conversion formula was entered first because mcg were needed in the first numerator.

RAPID PRACTICE 10-7 (p. 369)

1 **a.** 0.8 mL

$$\frac{mL}{dose} = \frac{1\,mL}{\underset{5}{\cancel{75\,mg}}} \times \frac{\overset{4}{\cancel{60\,mg}}}{dose} = \frac{0.8\,mL}{dose}$$

b. 5 mL
c. 5 min
d. 1 mL per min
e. 25 calibrations

2 **a.** 0.8 mL

$$\frac{mL}{dose} = \frac{1\,mL}{\underset{13}{\cancel{130\,mg}}} \times \overset{10}{\cancel{100\,mg}}$$

$$= 0.76, \text{ rounded to } \frac{0.8\,mL}{dose}$$

b. 3 mL
c. 3 min
d. 1 mL per min
e. 15 calibrations in a 10-mL syringe
f. 180 seconds (3 minutes)
g. 12 seconds per calibration

$$\frac{seconds}{calibration} = \frac{180}{15} = \frac{12\,seconds}{calibration}$$

h. Equation is balanced. Only seconds per calibration remain.

3 **a.** 2 mL

$$\frac{mL}{dose} = \frac{1\,mL}{\underset{1}{\cancel{5\,mg}}} \times \frac{\overset{2}{\cancel{10\,mg}}}{dose} = \frac{2\,mL}{dose}$$

b. N/A; 2 mL undiluted is total amount
c. 2 min
d. 1 mL per min (5 mg per min)
e. 10 calibrations for 2 mL on a 10-mL syringe
f. 120 seconds
g. 12 seconds per calibration

$$\frac{seconds}{calibration} = \frac{120}{10} = \frac{12\,seconds}{calibration}$$

h. Equation is balanced. Only seconds per calibration remain.

4 **a.** 2 mL

$$\frac{mL}{dose} = \frac{1\,mL}{\underset{1}{\cancel{0.4\,mg}}} \times \frac{\overset{2}{\cancel{0.8\,mg}}}{dose} = \frac{2\,mL}{dose}$$

b. 5 mL
c. 1 minute
d. 5 mL per min
e. 25 calibrations for 5 mL in a 10-mL syringe
f. 60 seconds (= 1 min)

g. 2.4 seconds per calibration

$$\frac{seconds}{calibration} = \frac{60}{25} = 2.4 \text{ seconds per calibration}$$

h. Equation is balanced. Only seconds per calibration remain.

5 **a.** 4 mL
b. N/A
c. 10 min (4 mg per min)
d. 0.4 mL per min
e. 20 calibrations in a 10-mL syringe
f. 600 (10 × 60) seconds
g. 30 seconds per calibration

$$\frac{seconds}{calibration} = \frac{600}{20} = \frac{30\,seconds}{calibration}$$

h. Equation is balanced. Only seconds per calibration remain.

CHAPTER 10 MULTIPLE-CHOICE REVIEW (p. 376)

1 b

$$\frac{mg}{hr} = \frac{\overset{1}{\cancel{500\,mg}}}{\underset{2}{\cancel{1000\,mL}}} \times \frac{10\,\cancel{mL}}{1\,hr} = \frac{10}{2} = \frac{5\,mg}{hr}$$

2 d

$$g\,Dextrose = \frac{25\,g}{\underset{1}{\cancel{100\,mL}}} \times \frac{\overset{10}{\cancel{1000\,mL}}}{1} = 250\,g\,Dextrose$$

$$kcal = \frac{4\,kcal}{1\,\cancel{g}} \times \frac{250\,\cancel{g}}{1} = 1000\,kcal\,Dextrose$$

3 d

$$\frac{mL}{hr} = \frac{500\,mL}{\underset{4}{\cancel{40\,mEq}}} \times \frac{\overset{1}{\cancel{10\,mEq}}}{1\,hr} = \frac{500}{4} = \frac{125\,mL}{hr}$$

4 b

$$\frac{drops}{min} = \frac{60\,drops}{1\,\cancel{mL}} \times \frac{\overset{1}{\cancel{30\,mL}}}{\underset{1}{\cancel{30\,min}}} = \frac{60\,drops}{min}$$

5 a

$$\frac{mg}{mL} = \frac{\overset{4}{\cancel{1000\,mg}}\,(1\,g)}{\underset{1}{\cancel{250\,mL}}}\;mg = \frac{4\,mg}{mL}$$

6 a
The diluted volume is used for the calculation:
5 mL in 5 min = 1 mL in 1 min

7 d

8 c

1 mg for each mL is the most concentrated solution.

9 b

$$\frac{500 \text{ mL remaining}}{3 \text{ hr remaining}} = \frac{167 \text{ mL}}{\text{hr}}$$

10 d

$$(2 \text{ mL} \times 60 \text{ min per hr})$$

$$\left(\frac{2 \text{ mL}}{1 \text{ min}} \times \frac{60 \text{ min}}{1 \text{ hr}} = \frac{120 \text{ mL}}{\text{hr}} \right)$$

CHAPTER 10 FINAL PRACTICE (p. 377)

1 a. 5 mL (ampules)

$$\frac{\text{mL}}{\text{dose}} = \frac{1 \text{ mL}}{0.4 \text{ mg}} \times \frac{2 \text{ mg}}{\text{dose}} = \frac{5 \text{ mL}}{\text{dose}}$$

b. 8 mL per hr

$$\frac{\text{mL}}{\text{hr}} = \frac{\overset{250}{\cancel{500}} \text{ mL}}{\underset{1}{\cancel{2} \text{ mg}}} \times \frac{0.03 \text{ mg}}{1 \text{ hr}} = \frac{7.5 \text{ mL}}{\text{hr}}$$

Equation is balanced. Only mL per hr remains.

2 125 mL per hr

$$\frac{\text{mL}}{\text{hr}} = \frac{500 \text{ mL}}{\underset{4}{\cancel{40} \text{ mEq}}} \times \frac{\overset{1}{\cancel{10} \text{ mEq}}}{1 \text{ hr}} = \frac{125 \text{ mL}}{\text{hr}}$$

Equation is balanced. Only mL per hr remains.

3 a. 11.3 mL per hr

$$\frac{\text{mL}}{\text{hr}} = \frac{\overset{1}{\cancel{250}} \text{ mL}}{\underset{2}{\cancel{500} \text{ mg}}} \times \frac{0.3 \text{ mg}}{\text{kg} \times \text{hr}} \times \frac{75 \text{ kg}}{1} = \frac{22.5}{2}$$

$$= 11.25, \text{ rounded to } \frac{11.3 \text{ mL}}{\text{hr}}$$

Equation is balanced. Only mg per hr and mL per hr remain.

b. 15 mL per hr

$$\frac{\text{mL}}{\text{hr}} = \frac{\overset{1}{\cancel{250}} \text{ mL}}{\underset{2}{\cancel{500} \text{ mg}}} \times \frac{0.4 \text{ mg}}{\text{kg} \times \text{hr}} \times \frac{75 \text{ kg}}{1}$$

$$= \frac{30}{2} = \frac{15 \text{ mL}}{\text{hr}}$$

Equation is balanced. Only mg per hr and mL per hr remain.

4 a. yes

b. 125 mL per hr

$$\frac{\text{mL}}{\text{hr}} = \frac{\overset{25}{\cancel{1000}} \text{ mL}}{\underset{1}{\cancel{40} \text{ mEq}}} \times \frac{5 \text{ mEq}}{\text{hr}} = \frac{125 \text{ mL}}{\text{hr}}$$

Equation is balanced. Only mL per hr remains.

c. 8 hr

$$\text{hr} = \frac{1 \text{ hr}}{\underset{1}{\cancel{125} \text{ mL}}} \times \frac{\overset{8}{\cancel{1000} \text{ mL}}}{1} = 8 \text{ hr}$$

5 a. 2.5 mL

$$\frac{\text{mL}}{\text{dose}} = \frac{1 \text{ mL}}{0.4 \text{ mg}} \times \frac{1 \text{ mg}}{\text{dose}} = \frac{2.5 \text{ mL}}{\text{dose}}$$

b. 6 sec per mL

$$\frac{\text{seconds}}{\text{mL}} = \frac{60 \text{ seconds}}{10 \text{ mL}} = \frac{6 \text{ seconds}}{\text{mL}}$$

Equation is balanced. Only seconds per mL remains.

6 a. 0.5 mg per mL

$$\frac{\text{mg}}{\text{mL}} = \frac{250 \text{ mg}}{500 \text{ mL}} = 0.5 \text{ mg per mL}$$

b. 19 mL per hr

$$\frac{\text{mL}}{\text{hr}} = \frac{\overset{1}{\cancel{500}} \text{ mL}}{\underset{25}{\underset{\cancel{125}}{\cancel{250} \text{ mg}}}} \times \frac{1 \text{ mg}}{\underset{1}{\underset{2}{\cancel{1000} \text{ mcg}}}} \times \frac{2.5 \text{ mcg}}{\text{kg} \times \text{min}}$$

$$\times \frac{\overset{6}{\cancel{64} \text{ kg}}}{1} \times \frac{\overset{\overset{6}{\cancel{30}}}{\cancel{60} \text{ min}}}{1 \text{ hr}} = \frac{480}{25} = \frac{19.2 \text{ mL}}{\text{hr}}$$

Equation is balanced. Only mL per hr remain.

7 a. 3 mL

$$\frac{\text{mL}}{\text{dose}} = \frac{4 \text{ mL}}{\underset{4}{\cancel{40} \text{ mg}}} \times \frac{\overset{3}{\cancel{30} \text{ mg}}}{\text{dose}} = \frac{12}{4} = \frac{3 \text{ mL}}{\text{dose}}$$

b. 15 calibrations

c. 450 seconds

$$\text{seconds} = \frac{\overset{15}{\cancel{60}} \text{ seconds}}{1 \text{ min}} \times \frac{1 \text{ min}}{\underset{1}{\cancel{4} \text{ mg}}} \times \frac{30 \text{ mg}}{1}$$

$$= 15 \times 30 = 450 \text{ seconds}$$

d. 30 seconds per calibration

$$\frac{\text{seconds}}{\text{calibration}} = \frac{450 \text{ seconds}}{15 \text{ calibrations}} = \frac{30 \text{ seconds}}{\text{calibration}}$$

Equation is balanced. Only seconds per calibration remains.

8 **a.** 8 mL

$$\frac{mL}{dose} = \frac{1\,mL}{\cancel{500\,mg}\,_1} \times \frac{\overset{2}{\cancel{1000\,mg}}}{1\,\cancel{g}} \times \frac{4\,\cancel{g}}{dose} = \frac{8\,mL}{dose}$$

b. 150 mL per hr

$$\frac{mL}{hr} = \frac{2.5\,mL}{1\,\cancel{min}} \times \frac{60\,\cancel{minute}}{1\,hr} = \frac{150\,mL}{hr}$$

Equation is balanced. Only mL per hr remains.

c. 4 g = 4000 mg

$$\frac{mg}{min} = \frac{4000\,mg}{250\,\cancel{mL}} \times \frac{2.5\,\cancel{mL}}{1\,min} = \frac{1000}{25} = \frac{40\,mg}{min}$$

Equation is balanced. Only mg per min remains.

Note: mg is the approved abbreviation for milligram. Do not abbreviate magnesium.

9 **a.** 15 mg per hr

$$\frac{mg}{hr} = \frac{1\,mg}{1000\,\cancel{mcg}} \times \frac{3\,\cancel{mcg}}{\cancel{kg} \times \cancel{min}}$$

$$\times \frac{82\,\cancel{kg}}{1} \times \frac{60\,\cancel{min}}{1\,hr}$$

$$= \frac{14{,}760}{1000} = 14.76,\text{ rounded to } \frac{15\,mg}{hr}$$

Equation is balanced. Only mg per hr remains.

b. 18.5 mL per hr

$$\frac{mL}{hr} = \frac{\overset{1}{\underset{5}{\cancel{250}}}\,mL}{\underset{4}{\cancel{200\,mg}}} \times \frac{1\,\cancel{mg}}{\underset{200}{\cancel{1000\,mcg}}}$$

$$\times \frac{3\,\cancel{mcg}}{\cancel{kg} \times \cancel{min}} \times \frac{82\,\cancel{kg}}{1} \times \frac{60\,\cancel{min}}{1\,hr}$$

$$= \frac{1476}{80} = 18.45,\text{ rounded to } \frac{18.5\,mL}{hr}$$

Equation is balanced. Only mL per hr remains.

Note: The nurse assesses the patient, contacts the prescriber, obtains an order to adjust the flow rate gradually to the ordered rate, and documents the incident.

10 **a.** 0.2 mg per mL

$$\frac{mg}{mL} = \frac{\cancel{50}\,mg}{\underset{1}{\cancel{250\,mL}}} = \frac{1}{5} = \frac{0.2\,mg}{mL}\text{ concentration}$$

Equation is balanced. Only mg per mL remain.

b. 5.4 mL per hr

$$\frac{mL}{hr} = \frac{\overset{5}{\cancel{250}}\,mL}{\underset{1}{\cancel{50\,mg}}} \times \frac{0.3\,\cancel{mcg}}{kg \times \cancel{min}} \times \frac{1\,\cancel{mg}}{1000\,\cancel{mcg}}$$

$$\times \frac{60\,kg}{1} \times \frac{60\,min}{1\,hr} = \frac{54}{10} = 5.4\text{ mL per hr}$$

Equations are balanced. Only mcg per min and mL per hr remain.

Suggestions for Further Reading

Gahart BL, Nazareno AR: *2021 Intravenous medications: a handbook for nurses and health professionals*, ed. 34, St. Louis, 2017, Mosby.

Lilley LL, Collins SR, Harrington S, Snyder JS: *Pharmacology and the nursing process*, ed. 9, St. Louis, 2021, Mosby.

Perry AG, Potter PA: *Clinical nursing skills and techniques*, ed. 10, St. Louis, 2021, Mosby.

www.baxter.com

www.globalrph.com/tpn.htm

www.hospira.com

www.safemedication.com

http://www.ismp.org/tools/highalertmedications.pdf

http://phys.org/news/2013-09-real-time-detector-iv-drugs-life-threatening.html

Evolve For additional practice problems, refer to the Critical Care Dosage section of the Elsevier's Interactive Drug Calculation Application, Version 1 on Evolve.

Now that you have mastered the principles and contents of this chapter, you will be on the road to safer practice and will also find Chapter 11, Antidiabetic Medications, and subsequent chapters relatively easy to learn.

PART V

Common High-Alert Medications

11 Antidiabetic Medications

ESTIMATED TIME TO COMPLETE CHAPTER: 3 hours

The prevalence of diabetes is increasing all over the world, including the United States, at an alarming rate. The increase of diabetes in the United States corresponds to changes in lifestyle leading to a very high incidence of obesity. This has generated many new medicines for treatment.

Measuring an ordered insulin dose in a syringe for subcutaneous administration is a basic skill that does not require math. However, IV insulin administration does require math calculations. To administer antidiabetic medications *safely*, the nurse must understand frequently encountered terms, know how to interpret orders and labels, differentiate blood glucose laboratory levels, distinguish the various pharmacological products ordered for treatment, identify manifestations of hypoglycemia and hyperglycemia, understand emergency treatment for those manifestations, and know when to withhold medication and seek further orders. Insulin is a high-alert medication, meaning that it has higher than average potential to cause harm if used in error.* This chapter focuses on basic concepts related to safe administration of insulin.

Many new medications for diabetes have been developed to meet this epidemic and are commonly encountered in the patient care setting. The doses must be individualized based on frequent current capillary or venous blood glucose results.

> ▲ **Cultural Note**
>
> Native American populations have been afflicted with very high rates of diabetes.
>
> In addition to studies of lifestyle changes imposed upon Native Americans leading to dietary and exercise changes over the decades, scientists have been exploring genetic influences on large weight gains within the U.S. Pima tribe. One-half of the U.S. Pima population has diabetes.

---

*Refer to the ISMP list of high-alert medications (see Appendix B).

VOCABULARY

Diabetes Mellitus (DM)	Chronic metabolic diseases due to insufficient insulin secretion and/or utilization, characterized by elevated blood glucose levels and abnormal carbohydrate metabolism. Also affects protein and fat metabolism.
Diabetes Mellitus type 1 (DM type I)	Characterized by elevated blood glucose levels due to insufficient insulin production and/or destruction of beta cells in the pancreatic islets of Langerhans. More frequent onset in young people. Requires lifelong insulin hormone replacement. Occurs in less than 10% of cases. Causal factors theorized to be autoimmune, genetic, and/or environmental. Formerly known as insulin-dependent diabetes mellitus or juvenile-onset diabetes.
Diabetes Mellitus type 2 (DM type 2)	The most common (and still increasing) form of diabetes (85% to 95% cases), characterized by elevated blood glucose levels due to insufficient insulin utilization (resistance) and/or insufficient insulin production. If not controlled with diet and lifestyle changes, it is treated with oral antidiabetics. Insulin may be added for better glucose control, particularly during stressful events such as infections and pregnancy. Causal factors are associated with sedentary lifestyle, genetics, obesity, and diet. Formerly known as adult-onset diabetes but increasingly seen in children. Patients may have the disease for several years before diagnosis. Formerly known as non-insulin-dependent diabetes or adult-onset diabetes.
Diabetic Ketoacidosis (DKA)	Emergency condition and complication of diabetes diagnosed by elevated blood glucose levels (>250 mg per dL), blood pH less than 7.3, elevated ketones in blood and urine, and often coma. Requires hospitalization and insulin therapy as well as other medications.
Glucagon	Blood glucose-*raising* hormone secreted by alpha (α) cells in the pancreatic islets of Langerhans, released in response to a fall below normal blood glucose levels. May be administered as a treatment for severe hypoglycemia levels (e.g., blood glucose level <60 mg per dL).
Hyperglycemia	Elevated glucose level in blood. Levels vary for diabetes diagnosis, postprandial (after meal) norms, and treatment and control needs. Refer to agency laboratory norms.
Hyperglycemic Hyperosmolar Nonketotic Coma (HHNK)	Fasting blood glucose level is greater than 600 mg/dL yet serum ketone levels are normal or only slightly elevated.
Hypoglycemia	Decreased level of glucose in blood (<70 mg per dL). May be caused by several factors: *skipped or delayed meal after insulin and/or some oral antidiabetic agents, or insulin overdose.* Usually more severe in insulin-dependent patients. The major potential adverse effect of insulin administration.
	Symptoms are variable among individuals and range from mild confusion, irritability, and sweating to impaired functioning to loss of consciousness and death. It should be treated early and promptly.
Insulin	Blood glucose-*lowering* hormone produced by the beta cells of the islets of Langerhans in the pancreas. It facilitates entry of glucose into muscle cells and other sites for storage as an energy source, thus lowering blood glucose levels. A high-alert medication.*
	Mnemonic: INsulin helps glucose get IN to cells.
Insulin Resistance	Diminished tissue ability to respond to insulin. Glucose levels continue to rise. Insulin production and levels then rise (hyperinsulinemia) in response, in an attempt to maintain normal glucose levels. Associated with DM type 2, obesity, and hypertension.
Insulin "Shock"	Urgent hypoglycemic condition (blood glucose <60 mg per dL). May be caused by an overdose of insulin for current glucose level or as a result of taking usual dose of insulin followed by inadequate or delayed dietary intake. Must be treated promptly with immediate form of glucose administration; oral if the patient is conscious or IV if the patient is unconscious or unable to swallow, followed up by *complex carbohydrate* to cover possible hypoglycemic rebound. Brain cells begin to be deprived of glucose when the blood glucose level falls below normal. (See "Hypoglycemia.")
Units	Standardized dose measurement of therapeutic effectiveness. Insulin is provided in units.

LABORATORY TEST TERMINOLOGY

Blood Glucose (BG)	Laboratory serum venous blood glucose test. Prescribers may order this test to verify capillary BGM and SMBG test results.
Blood Glucose Monitor (BGM)	Blood capillary handheld finger-stick device administered at the bedside by nurses or at home by patients.
Deciliter (dL)	One-tenth of a liter. Used to report number of milligrams in blood glucose laboratory test results (e.g., 100 mg per dL).
Fasting Blood Sugar (FBS)	Fasting (8-12 hr) reveals baseline blood glucose level (normal level, 70-100 mg per dL).*
Fructosamine	Determines average blood glucose level over a 2- to 4-week period.
Glycosylated Hemoglobin (A1c or HbA1c)	Determines average blood glucose level over the *past 2-3 months* by measuring the amount of glucose attached to hemoglobin in the red blood cells. Helpful in assessing newly diagnosed patients, severity of disease, home maintenance in those being treated, and risk for complications. A normal HbA1c level is 3.5% to 5.5% in nondiabetics.*
Postprandial Glucose Test	"After-meals" blood glucose test. Usually performed 2 hr after meals to determine individual ability to metabolize glucose, and to evaluate treatment. Two-hour postprandial blood glucose level is usually normal in nondiabetics and elevated in diabetics.*
Self-Monitored Blood Glucose (SMBG)	Obtained by patients with the blood glucose monitor. The result is reported by the patient.

*Normal values vary slightly from laboratory to laboratory. Glucose goal levels for diabetics may be slightly higher than for nondiabetics because of the risk of hypoglycemia.

➤ If blood glucose levels are reported by a laboratory in millimoles per liter, *multiply* by 18 to convert to milligrams per deciliter. Divide milligrams per deciliter by 18 to obtain the equivalent millimoles per liter.

Oral and Injectable Non-Insulin Antidiabetic Medications

➤ All antidiabetic medications are ISMP high-alert medications (see Appendix B).

Oral and injectable non-insulin antidiabetic medications are a growing number of hypoglycemic agents with varying pharmacologic properties that target specific problems of glucose metabolism for patients with type 2 diabetes mellitus. Many are available in more than one concentration. Some examples of these agents follow:

Class

Biguanides
- Glucophage, Glucophage XR, Fortamet, Riomet (metformin)

Meglitinides
- Repaglinide
- Starlix (nateglitinide)

Sulfonylurea
- Amaryl (glimepiride)
- Diabeta, Micronase (glyburide)
- Glucotrol, Glucotrol XL (glipizide)

DPP-4 inhibitors
- Januvia (sitagliptin)
- Onglyza (saxagliptin)

Alpha-glucosidase inhibitors
- Glyset (Miglitol)
- Precose (Acarbose)

Class

Thiazolidinediones
- Actos (pioglitazone)

Sodium Glucose Co-Transporter 2 inhibitors (SGLT 2) (oral products)
- Invokana (canagliflozin)
- Farxiga (dapagliflozin)
- Jardiance (empaglifozin)

Injectable Non-Insulin Products

GLP-1 Agonist (given for type 2 diabetes as an injection)
- Adlyxin (lixisenatide)
- Bydureon BCise, Bydureon (exenatide)
- Byetta (exenatide)
- Rybelsus, Ozempic (semaglutide)
- Trulicity (dulaglutide)

Class	Class

Class (right column):
- Tanzeum (albiglutide)
- Victoza (liraglutide)

Amylinomimetics (given for type 1 and type 2 diabetes as an injection)
- Symlin (pramlintide acetate)

➤ Note carefully the similarities of generic names. Confusion of look-alike drug names has resulted in medication errors.

Some of these drugs are available in several dosages. They may be combined with other drugs to enhance the effectiveness of treatment. Refer to the PrandiMet label, which is a combination of repaglinide and metformin.

EXAMPLES

Following are some examples of prescribers' orders for oral antidiabetics, along with the drug labels:

Glucophage 500 mg PO twice daily with meals

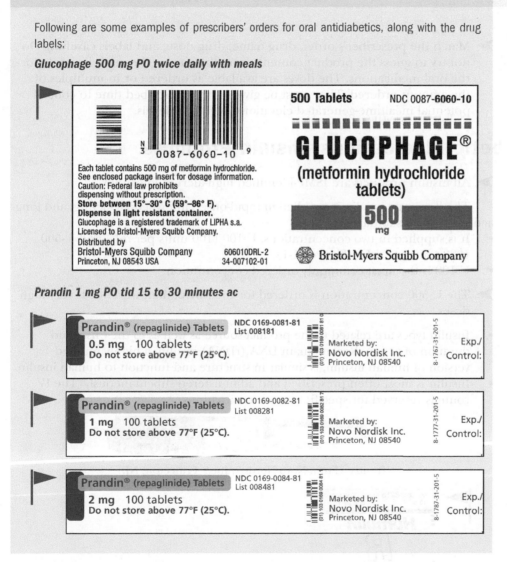

Prandin 1 mg PO tid 15 to 30 minutes ac

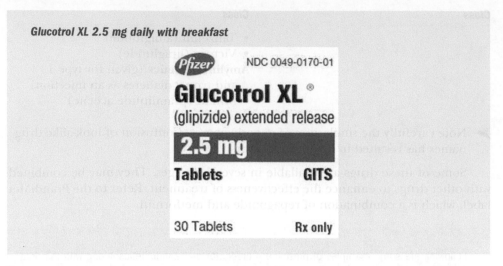

Glucotrol XL 2.5 mg daily with breakfast

➤ Match the prescriber's order, drug name, drug dose, and labels carefully. Do not try to guess the product contents from the name. The math is simple for the oral medications. The doses are available as ordered or in multiples of the amount ordered. They must be given at the prescribed time to control potential mealtime-generated elevations of glucose levels.

Parenteral Antidiabetic Medications: Insulin Products

⚑ ➤ All insulin products are ISMP-identified high-alert medications.

The hormone insulin is supplied in rapid-onset, intermediate-acting, and long-acting forms in standardized units.
* It is supplied in two concentrations: U-100 (100 units per mL) and U-500 (500 units per mL) (Figure 11-1).
* U-100 is the most commonly ordered concentration.

➤ The U-500 concentration is ordered for the *rare* patient who needs very high doses.

* Insulin types are related to the product source as well as to the onset and duration of action. Recombinant DNA (rDNA) insulin, a highly purified version of human insulin, is similar in structure and function to human insulin.
* Insulin is most often prescribed and administered subcutaneously. The IV route is reserved for specific acute-care situations.

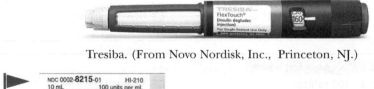

Tresiba. (From Novo Nordisk, Inc., Princeton, NJ.)

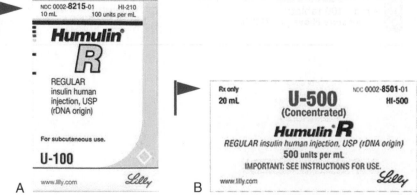

FIGURE 11-1 A, U-100 (100 units per mL) insulin. **B,** U-500 (500 units per mL) insulin.

➤ Do not confuse U-100 with the total amount in the vial. U-100 refers to the concentration per milliliter (100 units per mL).

➤ The most common adverse effect of insulin therapy is *hypoglycemia.*

➤ Spell out "units" even though the abbreviation U may be seen in some orders and preprinted MARs. It can be mistaken for zero and is on the "Do Not Use" list of the Joint Commission.

➤ Warning: Insulin activity varies among individuals. Monitor blood glucose levels closely.

➤ Prescribed timing of insulin administration and timing of meals are linked to the time of onset of the insulin activity. *Hypoglycemic* reactions may occur at any time, but insulin onset and peak activity times warrant close observation for potential hypoglycemic reactions.

➤ Consult manufacturer literature regarding mixing with other insulins and oral antidiabetic products. There are important differences and interactions among the products.

Examine the insulin activity chart in Table 11-1. Insulin fixed-combination mixes are supplied for patients who experience patterns of mealtime elevations.

TABLE 11-1   Insulin Activity Chart for Subcutaneous Administration, in Order of Onset of Action

Type	Brand Name	Onset of Action	Peak	Duration
Rapid Acting				
Insulin aspart	Novolog	10–20 min	40–50 min	3–5 hr
Insulin lispro	Humalog	15–30 min	1 hr	3–5 hr
Insulin glusiline	Apidra	20–30 min	1–1.5 hr	less than 6 hr
Short Acting				
Insulin injection regular	Novolin R	30–60 min	1.5–5 hr	8 hr
	Humulin R	30–60 min	1–5 hr	6–8 hr
Intermediate Acting				
Insulin isophane suspension	Novolin N	1.5 hr	4–12 hr	Up to 24 hr
(NPH)	Humulin N	1–2 hr	6–12 hr	18–24 hr
Long Acting (➤ do not mix with other insulins)				
Insulin glargine	Lantus	1 hr	None	24 hr or more
Insulin detemir	Levemir	0.8–2 hr	None	24 hr
Mixed Insulins				
70% insulin aspart protamine suspension + 30% insulin aspart (fixed premix)	Novolog Mix 70/30	10–20 min	2.4 hr	24 hr
75% insulin lispro protamine + 25% insulin lispro (fixed premix)	Humalog Mix 75/25 Humalog Mix 50/50	15 min	30–90 min	24 hr
Insulin isophane suspension (NPH) + regular insulin combination	Novolin 70/30	30 min	2–12 hr	24 hr
	Humulin 70/30	30 min	2–12 hr	24 hr

The mixes contain rapid-acting or short-acting insulin mixed with a longer-, slower-acting insulin, which reduces the fluctuations and elevations in blood glucose patterns. The intermediate- and longer-acting insulins contain additives that extend the action but render them unsuitable for IV administration.

<table>
<tr><td>**Q & A**</td><td>**ASK YOURSELF**</td><td>1</td><td>What are the five column headings in Table 11-1 that reveal key pieces of information that the nurse must understand about each type of insulin?</td></tr>
<tr><td></td><td>**MY ANSWER**</td><td></td><td>_____</td></tr>
<tr><td></td><td></td><td>2</td><td>Which type of insulin does not have a peak?</td></tr>
<tr><td></td><td></td><td></td><td>_____</td></tr>
</table>

FAQ *How are insulin types and amounts selected?*

ANSWER Types and amounts are selected on the basis of patterns in the patient's recent blood glucose levels, including the timing of elevations, particularly related to mealtime and activity patterns. The patient's motivation and compliance are also factored into insulin prescriptions.

CLINICAL RELEVANCE

- If the patient is hospitalized with extremely high blood levels of glucose, a rapid-acting insulin may be administered subcutaneously or intravenously to stabilize the patient.
- Some patients exhibit elevations only after meals, some have nighttime or early-morning spikes, and others have constant elevations.
- A small amount or **basal** (slow, low, continuous release) dose of long-acting insulin, such as insulin glargine, may be ordered with weekly dose adjustments. This amount does not cover mealtime elevations. The dose will be low enough to avoid *hypo*glycemic reactions. **Bolus** (single, concentrated) doses of insulin aspart and lispro, or regular insulins, may be ordered and administered separately to cover mealtime and/or other elevations.
- When a pattern of blood glucose levels in relation to meals emerges, the type and amount of insulin can be customized.
- Insulin mixes may be ordered twice a day to cover a patient's basal needs and mealtime elevations when a pattern is known.
- Intermediate- and long-acting insulins are *not* used to treat *acute hyper*glycemia.

<table>
<tr><td>**Q & A**</td><td>**ASK YOURSELF**</td><td>1</td><td>What is a basal dose of insulin?</td></tr>
<tr><td></td><td>**MY ANSWER**</td><td></td><td>_____</td></tr>
<tr><td></td><td></td><td>2</td><td>What are two reasons that bolus doses would be added to basal doses?</td></tr>
<tr><td></td><td></td><td></td><td>_____</td></tr>
</table>

Insulin Labels

Take a few minutes to examine the insulin product labels and identify the following:
- Name
- Type
- Concentration: U-100 or U-500 (U-500 is *rarely* ordered)
- Product source: rDNA

- Storage of insulin products, opened and unopened, is controversial. Some say refrigerate all. Others say the current bottle can be at room temperature and unopened bottles must be refrigerated. Check agency policy.
- Write the date opened on the label and discard the bottle according to the manufacturer guidelines, usually a month after opening.
- Expiration date.

CLINICAL RELEVANCE

Teach the patient to place insulin in an insulated cooler for travel (not on dry ice) and to carry it on his or her person. If insulin is warm, it may develop particles or crystals, may become discolored, and will not be effective in lowering the blood glucose level.

Short- and Rapid-Acting Insulins

There are several types and brands of rapid- or short- acting insulins on the market. Rapid- and short-acting insulins are administered to treat a current blood glucose elevation or an anticipated elevation in the near future, such as after the next meal. Figures 11-2 to 11-5 illustrate product labels of various rapid- and short-acting insulins.

Humalog and NovoLog insulin are to be given 10 to 15 minutes *before* a meal or with the meal, whereas Humulin R and Novolin R must be given 30 minutes before a meal (see Figures 11-2 to 11-4).

➤ If there is any chance that mealtime may be delayed, such as might occur in a hospital, do *not* give Humalog or NovoLog until the meal arrives.

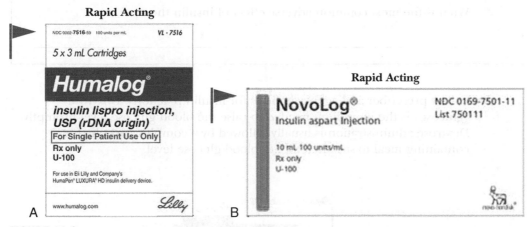

FIGURE 11-2 **A,** Humalog insulin. **B,** NovoLog insulin.

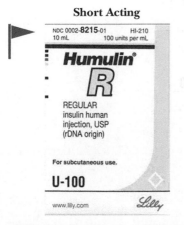

FIGURE 11-3 Humulin R insulin.

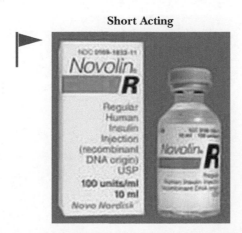

FIGURE 11-4 Novolin R insulin. (From Novo Nordisk, Inc., Princeton, NJ.)

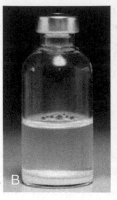
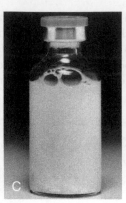
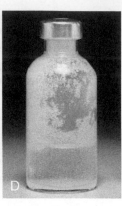

FIGURE 11-5 A, Humalog insulin should always look clear. **B,** Insulin at the bottom of the bottle. Do not use if insulin stays on the bottom of the bottle after gentle rolling. **C,** Clumps of insulin. Do not use if there are clumps of insulin in the liquid or on the bottom of the vial. **D,** Bottle appears frosted. Do not use if particles of insulin are on the bottom or sides of the bottle and give it a frosty appearance. (Copyright Eli Lilly and Company. All rights reserved. Used with permission.)

Q & A   **ASK YOURSELF**   **1**   What does U-100 on the label of the insulin vial mean?

   MY ANSWER   _____

   2   What is the most common adverse effect of insulin therapy?

   _____

➤ Follow prescriber and agency policies for insulin reactions. Dextrose (glucose) is the ingredient needed to raise the blood glucose level promptly. Dextrose administration is usually followed by a complex carbohydrate-containing meal to sustain a higher blood glucose level.

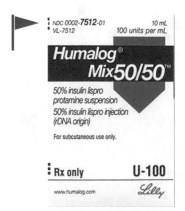

To treat a hypoglycemic episode, all patients with diabetes (especially those taking insulin) should:
- Take 15 to 20 grams of a simple carbohydrate such as: glucose tablets, glucose gel, a handful of raisins, 8 ounces of nonfat milk, or hard candies, jellybeans, or gumdrops (see package to determine how many to consume).
- This should be followed by a complex carbohydrate and protein snack such as peanut butter crackers or cheese and crackers, or half of a sandwich to prevent a possible hypoglycemic rebound from occurring.

CLINICAL RELEVANCE

ASK YOURSELF **Q & A**

1 What is the difference among each of these four types of Humulin insulin? Which are short-acting, intermediate-acting, or both?

MY ANSWER

_____

2 When reading two different numbers on the mixes, which number is the fast acting: the first or the second?

_____

RAPID PRACTICE 11-1 | Rapid- and Short-Acting Insulin Label Interpretation

ESTIMATED COMPLETION TIME: 10 to 15 minutes   **ANSWERS ON:** page 430

DIRECTIONS: *Read the information presented in the previous sections, examine the short-acting insulin labels on p. 393, and answer the questions briefly.*

1 If the patient is experiencing a *hypo*glycemic episode, why should diet beverages and sugar alcohols not be given?

_____

_____

2 **a.** What is the concentration of insulin on the labels? _____
   b. How many total units of insulin are contained in each vial? _____

3 What is the name of the ingredient needed to raise blood sugar levels promptly? _____

4 If there is a chance that a meal will be delayed, which two of the fast-acting insulins should be held and given *with* the meal? _____

5 Which two of these insulins must be given 30 minutes before a meal?
   a. Novolin R
   b. NovoLog (insulin aspart)
   c. Humulin R
   d. Humalog (insulin lispro)

➤ Only regular (R) insulins, insulin aspart (NovoLog), and insulin glulisine (Apidra) can be administered *intravenously as well as subcutaneously.* They must be *clear,* without precipitates, for IV administration. They do not need to be rolled or shaken because they are not suspensions (see Figure 11-5).

➤ Humalog must be diluted for IV use, but it is not commonly used. Always check the label for the permitted routes of administration.

As with all multiuse vials, write the *date and time opened* and initial the label. Discard the opened vial according to the product insert directions, after approximately a month. Consult product labels and inserts for more detailed information about storage, activity, expiration dates, and incompatibilities.

➤ Some of the labels say "Human Insulin" injection. They are not made from human pancreas. They are identical in structure to human insulin but are of rDNA origin.

➤ Do not confuse the capital letter *R* for *Regular* insulin with the small superscript ® indicating a registered product.

Q & A **ASK YOURSELF** 1 What would be expected to happen to the patient's blood glucose level if Humulin R, Novolin R, insulin lispro, or insulin aspart were given and the meal was delayed?

MY ANSWER _____

Intermediate-Acting Insulins

Usually patients receiving intermediate-acting products, including insulin mixes, receive *two* injections a day—one in the morning and one in the evening—plus a bedtime snack of complex carbohydrate, such as half a cheese sandwich or milk, to cover a potential hypoglycemic reaction from overlapping duration. Insulin mixes are usually prescribed for specified periods of time before breakfast and dinner. Some are ordered AM and PM without time specification.

➤ Clarify AM and PM orders with the prescriber as to precise time desired.

Isophane Insulin Human (abbreviated as NPH or N) is a modified insulin suspension that provides delayed basal insulin release. It has a longer duration than the short-acting insulins. The additives that extend the action make the solutions cloudy, rendering them inappropriate for IV administration. Suspension label directions call for gently rolling the vial to mix the ingredients before drawing up in a syringe. Read the manufacturer's label.

The insulin must then be given promptly. The additives extend the duration of coverage up to 26 hours, depending on the preparation (Figure 11-6).

Q & A **ASK YOURSELF** 1 What would happen to the solution in the syringe if there were a delay between drawing up the suspension and administering it?

MY ANSWER _____

2 Why might people whose employment regularly or irregularly requires second- or third-shift hours need special assistance with their antidiabetic medication schedule?

_____

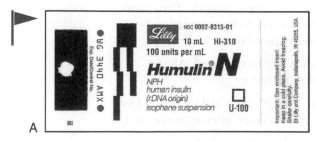 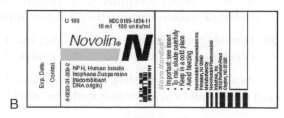

FIGURE 11-6 Intermediate-acting modified insulin suspensions.

| **RAPID PRACTICE 11-2** | Intermediate-Acting Insulin Suspensions |

ESTIMATED COMPLETION TIME: 5 to 10 minutes   **ANSWERS ON:** page 430

DIRECTIONS: *Read the material pertaining to intermediate-acting insulin products and answer the questions with brief phrases.*

1   Would these intermediate-acting products be clear or cloudy? _____

2   How many injections of intermediate-acting insulins per day do people usually receive? _____

3   Can a suspension be administered intravenously in an emergency? _____

4   Why do patients on insulin mixes and bedtime intermediate-acting insulins require a bedtime snack of a complex carbohydrate? What potential adverse effects are they trying to avoid?

_____

_____

5   What is the units-per-mL concentration on each intermediate product label in Figure 11-6?

_____

Short- and Intermediate-Acting Insulins: Insulin Fixed-Combination Mixes

Various insulin mixes combine rapid-acting or short-acting with a slower-acting insulin that can help control insulin and glucose levels through the fluctuations that follow two meals and reduce the number of injections the patient takes. Fixed-combination premixes, such as those shown below, spare the patient from having to self-prepare two types of insulin separately and then combine them. The concentration of mix selected depends on the patient's usual blood glucose patterns and levels. Patients with unstable levels and patterns cannot use premixed insulins. They must adjust their insulin doses to a current blood glucose test for better glycemic control. Most patients take a larger amount of intermediate-acting (slower release) insulin and *less* of the short rapid-acting, thus the 75/25 and 70/30 premixes.

Mixed insulins are taken twice a day at a *specific* number minutes before the morning and evening meals so that the short-acting part covers the first meal. Each injection covers two meals (or one meal and a bedtime controlled balanced snack).

➤ The timing of the injection depends on the type and specific onset of the *short-acting* insulin.

➤ The intermediate- and long-acting insulins contain additives that make them unsuitable for IV administration.

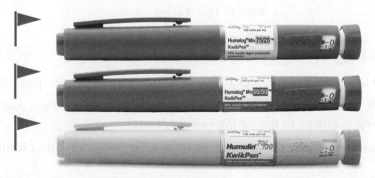

Long-Acting Insulins

Long-acting insulin contains additives that cause it to be released more slowly than the rapid-, short-, and intermediate-acting insulins. Long-acting insulin products are administered *subcutaneously* to patients with type 1 or 2 diabetes whose blood glucose levels are unresponsive to intermediate-acting insulins, such as patients with early-morning fasting elevations and/or to patients who cannot tolerate more than one injection per day (Figure 11-7).

➤ Long-acting insulins cannot be given intravenously because they contain additives to extend the action. These additives are not suitable for IV use.

Insulin glargine (Lantus) and insulin detemir (Levemir) are clear. They do *not* have a peak. They provide a steady release of insulin throughout the duration of 24 to 26 hours. For this reason, they are known as *basal* long-acting insulins.

➤ Insulin glargine and insulin detemir *cannot* be mixed with any other insulin even though they are clear solutions. They may be given at any hour but must be given at the *same* time each day to provide a steady release of basal (low-dose) insulin for 24 hours without a peak. If additional short-acting insulin is needed, it is administered subcutaneously as a bolus in a *separate* syringe.

Read the instructions on the Lantus label shown in Figure 11-7.

➤ It is safest to assume that insulin products *cannot be mixed* until you read the drug literature for each order. Nurses who do not regularly work with patients with diabetes cannot rely on memory. It is best to make a habit of always checking compatibilities with current drug literature and/or the pharmacy.

➤ Patients on evening rapid- or short-acting or any intermediate- or long-acting insulin should have a bedtime snack.

> ✳ *Mnemonic*
>
> *Lantus* begins with an *L* and has a *Long* duration.

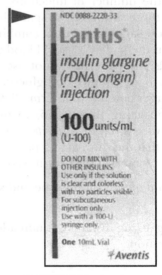

FIGURE 11-7 Lantus insulin.

RAPID PRACTICE 11-3	Long-Acting Insulin

ESTIMATED COMPLETION TIME: 5 to 10 minutes   **ANSWERS ON:** page 430

DIRECTIONS: *Read the information about long-acting insulin products and answer the following questions in two- or three-word phrases.*

1   Can insulin glargine or insulin detemir be mixed with any other insulin?

2   What is the concentration of the insulin glargine label shown in Figure 11-7?

_____

3   What is a unique feature of insulin glargine and insulin detemir?

_____

4   Can long-acting insulins be administered intravenously? _____

5   What is the generic name for Lantus insulin? _____

Steps to Prepare Doses for Insulin Syringes

1   Obtain and/or interpret the current blood glucose value. Follow the prescriber's directions for blood glucose values. Withhold insulin if the blood glucose level is low according to the prescriber's directions and agency policy. Contact the prescriber promptly if directions for low values are not written in the orders, and document the verification.

2   Read the order for name, type, dose, time, and route. If you are using an opened bottle, check the discard date, as with all multidose vials.

3   Select the appropriate insulin and an insulin syringe that is calibrated for the *same* concentration (e.g., 100 units per mL).

4   Examine all medication vials for clumps and precipitates. Insulin may develop precipitates if the temperature is too warm, if the vial has been contaminated, or if it has passed the expiration date.

5   If the insulin is a suspension, *gently roll* to disperse the contents, according to the manufacturer's current recommendations. Never shake insulin, it will cause air bubbles, which will alter the dose. Draw the appropriate amount of units in the insulin syringe using the technique learned for withdrawal of injectables from a vial.

Calculations are not needed for single insulin injections.

➤ Some agencies require two nurses for the *entire* preparation of all orders for insulin and other high-risk medications. They must co-sign the MAR indicating that each step of the preparation of the ordered insulin dose is correct. Check agency policy.

> ▲ *Cultural Note*
>
> In many countries, insulin preparations and syringe types vary. Remind patients to carry a generous supply of their own equipment in a small cooler for travel in their carry-on luggage.

Matching Insulin Concentration and Syringes

➤ The insulin syringe matches the number of units per mL on the label of the insulin bottle; for example, U-100 and 100 units per mL on the insulin bottle label and 100 units per mL on the syringe label. This is the most commonly used concentration in the United States.

Examine the following order: Give Novolin R 10 units subcut stat.

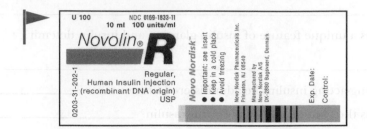

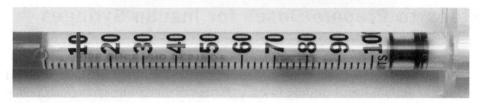

Examine the label. What is the brand name? *Novolin R*

What is the type (action)? *Short-acting (regular)*

Are there any terms not understood? Check current references and call the pharmacy if necessary.

How many total milliliters are there in the vial? *10 mL*

What is the concentration of drug to solution? *100 units per mL (U-100)*

How many total units in the vial? *10 mL × 100 units = 1000 units, a multidose vial*

Does this type of insulin need to be mixed or rolled? *No, because it is not a suspension.*

➤ Prepare insulin with an insulin syringe only.

Reading Units on Insulin Syringes

Insulin is manufactured, prescribed, and administered in units. The insulin syringe is calibrated in units.

Examine the syringes in Figure 11-8. The calibrations are for even amounts of insulin. Always note the total capacity of the syringe (1 mL, 100 units for this syringe), then ensure that the syringe calibrations are units, and finally note the number of calibrations between the markings. Reading the calibrated units on the insulin syringe is straightforward.

Each calibration represents *two* units on these 100-unit-per-1-mL syringes.

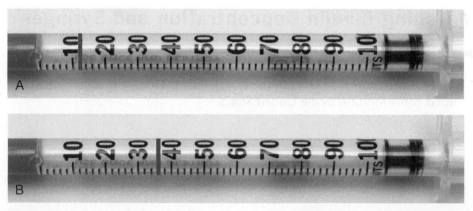

FIGURE 11-8 A, 100-unit insulin syringe marked at 12 units. **B,** 100-unit insulin syringe marked at 36 units.

Even- and Odd-Numbered Scales on Insulin Syringes

Syringes are available with calibrations in even numbers on one side and odd numbers on the other. There are also syringes available with either even or odd calibrations (Figure 11-9).

The dose administered must be in the *precise* number of units ordered. Each calibration is worth *2* units on the even- and on the odd-numbered scale.

➤ The standard insulin syringe calibrated in units, designed for a concentration of 100 units per mL, must be distinguished from the tuberculin syringe, which is also a 1-mL syringe calibrated in 0.01 mL (Figure 11-10).

---

1 How will you know the difference between an insulin syringe and a tuberculin syringe?	**ASK YOURSELF** **Q & A**
_____	**MY ANSWER**

CLINICAL RELEVANCE

Several drugs, but not all, must be given at very precise times.

➤ Insulin is one of those drugs that must be *prioritized* to be given on time. Check insulin orders one or two times per shift. The orders change rapidly with the patient's response to treatment. Always know the patient's most recent blood glucose level.

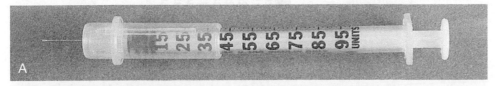

100 units per mL
(odd numbers)

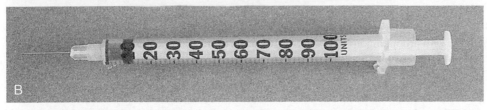

100 units per mL
(even numbers)

FIGURE 11-9 **A,** Insulin Safety-Lok syringe calibrated in 100 units per mL with odd number markings up to 95 units. **B,** Insulin syringe calibrated in 100 units per mL with even markings up to 100 units. (From Becton, Dickinson, and Company, Franklin Lakes, NJ.)

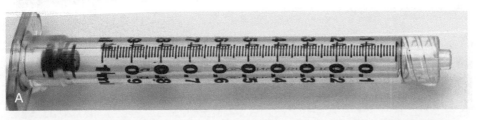

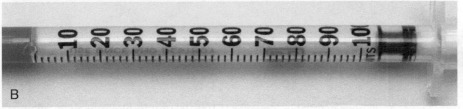

FIGURE 11-10 **A,** 1-mL tuberculin syringe calibrated in hundredths of a mL. **B,** 1-mL 100-units-per-mL insulin syringe calibrated in 2-unit increments.

Lo-Dose Syringes

Elderly people and patients with complications of diabetes often have diminished vision. Syringes are designed for individuals with special visual needs. They allow for better visualization of the smaller doses and are available in 30-unit, 50-unit, and 100-unit syringes (Figure 11-11).

➤ Syringes are calibrated in 1-unit increments.

➤ They are calibrated for U-100 insulin (100 units per mL).

Q & A	**ASK YOURSELF**	**1**	What is the difference between the calibration of units on the 1-mL insulin syringe and that on the Lo-Dose syringe?
	MY ANSWER		_____

Note the difference in visualization of 30 units of insulin drawn in each of the syringes in Figure 11-12.

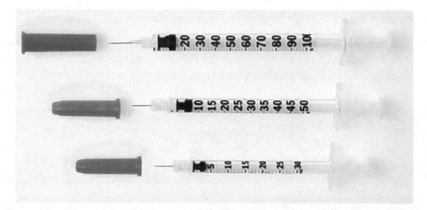

FIGURE 11-11 The syringe volume occupies 30, 50, or 100 units and can be used by patients who are taking up to 30, 50, or 100 units of insulin per dose. (From Becton, Dickinson, and Company, Franklin Lakes, NJ

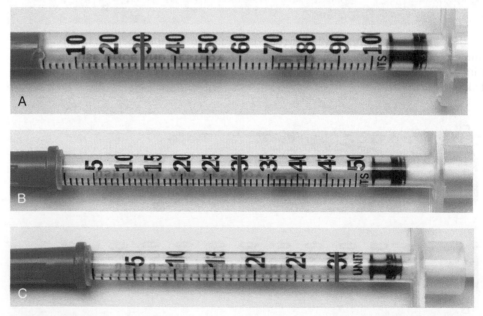

FIGURE 11-12 A, 30 units marked in a regular U-100 100-unit insulin syringe. **B,** 30 units marked in a U-100 50-unit Lo-Dose insulin syringe. C, 30 units drawn in a U-100 30-unit insulin syringe.

RAPID PRACTICE 11-4 | Reading Units on an Insulin Syringe

ESTIMATED COMPLETION TIME: 10 minutes   **ANSWERS ON:** page 430

DIRECTIONS: *Read the syringe dose measurement in units and write the number of units in the space supplied for problems 1 and 2. For problems 3 through 5, mark the syringe with the ordered number of units. All of the syringes are calibrated for U-100 insulin.*

1 **Ordered:** Humulin N insulin 28 units subcut AM and PM. Mark the dose ordered.

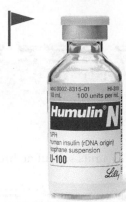

Copyright ©Eli Lilly and Company. All rights reserved. Used with permission.

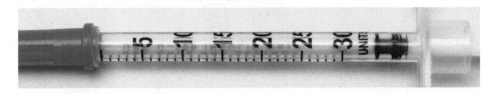

2 _____ units

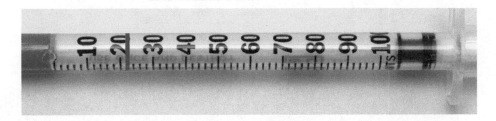

3 **Ordered:** insulin glargine 32 units subcut at bedtime daily. Mark the dose ordered.

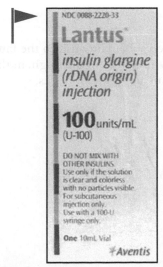

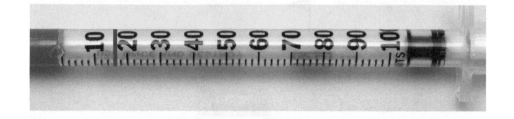

4 _____ units

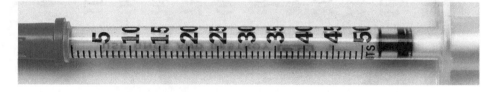

5 **Ordered:** Humulin R insulin 7 units subcut ac breakfast. Mark the dose ordered.

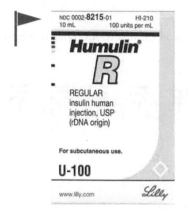

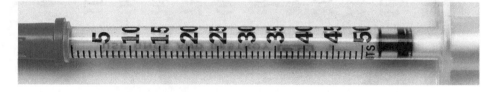

Sites for Insulin Injection

Insulin may be administered subcutaneously in the fatty tissue of the abdomen in a radius 2 *inches away from the umbilicus*, in the thigh, in the fatty tissue of the posterior upper arm, or in the fatty tissue of the buttocks.

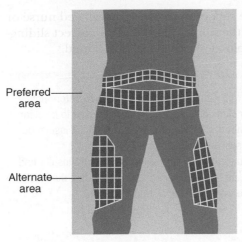
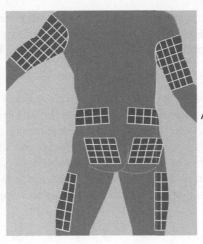

Preferred area

Alternate area

Alternate areas

★ *Communication*

"Which sites do you usually use for injection at home?"

➤ Use and rotate sites that the patient does not use at home (Figure 11-13). Document the site on the MAR.

FIGURE 11-13 Insulin injection areas. (Copyright ©Eli Lilly and Company. All rights reserved. Used with permission.)

Sliding-Scale Insulin

Sliding-scale short-acting insulins are titrated to *patients' current blood glucose* levels. They are usually ordered q6h for hospitalized patients on continuous liquid gastrointestinal tube feedings, or TPN.

They may also be ordered ac and bedtime to cover meal and bedtime glucose elevations for newly diagnosed patients until the patient can be stabilized on longer-acting insulins. The insulin dose "slides," or changes, with the most recent glucose levels. The scale is customized for each patient. Patterns of glucose elevations usually emerge.

Patients who experience difficult control of blood glucose levels may continue to cover elevated levels at mealtime on a sliding scale with bolus doses of short-acting insulin orders at home in addition to the longer-acting variety. The term *brittle diabetic* has been used to describe a patient who experiences poorly controlled blood glucose levels despite insulin therapy.

Examples of handheld glucose monitors for bedside and home finger stick draws of capillary blood are shown in Figure 11-14.

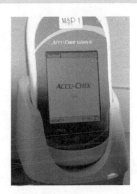

Accu-chek Informii does point-of-care testing and transfers the data to the electronic health record wirelessly.

CLINICAL RELEVANCE

- All diabetics should carry some sort of identification that states they are diabetic.
- Medic-Alert bracelets or necklaces are recommended. Traditionally these are etched with basic, key health information regarding diabetes, allergies, need for insulin, and so on. Newer versions include compact USB drives that can carry a person's full medical record for use in an emergency.
- Emergency medical personnel are trained to look for a medical identification when they are caring for people who can't speak for themselves.

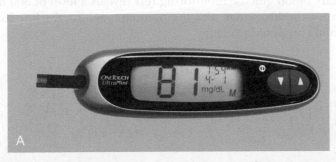
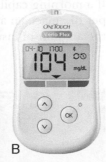

FIGURE 11-14 A, Life Scan One Touch® Ultra Mini®. **B,** LifeScan OneTouch Verio® meter. Handheld blood glucose monitors for finger or forearm stick with 50 test result memory. (**B,** ©LifeScan, Inc. (2017). Reproduced with permission.)

The patient may draw blood under the supervision of an experienced nurse or may self-monitor and report the result to the nurse (SMBG). The correct sliding-scale amount is drawn promptly after the blood glucose level is obtained.

CLINICAL RELEVANCE

Recheck a very low or high blood glucose level with a different monitoring device before acting on the reading. Examine the insulin bottle for discoloration if the product is supposed to be clear, and check it for particles. Ensure that a bottle that is supposed to be clear (regular, insulin detemir, or insulin glargine) is clear, not cloudy. Suspensions will be cloudy.

There have been some cases where hospitalized patients who self-administered insulin had unexplainable elevations of blood glucose and were finally observed to be discarding the insulin rather than taking it. Observe patients' technique when they are self-administering.

EXAMPLES

Examine the following sample sliding scale for a hospitalized patient.

Ordered: Humulin R subcut per sliding scale q6h, for a patient on TPN.

Sliding Scale for Subcutaneous Short-Acting Insulin Administration

Blood Sugar (mg per dL)	Insulin Amount
70–150	0 units
151–200	4 units
201–250	6 units
251–300	10 units
301–350	12 units (Recheck blood glucose level 1 hr after administration.)
351–400	15 units (Recheck blood glucose level 1 hr after administration.)
>400	Call physician and draw plasma blood glucose.

Monitor the results. The blood glucose level is checked by the nurse with the handheld device at the bedside unless a serum blood glucose lab test is ordered. This may be done to verify an abnormal blood glucose level.

➤ Note the *small amounts* of fast-acting insulin to be given.

➤ The trend is to replace sliding-scale insulin with customized bolus-basal, weight-based doses.

RAPID PRACTICE 11-5　Interpreting Sliding-Scale Orders

ESTIMATED COMPLETION TIME: 10 minutes　　　**ANSWERS ON:** page 430

DIRECTIONS: *Read the sliding scale in the example above and answer the questions with brief phrases.*

✷ **Communication**

"Mr. Y, your blood glucose level is 180. Your physician has ordered 2 units of Novalin R for this blood glucose level." Always keep your patient informed about blood glucose levels and type and dose of insulin. This is not only a teaching mechanism—it may prevent administration of a type or dose with which the patient has had an adverse event.

1　If a morning capillary blood glucose monitoring test reveals a level of 300 mg per dL, place an arrow on the syringe with the pointer touching the line for the amount of insulin you would prepare.

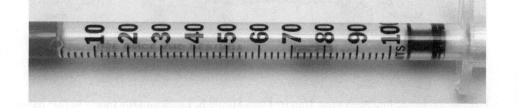

2 If the bedtime capillary blood glucose monitoring level was 330 mg per dL, what two actions would you take?*

_____

_____

3 What might be a reason that a plasma blood glucose test would be ordered from the laboratory instead of another capillary blood glucose test using the monitor at the bedside?

_____

4 If the sliding-scale blood glucose level was 140 mg per mL, what would the nurse do?

_____

_____

5 If a blood glucose monitoring test before dinner indicated a blood glucose level >400 mg per dL, what two actions would you take?

_____

_____

---

1 If the sliding scale was written 70–150, 150–200, 200–250, 250–300, 300–350, how much insulin would you give if the patient's blood glucose level was 150 mg per dL? With whom would you clarify this entire scale?

ASK YOURSELF

_____ MY ANSWER

➤ Separate flow sheets are usually maintained on the MAR for insulin administration. Table 11-2 provides examples of the information that may be contained on such a record.

_____

*➤ Take care if the abbreviation HS (bedtime) is encountered. It can be mistaken for half strength.

TABLE 11-2   Subcutaneous Insulin Administration Flow Sheet

GENERAL HOSPITAL						
John Doe #528995						
Date	Test Time	Test Result	Type of Test (BGM; SMBG; serum)	Insulin Type/Dose	Route/Location	Signature/ Title
1/1/22	0630	195	BGM	Novolog 4 units	subcut LA	Mark Smith, RN
1/1/22	1100	95	SMBG	0		Mark Smith, RN
1/1/22	1700	210	BGM	Novolog 5 units	subcut RA	Jan Carter, RN
1/1/22	2100	90	BGM	0		Jan Carter, RN
1/2/22	0630	200	Serum FBS	Novolog 4 units	subcut RT	Cal Pace, RN

BGM, Blood glucose monitor (capillary sample) performed by nurse; *LA*, left arm; *RA*, right arm; *RT*, right thigh; *Serum FBS*, fasting blood sugar (by lab or RN) (venous [serum] sample); *SMBG*, self-blood glucose monitoring (by patient) (capillary sample).

> **FAQ**   *Why is insulin not given for all blood glucose levels that are above normal?*
>
> **ANSWER**   Smaller elevations may not be treated with insulin to avoid hypoglycemic reactions. Dietary and lifestyle adjustments may be ordered to control lower elevations.

RAPID PRACTICE 11-6	Interpreting Insulin Orders

ESTIMATED COMPLETION TIME: 10 to 15 minutes   **ANSWERS ON:** page 431

DIRECTIONS: *Examine the answers given to problem 1. Read and interpret the insulin orders in problems 2 through 5. Refer to the vocabulary list and the insulin activity chart in Table 11-1 if needed. Mark the syringes with the dose ordered.*

1   Ordered: Humalog insulin lispro 6 units subcut tid 15 min ac for a patient with DM type 1.

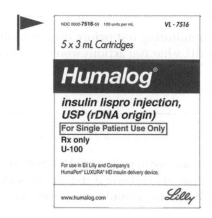

    a. What is the recommended time to administer this dose in the hospital? <u>With the arrival of the meals.</u>

    b. Why is this time recommended? <u>Because it is difficult to ensure the meal delivery within a 15-minute time frame.</u>

    c. What is the concentration of the product as shown on the label? <u>U-100, 100 units per mL.</u>

    d. Will the solution be clear or cloudy? <u>Clear.</u>

    e. Which of the following syringes is shaded to the correct amount? <u>Syringe number A.</u>

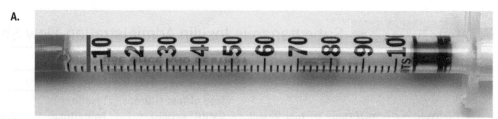

2 **Ordered:** Humulin N (NPH) 28 units subcut in AM daily for a patient with DM type 1.

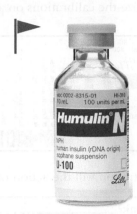

a. Is this a rapid- or intermediate-acting product? _____
b. Is it clear, or is it a suspension? _____
c. Does it need to be agitated before being withdrawn from the vial? _____
d. In how many hours will it peak? _____
e. By what route will it be administered? _____
f. Mark the syringe with the ordered dose.

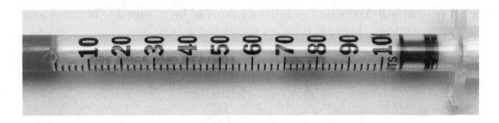

3 **Ordered:** Novolin N 42 units subcut AM daily for a patient with DM type 1 maintenance.

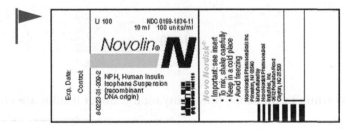

a. What route will be used to administer this order?
b. Mark the syringe with the ordered amount.

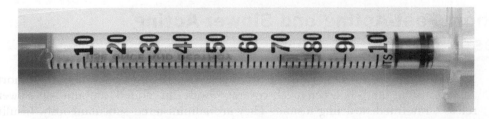

4 **Ordered:** Novolin R 10 units tid subcut ac, for a patient with a severe infection who has type 2 diabetes and poor vision. The nurse plans to assess the patient's ability to visualize the calibrations on a Lo-Dose syringe.

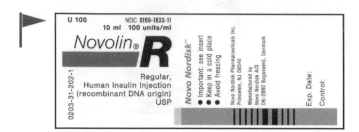

a. How long after administration will the action of this insulin action begin (onset)? _____

b. When will the action peak? _____

c. How long will it last? _____

d. Mark the syringe with the ordered dose.

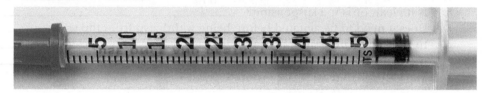

5 A patient with DM type 1 who has a history of high, unstable blood glucose levels is taking Humulin R before meals and at bedtime.

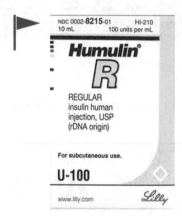

a. According to the label, how many total units of insulin are contained in the vial? _____

b. Is this a short- or intermediate-acting product? _____

c. What is the concentration? _____

Mixing Insulins: Short Fast-Acting and Slower-Acting Intermediate Mixes

Mixed insulins provide blood glucose coverage for meals with a small amount of short-acting insulin and between-meal coverage with an added amount of slower-release, intermediate-acting insulin. They are administered subcutaneously. Insulin mixes may be ordered twice a day for patients until their blood glucose pattern is established or to provide additional coverage for postprandial blood glucose elevations.

As with all insulins, initial orders for intermediate mixes are conservative to prevent hypoglycemic episodes. The trend is to prescribe one of the *fixed premixed* combinations available on the market.

Fixed premixed intermediate- and short-acting combination insulins

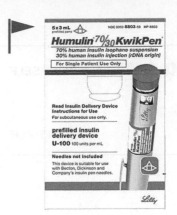

The *first* number of a fixed combination insulin mix indicates the *percentage* of slower-, *intermediate*-acting insulin. The second number indicates the *percentage* of short-, or *rapid*-acting insulin. The product label in Figure 11-15 illustrates this information.

▶ If the order is for *10* units, 7 units (70% of 10 units) would contain NPH, the intermediate-acting insulin, and 3 units (30% of 10 units) would contain the fast-acting insulin.

These mixes are offered as a safe and convenient method for patients who would have difficulty drawing up injectable mixtures in a syringe. The amounts are small, and an error of even 1 unit can make a difference. In addition to ease of preparation, the premixed combinations reduce chance of error and save time. Most patients receive a larger amount of intermediate-acting insulin and a smaller amount of short-, rapid-acting insulin. Some patients need a 50/50 mix because of very high mealtime blood glucose elevations.

A premix order specifies the number of units based on the patient's need for each type. For example:

Humalog Mix 50/50, 10 units subcut 30 min ac breakfast and dinner.

FIGURE 11-15 Humulin 70/30 insulin. (Copyright ©Eli Lilly and Company. All rights reserved. Used with permission.)

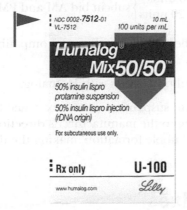

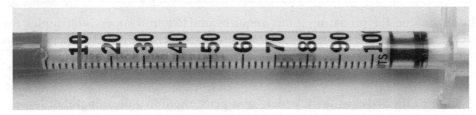

Novolin Mix 70/30, 18 units subcut 30 min ac breakfast and dinner.

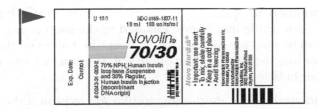

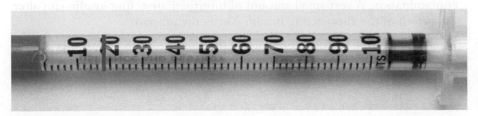

➤ Note that the order for a premixed insulin mix is in *total* number of units.

 Q & A **ASK YOURSELF** **1** If you were giving 8 units of Novolin 70/30 insulin, how many units would contain short-acting NPH insulin and how many units would contain fast-acting insulin?

MY ANSWER _____

➤ ISMP recommends that two nurses perform an independent check of drug and dose for all high-risk medications *before* administration.

When the Mix Must Be Prepared by the Nurse

Occasionally, the nurse must prepare an insulin mix, drawing up two different insulins in one syringe. Regular and intermediate-acting insulins are the most common combination. They are bracketed or designated "Mix" in the order:

Humulin R 6 units
Humulin N 20 units } subcut bid AM and PM 30 min ac

Read both product labels to be sure they are compatible. Not all insulin brands can be mixed with others.

➤ Do not confuse Humulin products with Humalog.

Similar to intermediate suspensions, the mixes need to be rolled adequately until well mixed, according to the manufacturer's directions. Too vigorous shaking will result in extensive air bubble formation, making the dose inaccurate. The dose is less than 1 mL.

Technique for Preparing Insulin Mixes

The technique for preparing a mix requires practice and supervision under the direction of an instructor or experienced nurse. (See Figure 8-6 and Chapter 8 for technique of mixing medications from two vials.)

1 Check the order and compatibility of the two types of insulin.

2 Identify the vials, verify the orders, and place them in a meaningful order in front of you. Roll the intermediate suspension. Clean the tops of each vial with an alcohol swab.

3 Measure and insert air *equal* to the amount of ordered insulin into each vial, the intermediate-acting insulin *first*, followed by the short-acting insulin, with the syringe to be used for administration. Keep the bottles on the counter to insert the air into the air at the top of the vial. Inserting air into the liquid will create air bubbles.

➤ 4 Always withdraw the clear, short-acting insulin *first* to protect the vial from contamination. A very small amount of intermediate-acting insulin can alter the action of the short-acting insulin. Verify the amount.

5 After withdrawing the ordered amount of regular insulin, gently mix the suspension according to label directions and withdraw exactly the amount ordered. Gently tap out any air bubbles and verify the precise combined

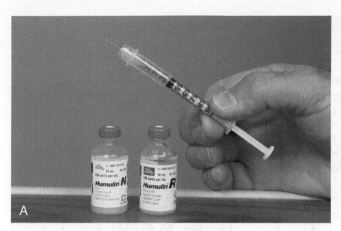
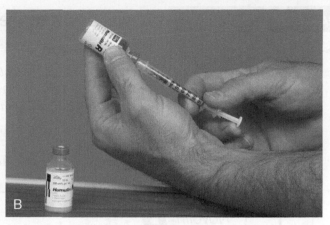

FIGURE 11-16 **A,** Vials of intermediate- and rapid- or short-acting insulin and syringe with air injected into vial. **B,** Withdrawal of regular insulin. Always withdraw the regular insulin first after the vials have been prepared. (From Perry AG, Potter PA, Ostendorf WR: *Clinical nursing skills and techniques,* ed. 9, St. Louis, 2018, Mosby.)

amount. If the total amount is incorrect, discard the syringe and start over. One extra unit is one unit too much.

➤ Protect the short-acting insulin vials from contamination by withdrawing from them first. Do not allow distractions during this procedure (Figure 11-16).

In addition to verifying labels, it may be helpful to remember the sequence with the following table, keeping in mind that *cloudy* refers to intermediate suspension preparations and *clear* refers to short-acting preparations:

Step 1	Step 2	Step 3	Step 4
Air in Cloudy	Air in Clear	Withdraw short-acting Clear	Withdraw intermediate-acting Cloudy

This sequence permits the nurse to proceed from step 2 to step 3 with the short-acting preparation without removing the needle from the vial.

The following is an example of a mixture of 24 units of Humulin N plus 6 units of Humulin R, for a total dose of 30 units.

> ✳ *Mnemonic*
>
> **Clear before Cloudy.**
> The weather is clear, and then it becomes cloudy. Draw up clear insulin first, then cloudy insulin.

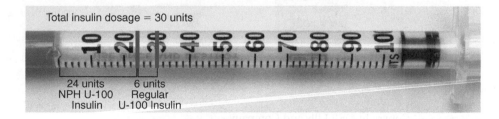

Total insulin dosage = 30 units

24 units NPH U-100 Insulin   6 units Regular U-100 Insulin

FAQ   *How can I remember which insulin products can be mixed and which cannot?*

ANSWER ➤ Always read the product label and inserts. Consult the pharmacy if necessary. Do not rely solely on the prescriber's order. In general, remember that a mix consists of a short-acting and an intermediate-acting insulin of the same brand, and that the long-acting insulin glargine and insulin detemir cannot be mixed with any other insulin.

RAPID PRACTICE 11-7 | Short- and Intermediate-Acting Insulin Mixes

ESTIMATED COMPLETION TIME: 15 minutes   **ANSWERS ON:** page 431

DIRECTIONS: *Read the explanation of short-acting and intermediate-acting insulin mixes. Examine the answers provided for problem 1 and complete problems 2 through 5 in a similar manner.*

1 **Ordered:** Novolin R 6 units and Novolin N 20 units subcut bid AM and PM. Mark the syringe with the total amount. Place an arrow touching the intermediate-acting dose calibration.

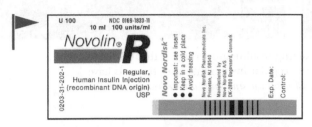 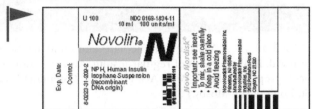

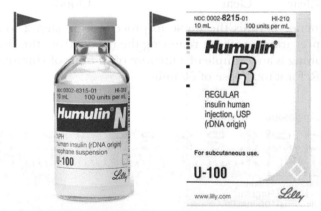

2 **Ordered:** Humulin N 30 units and Humulin R 4 units subcut bid AM and PM. Mark the syringe with the total amount. Place an arrow touching the intermediate-acting dose calibration.

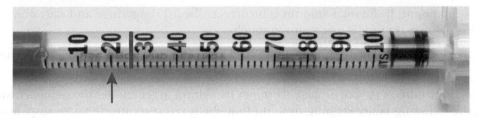

Copyright ©Eli Lilly and Company.
All rights reserved. Used with permission.

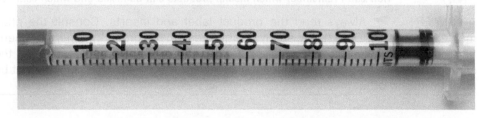

3   **Ordered:** Humulin R 8 units and Humulin N 24 units subcut 30 min ac breakfast and dinner. Mark the syringe with the total amount. Place an arrow touching the intermediate-acting dose calibration.

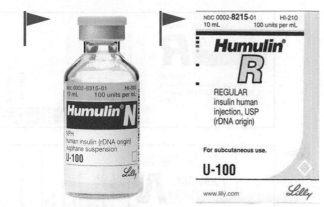

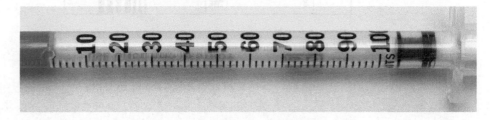

4   **Ordered:** Novolin R 2 units and Novolin N 16 units subcut AM and PM. Mark the syringe with the total amount. Place an arrow touching the intermediate-acting dose calibration.

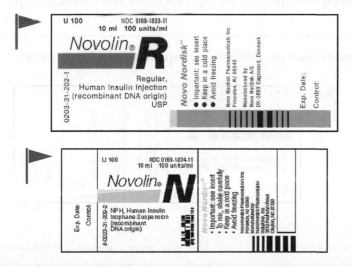

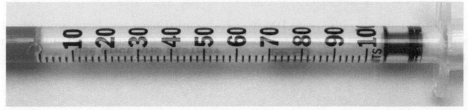

5 **Ordered:** Novolin R 10 units and Novolin N 42 units subcut 30 min ac breakfast and dinner. Mark the syringe with the total amount. Place an arrow touching the intermediate-acting dose calibration.

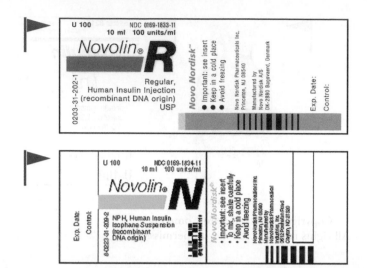

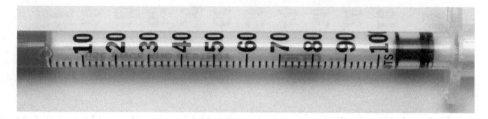

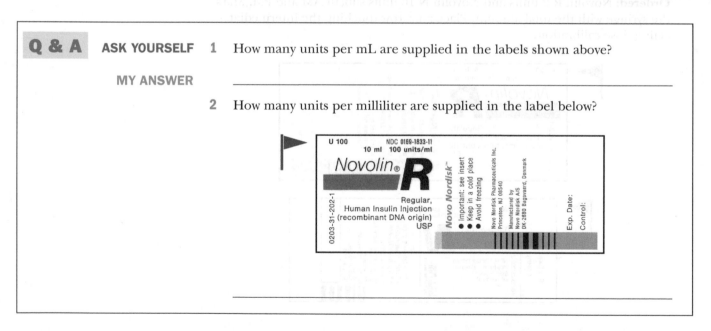

<table>
<tr><td>**Q & A**</td><td>**ASK YOURSELF**</td><td>1</td><td>How many units per mL are supplied in the labels shown above?</td></tr>
<tr><td></td><td>**MY ANSWER**</td><td></td><td>_____</td></tr>
</table>

2 How many units per milliliter are supplied in the label below?

A few patients with severe DM type 1 who must have very large amounts of insulin, over 100 units per dose, may be prescribed U-500 insulin (500 units per mL) to reduce the volume of the injections and reduce the number of the injection sites. This is not a common order and is usually administered only in the hospital.

Intravenous Insulin Infusions

➤ Insulin infusions are administered in the hospital for acute hyperglycemia. Many agencies publish their own standard for the concentration of an insulin infusion, either 1 unit per mL or 0.5 unit per mL, in 0.9% NaCl solution. These infusions are either factory pre-mixed or mixed in the pharmacy by the pharmacist.

➤ On the rare occasion a nurse would mix this IV solution he or she should use a fresh, unopened bottle of Regular or Humalog insulin, whichever is ordered, to prepare the infusion.

➤ A label with the number of units and concentration needs to be attached to the IV solution, as with all other medicated IV solutions. Insulin should be administered on its own separate line.

When the concentration is 100 units in 100 mL of 0.9% NaCl (1 unit per mL) or 50 units in 100 mL of 0.9% NaCl (0.5 unit per mL), it is *very helpful* to estimate the flow rate in milliliters per hour using mental arithmetic. Remember that the flow rate cannot be calculated until the concentration of the solution in units per milliliter is known. Verify the estimate with a DA equation.

EXAMPLES

Infuse	Concentration	Flow Rate
0.5 unit per hr	100 units per 100 mL, or 1 unit per 1 mL	0.5 mL per hr
3 units per hr	100 units per 100 mL, or 1 unit per 1 mL	3 mL per hr
1 unit per hr	50 units per 100 mL, or 0.5 unit per 1 mL	2 mL per hr
3 units per hr	50 units per 100 mL, or 0.5 unit per 1 mL	6 mL per hr

The flow rates are very low, and with a 1:1 (1 unit to 1 mL, or 100 units to 100 mL) concentration, the number of units ordered per hour is equal to the mL per hr flow rate.

➤ Use an IV pump for IV insulin administration.

EXAMPLES

Ordered: Humulin R IV infusion 5 units per hr, recheck BG 1 hr and call office.

$$\frac{mL}{hr} = \frac{\cancel{100}\ mL}{\cancel{100\ units}} \times \frac{5\ \cancel{units}}{1\ hr} = 5\ mL\ per\ hr$$

CLINICAL RELEVANCE

➤ Check orders frequently for changes. Changes are common in acute-care situations.

Monitor blood glucose levels at least every hour or more often, according to agency protocol.

Report low and high blood glucose levels and unusual changes promptly. Follow the prescriber's and agency's directions for treatment. Document the instructions. Know where a 50% dextrose injection and/or a glucagon injection is available for hypoglycemic emergencies (Figure 11-17).

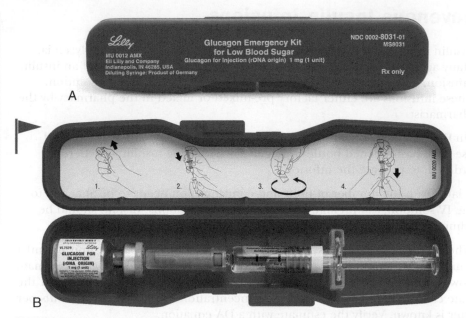

FIGURE 11-17 A, Glucagon emergency kit. **B,** Dextrose 50%. (**A,** Copyright ©Eli Lilly and Company. All rights reserved. Used with permission.)

RAPID PRACTICE 11-8 | **IV Infusions**

ESTIMATED COMPLETION TIME: 20 minutes   **ANSWERS ON:** page 431

DIRECTIONS: *Study the examples. Calculate the flow rate. Label answers.*

1 **Ordered:** IV at 4 units per hr, for a patient with a glucose level of 325 mg per dL. Available: 50 units Novolin R insulin in 100 mL 0.9% NaCl solution.

    a. Estimated flow rate in mL per hr? _____

    b. Ordered flow rate in mL per hr? _____

    DA equation:

    c. Evaluation: _____

2 **Ordered:** Humulin R insulin IV at 3 units per hr. Available: Humulin R insulin 100 units in 100-mL 0.9% NaCl solution.

    a. Estimated flow rate in mL per hr? _____

    b. Ordered flow rate in mL per hr? _____

    DA equation:

    c. Evaluation: _____

3 **Ordered:** to wean the patient (refer to example in problem 3) and reduce the flow rate by 50% because the blood glucose level has dropped to 185 mg per dL.

  a. Estimated flow rate in mL per hr? _____

  b. Ordered flow rate in mL per hr? _____

  DA equation:

  c. Evaluation: _____

4 **Ordered:** Novolin R insulin IV at 2 units per hr. Infusing: IV of D5W 100 mL with 50 units Novolin II R insulin added. It is flowing at 2 mL per hr.

  a. Estimated flow rate ordered: _____

  b. Ordered flow rate in mL per hr? _____

  DA equation:

  c. Evaluation: _____

  d. What nursing actions, if any, should be taken? _____

5 **Ordered:** Humulin R insulin IV at 6 units per hr, for a patient with a glucose level of 400 mg per dL. Draw a plasma glucose test stat to verify the capillary monitor level and recheck in 1 hour. Available: 50 units Humulin R insulin in 100 mL 0.9% NaCl solution.

  a. Estimated flow rate in mL per hr? _____

  b. Ordered flow rate in mL per hr? _____

  DA equation:

  c. Evaluation: _____

RAPID PRACTICE 11-9 Insulin Differences

ESTIMATED COMPLETION TIME: 10 to 15 minutes   **ANSWERS ON:** page 432

DIRECTIONS: *Answer the questions pertaining to the differences among the insulin solutions available.*

1 **a.** What are the two concentrations of insulin supplied? _____

  b. Of the two, which one is more commonly used? _____

2 **a.** Which are the only types of insulin that may be given intravenously?

  _____

  b. Are they clear or cloudy in the bottle? _____

3 Which two types of insulin within the same brand are most frequently given in mixed combination: short-, intermediate-, or long-acting? _____

4 **a.** When short- and intermediate-acting insulin are combined, which of the two is usually given in the larger dose? _____

  b. Why do you think this is so? _____

Insulin Administration Devices

New products on the market are developed to make insulin administration more convenient, easier, and less painful.

Prefilled pens

Prefilled insulin pens contain regular insulin, intermediate-acting insulin, and mixtures of the two for ease of use by patients who have difficulty manipulating syringe equipment. They are also used for patients with poor vision. The dose can be dialed easily. Pens are less noticeable than are syringes for injection in public places (Figure 11-18).

These devices require needles that are separate from the pen itself to administer the insulin.

CLINICAL RELEVANCE

Teaching patients how to manage diabetes is a challenge. Consider all the content in this chapter, which is limited to medication administration only. The patient with diabetes has a great deal more to learn about the disease than just medication administration. The patient usually is not a health-care professional. It is helpful to plan the teaching around the reason for hospitalization: Is this a newly diagnosed patient, or did illness, travel, or noncompliance with the medication regimen cause the hospitalization in a person who has had diabetes for a long time? What is the patient's assessment of the reason for hospitalization?

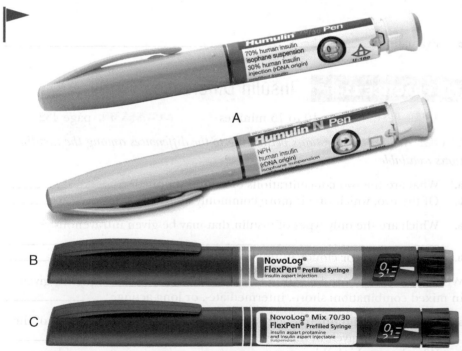

FIGURE 11-18 Prefilled pens are convenient for work and travel. They are also used for patients with poor vision. **A,** Humulin® 70/30 and Humulin® N insulin pens. **B,** NovoLog® FlexPen®. **C,** NovoLog® Mix 70/30 FlexPen®. (**A,** Copyright ©Eli Lilly and Company. All rights reserved. Used with permission. **B, C,** From Novo Nordisk, Inc., Princeton, NJ.)

Insulin pumps and continuous glucose monitoring (CGM)

Insulin pumps are devices worn by patients who need more frequent administration to maintain control of glucose levels. Two types are available: implantable and portable. A programmed, continuous, subcutaneous dose of rapid- or short-acting insulin is delivered through a subcutaneous access site throughout the day and night. Pumps deliver a continuous infusion of insulin throughout the day. Boluses of rapid- or short-acting insulins can be administered as needed such as at mealtimes.

➤ Only rapid- or short-acting insulins are used in insulin pumps. Frequent blood glucose monitoring is recommended for these patients to normalize their glucose levels.

➤ A continuous glucose monitoring device is now available. It allows rapid dosage adjustments for better glucose control. It is placed with a subcutaneous probe, and it periodically evaluates the blood glucose level. Glucose results are sent to a "smart phone" such as an iPhone or a device such as an Apple watch, and the results can also be sent to the devices of family members or caregivers. Some glucose monitors "talk" to the insulin pump and can trigger a bolus dose to be released if the glucose level is elevated.

> ✴ **Communication**
>
> "What brought you to the hospital?" "Has this happened before?" "What has been the most difficult part of this disease for you?" "What parts of the diet are difficult?" Be prepared to listen to the patient's answers to these questions. Then, assess the teaching needs and formulate a prioritized practical teaching plan that takes into account what the patient already knows and urgently needs to know.

CHAPTER 11 MULTIPLE-CHOICE REVIEW

ESTIMATED COMPLETION TIME: 30 minutes   **ANSWERS ON:** page 432

DIRECTIONS: *Select the best answer for the following questions.*

1 Which word best describes the major effect of insulin overdose? _____
   a. Hypotension   c. Hypoglycemia
   b. Hyperglycemia   d. Polyuria

2 Which types of insulin should be clear? _____
   a. Regular, insulin glargine, and insulin detemir
   b. Humulin N
   c. All insulin preparations
   d. Novolin N

3 What expectation is reasonable for nurses to have about most prescribed doses of rapid-acting insulin? _____
   a. They are usually high doses.
   b. They are usually low doses.
   c. They are always combined with intermediate-acting insulins.
   d. They contain additives to extend their action.

4 At which level of blood glucose may a patient be likely to experience symptoms of hypoglycemia? _____
   a. >400 mg per dL   c. 100 mg per dL
   b. 100-200 mg per dL   d. <70 mg per dL

5 Which explanation reflects the most likely serious and unwelcome result of reversing the dosage for an order for 6 units of regular insulin and 30 units of NPH? _____
   a. Early onset of hypoglycemic episode
   b. Late onset of hypoglycemic episode
   c. Early onset of hyperglycemic episode
   d. Late onset of hyperglycemic episode

6 How may a nurse's action be *most likely* to cause a hypoglycemic episode for a patient? _____

   a. Administer too low a dose of insulin for a patient of a particular weight.

   b. Give a dextrose-containing beverage to a patient.

   c. Administer a dose of regular or rapid-acting insulin that is not followed by a meal.

   d. Set up an insulin pump for a patient with the prescribed basal dose.

7 Which insulin schedule requires a bedtime snack? _____

   a. Regular insulin in the morning and before lunch

   b. Short-acting insulin before lunch

   c. Intermediate-, long-acting, and any evening insulins

   d. Insulin lispro before lunch

8 What does a prepared insulin mix such as Humulin N 70/30 contain? _____

   a. Lower doses than if each insulin was administered separately

   b. 70% rapid-acting insulin and 30% intermediate-acting insulin

   c. 100% Humulin N

   d. 70% intermediate-acting insulin and 30% rapid-acting insulin

9 Which route is most commonly prescribed for administering insulin? _____

   a. Intradermal   **c.** Intramuscular

   b. Subcutaneous   **d.** Intravenous

10 Which insulin must never be mixed with any other? _____

   a. Humulin N   **c.** Novolin R

   b. Humalog   **d.** Lantus

CHAPTER 11   FINAL PRACTICE

ESTIMATED COMPLETION TIME: 1 to $1\frac{1}{2}$ hours   **ANSWERS ON:** page 432

DIRECTIONS: *Answer the following questions using DA equations to verify doses and flow rates. Use a calculator for long division and multiplication. Label answers.*

1 **Ordered:** insulin lispro 12 units tid 10 min before meals.

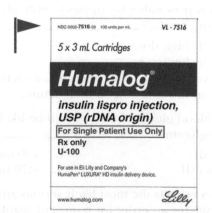

   a. Is this a rapid-, short-, intermediate-, or long-acting insulin?

_____

b. Place an arrow touching the calibration for the amount of the insulin.

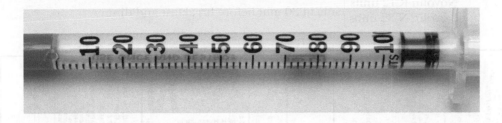

2 Ordered:

Humulin R 20 units ⎫
Humulin N 44 units ⎭ subcut 30 min before breakfast and dinner.

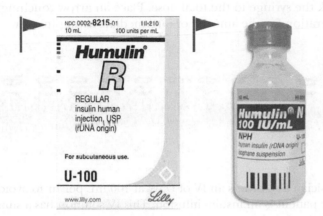

a. Which insulin will you withdraw first? _____

b. Mark the syringe to the total dose. Place an arrow touching the calibration for the amount of intermediate-acting insulin.

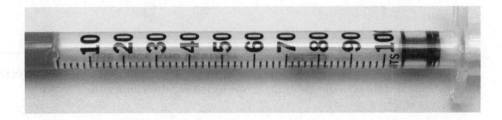

3 The patient referred to in problem 2 has a blood glucose level of 325 mg per dL. Refer to problem 8 flow rate sliding scale.

a. Using the sliding scale given in Problem 8, what flow rate in milliliters per hr will be administered? _____

b. Use a DA equation to back up mental arithmetic flow rate estimate. _____

DA equation:

c. Evaluation: _____

4 Ordered:

Novolin R 12 units ⎫
Novolin N 32 units ⎬ subcut 30 min before breakfast and dinner.

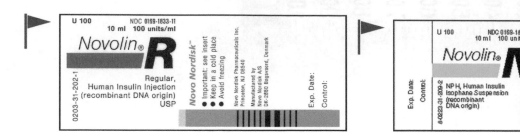

a. Which insulin will you withdraw first? _____

b. Mark the syringe to the total dose. Place an arrow touching the calibration for the amount of intermediate-acting insulin.

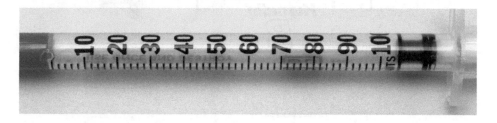

5 The physician also orders an IV of D5W at 100 mL per hr to avoid hypoglycemia while the patient is on insulin infusion. This IV solution has a small amount of glucose in it.

a. How many grams of glucose are contained in a 1000-mL container of D5W?

DA equation:

b. Evaluation: _____

6 Ordered: Novolin N 42 units subcut AM and PM, 30 min before meals. Select the appropriate syringe. Draw an arrow touching the calibration for the correct dose.

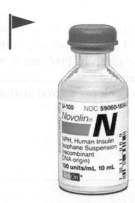

(From Norvo Nordisk, Inc., Princeton, NJ.)

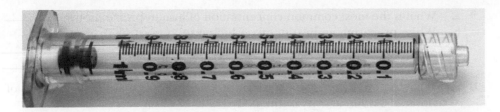

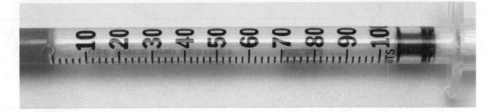

7 The next blood glucose level obtained for the patient in problem 2 is 210 mg per dL. The order calls for decreasing the flow rate by 50%.

   a. Using the sliding scale below, estimate the rate the nurse will set on the pump and verify with a DA equation. _____

Blood Glucose Level (mg per dL)	Infusion Rate (units per hr)
151–200	1
201–250	2
251–300	3
301–400	4
>400	5

   DA equation:

   b. Evaluation: _____

Problems 8 through 10 refer to the patient in problem 2.

8 **Ordered:** Humulin Regular insulin IV infusion in 0.9% NaCl to start at rate of 5 units per hr, for a patient with a blood level glucose >400 mg per dL. Available: Humulin Regular 100 units per 100 mL of 0.9% NaCl solution. Obtain blood glucose monitor test results every hour. Discontinue any other insulin orders.

   a. How many units per mL are contained in the available solution?

   _____

   b. Estimate the flow rate with mental arithmetic and verify with a DA equation. _____

   DA equation:

   c. Evaluation: _____
   d. Should the infusion be administered on an electronic infusion pump?

   _____

9 **a.** What is the most common concentration of insulin preparations? _____

   b. When preparing an insulin mix, which insulin must be protected and withdrawn first from the vial? _____

   c. Why? _____

10 **a.** What are the three major types of exogenous insulin available in terms of onset of insulin activity in the body?

   _____

   b. What type of nutrient will the nurse promptly administer if the patient is conscious, is symptomatic, and can swallow and the blood glucose level falls below 70 mg per dL?

   _____

CHAPTER 11 ANSWER KEY

RAPID PRACTICE 11-1 (p. 399)

1 Diet products do not contain dextrose.
2 **a.** 100 units per mL
   b. 1000 units (100 units × 10 mL)
3 Dextrose (glucose)
4 Humalog (insulin lispro), NovoLog (insulin aspart)
5 **a.** Novolin R; **c.** Humulin R

RAPID PRACTICE 11-2 (p. 401)

1 Cloudy
2 Two injections per day, one AM and one PM.
3 No
4 There is potential for overlapping duration. They are trying to avoid a hypoglycemic episode during sleep.
5 100 units per mL

RAPID PRACTICE 11-3 (p. 402)

1 No
2 100 units per mL
3 They have relatively flat action. They do not have a peak.
4 No. They contain additives.
5 Insulin glargine

RAPID PRACTICE 11-4 (p. 407)

1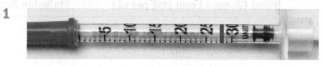

2 22 units
3

4 16 units
5

RAPID PRACTICE 11-5 (p. 410)

1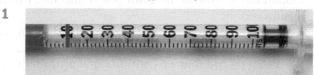

2 Give 12 units Humulin R subcut. Recheck BG in 1 hr.
3 To verify the accuracy of the finger stick blood glucose before instituting more aggressive treatment.
4 Hold insulin (0 units).
5 Call physician immediately. Draw plasma BG.

RAPID PRACTICE 11-6 (p. 412)

2 **a.** intermediate
b. suspension
c. Yes. Some manufacturers recommend *gentle shaking*. Others recommend *rolling the vial*. Read the directions on the product.
d. 6 to 12 hr
e. subcutaneously
f.

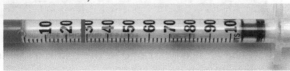

3 **a.** subcutaneous
b.

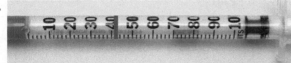

4 **a.** 30 min
b. $2\frac{1}{2}$ to 5 hr
c. 8 hr
d.

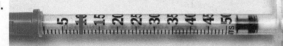

5 **a.** 1000 units
b. rapid
c. 100 units per mL

RAPID PRACTICE 11-7 (p. 418)

2

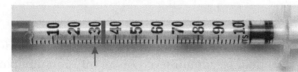

3

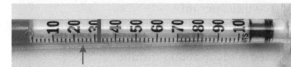

4

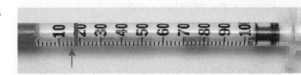

5

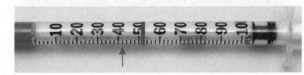

➤ Assess patient mental status, vision, and hand-eye coordination if self-administration will be needed at home.

RAPID PRACTICE 11-8 (p. 422)

1 **a.** 8 mL per hr, because concentration is 1 unit : 2 mL.
b. 8 mL per hr

$$\frac{mL}{hr} = \frac{\overset{2}{\cancel{100}\ mL}}{\underset{1}{\cancel{50}\ \cancel{units}}} \times \frac{4\ \cancel{units}}{1\ hr} = \frac{8\ mL}{hr}$$

c. Equation is balanced. Estimate equals answer.

2 **a.** 3 mL per hr, because concentration is 1 : 1.
b. 3 mL per hr

$$\frac{mL}{hr} = \frac{\overset{1}{\cancel{100}\ mL}}{\underset{1}{\cancel{100}\ \cancel{units}}} \times \frac{3\ \cancel{units}}{1\ hr} = \frac{3\ mL}{hr}$$

c. Equation is balanced. Estimate equals answer.
Note: A "U" for units can be misread as a zero (0).

3 **a.** 6 mL per hr (half of original order)
b. 6 mL per hr

$$\frac{mL}{hr} = \frac{\overset{2}{\cancel{100}\ mL}}{\underset{1}{\cancel{50}\ \cancel{units}}} \times \frac{3\ \cancel{units}}{hr} = \frac{6\ mL}{hr}$$

c. 6 mL per hr is 50% of original 12 mL ordered. Estimate supports answer.

4 **a.** 4 mL per hr, because concentration is 1 unit : 2 mL.
b. 4 mL per hr

$$\frac{mL}{hr} = \frac{\overset{2}{\cancel{100}\ mL}}{\underset{1}{\cancel{50}\ \cancel{units}}} \times \frac{2\ \cancel{units}}{1\ hr}$$

$$= \frac{4\ mL}{hr}\ \text{ordered flow rate}$$

c. Flow rate is incorrect. It is half the ordered rate.
d. Assess current blood glucose level. Consult with prescriber for flow rate order changes. Document. Check agency policy about an incident report.

5 **a.** 12 mL per hr, because concentration is 1 : 2.
b. 12 mL per hr

$$\frac{mL}{hr} = \frac{\overset{2}{\cancel{100}\ mL}}{\underset{1}{\cancel{50}\ \cancel{units}}} \times \frac{6\ \cancel{units}}{1\ hr} = \frac{12\ mL}{hr}$$

c. Evaluation: Equation is balanced. Estimate equals answer.

RAPID PRACTICE 11-9 (p. 423)

1 **a.** 100 units per mL and 500 units per mL
  b. U-100 is the most commonly used.
2 **a.** Regular insulins: insulin aspart (Novolog) and insulin glulisine (Apidra)
  b. clear
3 short- and intermediate-acting
4 **a.** The intermediate-acting insulin is usually the larger dose.
  b. It is a modified product to cover a longer duration.

CHAPTER 11 MULTIPLE-CHOICE REVIEW (p. 425)

1 c
2 a
3 b
4 d
5 a
6 c
7 c
  Note: This helps prevent hypoglycemic episodes during sleep.
8 d
9 b
10 d
  Note: If a short-acting insulin is needed, it can be given separately.

CHAPTER 11 FINAL PRACTICE (p. 426)

1 **a.** Insulin lispro is rapid acting.
  b.

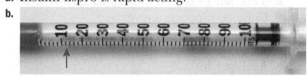

2 **a.** Humulin R insulin to prevent the regular insulin from contamination by the product.
  b.

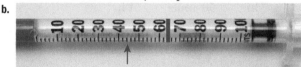

The nurse must focus to avoid confusing the doses.

3 **a.** 4 mL per hr to deliver $\dfrac{4 \text{ units}}{\text{hr}}$

  b. $\dfrac{\text{mL}}{\text{hr}} = \dfrac{\overset{1}{\cancel{100}} \text{ mL}}{\cancel{100} \text{ units}} \times \dfrac{4 \cancel{\text{ units}}}{1 \text{ hr}} = \dfrac{4 \text{ mL}}{\text{hr}}$

  c. Estimate equals answer.
4 **a.** Novolin R
  b.

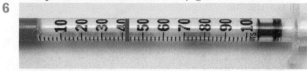

5 **a.** 50 g

$$g \text{ glucose} = \dfrac{5 \text{ g}}{\dfrac{\cancel{100} \text{ mL}}{1}} \times \dfrac{\overset{10}{\cancel{1000} \text{ mL}}}{1} = 50 \text{ g glucose}$$

  b. Equation is balanced. Only grams remain.
6

(The choice of syringe in the text is a 100-unit insulin syringe.)

7 **a.** $\dfrac{1}{2}$ of 4 mL per hr = 2 mL per hr

  50% = 0.5 or $\dfrac{1}{2}$

  $\dfrac{\text{mL}}{\text{hr}} = \dfrac{\overset{2}{\cancel{4}} \text{ mL}}{\text{hr}} \times \dfrac{1}{\underset{1}{\cancel{2}}} = \dfrac{2 \text{ mL}}{\text{hr}}$

  b. Estimate equals answer.
8 **a.** 1 unit per mL

  $\dfrac{\text{units}}{\text{mL}} = \dfrac{\overset{1}{\cancel{100}} \text{ units}}{\underset{1}{\cancel{100}} \text{ mL}} = \dfrac{1 \text{ unit}}{\text{mL}}$

  b. 5 mL per hr of a 1:1 solution (for 5 units per hr)

  $\dfrac{\text{mL}}{\text{hr}} = \dfrac{\overset{1}{\cancel{100}} \text{ mL}}{\underset{1}{\cancel{100} \text{ units}}} \times \dfrac{5 \cancel{\text{ units}}}{\text{hr}} = \dfrac{5 \text{ mL}}{\text{hr}}$

  c. Estimate equals answer.
  d. Yes. Insulin solutions for IV administration should be administered on an infusion pump on a separate line.
9 **a.** 100 units per mL
  b. Regular insulin must be withdrawn first to protect it from contamination from an intermediate-acting insulin.
  c. Contamination would alter (lengthen) the action of the regular insulin.
10 **a.** Short-, intermediate-, and long-acting commercial preparations
  Note: Endogenous insulin refers to insulin produced by the individual's own beta cells. Exogenous and endogenous insulin can be differentiated by a C peptide assay test.
  b. Glucose, followed by a complex carbohydrate

Suggestions for Further Reading

http://www.cdc.gov/diabetes
http://diabetes.niddk.nih.gov
http://www.bd.com/us/diabetes

⊖volve   For additional practice problems, refer to the Dosages Measured in Units section of the Elsevier's Interactive Drug Calculation Application, Version 1 on Evolve.

Chapter 12 focuses on anticoagulants, high-alert drugs that are also delivered in units. Many of the principles learned in this chapter can be applied to Chapter 12.

12 ⚑ Anticoagulant Medications

OBJECTIVES

- Differentiate oral and parenteral anticoagulants and their related tests.
- Calculate doses for oral and parenteral anticoagulants.
- Evaluate and titrate anticoagulant doses based upon relevant laboratory tests.
- Identify antidotes for anticoagulant therapy.
- Identify critical patient safety issues related to anticoagulant therapy.

ESTIMATED TIME TO COMPLETE CHAPTER: 2 hours

All anticoagulant products are high-alert medications. The nurse must understand the underlying theory of action of the medications, the differences, the antidotes, related pathophysiologic conditions, and relevant clinical assessments including interpretation of laboratory results.

There have been many preventable adverse drug events (ADEs)/sentinel events with anticoagulants. Because of variations in patients' dose response, the dose must be carefully titrated based on results of frequent patient-based laboratory testing. The goal is to extend clotting time sufficiently to prevent adverse clotting events. Normal clotting time poses a risk of thromboembolic events for a variety of conditions.

Anticoagulants are prescribed for many conditions, including:
- Prolonged immobility
- Preoperative, intraoperative, and postoperative surgery
- Potential, intra-, and post-cardiac events, such as arrhythmias (particularly atrial fibrillation), and myocardial infarction
- History of thromboembolic conditions, such as deep vein thromboses (DVTs), pulmonary emboli, and stroke
- Maintenance of patency of selected IV lines
- History of cardiac valve replacement

Nurses are expected to administer oral, subcutaneous, and IV anticoagulants.

VOCABULARY

Deep Vein Thrombus (DVT)	Blood clot usually located in the deeper veins of leg or pelvis. Has potential to travel.
Embolus	Blood clot that travels from its original location, usually a pelvic or leg vein. May block circulation in another vessel, such as a pulmonary artery (PE).
Petechiae	Pinpoint-sized hemorrhages seen on skin and mucous membranes, indicative of a bleeding disorder.
Pulmonary Embolus (PE)	Blood clot (often a DVT) that has traveled through the circulation and blocked an artery of the lung.
Thrombocytopenia	Decreased platelet count. Contraindication for heparin therapy.
Thrombus	Blood clot that forms in a blood vessel, usually a vein.

1 What is the difference between DVT and PE?

ASK YOURSELF **Q & A**

MY ANSWER

MEDICATIONS

Anticoagulants	Drugs that interfere with specific clotting factors, thus prolonging the coagulation time. They are used for patients with potential or current heart, lung, and vessel disease. They do *not* dissolve established clots, nor do they "thin" blood, although they are commonly referred to as blood thinners.
Clotting Factors	Proteins and enzymes in the blood that are essential for coagulation. ➤ Tests are performed to identify specific factor deficiencies as well as to monitor anticoagulant therapy.
Dabigatran (Pradaxa)	An oral anticoagulant that does not require frequent monitoring of the blood. No antidote available if effects need to be reversed.
Flush Solutions (Heplock Flush)	Heplock Flush: Low-dose heparin (10 to 100 units per mL) used to maintain patency of indwelling IV devices. Up to 500 units per mL may be ordered for central lines used for dialysis. Saline Flush: Used to maintain patency of some indwelling IV devices. Trend has been to replace the heparin flush with the less dangerous saline flush when it will do the job.
Fundaparinux sodium (Arixtra)	A Factor Xa inhibitor given subcutaneously once daily for DVT prophylaxis or PE treatment. Not interchangeable with heparin.
Low-Molecular-Weight Heparin (LMWH) **Dalteparin (Fragmin)** **Enoxaparin (Lovenox)**	Altered (fractionated) heparin with lower risk of thrombocytopenia than unfractionated heparins, thus lower risk of bleeding. Dose based on patient's *weight*. It is given by subcutaneous or IV route. Does *not* need to be monitored frequently, as with unfractionated heparin, which requires frequent monitoring with the activated partial thromboplastin time test. Can be administered at home with selected patients. Used for prevention of thromboemboli for high-risk patients, including orthopedic surgical patients.
Oral Anticoagulants: Warfarin Sodium (Coumadin) **Rivaroxaban (Xarelto)** **Dabigatran (Pradaxa)** **Apixaban (Eliquis)**	Frequently prescribed outpatient oral anticoagulant that inhibits vitamin K dependent clotting factors. Tests to monitor coagulation with warfarin are the international normalized ratio (INR) test and prothrombin time (PT). Interacts with many drugs and nutritional supplements.
Parenteral Anticoagulants **Heparin Sodium** **Heparin Calcium**	Heparin sodium or calcium acts on multiple coagulation factors. From bovine intestinal source, heparin is given by IV or subcutaneous route. Activated partial thromboplastin time (aPTT) test results must be monitored closely q4-6h until levels are stabilized, after dose adjustments, and then daily. Not suitable for home use. Anti-Xa is becoming more commonly used for monitoring patients on IV heparin therapy.
Protamine Sulfate	Antidote for heparin and heparinoid drugs.
Thrombolytic Agents	Drugs that "lyse," or dissolve, clots if given intravenously within a specified amount of time. Used for patients with acute stroke or pulmonary embolism. Also instilled to "de-clot" central line catheters, then aspirated so that patient does not receive the medication systemically.
Vitamin K (phytonadione)	Antidote for warfarin products.

1 What are some of the differences between heparin, warfarin, and LMWH products?

ASK YOURSELF **Q & A**

MY ANSWER

➤ To prevent drug interactions, patients need to inform their physician if they are taking other medications such as anticoagulants, aspirin, or nonsteroidal anti-inflammatory drugs (NSAIDs).

COAGULATION TESTS

Activated Partial Thromboplastin Time (aPTT)	A *newer* form of the PTT test with activators added, *preferred* for monitoring *heparin* therapy, *not* to be confused with PT test for warfarin. "Normal" control aPTT time is about 30 to 40 seconds (about $\frac{1}{2}$ minute), depending on test agents used.
Anti-Xa Assay	A newer test designed to measure heparin and low-molecular-weight heparin (LMWH) levels and monitor anticoagulant therapy effectiveness. There are target therapeutic ranges depending on the type of heparin used. Dosages are titrated to maintain target ranges.
Control Values	Laboratory-derived "average normal values" for specific test results. May vary from laboratory to laboratory, depending on agents used for testing. Determined daily by laboratory tests for prothrombin time, partial thromboplastin time, and activated partial thromboplastin time tests to ensure efficacy of agents used for each batch of tests for accurate measurement.
International Normalized Ratio (INR)	Standardized formula-derived laboratory value *preferred* for monitoring *warfarin* therapy. Normal blood has an INR of 1. Therapeutic target range for blood of anti-coagulated patients is 2.0 to 3.0 INR value, derived from patient-specific prothrombin time value.
Other tests that may be ordered for patients receiving anticoagulant therapy or those with coagulation disorders	Activated coagulation time (ACT) Bleeding time D-dimer test Hematocrit (Hct) Hemoglobin (Hgb) Liver function tests (LFTs) Renal function tests Specific clotting factor assays Stool test for occult blood Urine test for blood Whole blood clotting time (WBCT)
Platelet Count	Actual count of number of thrombocytes in blood (normal adult value, 150,000 to 400,000 per mcL). Less than 50,000 per mcL poses risk of bleeding from minor trauma and surgery. Less than 20,000 per mcL poses *great risk* of spontaneous hemorrhage.
Prothrombin Time (PT, or Pro Time)	Formerly used for monitoring warfarin therapy, it now may be used as an adjunct to INR. It is not as reliable as INR. Normal control values in *uncoagulated* patients vary from laboratory to laboratory by 11 to 15 seconds. This should not be confused with an aPTT test which is used to monitor heparin therapy.

Q & A **ASK YOURSELF**

1 What is the preferred test for patients receiving heparin products, as opposed to the test for those receiving warfarin products?

MY ANSWER _____

2 What is the main risk for patients who have thrombocytopenia?

_____

FAQ *What is the difference between a normal (control) value for a PT or an aPTT and a therapeutic level?*

ANSWER The normal control value is the coagulation time in seconds for a specific test, such as the aPTT, for a person who is *not* receiving anticoagulants. It varies from test to test and laboratory to laboratory, depending on the agents used for the test.

When patients receive anticoagulants, they receive a *"therapeutic amount"* of drug that will *extend* their coagulation time to reduce their risk of having a thromboembolic event. Anticoagulant doses are individualized for each patient, or "patient-specific," based on the patient's test results.

The therapeutic level is based on the laboratory daily control value. It is the desired *target* coagulation range in seconds that prevents clot formation in patients who are at risk. It is *longer than* the normal control finding for an aPTT coagulation test, which is 30 to 40 seconds for a person who is *not* receiving heparin.

The therapeutic level for an aPTT test is within *1.5 to 2.5 times the control value in seconds* (45-100 seconds), a narrow therapeutic range that will prolong clot formation but not be excessive enough to cause bleeding.

To evaluate a patient-specific coagulation test result:

- Obtain the therapeutic target range by multiplying the control value by the desired factors for the range.
- Compare the patient's test result to see if it falls within the range.

EXAMPLES

3/12/2018, Control value for aPTT: 30 seconds

Therapeutic target range: 1.5 to 2.5 times the control value (45 to 100 seconds)

aPTT results for Patient X, a patient receiving heparin: 130 seconds

Decision: Hold the anticoagulant. It is not within the desired therapeutic range. Notify the prescriber promptly. Obtain orders. Document. Monitor the patient for bleeding events.

Analysis: Patient's aPTT coagulation time has been *extended* too long with recent doses of anticoagulants. Patient is at risk for bleeding. Antidote may be prescribed.

Note that if the value was *below* the therapeutic range, the patient would be at risk for a thromboembolic event.

CLINICAL RELEVANCE

➤ Assess clients on anticoagulants for bleeding gums, bruises, and prolonged bleeding after injections. Always check current coagulation test results.

1 If a *control value* for a coagulation test is 12 seconds and the *therapeutic range* is 1.5 to 2.5 times the control value, would the patient's test result be within therapeutic range if it was *24 seconds*?

ASK YOURSELF   **Q & A**

_____ **MY ANSWER**

Oral Anticoagulants

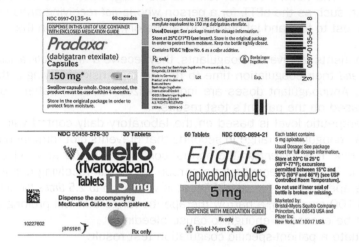

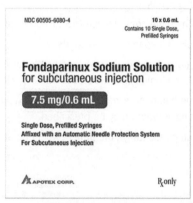

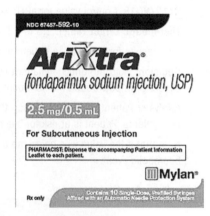

Some of the newer oral anticoagulants do not require the frequent lab work monitoring like warfarin.

Injectable Anticoagulants

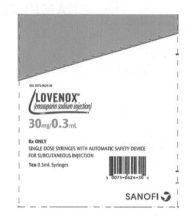

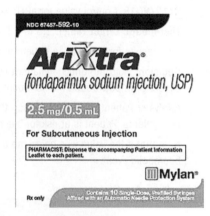

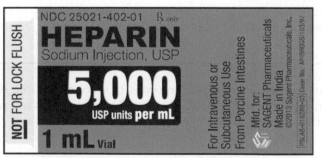

| RAPID PRACTICE 12-1 | Anticoagulants and Antidotes |

ESTIMATED COMPLETION TIME: 5 to 10 minutes   **ANSWERS ON:** page 460

DIRECTIONS: *Identify the correct agent, term, purpose, or antidote for anticoagulant therapy.*

1   The drug antidote for warfarin excess is _____

   a.   Blood transfusion   **c.**   Vitamin K (phytonadione)
   b.   Iron   **d.**   Protamine sulfate

2   Drugs that dissolve clots are classified as _____

   a.   Anticoagulants   **c.**   Thrombolytic enzyme agents
   b.   Hormones   **d.**   Salicylates

3   The drug antidote for heparin excess is _____

   a.   Blood transfusion   **c.**   Vitamin K (phytonadione)
   b.   Iron   **d.**   Protamine sulfate

4   The difference between a control value and a therapeutic value for a specific anticoagulant test is _____

   a.   The control value is the extended blood coagulation time in seconds needed to prevent clots, whereas the therapeutic desired value is the normal coagulation time in seconds for a patient not receiving anticoagulants.
   b.   The control value is the level that the prescriber orders for the patient to control his or her blood coagulation. The therapeutic coagulation levels or range is less time in seconds than the control value.
   c.   The control value is the laboratory-derived normal coagulation time in seconds for a particular test for a patient who is not receiving anticoagulants. The therapeutic value is the desired extended time in seconds for the patient receiving a specific anticoagulant.
   d.   The control value and the therapeutic time in seconds for coagulation are the same for all patients receiving a specific anticoagulant.

5   Intravenous flush solutions are used for which purpose? _____

   a.   Occult blood in stool and hematuria
   b.   Epistaxis
   c.   Petechiae and ecchymoses
   d.   Patency of IV access devices

FAQ   *What is the relationship between the PT value and the INR value?*

ANSWER   A current INR standardized test value introduced by the World Health Organization in 1983 is required to adjust or titrate warfarin doses. The patient's therapeutic INR range is determined daily by the individual laboratory based in part on the PT value. The INR is not a separate test. It is a formula-derived value:

$$INR = \left. \frac{\text{Patient's PT Value}}{\text{Mean Normal PT Value*}} \right\} ISI$$

The INR value is used to evaluate the patient's response to treatment. Some prescribers also require the PT to be reported with the INR.

*ISI: International Sensitivity Index, a value assigned to the thromboplastin reagent by the manufacturer of the specific laboratory test material.

TABLE 12-1 Comparison of Anticoagulant Products

	Rivaroxaban (Xarelto)	Warfarin (Coumadin)	Dabigatran (Pradaxa)	Apaxiban (Eliquis)	Heparin (unfractionated)	Low-Molecular-Weight Heparin (LMWH)
Route	Oral	Oral	Oral	Oral	Subcutaneous or IV	Subcutaneous or IV
Tests	Baseline creatinine	PT INR	None	Baseline creatinine	aPTT Anti-Xa	Anti-Xa aPTT
Drug antidote	None	Vitamin K	None	None	Protamine sulfate	Protamine sulfate

➤ All anticoagulant products are high-alert medications.

➤ Immediate treatment must be obtained if a patient assessment, including laboratory results, suggests any sign of a bleeding episode, allergic reaction, and/or interaction with other medications.

➤ Heparin and LMWH doses are *not* interchangeable.

➤ Do not confuse PT with aPTT.

➤ Plasma, plasma expanders, and blood also may be needed to counteract loss of blood from overdoses of anticoagulants.

RAPID PRACTICE 12-2 Interpreting PT and INR Results

ESTIMATED COMPLETION TIME: 20 minutes   **ANSWERS ON:** page 460

DIRECTIONS: *Examine the test results and provide the requested answers.*

1 Three days later, Mr. X's INR is 3. The physician lowers the Coumadin dosage to 2.5 mg per day. Mr. X's tablets are scored. He is instructed to buy a pill cutter at a local pharmacy and to keep a record of when he takes his nightly Coumadin dose. His next few laboratory tests will be scheduled weekly.

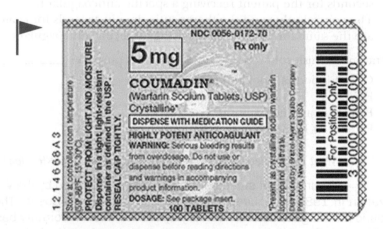

a. How many pills will Mr. X take daily? _____

b. Which of the following Coumadin doses would be safest for Mr. X to have prescribed for his next prescription, assuming that his INR remains stable? _____

CLINICAL RELEVANCE

➤ Assess patients for the variety of doses they may have on hand at home and the precautions they should take to avoid taking the wrong dose. It is not unusual to have doses adjusted. Keeping track of changing doses of the same medication can be challenging.

2 A few weeks later, Mr. X's INR result is 7, and he is complaining of bleeding when he brushes his teeth as well as dark-colored urine and stools, which test positive for presence of blood. The PT value is 49 seconds. The therapeutic INR value is 2 to 3 for Mr. X. The control PT is 12 seconds.

   a. What is the nurse's evaluation of the laboratory results? (Circle one.)
      1. Mr. X is in danger of forming thrombi or emboli.
      2. Mr. X is in danger of bleeding from excessive anticoagulation.
      3. Mr. X's results are within normal limits for anticoagulation.

The physician orders vitamin K 2 mg subcut stat to reverse the warfarin and lower the INR.

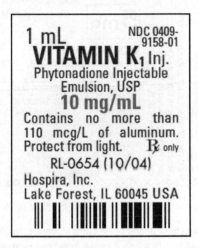

   b. How many mL of vitamin K will the nurse prepare for injection after the dilution? Use mental arithmetic, and verify with a DA equation. _____

   DA equation:

   Evaluation: _____

Mr. X is instructed to hold the Coumadin dosage until results of his next INR test.

3 What is the nurse's evaluation of Mr. X's PT time (25 seconds)? (Circle one.)
   a. 25 seconds is within the desired range for extended coagulation for Mr. X.
   b. Mr. X needs a higher dose of anticoagulant and is at risk for thrombus or embolus formation.
   c. Mr. X is receiving too much anticoagulant.
   d. Mr. X's PT value should be 11.5 seconds.

4 Mr. X, named in problem 1, has a PT test ordered in addition to the INR. PT was reported at 25 seconds. The laboratory control PT value was 11.5 seconds.

➤ The therapeutic PT time for an anticoagulated patient such as Mr. X is 2 to 2.5 times the laboratory control value.

What is the desired PT range for Mr. X in seconds? _____

5 A patient, Mr. X, was discharged post–myocardial infarction on Coumadin 5 mg PO bedtime daily. The patient has been requested to return to the office twice a week for INR test follow-up to ensure that the Coumadin dosage is within the therapeutic range. The medication is prescribed at bedtime so that, if the following morning laboratory test result requires dose adjustment, it can be made the same evening.

The prescription is for warfarin 5 mg #60 pills. "Take 5 mg at bedtime as directed." The tablets are scored, and if the dosage needs to be reduced, the patient can take 2.5 mg if prescribed without purchasing another prescription.

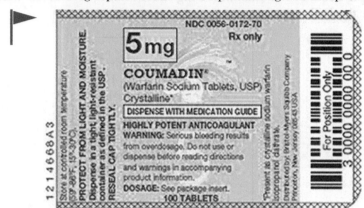

CLINICAL RELEVANCE

➤ Patient discharge teaching needs to be comprehensive, including the many foods that contain vitamin K, effects of alcohol intake, need to maintain consistent levels of foods with vitamin K (if prescriber recommended) to stabilize test results, recommendation not to omit doses, need for frequent follow-up lab testing, signs and symptoms of problems, and when to call the physician. Information on over-the-counter medicines to avoid is critical. Written instructions should be provided.

✴ Communication

Mrs. C.: (being discharged) "Get emergency medical help if you have any of these **signs of allergic reaction:** nausea, vomiting, sweating, hives, itching, trouble breathing, swelling of your face, lips, tongue, or throat, or feeling like you might pass out."

✴ Communication

"Mr. X, how do you keep track of your anticoagulant medications when you take them at home?"

The normal therapeutic range of INR for Mr. X on anticoagulant therapy is 2 to 3. For the first laboratory test in the office, the INR value was 2.6. What is the expected decision for Mr. X? (Circle one.)

a. Continue on 5-mg-per-day dose and return to office in 3 days for next INR.
b. Hold the Coumadin. Come in for vitamin K (phytonadione) injection.
c. Increase the Coumadin dose to 7.5 mg per day.
d. Order an aPTT test.

➤ Noncompliance with anticoagulant therapy can be fatal. Forgetting to take a medication or doubling up is not a rare occurrence, even in the most alert patient population. Remember, there is a difference between what is taught and what is learned.

Q & A **ASK YOURSELF** 1 Take a minute to browse your most comprehensive current pharmacology text for drug and food interactions with Coumadin. Besides aspirin, other NSAIDs, and antibiotics, what other medications do you recognize on the list? What effect do they have on the anticoagulant?

MY ANSWER _____

2 Does the length of the list illustrate the need to check the medications each patient is currently receiving?

_____

> ➤ Extensive patient teaching regarding anticoagulant therapy is critical. One example of a preventable tragedy was a patient who suffered lacerations in a relatively minor automobile accident and who died from loss of blood. The patient did not carry a wallet card with information about the medication (warfarin) nor the dosage, nor did the patient wear a Medic-Alert identification bracelet.

CLINICAL RELEVANCE

> ➤ A responsible family member needs to have all the priority information about the anticoagulant dosage, timing, testing, and follow-up visits. Patients need to be reminded to carry a list of their medications and dosages on their person at all times. Patients on long-term anticoagulant therapy should be encouraged to wear a Medic-Alert identification bracelet.

CLINICAL RELEVANCE

Injectable Anticoagulants

The most common parenteral anticoagulant is heparin sodium. It can be administered intravenously in the hospital, but it requires frequent titration based on laboratory results. Subcutaneous heparin is also frequently administered in the hospital. It is derived from pork and bovine intestinal mucosa, and it interacts with many drugs.

> ➤ If ordered IV, heparin must be administered on an infusion pump with a primary IV line dedicated for heparin administration only.

Take a moment to examine some examples of the varied doses of heparin available. It helps to have a general understanding of the purpose of the range of doses because the selection of the correct concentration is a critical nursing decision.

> ➤ As with most liquid injectables for adults, drug amounts in mL are usually rounded to the nearest tenth of a mL.

> ➤ Check agency policies regarding requirements for an independent nurse check of anticoagulants before each dose administration.

Heparin Flushes (Low-Dose Concentrations)

Occasionally flushes of very low-dose heparin are administered to maintain the patency of venous access sites. They are given far less frequently now than in the past, as saline is now more commonly used (Figure 12-1).

> ➤ The flush solution—saline or heparin—is selected according to agency protocol.

> ➤ Saline solution may be preferred as a flush for most venous access devices.

The prescriber does not write the volume in milliliters of the flush to be used. The volume of the flush depends on the fluid capacity of the indwelling device and institutional policy. The longer the catheter, the more volume will be needed to "flush" the line.

> ➤ There have been tragic consequences when the wrong dose (with a stronger concentration) has been used for a heparin flush.

> ➤ Consult agency guidelines and equipment literature for precise concentrations and volumes for each type of flush.

> ➤ Know the difference when you see these acronyms:

SASH, acronym for heparin flush: Saline, Administer (drug), Saline, Heparin
SAS, acronym for saline flush: Saline, Administer (drug), Saline

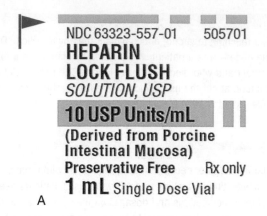

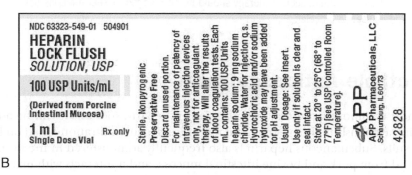

FIGURE 12-1 A, Heparin lock flush 10 units per mL. **B,** Heparin lock flush 100 units per mL.

Q & A	**ASK YOURSELF**	**1**	As I check my pharmacology reference for heparin drug interactions, why do I realize it would be critical to flush IV lines with saline solution *before* and *after* administering heparin?

MY ANSWER _____

2 Which incompatible drug is one I have most frequently seen or heard about?

_____

3 Why must IV heparin have a separate IV line and be administered using an infusion pump?

_____

Heparin for Subcutaneous and Intravenous Administration

Like many other drugs, heparin is supplied in several concentrations. Refer to Figures 12-2 and 12-3.

➤ These concentrations should *not* be used for flushes.

➤ Heparin has been identified as a high-alert drug by the Institute for Safe Medication Practices (ISMP) (see Appendix B). It is critical to select the correct ordered concentration of a powerful drug such as heparin.

1 What is the difference in the heparin product concentrations shown in Figures 12-2 and 12-3?

MY ANSWER

_____

_____

_____

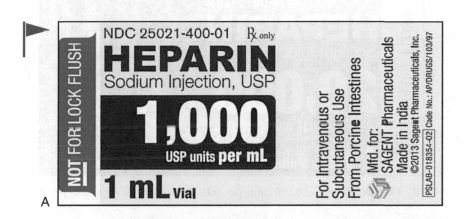

A, NDC 25021-400-01 Rx only

HEPARIN
Sodium Injection, USP

1,000 USP units **per mL**

NOT FOR LOCK FLUSH

1 mL Vial

For Intravenous or Subcutaneous Use From Porcine Intestines

Mfd. for: SAGENT Pharmaceuticals Made in India
©2013 Sagent Pharmaceuticals, Inc.

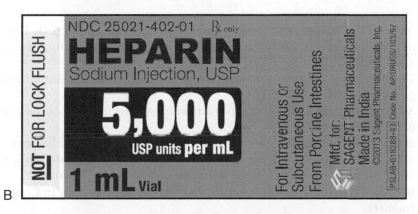

B, NDC 25021-402-01 Rx only

HEPARIN
Sodium Injection, USP

5,000 USP units **per mL**

NOT FOR LOCK FLUSH

1 mL Vial

For Intravenous or Subcutaneous Use From Porcine Intestines

Mfd. for: SAGENT Pharmaceuticals Made in India
©2013 Sagent Pharmaceuticals, Inc.

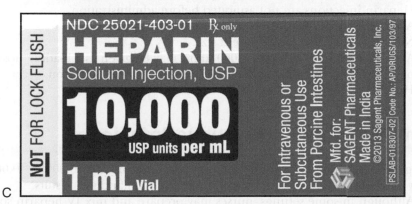

C, NDC 25021-403-01 Rx only

HEPARIN
Sodium Injection, USP

10,000 USP units **per mL**

NOT FOR LOCK FLUSH

1 mL Vial

For Intravenous or Subcutaneous Use From Porcine Intestines

Mfd. for: SAGENT Pharmaceuticals Made in India
©2013 Sagent Pharmaceuticals, Inc.

FIGURE 12-2 **A,** Heparin 1000 units per mL. **B,** Heparin 5000 units per mL. **C,** Heparin 10,000 units per mL.

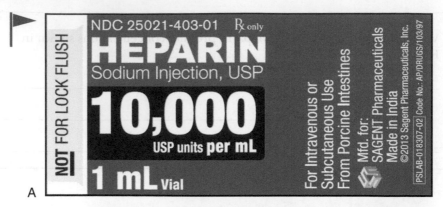

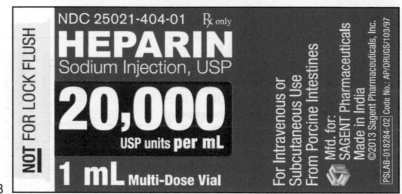

FIGURE 12-3 **A,** Heparin 10,000 units per mL. **B,** Heparin 20,000 units per mL.

- A dose of 5000 units per 1 mL is 5 times more concentrated than 1000 units per mL. A dose of 10,000 units per 1 mL is 10 times more concentrated than 1000 units per mL.
- The more concentrated the dose, the greater the anticoagulant effect and the greater the risk of bleeding.
- Adding or subtracting a zero from an order or misreading a *U* as a zero must be avoided.
- Many at-risk patients receive a standard dose of 5000 units of heparin subcutaneously q8h or q12h for DVT prevention. This dose does not require aPTT monitoring. Platelet counts may be ordered every few days.
- Injection sites are rotated. Refer to Sites for Insulin Injection in Chapter 11 (p. 404).
- Heparin injections are not aspirated before administration.
- Avoid massaging the site.
- Needle angle depends on patient size.
- A bolus of low-dose heparin, 5000 units, may be given as a loading dose and/or as a test for reactions such as allergies before an IV infusion.
- Heparin is never given via the IM route.

Heparin Concentrations Used for Intravenous Infusions

The general guidelines for continuous heparin infusions are 20,000 to 40,000 units every 24 hours, depending on the patient's condition and test results.

Although in some settings, nurses may prepare and mix IV heparin solutions, the trend is to use premixed preparations or have the pharmacy mix the solution to ensure the patient's safety.

There are also premixed preparations of heparin of 12,500 units per 250 mL NS and 25,000 to 40,000 units in 250 or 500 mL NS. Heparin is also available premixed in ADD-Vantage vials to accompany ADD-Vantage IV solution containers. Refer to Chapter 9 for a review of the ADD-Vantage® System.

RAPID PRACTICE 12-3	Heparin Preparations and Preventing Errors

ESTIMATED COMPLETION TIME: 10 minutes   **ANSWERS ON:** page 460

DIRECTIONS: *Examine the preceding information about heparin and the labels and review the vocabulary to answer the following questions 1 through 10.*

CLINICAL RELEVANCE

Contrast the concentration on the label below and the last label on p. 442. Three infants died in one agency as a result of being given a dose from the 10,000 units per mL label instead of the 10 units per mL label.

Most medicines today have more than one form and more than one concentration, whether oral or injectable. Pharmaceutical companies have been requested to avoid similarly appearing labels.

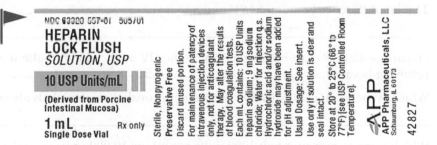

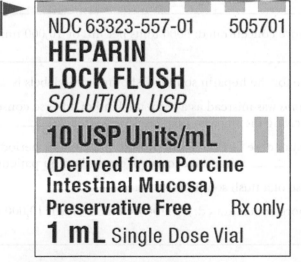

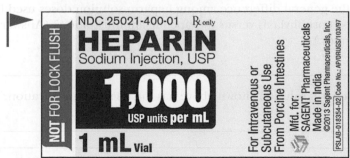

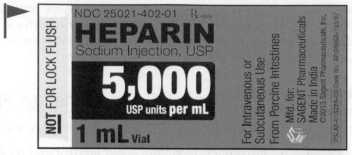

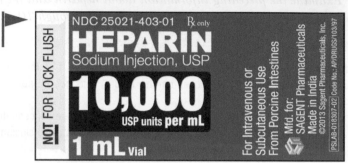

1 The key difference between SASH and SAS is _____

_____.

2 Heparin solutions must be isolated from other IV medications a patient is receiving because _____.

3 Which is the *lowest* concentration of solution provided on the labels above?

_____

4 Which is more concentrated: 1000 units per mL or 10,000 units per mL?

_____

5 Which is more concentrated: 5000 units per mL or 10,000 units per mL?

_____

6 The volume for the heparin solutions shown on the labels is _____.

7 If a *U* for *units* was misread as a zero, the kind of adverse consequence to the patient receiving the heparin dose could be _____

8 The maximum dose of IV heparin units over a 24-hour period is about _____ (can be exceeded, depending on patient's condition).

9 The purpose of a flush solution is _____.

10 Which is more concentrated: a 1:1000 solution or a 1:10,000 solution? _____

Q & A   **ASK YOURSELF**   1   What is the general difference among heparin solution doses used for flush versus prophylaxis versus therapeutic administration? (Answer in brief phrases.)

   MY ANSWER   _____

2   Which heparin solution shown above has the *highest* concentration?

_____

Calculating Heparin Flow Rates

Calculations are the same as for any other DA-style equation.

Determine mL per Hour

Weight-based orders based on kg weight are recommended by TJC for all drugs to reduce dosing errors. In addition, it is recommended that the prescriber calculate the dose and show the calculations. The nurse still has to do an independent math check of the flow rate based on the order and the IV solution (label) even if the flow rate was supplied by the prescriber, pharmacy, or programmed electronic infusion pump.

EXAMPLES

Ordered: heparin 24 units per kg per hr. Patient weight is 50 kg.

Available: heparin 25,000 units in 500 mL D5W (500 mL per 25,000 units)

How many milliliters per hour (to the nearest tenth of a mL per hr) should be administered?

Step 1	=	Step 2	×	Step 3	=	Answer
Desired Answer Units	=	Starting Factor	×	Given Quantity and Conversion Factor(s)* *as needed	=	Estimate, Multiply, Evaluate

$$? \frac{mL}{hr} = \frac{\overset{1}{\cancel{500}}\ mL}{\underset{\underset{1}{50}}{\cancel{25,000\ units}}} \times \frac{24\ \cancel{units}}{\cancel{kg} \times 1\ hr} \times \frac{\overset{1}{\cancel{50\ kg}}}{1} = 24\ mL\ per\ hr$$

The final equation will be written like this:

$$? \frac{mL}{hr} = \frac{\overset{1}{\cancel{500}}\ mL}{\underset{\underset{1}{50}}{\cancel{25,000\ units}}} \times \frac{24\ \cancel{units}}{\cancel{kg} \times 1\ hr} \times \frac{\overset{1}{\cancel{50\ kg}}}{1} = \frac{24\ mL}{hr}$$

Analysis: This equation has a required numerator and denominator containing the desired answer units. The selected starting factor is positioned with mL in the numerator. Hr appear in the denominator of step 3. Reduction and cancellation before multiplication simplifies the math.

Evaluation: The answer matches the desired answer. The order of 1200 units per hr is within the recommended heparin continuous adult infusion rate of 20,000 to 40,000 units per 24 hr. My estimate after all the data are entered is that the flow rate will be low—about 1/50 of 1200 (500 divided by 25,000 = 1/50) (1200 ÷ 50 = 24). The estimate supports the answer.

➤ Remember that IVs for high-alert drugs must be administered on an electronic infusion pump.

Determine Units per Hour

The nurse often comes on shift duty to find IVs infusing. The nursing responsibility is to ensure that each flow rate is correct for the dose ordered and solution concentration (label) provided, and to be able to report how many units per hr are infusing. Are the units per hr being administered the same as ordered by the prescriber? Is the dose within adult SDR (20,000 to 40,000 units) for continuous IV for 24 hr? If not, why not?

➤ A standard heparin solution concentration on many units is 25,000 units in 250 mL of D5W.

➤ Contrast the mL-per-hr flow rate with the number of heparin units per hr.

EXAMPLES

Existing infusion: heparin flowing at 10 mL per hr

Infusion labeled 25,000 units heparin in 250 mL D5W

How many units per hour (to the nearest 100 units per hour) are being administered?

Step 1	=	Step 2	×	Step 3	=	Answer
Desired Answer Units	=	Starting Factor	×	Given Quantity and Conversion Factor(s)* *as needed	=	Estimate, Multiply, Evaluate
$? \dfrac{\text{units}}{\text{hr}}$	=	$\dfrac{\overset{100}{\cancel{25{,}000}} \text{ units}}{\underset{1}{\cancel{250 \text{ mL}}}}$	×	$\dfrac{10 \text{ } \cancel{\text{mL}}}{1 \text{ hr}}$	=	$1000 \dfrac{\text{units}}{\text{hr}}$

Analysis: Convert the flow rate from volume per hr (mL per hr) to medication per hr (units per hr). *The selected starting factor, obtained from the labels on the IV bottle, permitted a match with units, one of the two desired answers. The flow rate provided a match with the second desired answer unit, hr, in the denominator (hr must appear in the denominator under the dividing line). Reduction and cancellation make the math easy in this simple equation.

Evaluation: My estimate after the data are entered in the equation is 50 × 20, and the estimate supports the answer. The equation is balanced. 1000 units per hr is within the recommended continuous heparin infusion rate of 20,000 to 40,000 units per 24 hr.

| RAPID PRACTICE 12-4 | Titrating Heparin Doses to aPTT Values |

ESTIMATED COMPLETION TIME: 20 to 30 minutes   **ANSWERS ON:** page 460

DIRECTIONS: *Read the following case history information for the patient on heparin therapy. Calculate the doses and provide the requested nursing evaluations. Round all doses to the nearest 100 units. Label all work.*

Mr. Y has been hospitalized with atrial fibrillation, a condition that predisposes him to thromboembolus formation. The physician has ordered a complete blood screening for clotting and bleeding times, including a baseline platelet count and aPTT. Mr. Y's baseline aPTT is 30 seconds. He is not receiving anticoagulants yet. The platelet count is 250,000 per microliter.

Because both of Mr. Y's values are within the normal range, the physician institutes heparin therapy to extend coagulation time.

> Initial order for Mr. Y: heparin 5000 unit bolus loading test dose IV slowly. Pharmacology references state to infuse the first 1000 units over 1 minute, then give the rest of the IV loading dose before starting a continuous infusion. Follow with continuous infusion at 1000 units per hr. Obtain an aPTT in 4 hours.

Thus, the slow bolus test dose is ordered.

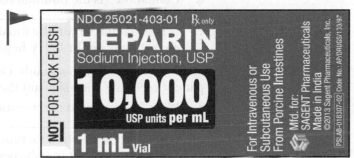

1 The physician writes the following order: Start heparin infusion at 1000 units per hr. Available: heparin 25,000 units per 250 mL of NS. Heparin infusions are administered on infusion pumps.

   a. The nurse will set the flow rate at how many mL per hr?

   DA equation:

   b. Evaluation: _____

   Prescriber orders IV heparin schedule for Mr. Y, whose weight is 80 kg. Titrate (adjust) heparin q4h to maintain aPTT. Up to **44 seconds,** increase infusion by 1 unit per kg per hr. **45 to 75 seconds:** no adjustment. **76 to 80 seconds:** decrease infusion by 1 unit per kg per hr. aPTT greater than **80 seconds:** hold infusion. Call physician for orders. All rates are to be rounded to the nearest 100 units per hr.

   ➤ It is recommended to have a responsible family member present for patient teaching.

2 Mr. Y's next aPTT is 50 seconds. Control is 30 seconds. Desired aPTT for patient receiving heparin anticoagulant therapy is 1.5 to 2.5 times control.

   a. Desired therapeutic range in seconds for Mr. Y: _____

   b. Is Mr. Y's current result within the aPTT therapeutic range? (Yes/No) _____

    c. Does an adjustment need to be made in IV heparin units per hr and IV flow rate based upon the aPTT result and the titration schedule? (Use brief phrases.)

_____

_____

    DA equation if applicable:

    d. Evaluation: _____

3 The orders for a new patient read: Heparin infusion: 32 units per kg per hr. The nurse on the oncoming shift sees that the existing flow rate is 32 mL per hr. Patient weight is 50 kg.

    a. How many units per hr to the nearest 100 units is the patient receiving based on the existing concentration of heparin 12,500 units per 250 mL of NS? _____

    DA equation:

    b. Evaluation: (Is the flow rate correct or incorrect for the order?)

_____

    c. Is this amount within the usual recommended 24-hour range of 20,000 to 40,000 units per hr for IV heparin infusions? (Yes/No) _____

4 Mr. Y's next aPTT is 76 seconds. Control is 30 seconds.* Desired aPTT for patient receiving anticoagulant therapy is 1.5 to 2.5 times control.

    a. What is the desired therapeutic aPTT range in seconds for Mr. Y?

_____

    b. Is it within the desired therapeutic range? _____

    c. Will an adjustment in units per hr be needed based on the aPTT result and the titration schedule ordered in problem 2? (Answer briefly.)

_____

_____

    d. If so, how many units per hr should Mr. Y receive? Do not round.

    DA equation:

    e. Will there be an adjustment needed in Mr. Y's IV flow rate? _____

    f. If so, how many mL per hr should he receive?

    DA equation:

5 Why is thrombocytopenia, as measured by a platelet count under 100,000 per microliter, a contraindication to the institution of heparin therapy? Refer to Vocabulary if necessary. (Give a brief answer.)

_____

---

*Think of a _half-minute_ as a rough, approximate normal aPTT. The normal range is about 20 to 35 seconds. Use the precise range supplied by the individual laboratory for heparin administration.

RAPID PRACTICE 12-5	**Anticoagulant and Antidote Calculation Practice**

ESTIMATED COMPLETION TIME: 20 minutes   **ANSWERS ON:** page 460

DIRECTIONS: *Read each patient's history. Calculate the doses using a DA equation.*

1 A current drug reference states to administer the protamine sulfate IV ordered in problem 1 *slowly over 1 to 3 minutes.*

➤ Too-rapid administration can result in anaphylaxis, severe hypotension, hypertension, bradycardia, and dyspnea.

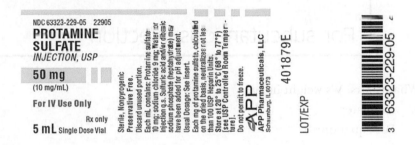

a. How many mL (to the nearest tenth) of protamine sulfate IV will be administered to Mr. M (problem 1)? _____
   DA equation:

b. Evaluation: _____

2 Mr. M is receiving heparin continuous infusion of 12 units per kg per hr.
   Available: premixed heparin 25,000 units in 500 mL. Mr. M's weight is 90 kg.

   a. How many units per hour of heparin should Mr. M receive to the nearest 100 units? _____

   b. What rate will the nurse set on the infusion pump to the nearest mL?
      DA equation:

   c. Evaluation: _____

3 Fragmin 80 international units per kg is ordered prophylactically q12h subcut for Mrs. V, a patient with unstable angina. Mrs. V weighs 110 lb.

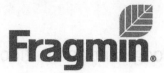

10 x 0.2 mL single dose syringes, preassembled with needle guards
NDC 0013-2426-91

Fragmin®

dalteparin sodium injection

5000 IU (anti-Xa) per 0.2 mL

For subcutaneous injection

What is Mrs. V's weight in kg?

a. Estimate:

DA equation:

b. Evaluation: _____
c. How many units will the nurse prepare for Mrs. V.?

DA equation:

d. Evaluation: _____
e. How many mL will the nurse prepare to the nearest hundredth of a mL?
Estimate:

DA equation:

f. Evaluation: _____

➤ Do *not* interchange units with milligrams for dose. Check the order and label, and compare units ordered to units supplied.

4 Mrs. J is scheduled for a hip replacement. She is placed on prophylactic anticoagulation with an LMWH agent, dalteparin (Fragmin):

2500 international units subcut 2 hours before surgery
2500 international units subcut 8 hours after surgery
5000 international units subcut daily for 14 days postoperatively in the
    hospital and at home

CHAPTER 12

Periodic complete blood count, platelet count, and stool test for occult blood were ordered.

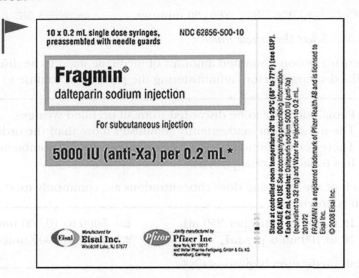

How many mL will Mrs. J need to receive preoperatively (to the nearest tenth of a mL)?

a. Estimated dose.

b. DA equation:

c. Evaluation: _____

Anticoagulant NGN

Janelle Martin, a 68 year old was admitted to the ICU with a pulmonary embolism. She is 10 days post hip arthroplasty. She is short of breath, and says "I feel like I am dying". Her weight is 148 pounds. Here are her orders:
- Admit to ICU: Diagnosis pulmonary embolus
- O2 at 6 liters per minute via non-rebreather mask
- IV 0.9 NS at 100 mL per hour
- Heparin IV – bolus 80 units/kg now and then run it at 2200 units/hour
- CBC with platelet count, PT and aPTT now.
- Repeat aPTT in 4 hours and after each dosage change.

1. How many kilograms does Janelle Martin weigh?_____
   *67.13 kilograms

2. How many units will be in the heparin bolus that will be given?_____
   *5371 units

3. Your Heparin infusion is a premixed 500 mL D5W with 20,000 units of heparin. How many units are in each mL?_____
   *40mL

4. How many mL will be in your bolus dose?
   *134 mL

5. How many mL/hour will you administer to deliver 2200 units/hour?
   *55 mL/hour

6. Janelle Martin's aPTT was returned and was 36 seconds which necessitates a dosage increase of 200 units per hour. How many mL/hour do you need to set the IV pump in order to deliver 2400 units per hour?
   *60 mL/hour

CHAPTER 12   MULTIPLE-CHOICE REVIEW

ESTIMATED COMPLETION TIME: 20 to 30 minutes   ANSWERS ON: page 461

DIRECTIONS: *Select the correct answer.*

1 The main reason unwanted amounts of medicine need to be discarded from prefilled syringes before administering the prescribed volume to the patient is _____

   a. Remainders are to be discarded from all prefilled syringes.
   b. The nurse might inadvertently administer more than the ordered amount.
   c. There is risk of undermedication and a potential thromboembolic event.
   d. It is usually hospital policy.

2 Which of the following dose concentrations are commonly used if a heparin flush is ordered? _____

   a. 10 to 25,000 units per 250 mL   c. 5000 to 10,000 units per mL
   b. 10 to 100 units per mL   d. 1000 to 5000 units per mL

3 Which medication is given orally? _____

   a. Warfarin   c. Heparin sodium
   b. Heparinoids   d. Heparin calcium

4 Which antidote should be on hand for patients receiving heparin therapy? __

   a. Activated charcoal   c. Potassium chloride
   b. Vitamin K   d. Protamine sulfate

5 Which of the following medication(s) require(s) INR testing? _____

   a. Streptokinase   c. Heparin sodium or calcium
   b. Heparinoids   d. Warfarin products

6 The general recommended flow rate for initial continuous heparin infusions for adults, which can vary widely depending on the patient's condition and test results, is approximately _____

   a. 1000 to 1700 units per hr   c. 5000 units per hr
   b. 5 to 10 units per hr   d. 25,000 units per hr

7 Which of the following statements is true about the relationship between international units and milligrams? _____

   a. Milligrams are a measure of weight, and international units are a standardized amount that produces a particular biologic effect.
   b. Milligrams and corresponding units can be determined by the nurse using a standard formula for all drugs.
   c. The effect of 1 mg is equal to the effect of 1 international unit of the same product.
   d. Milligrams, milliliters, and international units can be used interchangeably.

8 Which bests describes the "control value" for aPTT and PT testing? _____

   a. It reflects the patient's current laboratory value before treatment.
   b. It is a measure of therapeutic response to anticoagulation.
   c. It reflects the current laboratory norm based on the batch of materials used for testing that day.
   d. It is the general range of norms for all patients receiving anticoagulants.

9 When may a physician have to consider the danger of prescribing anticoagulants for a patient? _____

   a. The patient is at high risk for DVT.
   b. The patient is at very high risk for developing clots.
   c. The patient is noncompliant with medication and test regimens.
   d. The patient is elderly and lives with children.

10 The preferred test for monitoring heparin therapy is _____

   a. PT   **c.** PTT

   b. aPTT   **d.** INR

CHAPTER 12   FINAL PRACTICE

ESTIMATED COMPLETION TIME: 1 to 2 hours   **ANSWERS ON:** page 461

DIRECTIONS: *Answer the anticoagulant-related questions. Evaluate your equations. Label all answers.*

1 A nurse checks an infusion of heparin 25,000 units per 500 mL Ringer's solution. It is flowing at 40 mL per hr.

   a. How many *units* of heparin per hour are being delivered?

      DA equation:

   b. Evaluation: _____

   c. Is this order within the recommended 24-hour dose for heparin infusions? _____

2 The order for the infusion solution in problem 5 is for 1200 units per hr based on kg weight.

   a. For how many mL per hr will the nurse set the infusion?

      DA equation:

   b. What adverse effect will the nurse monitor for, in addition to obtaining another aPTT? _____

3 Ordered: heparin infusion of 2000 units per hr based on patient's weight. A heparin infusion of 25,000 units in 250 mL is being administered at 20 mL per hr.

   a. How many *units per hour,* to the nearest 100 units, are being infused?

      DA equation:

   b. Evaluation: _____

4 a. What does "extended coagulation time" mean to you?

      _____

   b. Why should a heparin infusion be administered on an infusion pump?

      _____

5 Ordered: heparin 18 units per kg per hr in a continuous infusion. Available: heparin 25,000 units in 500 mL D5W. Patient's weight: 70 kg.

   a. How many units per hr are ordered? (Round to the nearest 100):

      DA equation:

   b. Evaluation: _____

   c. The nurse will set the flow rate at how many mL per hr: _____

      DA equation:

   d. Evaluation: _____

6 **Ordered:** Enoxaparin 30 mg subcut daily at bedtime: It is supplied in a prefilled syringe.

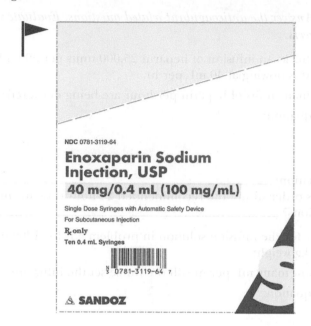

NDC 0781-3119-64

Enoxaparin Sodium Injection, USP

40 mg/0.4 mL (100 mg/mL)

Single Dose Syringes with Automatic Safety Device

For Subcutaneous Injection

R_x only

Ten 0.4 mL Syringes

0781-3119-64 7

△ **SANDOZ**

   a. What type of drug is enoxaparin: heparin, LMWH, warfarin, or thrombolytic derivative? _____

   b. How many mL will the nurse prepare?

      DA equation:

   c. Evaluation: _____

7 The patient described in problem 1 has another aPTT drawn 6 hours later. The result is 65 seconds.

   a. Adjustment in mL per hr if applicable. _____

      DA equation:

   b. Evaluation: _____

8 **Ordered:** Coumadin (warfarin sodium) 5 mg at bedtime for an elderly patient for discharge post–mitral valve replacement. INR values are ordered twice weekly for the first month. The target therapeutic INR is 2 to 3 for this patient. The laboratory reports the patient's INR result at 5.

   a. What will the physician probably do regarding the dosage of Coumadin—*raise* it or *lower* it? (Circle one.)

b. If the patient has several different strengths of Coumadin at home because of dosage adjustments, what sort of advice would be advisable to give the patient regarding drug storage?

_____

_____

9 **Ordered:** continuous heparin infusion to maintain the aPTT between 60 and 70 seconds, for a patient with atrial fibrillation. After the initial slow bolus loading dose of 5000 units IV, draw a stat aPTT and begin the infusion at 1000 units per hr. Obtain the aPTT q6h. Patient weight is 70 kg. The following sliding scale is given to titrate the heparin infusion:

aPTT	Action
30 to 45 seconds	Increase the drip by 3 units per kg per hr.
46 to 70 seconds	No change.
71 to 85 seconds	Reduce the drip by 2 units per kg per hr.
Over 85 seconds	Hold the infusion for 1 hr. Call the physician for orders.

Available: 25,000 units of heparin in 250 mL D5W. The first aPTT drawn is 40 seconds.

a. Initial flow rate in mL per hr at 1000 units per hr should be set at:

DA equation:

b. Evaluation: _____
c. Nurse's evaluation of the first aPTT. (Give a brief answer.) _____
d. Adjusted number of units per hr if applicable. (Round to the nearest 100 units):

DA equation:

e. Evaluation: _____
f. Adjusted number of mL per hr if applicable: _____

DA equation:

g. Evaluation: _____

10 **Ordered:** heparin infusion of 1500 units per hr based on an order of 20 units per kg per hr for a patient weighing 75 kg. Available: heparin 25,000 units per 500 mL NS. The IV is infusing at 20 mL per hr when the nurse arrives on the shift.

a. Is the existing flow rate correct? If not, what should it be?

DA equation:

b. Evaluation: _____

RAPID PRACTICE 12-1 (p. 439)

1 c   4 c
2 c   5 d
3 d

RAPID PRACTICE 12-2 (p. 440)

1   a. one-half tablet using a pill cutter
     b. 2.5 mg
2   a. 2
     b. 0.2 mL

$$\frac{mL}{dose} = \frac{1\,mL}{\underset{5}{\cancel{10\,mg}}} \times \frac{\overset{1}{\cancel{2\,mg}}}{dose} = \frac{0.2\,mL}{dose}$$

     Equation is balanced. Only mL remain.
3   a
4   23-29 seconds (2×11.5 seconds and 2.5×11.5 seconds)
5   a

RAPID PRACTICE 12-3 (p. 447)

1   SASH includes Heparin in addition to saline
2   of possible adverse interactions
3   10 units per mL
4   10,000 units per mL
5   10,000 units per mL
6   1 mL
7   bleeding or hemorrhage
8   20,000 to 40,000 units
9   to maintain patency of venous access devices
10   1:1000 (one part drug per 1000 mL)

➤ Understanding questions 4, 5, and 10 is critical for patient safety.

RAPID PRACTICE 12-4 (p. 451)

1   a. 10 mL per hr

$$\frac{mL}{hr} = \frac{\overset{1}{\cancel{250}}\,mL}{\underset{1}{\underset{100}{\cancel{25,000\,units}}}} \times \frac{\overset{10}{\cancel{1000\,units}}}{1\,hr} = \frac{10\,mL}{hr}$$

     b. Equation is balanced. Only mL per hr remains.
2   a. 45 to 75 seconds ($1.5 \times 30 = 45$ seconds) ($2.5 \times 30 = 75$ seconds)
     b. Yes
     c. No. Between 45 and 75, no adjustment is necessary.
     d. N/A

3   a. 1600

$$\frac{units}{hr} = \frac{\overset{50}{\cancel{12,500}}\,units}{\underset{1}{\cancel{250\,mL}}} \times \frac{32\,\cancel{mL}}{hr} = \frac{1600\,units}{hr}$$

     b. Flow rate is correct.
     c. Yes ($1600 \times 24 = 38{,}400$ units in 24 hr).
4   a. 45 to 75 seconds
     b. No
     c. Yes. The units per hr need to be reduced by 1 unit per kg per hr.
     d. 50 units per hr

$$\frac{units}{hr} = \frac{1\,unit}{1\,\cancel{kg}} \times \frac{50\,\cancel{kg}}{hr}$$
$$= 50 \text{ units reduction/hour}$$

     1600 units/hour − 50 units/hour = 1550 units/hour

     e. Yes
     f. 9 mL per hr

$$\frac{mL}{hr} = \frac{\overset{1}{\cancel{250}}\,mL}{\underset{1}{\underset{100}{\cancel{25,000\,units}}}} \times \frac{\overset{15.5}{\cancel{1550\,units}}}{1\,hour} = \frac{15.5\,mL}{hr}$$

5   Thrombocytopenia predisposes to bleeding. The addition of heparin would increase the risk.

RAPID PRACTICE 12-5 (p. 453)

1   a. 0.6 mL

$$\frac{mL}{dose} = \frac{1\,mL}{10\,\cancel{mg}} \times \frac{5.5\,\cancel{mg}}{1}$$
$$= 0.55\,mL, \text{ rounded to } \frac{0.6\,mL}{dose}$$

     b. Equation is balanced. Only mL remain.
2   a. 1100 units per hr (1080, rounded to 1100)
     b. 22 mL per hr

$$\frac{mL}{hr} = \frac{\overset{1}{\cancel{500}}\,mL}{\underset{50}{\cancel{25,000\,units}}} \times \frac{110\cancel{0\,units}}{1\,hr}$$
$$= \frac{110}{5} = \frac{22\,mL}{hr}$$

     c. Equation is balanced. Only mL per hr remains.

3 a. 55 (110 ÷ 2)

$$kg = \frac{1\ kg}{2.2\ lb} \times \frac{\overset{50}{\cancel{110\ lb}}}{1} = 50\ kg$$

b. Equation is balanced. Estimate supports answer.
c. 4000 units

$$units = \frac{80\ units}{1\ \cancel{kg}} \times 50\ \cancel{kg} = 4000\ units$$

d. Equation is balanced. Only units remain.
e. less than 1 mL

$$\frac{mL}{dose} = \frac{0.2\ mL}{\underset{5}{\cancel{5000\ units}}} \times \overset{4}{\cancel{4000\ units}}$$

$$= \frac{0.8}{5} = \frac{0.16\ mL}{dose}$$

Note: Whether you give 0.16 or 0.2 mL depends on the calibration of the available syringe and agency and prescriber protocols.
f. Equation is balanced. Estimate supports answer.

4 a. half of 0.2 mL = 0.1 mL

b. $$\frac{mL}{dose} = \frac{0.2\ mL}{\underset{2}{\cancel{5000\ units}}} \times \frac{\overset{1}{\cancel{2500\ units}}}{dose}$$

$$= \frac{0.2}{2} = \frac{0.1\ mL}{dose}$$

c. Equation is balanced. Estimate supports answer.

CHAPTER 12 MULTIPLE-CHOICE REVIEW (p. 456)

1	b	6	a
2	b	7	a
3	a	8	c
4	d	9	c
5	d	10	b

CHAPTER 12 FINAL PRACTICE (p. 457)

1 a. 2000 units per hr

$$\frac{units}{hr} = \frac{\overset{50}{\cancel{25,000}}\ units}{\cancel{500\ mL}} \times \frac{40\ \cancel{mL}}{1\ hr} = \frac{2000\ units}{hr}$$

b. Equation is balanced. Only units per hr remains.
c. No. 48,000 units for 24 hours (2000 units × 24) exceeds recommendations for up to 40,000 units per 24 hr. Contact prescriber promptly about the order and document the response.

2 a. 24 mL per hr

$$\frac{mL}{hr} = \frac{\overset{1}{\cancel{500}}\ mL}{\underset{50}{\cancel{25,000\ units}}} \times \frac{1200\ \cancel{units}}{hr} = \frac{1200}{50}$$

$$= \frac{24\ mL}{hr}$$

b. Monitor for bleeding
3 a. 2000 units per hr. The infusion rate is correct.

$$\frac{units}{hr} = \frac{\overset{100}{\cancel{25,000}}\ units}{\underset{1}{\cancel{250\ mL}}} \times \frac{20\ \cancel{mL}}{hr} = \frac{2000\ units}{hr}$$

b. The equation is balanced. The ordered units per hr are being infused.
4 a. "Delayed coagulation," "delayed clotting time," an effect of anticoagulants
b. It is a high-risk drug with potential for serious adverse effects of bleeding and hemorrhage. An infusion pump delivers a controlled rate.
5 a. 1300 units per hr

$$\frac{18\ units}{1\ \cancel{kg}} \times \frac{70\ \cancel{kg}}{1\ hr} = \begin{matrix}1260,\ rounded\ to\\1300\ units\ per\ hr\end{matrix}$$

b. Equation is balanced. Only units per hr remains.
c. 26 mL per hr

$$\frac{mL}{hr} = \frac{\overset{1}{\cancel{500}}\ mL}{\underset{50}{\cancel{25,000\ units}}} \times \frac{1300\ \cancel{units}}{1\ hr}$$

$$= \frac{1300\ mL}{50\ hr} = \frac{26\ mL}{hr}$$

d. Equation is balanced. Only mL per hr remains.
6 a. LMWH
b. 0.3 mL

$$\frac{mL}{dose} = \frac{0.4\ mL}{\underset{4}{\cancel{40\ mg}}} \times \frac{\overset{3}{\cancel{30\ mg}}}{dose} = \frac{1.2}{4} = \frac{0.3\ mL}{dose}$$

c. Equation is balanced. Only mL remain.
7 a. No adjustment is needed.
b. N/A
8 a. Lower it
b. Keep all the unused dosages (prescriptions) stored separately from the current dose strength.

9 a. 10 mL per hr

$$\frac{mL}{hr} = \frac{\overset{1}{\cancel{250}\ mL}}{\underset{1}{\underset{100}{\cancel{25{,}000\ units}}}} \times \frac{\overset{10}{\cancel{1000\ units}}}{hr} = \frac{10\ mL}{hr}$$

b. Equation is balanced. Only mL per hr remains.

c. The aPTT is too low at 40 seconds. Rate needs to be increased by 3 units per kg per hr.

d. 200 units increase per hr

$$\frac{units}{hr} = \frac{3\ units}{1\ \cancel{kg}} \times \frac{70\ \cancel{kg}}{1\ hr}$$
$$= 210\ units\ per\ hr\ increase\ needed$$
$$(rounded\ to\ 200\ units\ increase\ per\ hr)$$

e. Equation is balanced. Only units per hr remains.

f. 12 mL per hr

$$\frac{mL}{hr} = \frac{\overset{1}{\cancel{250}\ mL}}{\underset{1}{\underset{100}{\cancel{25{,}000\ units}}}} \times \frac{\overset{12}{\cancel{1200\ units}}}{hr} = \frac{12\ mL}{hr}$$

g. Equation is balanced. Only mL per hr remains. Flow rate needs to be increased to 12 mL per hr.

10 a. IV rate is too slow and needs to be adjusted to 30 mL per hr. Assess patient. Document. Check agency policy for IV rate adjustments. Contact prescriber.

$$\frac{mL}{hr} = \frac{\overset{1}{\cancel{500}\ mL}}{\underset{1}{\underset{50}{\cancel{25{,}000\ units}}}} \times \frac{\overset{30}{\cancel{1500\ units}}}{1\ hr} = \frac{30\ mL}{hr}$$

b. Equation is balanced. Only mL per hr remain.

Suggestions for Further Reading

http://clotcare.com
http://www.ismp.org/highalertmedications
http://www.jointcommission.org/sentinel_event.aspx

⊖volve For additional practice problems, refer to the Dosages Measured in Units section of the Elsevier's Interactive Drug Calculation Application, Version 1 on Evolve.

Chapter 13 focuses on pediatric dose calculations. These determinations are often multi-step calculations of fractional doses of medications using the familiar techniques of dimensional analysis.

PART VI

Medications for Infants and Children

CHAPTER 13 Pediatric Medications

13 Pediatric Medications

OBJECTIVES

- Distinguish the milligram (mg), microgram (mcg), gram (g), and square meter (m^2) units of measurement.
- Evaluate orders for minimum and maximum pediatric safe dosage range (SDR) doses.
- Calculate pediatric weight-based doses for oral and parenteral routes.

- Define body surface area (BSA) and distinguish m^2 from mg and mcg metric measurements.
- Calculate flow rates for IV volume-control devices.
- State measures to prevent medication errors for pediatric patients.

ESTIMATED TIME TO COMPLETE CHAPTER: 3 hours

Introduction

To avoid injury, yet retain therapeutic value, medication doses must be highly individualized for the pediatric population. Body fluid and electrolyte balance, as well as immature renal and liver function, dictate a need for great care with fluid and medication administration in infants and children. Medication dosages must be specifically tailored in order to avoid medication errors in this vulnerable population.

Doses for children are usually based on *weight*—micrograms, milligrams, or grams per kilogram of body weight—or on *surface area:* micrograms or milligrams per square meter of body surface area. Therapeutic doses for children are included in most current medication references. The trend is for the pharmacy to supply more pediatric-specific pre-prepared medications to reduce the chance of calculation error.

➤ Occasionally, young patients receive an adult dose because of the severity of illness, the threat to life, or the lack of response to lower doses.

➤ Safe medication administration with pediatric population must include:

1. Verifying that the order is within the SDR for the target population
2. Distinguishing microgram, milligram, and square meter units of measurement
3. Calculating accurate individual doses and fluid needs for all routes
4. Identifying the correct patient when the patient cannot speak (using multiple identifiers)
5. Assessing side effects and complications in nonverbal patients

The nurse has extra responsibilities to protect the safety of the pediatric patient.

➤ Pediatric patients cannot protect themselves from medication errors. Many cannot identify themselves and are not in a position to question medications and medication orders or to verbalize physical complaints. In addition to using printed identification bracelets, bar codes, and other methods, the nurse should have a family member verify the identity of a pediatric patient.

➤ Pediatric patients suffer a much higher rate of medication errors than adults.

The preceding chapters provide a considerable foundation for mastering the calculations in this chapter. Weight-based orders and safe dose ranges for adults have been covered in Chapters 5 and 10.

> ▲ **Cultural Note**
>
> Cultural awareness of naming practices is important in avoiding mis-identification of a patient who is to receive medications and treatments. When identifying a pediatric patient, keep in mind that naming practices of parents and children vary widely among cultures. Family members may have different last names, based on particular paternal and maternal naming practices.

VOCABULARY

Body Surface Area (BSA)	Area covered by the skin, measured in square meters. Used for accurate dosing of powerful drugs such as drugs for chemotherapy and for adult and pediatric at-risk populations.
Milligrams per Kilogram (mg per kg)	Drug amount in milligrams based on kilograms of body weight. The most common unit of measurement for prescribed doses of medications for pediatric and frail patients and for powerful drugs.
Nomogram	Graphic representation of numerical relationships. A BSA nomogram is used to estimate square meters of body surface area. This is the least accurate method of calculating BSA.
Safe Dose Range (SDR)	Minimum-to-maximum therapeutic dose range for a target population: adult, child, infant, neonate, or elderly.
Square Meter (m²)	Metric unit of area measurement. Powerful medications, particularly anti-cancer medications, may be based on square meters of BSA.

Comparing Adult and Pediatric Medication Doses and Schedules

➤ Examine the selected examples in Table 13-1, and note the differences in dosing and units of measurement for adults and children.

There may be multiple drug dosage recommendations based on precise age groups and on various disease conditions for which one drug may be prescribed.

1 Which of the recommended SDRs for amoxicillin is weight-based: the adult or the child? (Refer to Table 13-1.)	**ASK YOURSELF** **Q & A**
_____	**MY ANSWER**

Taking 2 or 3 minutes to verify a safe dose order with a current pediatric drug reference and/or pharmacy may prevent a tragic error.	**CLINICAL RELEVANCE**

TABLE 13-1	Drug Dosage Comparison by Age Group
Name of Drug	**Dose Comparison**
▶ **Potassium Chloride Infusions (KCl)***	SDR, **Adult,** Individualized: IV 20–60 mEq q24h 200 mEq per 24 hr for hypokalemia is usually not exceeded. 40 mEq dilution per liter preferred SDR, **Child,** Individualized: IV 1–4 mEq per kg of body weight per 24 hr *or* 10 mEq per hr, whichever is <u>less</u>, not to exceed 40 mEq per 24 hr. Must be at least 40 mEq dilution per liter. Monitor serum potassium levels. Contact prescriber if patient is fluid restricted. Monitor ECG for symptoms of hypokalemia and hyperkalemia. Pediatrics: KCl must be infused on electronic infusion pump. Obtain written order for *each* infusion.
▶ **Morphine Sulfate** Pain relief Postoperative analgesia Severe chronic cancer pain	**Adult,** IV: 2.5-15 mg q4h **Child,** IV: 0.01-0.04 mg per kg per hr **Neonate,** IV: 0.015-0.02 mg per kg per hr* **Child,** IV: 0.025-2.6 mg per kg per hr
Amoxicillin	**Adult,** PO: 250-500 mg q8h **Child,** PO: 25-50 mg per kg per day (max 60-80 mg per kg per day divided q8h)
▶ **Digoxin IV Injection**	Initial loading (digitalizing dose) **Premature:** 15-25 mcg per kg; **2–5 yrs:** 25-35 mcg per kg; **over 10 years:** 8-12 mcg per kg

*A neonate refers to an infant in the first 4 weeks of life. Consult drug references for child age-related dose guidelines. They vary.

➤ Slashes (/) will be seen in printed drug references. Write out "per" for slashes to avoid misinterpretation and medication errors.

RAPID PRACTICE 13-1	Medication Dosing Differences for Children and Adults

ESTIMATED COMPLETION TIME: 10 to 15 minutes   **ANSWERS ON:** page 504

DIRECTIONS: *Examine Table 13-1 to answer the questions pertaining to SDR guidelines.*

1 What action must be taken if a patient is fluid restricted and potassium is ordered?

_____

2 What is the difference in the *maximum* doses of morphine sulfate for a child with postoperative pain and a child with severe chronic cancer pain?

_____

3 What is the *maximum* recommended initial loading dose of Digoxin IV injection for a child over 10 yrs? _____; A premature infant? _____

Calculating Kilograms From Pounds and Ounces

A patient's body weight in pounds or kilograms is usually calculated to the nearest tenth for determining pediatric doses.

➤ It is important to note that ounces must be converted to tenths of a pound *before* kilograms are calculated. For example, 5 lb 4 oz is *not* equal to 5.4 lb.

EXAMPLES

How many kilograms are equivalent to 5 lb 4 oz?

First: Convert 5 lb 4 oz to pounds.

Conversion factor: 16 oz = 1 lb

➤ Ounces must be converted to tenths of a pound *before* kilograms are calculated. 5 lb 4 oz is *not* equal to 5.4 pounds.

Step 1	=	Step 2	×	Step 3	=	Answer
Desired Answer Units	=	Starting Factor	×	Given Quantity and Conversion Factor(s)	=	Estimate, Multiply, Evaluate
lb	=	$\dfrac{1\ lb}{\dfrac{16\ oz}{4}}$	×	$\dfrac{\overset{1}{\cancel{4\ oz}}}{1}$	=	$\dfrac{1}{4} = 0.25\ lb$

Pediatric doses are frequently calculated to the hundredths place.

The equation to convert ounces to pounds will be written like this:

$$lb = \frac{1\ lb}{\dfrac{16\ oz}{4}} \times \frac{\overset{1}{\cancel{4\ oz}}}{1} = 0.25\ lb$$

Total pounds = 5 lb + 0.25 lb = 5.25 lb, which is rounded up to 5.3 lb

Next: Convert 5.3 lb to kilograms.

Conversion factor: 2.2 lb = 1 kg.

Step 1	=	Step 2	×	Step 3	=	Answer
Desired Answer Units	=	Starting Factor	×	Given Quantity and Conversion Factor(s)	=	Estimate, Multiply, Evaluate
kg	=	$\dfrac{1\ kg}{2.2\ \cancel{lb}}$	×	$\dfrac{5.3\ \cancel{lb}}{1}$	=	2.4 kg

The final equation will be written like this:

$$kg = \frac{1\ kg}{2.2\ \cancel{lb}} \times \frac{5.3\ \cancel{lb}}{1} = 2.4\ kg$$

Analysis: Two simple conversion equations were used for this problem. Ounces needed to be changed to lb and then added to the 5 lb.

Evaluation: The answer unit is correct: kg. A rough estimate of (lb ÷ 2) supports the answer. (Math check: 5.3 ÷ 2.2 = 2.4.) The equation is balanced.

➤ Estimates can alert you to major math errors. Always verify your estimates.

RAPID PRACTICE 13-2 Converting Pounds to Kilograms

ESTIMATED COMPLETION TIME: 20 to 25 minutes   ANSWERS ON: page 504

DIRECTIONS: *Estimate and calculate the weight in kg. Calculate the weight in kg to the nearest tenth of a kilogram using DA-style equations. Verify the result with a calculator. Remember to change ounces to pounds if necessary.*

1   12 lb 3 oz
   a.   Estimated kg wt: _____
   b.   Actual wt in kg:
         DA equation:

   c.   Evaluation: _____

2   20 lb 6 oz
   a.   Estimated kg wt: _____
   b.   Actual wt in kg:
         DA equation:

   c.   Evaluation: _____

3   4 lb 8 oz
   a.   Estimated kg wt: _____
   b.   Actual wt in kg:
         DA equation:

   c.   Evaluation: _____

4   25 lb 9 oz
   a.   Estimated kg wt: _____
   b.   Actual wt in kg:
         DA equation:

   c.   Evaluation: _____

5   18 lb 12 oz
   a.   Estimated kg wt: _____
   b.   Actual wt in kg:
         DA equation:

   c.   Evaluation: _____

Calculating Safe Dose Range (SDR)

➤ Review the logic and example of the multi-step process for evaluating an order for safe dose. A calculator is helpful.

STEPS

1 Obtain the total body weight in the desired terms.
2 Calculate the SDR.
3 Compare and evaluate the order with the SDR. Contact the prescriber if the order is not within the SDR.
➤ 4 If the order is safe, estimate, calculate, and evaluate the dose.

EXAMPLES

Ordered: Drug Y, 60 mg PO per day in AM

Patient's wt: 26 lb 6oz

SDR: 5-10 mg per kg per day in a single dose

Supplied: Drug Y, 100 mg per 5 mL

Conversion factors: 16 oz = 1 lb and 2.2 lb = 1 kg

Steps

1. **Total lb** $= \dfrac{1 \text{ lb}}{16 \text{ oz}} \times \dfrac{6 \text{ oz}}{1} = 0.375$, rounded to 0.4 lb.

   $26 + 0.4 \text{ lb} = 26.4 \text{ total lb}$

Total kg: *(not needed for order; total lb to kg will be entered within SDR equation)**

2. **SDR for this child:**

   $$\frac{\text{mg}}{\text{day}} = \frac{5 \text{ mg}}{\text{kg} \times \text{day}} \times \frac{1 \text{ kg}}{2.2 \text{ lb}} \times \frac{26.4 \text{ lb}}{1} = 60 \text{ mg per day low safe dose}$$

   $$\frac{\text{mg}}{\text{day}} = \frac{10 \text{ mg}}{\text{kg} \times \text{day}} \times \frac{1 \text{ kg}}{2.2 \text{ lb}} \times \frac{26.4 \text{ lb}}{1} = 120 \text{ mg per day high safe dose}$$

3. **Evaluation:** It can be seen at a glance that the dose ordered is within the SDR for the total amount and the schedule. Medication is safe to give.

4. **Dose Calculation:**

Estimate: Will be giving less than 5 mL

   $$\frac{\text{mL}}{\text{dose}} = \frac{\frac{1}{5} \text{ mL}}{\frac{100 \text{ mg}}{2}} \times \frac{60 \text{ mg}}{\text{dose}} = 3 \text{ mL per dose}$$

Analysis and evaluation: The equation is balanced. This is a reasonable dose because the order was for slightly more than one-half the number of mg supplied in 5 mL.

———————
*Had the order been for mg per kg or mcg per kg, the lb-to-kg conversion would have been done separately first.

• Note that once the *total number of pounds* is determined, it is entered in the SDR equations with the conversion formula to kilograms.

➤ Do not confuse the SDR doses with the ordered dose.

---

1 What are the four main steps in the sequence for evaluating and calculating the recommended safe dose? (State your answer using one to three key words for each step.)

ASK YOURSELF

_____ **MY ANSWER**

RAPID PRACTICE 13-3 Evaluating Medication Orders for SDR

ESTIMATED COMPLETION TIME: 25 minutes   **ANSWERS ON:** page 504

DIRECTIONS: *Obtain total lb and change to kg if needed. Calculate the SDR. Compare the ordered dose with the SDR in same units of measurement (compare mcg to mcg, mg to mg, and g to g using metric conversion formulas). Evaluate the order for safe dose.*

1   **Ordered:** Drug Y, 250 mg PO 4 times daily. SDR for children: 1–1.5 g per day in 4 divided doses.

    a. SDR for children: _____

    b. Evaluation of order: _____

    c. Evaluation: *Safe to give* or *Hold and clarify promptly with prescriber?* (Circle one.)

2   **Ordered:** Drug Y, 35 mg IM stat

    SDR for children: 1–3 mg per kg q4-6h

    Patient wt: 20 lb 4 oz

    a. Estimated kg wt: _____ Actual kg wt: _____

    b. SDR for this child: _____

    DA equation:

    c. Evaluation: *Safe to give* or *Hold and clarify promptly with prescriber?* (Circle one.)

3   **Ordered:** Drug Y, 5 mg IV q8h. SDR for children: 200–500 mcg per kg per day in 3 divided doses. Patient's weight: 12 lb.

    a. Estimated kg wt: _____ Actual kg wt: _____

    b. SDR for this child: _____

    DA equation:

    c. Evaluation: *Safe to give* or *Hold and clarify promptly with prescriber.* (Circle one.)

4   **Ordered:** Drug Y, 2 mg PO q6h. SDR for children: 500–800 mcg per kg per day in 4-6 divided doses. Patient's weight: 22 lb.

    a. Estimated kg wt: _____ Actual kg wt: _____

    b. SDR for this child: _____

    DA equation:

    c. Evaluation: *Safe to give* or *Hold and clarify promptly with prescriber?* (Circle one.)

5 **Ordered:** Drug Y, 500 mcg IV per hr. SDR for children: 10–20 mcg per kg per hr. Patient's weight: 66 lb.

  a. Estimated kg wt: _____ Actual kg wt: _____

  b. SDR for this child: _____

      DA equation:

  c. Evaluation: *Safe to give* or *Hold and clarify promptly with prescriber?* (Circle one.)

Body Surface Area (BSA)

The weight-based medication orders for mg per kg and mcg per kg are the most frequently encountered units of measurement found in medication orders for children. Occasionally, the nurse will encounter an order for a child or an adult based on body surface area (BSA) in square meters (m²) of skin. BSA-based dosing is considered superior to weight-based dosing for specific medications, particularly doses that can easily be toxic such as chemotherapy agents.

Most medications ordered in square meters of BSA are calculated by the pharmacist or prescriber and frequently are antineoplastic drugs administered by a nurse who has chemotherapy certification. Square meters of BSA may also be used for the SDR of drugs other than anticancer agents, particularly for infants, children, and geriatric patients.

The BSA nomogram is an *estimation* of BSA (and the least accurate) and is faster to use than the formulas. Figure 13-1 is an example of a nomogram of a BSA-derived medication dose.

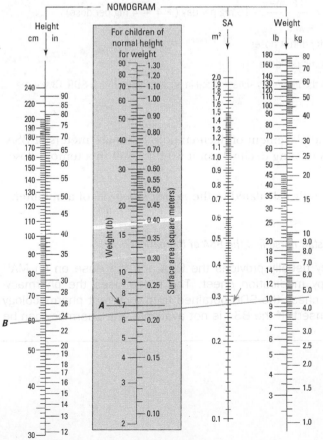

FIGURE 13-1 Modified West Nomogram for Body Surface Area Estimation. The red line denoted by arrow *A* in the highlighted column, "Children of Normal Height for Weight," illustrates a BSA of 0.22 m² for a child weighing 7 pounds. Calculations for children who are *not* at normal height for weight as determined by pediatric standard growth charts will have a different BSA for their weight. The outside columns are used to plot their height and weight. The BSA, 0.28 m² is read at the intersection as indicated by the red arrow over line *B* on the column titled "*SA*" by connecting the two plotted measurements with a straight line *B*. There are additional nomograms for adults. (Nomogram modified with data from Kliegman RM, St. Geme JW, Blum NJ, Shah SS, Tasker RC, Wilson KM: *Nelson textbook of pediatrics*, ed 21, Philadelphia, 2020, Saunders.)

The nurse is expected to be able to define BSA, identify square meters, and, *most important*, distinguish among m² and mg and mcg metric measurements when reading orders, medication records, and current drug references and when calculating SDR. The nurse rarely calculates the BSA. Pharmacy usually calculates this, mixes the dose, and delivers the drug to the unit in the prescribed amount to be administered.

The BSA is derived from formulas based on the patient's weight and height. There are two BSA formulas, one for the metric system and one for the English (or imperial) system.

Metric Formula	English Formula
$$\sqrt{\frac{\text{weight (kg)} \times \text{height (cm)}}{3600}} = \textbf{BSA}\ (m^2)$$	$$\sqrt{\frac{\text{weight (lb)} \times \text{height (inches)}}{3131}} = \textbf{BSA}\ (m^2)$$

Calculating milligrams per square meter (mg per m²)

In calculating the mg per m² of BSA, the sequence is the same as that used in mcg- and mg-based SDR calculations.

➤ The calculation of milligrams per square meter is performed using a DA-style equation or simple multiplication, just as it is for calculating milligrams per kilogram (e.g., 2 mg per m² means "2 milligrams of medicine for each square meter of body surface area").

EXAMPLES

Examine the following example.

Ordered: Drug Y, 4 mg PO qid

Patient's BSA: 0.8 m². SDR: 20 mg per m² daily in 4 divided doses.

$$\frac{\text{mg}}{\text{day}} = \frac{20\ \text{mg}}{\text{m}^2\ \text{day}} \times \frac{0.8\ \text{m}^2}{1} = 16\ \text{mg per day}\ (\div\ 4 = 4\ \text{mg per dose})$$

SDR: 16 mg total per day divided in 4 doses

Order: 16 mg total per day, 4 mg per dose

Evaluation: The total dose and the frequency schedule are in accordance with the SDR. Give 4 mg.

➤ Pay close attention to the placement of decimal points. Square meters of BSA are *very small amounts*. A missing decimal point would result in a tenfold dose error.

➤ Pediatric doses are generally calculated to the *nearest hundredth* of a milliliter. Check agency policies.

FAQ   *Where will the staff nurse find the BSA of the patient?*

ANSWER   The pharmacy usually provides the BSA and the dose on an MAR or a separate chemotherapy medication sheet. The nurse uses the pharmacy-provided BSA calculation to check the SDR obtained from a current pharmacology reference or drug package insert. If the BSA is not available, the pharmacy can be contacted.

RAPID PRACTICE 13-4	Evaluating Pediatric SDR

ESTIMATED COMPLETION TIME: 15 to 20 minutes   **ANSWERS ON:** page 505

DIRECTIONS: *Evaluate the following orders. For BSA in square meters (m², read the nomogram in Figure 13-1 and calculate the safe dose. Set up a DA equation, and verify your answer with a calculator. State the reason for giving or withholding the medication.*

1 **Ordered:** gentamicin 125 mg q8h IV, for a child with a severe infection weighing 50 kg. SDR: 2–2.5 mg per kg q8h.

    a. Is BSA needed? Why or why not? _____

    b. SDR for this patient: _____

    DA equation:

    c. Evaluation: *Safe to give* or *Hold and clarify promptly with prescriber?* (Circle one and state reason.) _____

2 **Ordered:** An IV infusion of heparin 225 units per hr for a baby of normal height for weight of 10 lb.

    SDR: 20,000 units per m² q24h continuous IV infusion

    a. BSA for this child: _____

    b. SDR for this patient: _____

    DA equation:

    c. Evaluation: *Safe to give* or *Hold and clarify promptly with prescriber?* (Circle one and state reason.) _____

3 **Ordered:** methotrexate 15 mg PO daily, for a child with leukemia who is of normal height for weight of 70 lb. SDR: 3.3 mg per m² per day.

    a. BSA for this child: _____

    b. SDR for this patient: _____

    DA equation:

    c. Evaluation: *Safe to give* or *Hold and clarify promptly with prescriber?* (Circle one and state reason.) _____

➤ There may be a good reason for a very high dosage order, such as severity of illness or nonresponsiveness to a lower dosage. The nurse must clarify and document the response from the prescriber, as in the following example:

"4/25/2018, 1800: Dose of Drug Y, 5 mg per hr IV for 22-kg child, verified with prescriber per TC. John Smith, R.N."

4 **Ordered:** vincristine 1 mg IV once a week, for a child with Hodgkin's disease who is of normal height for weight of 30 lb. SDR: 1.5–2 mg per m^2 per week.

   a. BSA for this child: _____

   b. SDR for this patient: _____

   DA equation:

   c. Evaluation: *Safe to give* or *Hold and clarify promptly with prescriber?* (Circle one and state reason.) _____

5 **Ordered:** dopamine 20 mcg per min IV, for an infant with respiratory distress syndrome who weighs 5 kg. SDR: starting dose 1–5 mcg per kg per min.

   a. Is BSA needed? Why or why not? _____

   b. SDR for this patient: _____

   DA equation:

   c. Evaluation: *Safe to give* or *Hold and clarify promptly with prescriber?* (Circle one and state reason.) _____

Medication Administration Equipment

In addition to dose modifications, the equipment used to deliver medication to a child may be different from that used for an adult. Droppers, bottle nipples, measuring teaspoons, special oral syringes, and regular syringes **with the needle removed,** with or without a short tubing extension, may be used.

CLINICAL RELEVANCE

The medications may be administered with pleasant-tasting, nonessential foods (such as applesauce or pudding) to disguise an unfamiliar or unwelcome taste. A pill-crushing device or mortar and pestle may be needed to grind and mix tablets as long as they are not enteric coated (Figure 13-2). Water, applesauce, or sherbet may be used to mix the medication or to follow the medication, depending on diet orders, swallowing ability, and age. Popsicles may be permitted immediately after a medicine to offset the taste. Some children prefer to drink from a 1-oz medicine cup.

➤ If a nipple is used to deliver medication, rinse the nipple with water first so that the medicine will flow rather than stick to the nipple.

➤ Follow the medicine with water or formula *within the fluid limitations* permitted for the patient (Figure 13-3).

When family members are present, they can be very helpful by holding the child and/or giving the oral medication and something more pleasant-tasting to follow.

Remember that medications can be measured accurately with a syringe and then transferred to another receptacle such as a cup or a bottle.

➤ Do NOT mix medicines in milk or formula. If the child consumes only part of the liquid, the amount of the dose received is uncertain.

➤ Take extra measures to assess swallowing ability before attempting to give any medications by mouth to at-risk populations. This may include checking the gag reflex with a tongue blade.

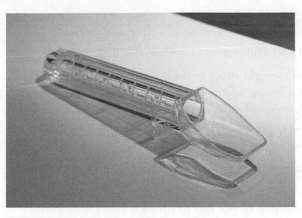
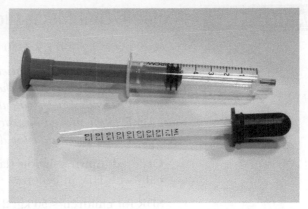

FIGURE 13-2 A, Pediatric oral medication device. **B,** Additional pediatric oral medication devices.

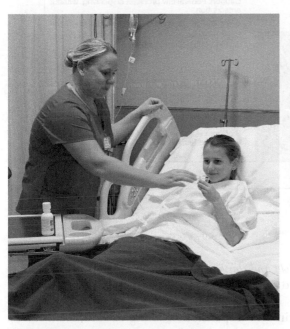
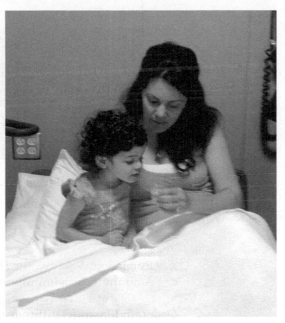

FIGURE 13-3 A, Child receiving liquid oral medications. **B,** Assistance from a parent for nonpainful procedures is desirable.

➤ The presence of a gag reflex alone is not enough to assume swallowing ability. Follow up with a test of swallowing some sips of water. Do not assume that a baby can always drink from a bottle. Infants and children can have swallowing problems, just as adults can.

➤ Reminder: Never cut unscored tablets. Never crush enteric-coated, ER, SR, or gel-coated medications. Do not crush capsules. Check with pharmacy and/or prescriber if it is deemed necessary to alter the ordered form of medication.

CLINICAL RELEVANCE

Giving medications to pediatric patients can be a challenge. Some nurses have the intuitive skills necessary to obtain cooperation, and others acquire skills through experience. It helps the pediatric nursing student to shadow an experienced pediatric nurse. Patient charting records and handoff report should provide clues as to the child's behaviors and preferences.

| **RAPID PRACTICE 13-5** | Pediatric Oral Medications |

ESTIMATED COMPLETION TIME: 30 to 60 minutes   **ANSWERS ON:** page 505

DIRECTIONS: *Determine the patient's weight in kg to the nearest tenth if needed. Calculate SDR, and evaluate the order for appropriate dose and schedule. If the order is safe to administer, calculate liquid doses to the nearest tenth and doses less than 1 mL to the nearest hundredth of a mL. If the drug is to be held, state the reason but do not calculate the dose.*

1 **Ordered:** Epivir solution (lamivudine), an antiviral agent, 18 mg PO tid for a baby with HIV infection

   SDR for children <50 kg: 2 mg per kg per day in divided doses q8h with zidovudine

   Patient's weight: 20 lb

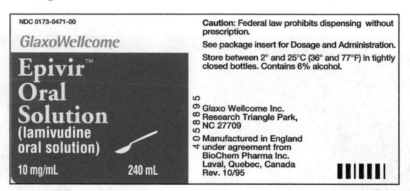

   a. SDR for this child: _____

   DA equation:

   b. Evaluation: *Safe to give* or *Hold and clarify promptly with prescriber?* (Circle one.)
   c. Amount to be administered if safe dose: _____

2 **Ordered:** Biaxin (clarithromycin oral suspension) 150 mg PO bid, for a child with otitis media.

   SDR for this child: 15 mg per kg per day in 2 divided doses

   Patient's weight: 44 lb

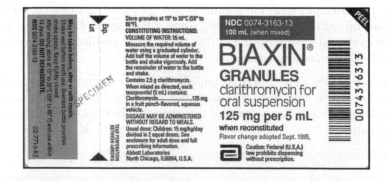

   a. SDR for this child: _____

   DA equation:

   b. Evaluation: *Safe to give* or *Hold and clarify promptly with prescriber?*
   (Circle one and state reason.) _____
   c. Dilution directions: _____
   d. Amount to be administered if safe dose: _____

3 **Ordered:** leucovorin 20 mg PO 6 hr after administration of the antineoplastic methotrexate today to prevent toxicity.

SDR: 10 mg per m^2 per dose

Patient's weight: 70 lb (31.8 kg). BSA: 1.10 m^2*

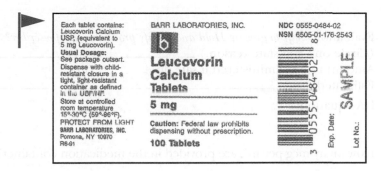

   a. SDR for this child: _____

   DA equation:

   b. Evaluation: *Safe to give* or *Hold and clarify promptly with prescriber?*
   (Circle one and state reason.) _____
   c. Amount to be administered if safe dose: _____

   DA equation:

   d. Evaluation: _____

4 **Ordered:** Lanoxin (digoxin) elixir 0.1 mg PO bid maintenance dose, for a 4-year-old child with congestive heart failure who has already received a loading dose.

SDR for children >2 years: loading dose 0.02–0.04 mg per kg divided q8h over 24 hr; maintenance dose 0.006–0.012 mg per kg in divided doses q12h

Patient's weight: 18 kg

_____

*Trailing zeros (e.g., 1.10 m^2) are not permitted (per TJC) in patient medication-related documents. They are encountered in printed laboratory, drug, and scientific references and are appropriate for BSA nomograms.

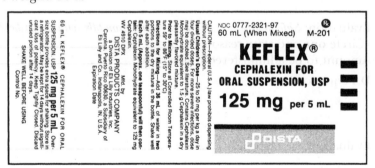

a. SDR for this child to nearest hundredth of a mg: _____

DA equation:

b. Evaluation: *Safe to give* or *Hold and clarify promptly with prescriber?*
(Circle one and state reason.) _____

c. Amount to be administered if safe dose:

Estimated dose: _____

DA equation:

d. How many mcg per mL are provided in the medication container? _____

5 **Ordered:** Keflex (cephalexin for oral suspension) 150 mg PO qid for a child
with a mild upper respiratory infection.

Read the label to obtain the SDR.

Patient's weight: 36 lb

a. SDR for this child: _____

DA equation:

b. Evaluation: *Safe to give* or *Hold and clarify promptly with prescriber?*
(Circle one and state reason.) _____

c. Total number of mg in container: _____

d. Dilution directions (use brief phrases): _____

e. Volume to be administered if safe dose: _____

Q & A	**ASK YOURSELF**	1	What amount would have been administered if the nurse was unfamiliar with square meters and used the weight in kilograms or pounds instead of square meters in problem 2 to calculate the dose?
	MY ANSWER		_____

Injection Sites

Injections are traumatic for pediatric patients. IV Saline Lock ports are often used to administer medications.

Check agency policies regarding injection sites. With all injections, the potential site must be fully visible and carefully assessed.

The vastus lateralis muscle can be used from birth to adulthood but is a *preferred injection site* for babies younger than 7 months of age (Figure 13-4).

These three injection sites are best for pediatric patients:

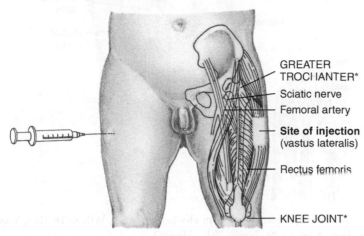

GREATER
TROCHANTER*
Sciatic nerve
Femoral artery
Site of injection
(vastus lateralis)
Rectus femoris
KNEE JOINT*

FIGURE 13-4 Injection site for vastus lateralis. (From Hockenberry MJ, Wilson D: *Wong's nursing care of infants and children,* ed 11, St. Louis, 2019, Mosby.)

➤ The ventrogluteal muscle is an *alternative site* for children over 7 months of age and adults (Figure 13-5).

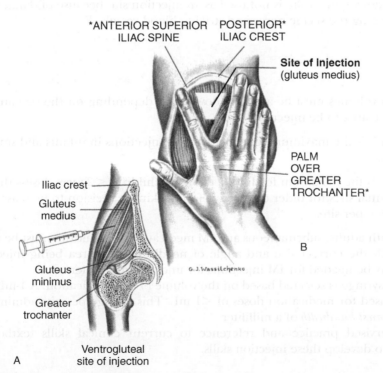

ANTERIOR SUPERIOR   POSTERIOR
ILIAC SPINE   ILIAC CREST

Site of Injection
(gluteus medius)

PALM
OVER
GREATER
TROCHANTER*

B

Iliac crest
Gluteus
medius
Gluteus
minimus
Greater
trochanter

G.J.Wassilchenko

Ventrogluteal
A   site of injection

FIGURE 13-5 A, Ventrogluteal injection site. **B,** Gluteus medius injection site. (From Hockenberry MJ, Wilson D: *Wong's nursing care of infants and children,* ed 11, St. Louis, 2019, Mosby.)

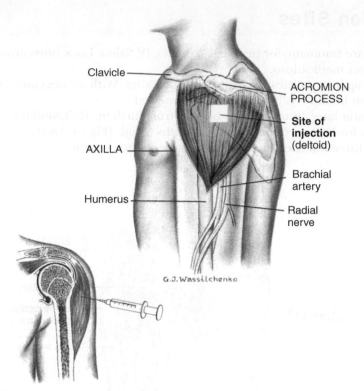

Clavicle

ACROMION PROCESS

Site of injection (deltoid)

AXILLA

Brachial artery

Humerus

Radial nerve

G.J.Wassilchenko

FIGURE 13-6 Deltoid injection site. (From Hockenberry MJ, Wilson D: *Wong's nursing care of infants and children,* ed 11, St. Louis, 2019, Mosby.)

➤ The deltoid site may be used for small-volume, non-irritating medications (0.5 to 1 mL) in older children and adults with well-developed deltoid muscles (Figure 13-6).

➤ The dorsogluteal site is not used as an injection site because of danger of damaging the sciatic nerve and striking blood vessels.

Safe Injection Volumes

Injection volumes must be adjusted downward, depending on the size and condition of the area to be injected.

➤ 0.5 mL is the maximum for subcutaneous injections in infants and small children.

➤ 1 mL is the maximum for IM injections in children <2 years. Assess the potential sites for older children before making a decision to increase the volume per site.

As with adults, subcutaneous and IM medications in children must be administered with the correct size and angle of needle for the area being injected. An angle may be needed for IM injections for underweight patients.

The syringe is selected based on the volume of the medication. A 1-mL syringe may be used for medication doses of <1 mL. This syringe permits administration to the *nearest hundredth* of a milliliter.

Supervised practice and reference to current clinical skills textbooks are needed to develop these injection skills.

| **RAPID PRACTICE 13-6** | Subcutaneous and Intramuscular Injections |

ESTIMATED COMPLETION TIME: 25 to 30 minutes   **ANSWERS ON:** page 506

DIRECTIONS: *Evaluate the following orders. If the dose is safe to administer, calculate the dose. Evaluate all your equations. Indicate the nearest measurable dose with an arrow on the syringe provided.*

1   **Ordered:** epinephrine injection 1.2 mg subcut stat, a bronchodilator for a child with asthma.

SDR for children: IM or SC 0.01–0.03 mg per kg q5min if needed

Patient's weight: 66 lb.

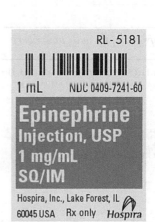

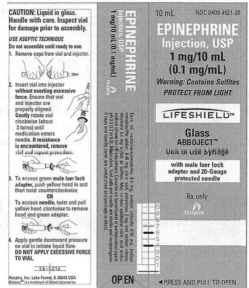

a.   SDR for this child: _____

DA equation:

b.   Evaluation: *Safe to give* or *Hold and clarify promptly with prescriber?*
        (Circle one and state reason.) _____

c.   What is the amount of difference in concentration between the two
        labels? _____

d.   Which of the two labels is more concentrated? _____

e.   Amount to be administered if safe to give:

DA equation:

f.   Evaluation: _____

2   **Ordered:** Humalog insulin 3 units subcut 4 times daily ac and at bedtime, for a newly diagnosed 10-year-old child with diabetes type 1.

SDR for children: initial 2-4 units subcut 4 times daily ac and at bedtime

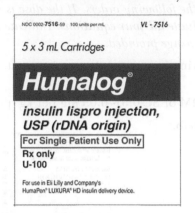

NDC 0002-**7516**-59   100 units per mL   **VL - 7516**

5 x 3 mL Cartridges

Humalog®

insulin lispro injection, USP (rDNA origin)

For Single Patient Use Only
Rx only
U-100

For use in Eli Lilly and Company's
HumaPen® LUXURA® HD insulin delivery device.

a.   SDR for this child: _____

b.   Evaluation: *Safe to give* or *Hold and clarify promptly with prescriber?* (Circle one and state reason.) _____

c.   Draw an arrow pointing to the dose on the syringe that would be easier to read for this dose.

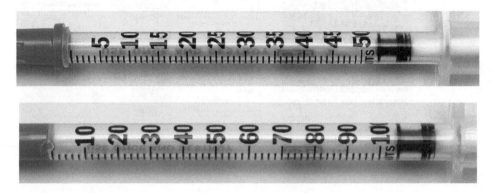

d.   Would a bedtime snack be needed? If so, why?

_____

➤ Remember that you may encounter *SC* and *HS* as abbreviations for "subcutaneous" and "bedtime." Do not write these abbreviations because they can be misinterpreted. The word *subcutaneous* or the abbreviation *subcut* should be used. *Hour of sleep* or *bedtime* should be written rather than *HS*.

3   **Ordered:** buprenorphine hydrochloride 80 mcg IM, an analgesic for a child with pain

SDR for children: IM 0.004 mg/kg IM q4-6h

Patient's weight: 44 lb.

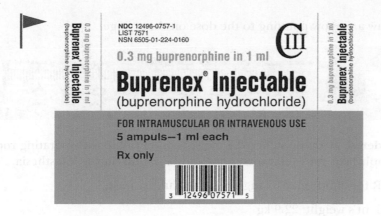

NDC 12496-0757-1
LIST 7571
NSN 6505-01-224-0160

C III

0.3 mg buprenorphine in 1 ml

Buprenex® Injectable
(buprenorphine hydrochloride)

FOR INTRAMUSCULAR OR INTRAVENOUS USE
5 ampuls—1 ml each

Rx only

a. SDR for this child: _____

   DA equation:

b. Evaluation: *Safe to give* or *Hold and clarify promptly with prescriber?*
   (Circle one and state reason.) _____

c. Amount to be administered if safe to give to nearest hundredth of a mL:

   DA equation:

d. Evaluation: _____

4 **Ordered:** phytonadione (vitamin K) 4 mg IM once a week prophylactically
for hypothrombinemia, for a child on prolonged TPN therapy who has not
walked in several months.

SDR for children: 2-5 mg once weekly IM

1 mL   NDC 0409-
              9158-01
VITAMIN K₁ Inj.
Phytonadione Injectable
Emulsion, USP
10 mg/mL
Contains no more than
110 mcg/L of aluminum.
Protect from light.   ℞ only
RL-0654 (10/04)
Hospira, Inc.
Lake Forest, IL 60045 USA

a. SDR for this child: _____

b. Evaluation: *Safe to give* or *Hold and clarify promptly with prescriber?*
   (Circle one and state reason.) _____

c. Amount to be administered if safe to give:

   DA equation:

d. Evaluation: _____

Draw an arrow pointing to the dose on the syringe.

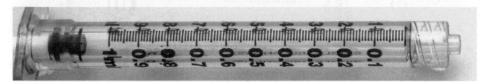

5 **Ordered:** atropine sulfate 0.2 mg subcut on call to the operating room, as prophylaxis for excess secretions and salivation during anesthesia.

SDR for children: 0.01 mg per kg subcut per dose

Patient's weight: 22.9 kg

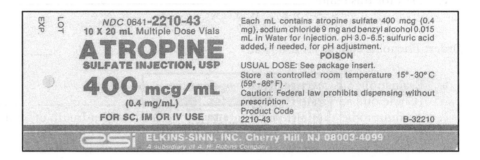

a. SDR for this child: _____

DA equation:

b. Evaluation: *Safe to give* or *Hold and clarify promptly with prescriber?*
(Circle one and state reason.) _____

c. Amount to be administered if safe to give:

DA equation:

d. Evaluation: _____

Draw an arrow pointing to the dose on the syringe.

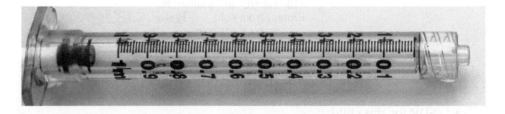

Fluid Requirements

Volume needs vary and need to be adjusted for the weight and age of the child. Infants have a larger percentage of fluid volume as a percentage of body weight than do older children and adults. They also have a greater BSA in relation to body mass, which causes them to lose more water through the skin than do older children and adults. They lose a higher percentage of fluids from the lungs because of their more rapid respirations and excrete more urine because it is less concentrated.

➤ Overhydration and dehydration can present a grave risk to pediatric patients. There are several formulas for calculating fluid requirements. They

TABLE 13-2	Fluid Requirements of Healthy Children and Adults			
			AVERAGE FLUID INTAKE REQUIREMENT	
Weight	Normal Fluid Volume Need	Sample Weight (kg)	Daily	Hourly
Neonate	90 mL per kg per 24 hr	3 kg	270 mL	11 mL
Up to 10 kg	120 mL per kg per 24 hr after age 7 days	8 kg	960 mL	40 mL
11–20 kg	1000 mL + 50 mL per kg over 10 kg	15 kg	1250 mL	52 mL
Over 20 kg	1500 mL + 20 mL per kg over 20 kg	25 kg	1600 mL	67 mL
Average adult	2-3 liters per day	68 kg	2000-3000 mL	125 mL

are adjusted for maintenance and replacement as well as for conditions requiring *fluid restrictions*. Some formulas are based on caloric metabolism and others on BSA. Keep in mind these concepts and the data in Table 13-2, which follows, when administering any kind of fluids and oral or parenteral medications to pediatric patients.

Table 13-2 illustrates the average fluid requirements of *healthy* adults, babies, and children of various weights.

---

1 What would be the normal 24-hr fluid intake requirement for a baby weighing 8 kg (17.6 lb) compared with an adult weighing 68 kg?

ASK YOURSELF

MY ANSWER

_____

CLINICAL RELEVANCE

➤ A child with cardiac, respiratory, or renal dysfunction may have severe fluid restrictions imposed. Such restrictions would affect the amount of fluid to be administered with medications as well as IV solution flow rates.

➤ If a pediatric patient is receiving fluids from other sources, such as bottles and cups, the IV volume must be adjusted downward accordingly, per the health care provider orders. Oral liquid medications are counted as part of the 24-hour fluid limits set by the prescriber, as are liquids that accompany solid oral medications.

Intravenous Injections

➤ Infusion volumes for infants and children are much *smaller* and infusion rates *slower* than for average adults. Use of a volumetric infusion pump for IV fluids and medications is preferred for pediatric patients.

Using a volume-control device

The use of a volume-control device protects patients from accidental fluid and drug overload if the flow rate is programmed correctly. Volume-control devices may be used for four purposes:

1 Volume control devices are less commonly used now that sophisticated electronic IV infusion pumps "smart pumps" are available.

2 Volume control devices can be used with an electronic IV infusion pump or by gravity.

3 They protect from possible fluid overload from the main IV line. This is achieved by opening the clamp from the main IV line to fill the chamber with 1 or 2 hours worth of IV fluid, according to agency policy.

4 The medication may be added to the solution from the main IV bag or to a separate solution placed in the volume-control device. This would be an alternative to attaching a piggyback medicated solution to a port on a primary IV line. (Refer also to Chapter 9.)

Using Volume-Control Chambers to Protect Patients from Fluid and Drug Overload

EXAMPLES

Ordered: Drug Y in a continuous IV infusion at 1.5 mg per kg per hr

Available: 100 mg in 100 mL NS

Patient's weight: 8 kg

SDR: maximum 6 mg per kg per hr

Agency policy: 1 hour's worth of fluid volume is maximum amount permitted in volume control chamber.

$$\frac{mg}{hr} = \frac{1.5\ mg}{1\ \cancel{kg}} \times \frac{8\ \cancel{kg}}{hr} = 12\ mg\ per\ hr$$

To calculate the volume in mL per hr needed to deliver 12 mg per hr,

$$\frac{mL}{hr} = \frac{\overset{1}{\cancel{100}}\ mL}{\underset{1}{\cancel{100\ mg}}} \times \frac{12\ \cancel{mg}}{1\ hr} = 12\ mL\ per\ hr$$

The nurse opens the clamp on the main IV line, puts 1 hour's worth of medicated fluid (12 mL) in the volume-control device, and shuts the clamp to the main IV line (Figure 13-8). An alarm will be set off to alert staff to a need for chamber refill.

➤ Agency flush procedures must be followed.

Q & A ASK YOURSELF

1 An IV infusion contains 100 mg of drug in 250 mL of solution. What is the maximum amount of fluid and medicine that can flow into the patient very rapidly if the main IV line malfunctions (assuming there is no volume-control device in place)?

MY ANSWER _____

Using a Volume-Control Device to Administer Intravenous Medication The medication dose may be added with a syringe through the port to the chamber after the IV diluent is placed in the volume-control device (see Figure 13-7).

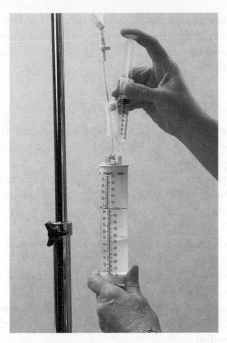

FIGURE 13-7 Adding medication to a volume control device. (From Perry AG, Potter PA, Ostendorf WR: *Clinical nursing skills and techniques,* ed 10, St. Louis, 2021, Mosby.)

➤ If a *different medication* than that shown on the label of the main IV fluid is added to a volume-control device, a medication label must be attached to the volume-control device.

For example, with a main IV solution of potassium in D5W and an ordered antibiotic of amikacin to be infused over 30 minutes, a label such as the following would be attached to the volume-control device:

> MEDICATION ADDED
>
> 1/11/2022, 1800, amikacin sulfate 50 mg per 50 mL D5W. Flow rate: 25 mL per hr.
>
> John Smith, R.N.

This label will alert the staff that a *flush* and possible flow rate change will be necessary after the medication infusion is completed.

Flushing a volume-control device

The volume-control device and tubing must be cleared of medication residue with a "flush" *before* and *after* the medication has been infused. If the flush solution is different from the main IV solution, a new label must be placed on the volume-control device to alert the staff that a flush is taking place. The label alerts the staff to *wait before* adding another medication to the system.

> FLUSH
>
> 1/11/2022, 1830, 15 mL D5W infusing
>
> John Smith, R.N.

Check agency policies for types and amounts of flushes. A flush may be indicated before and after a medication is administered and may consist of 5-10 mL or more of solution. It should be of an amount sufficient to clear the volume-control device and the rest of the IV line to the venous entry site.

Calculating for a volume-control device

- Calculate the *total amount of fluid* for the dose and diluent (e.g., 5 mL antibiotic to be diluted to 30 mL with NS) as stated in the drug insert or pediatric drug reference.
- Shut the clamp to the main IV line. Flush line according to agency policy. Place the diluent *minus* the amount of medicine in the calibrated chamber of the volume-control device (e.g., 30 mL − 5 mL medicine = 25 mL NS).
- Add the medicine and gently mix the medicine and diluent in the calibrated chamber.
- Administer the medicine at the ordered flow rate. Label the volume-control device.
- Flush the volume-control device with the needed amount and type of flush solution. Label the volume-control device for the flush. Reset the flow rate as needed.

➤ If an infusion pump is not available, a microdrip pediatric administration set with a DF of 60 is used with a volume-control device. Recall that the hourly drops per minute flow rate for a microdrip set is equal to the number of mL per hr ordered (Figure 13-8).

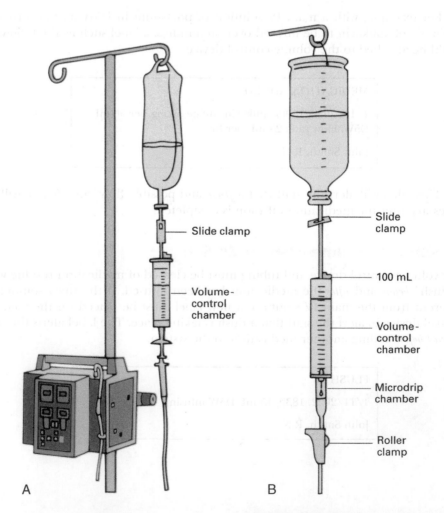

FIGURE 13-8 A, Electronic infusion pump with volume-control device. **B,** Gravity infusion with volume-control device and microdrip tubing.

RAPID PRACTICE 13-7	Volume-Control Device Flow Rates

ESTIMATED COMPLETION TIME: 10 minutes   **ANSWERS ON:** page 507

DIRECTIONS: *Examine the example in problem 1. Calculate the amount of medicine and flush to be administered. Refer to Intravenous Piggyback Solutions in Chapter 9 for review if necessary.*

1   **Ordered:** 2 mL medicine to be diluted to 25 mL D5W in a volume-control device on a volumetric pump and infused over 30 minutes.

   a. Amount of diluent to place in volume-control device:
   25 mL − 2 mL = 23 mL diluent
   b. Amount of medicine to place in volume-control device: 2 mL medicine
   c. IV flow rate to set on the pump: 50 mL per hr
   DA equation:

$$\frac{mL}{hr} = \frac{25\ mL}{\cancel{30\ min}\ 1} \times \frac{\cancel{60\ min}\ 2}{1\ hr} = 50\ mL\ per\ hr$$

   d. Evaluation: The equation is balanced. An IV flow rate of 50 mL over 60 minutes will deliver 25 mL in 30 minutes.

   Follow the medication with a 5- to 10-mL flush. Check agency policy for content and volume of flush.

2   **Ordered:** 25 mL of medicine to be diluted to 50 mL in NS in a volume-control device attached to a gravity infusion device with a pediatric microdrip tubing set to be administered over 1 hour. (Refer to Chapter 9 for a review of flow rate calculations for microdrip sets.)

   a. Amount of diluent to place in volume-control device: _____
   b. Amount of medicine to place in volume-control device: _____
   c. Flow rate to set on microdrip pediatric set: _____ drops per min

   Follow the medication with a 5- to 10-mL saline flush. Check agency policy.

3   **Ordered:** 10 mL medicine to be diluted to 20 mL NS in a volume-control device on a volumetric infusion pump and infused over 30 minutes.

   a. Amount of diluent to place in volume-control device: _____
   b. Amount of medicine to place in volume-control device: _____
   c. IV flow rate to set on pump: _____
   DA equation:

   d. Evaluation: _____

   Follow the medication with a 5- to 10-mL flush. Check agency policy.

4   **Ordered:** 3 mL of medication to be diluted to 15 mL in NS in a volume-control device on gravity infusion with microdrip tubing to be administered over 30 minutes.

   a. Amount of medicine to prepare for volume-control device: _____
   b. Flow rate to set on microdrip pediatric set: _____ drops per min
   DA equation:

   d. Evaluation: _____

   Follow the medication with a 5- to 10-mL flush. Check agency policy.

✳ *Communication*

Nurse A to Nurse B after calculating dose of IV heparin/insulin/vancomycin/potassium or other high-risk drugs for Baby B: *"Would you please double-check this order for me?"*

Nurse A: *"Yes. Let me see the patient record."* Nurse B verifies the baby's allergies and current weight, reads the order, checks the SDR in a current drug reference, checks the label, and calculates the dose.

Nurse B: *"The order is safe. This is the dose I calculated."*

Nurse A: *"I calculated a different dose. Let me recheck my numbers."* Nurse A finds an error in calculations and the corrected dose equals Nurse B's calculations.

Nurse B verifies the dose preparation by Nurse A. If it involved more than one drug, Nurse B verifies that the dose prepared from each container is correct.

What could be the consequence if any of these six steps were skipped: allergies, current weight, order, SDR, label, dose?

5 **Ordered:** 15 mL of medication to be diluted to 30 mL in D5W on a volumetric infusion pump to be administered over 20 minutes.

    a. Amount of diluent to place in volume-control device: _____

    b. Amount of medicine to place in volume-control device: _____

    c. Flow rate to set on infusion pump: _____

    DA equation:

    d. Evaluation: _____

Follow the medication with a 5- to 10-mL flush. Check agency policy.

Syringe pump infusers

A syringe pump system may be used to deliver *small-volume intermittent* infusions, which can also protect the patient from fluid and drug overload if the flow rate is programmed correctly. Syringe pump infusers can now be programmed for flow rates and alarms (Figure 13-9).

➤ To reduce errors, multiple national agencies are recommending independent double checks of high-risk drugs for pediatric and adult patients for *each* dose of the medication. Check your agency's policies also. Consult the pharmacist and/or prescriber if questions arise about the order.

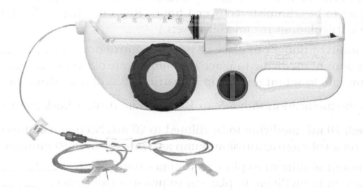

FIGURE 13-9 Freedom 60 syringe infusion pump system. (The FREEDOM60 is registered under KORU. We usually use this language in our marketing piece "The FREEDOM60® and FreedomEdge® Syringe Infusion Systems, Precision Flow Rate Tubing™ and HIgH-Flo Subcutaneous Safety Needle Sets™ are registered trademarks of KORU Medical Systems and are compliant with Medical Device Directive 93/42/EEC. KORU Medical Systems is ISO 13485 certified.")

Review of Infusion Rate Calculations

EXAMPLES

If the ordered dose is within the SDR, the nurse calculates the flow rate in mL per hr to the nearest measurable amount on the equipment.

Ordered: Drug Y continuous infusion at 30 mcg per hr

Patient's weight: 66 lb, or 30 kg

SDR for children: 20-35 mcg/kg per 24 hr in IV infusion

Available: 2 mg ampule in 250 mL.

SDR for this patient:	20 mcg × 30 kg = 600 mcg low safe dose q24h
(Use calculator)	35 mcg × 30 kg = 1050 mcg high safe dose q24h
Ordered dose:	30 mcg × 24 hr = 720 mcg per hr

(Use calculator)

Evaluation: The ordered daily dose is within the SDR and safe to give.

$$\frac{mL}{hr} = \frac{\overset{1}{\cancel{250}}\ mL}{\underset{1}{\cancel{2}\ mg}} \times \frac{1\ \cancel{mg}}{\underset{4}{\cancel{1000}\ mcg}} \times \frac{\overset{15}{\cancel{30}\ mcg}}{1\ hr} = \frac{15\ mL}{4\ hr} = 3.75\ mL\ per\ hr$$

Administer at 3.75 mL per hour.

➤ When using a calculator, always repeat the calculation twice.

Comparing Safe Dose Range and Order

➤ Remember to compare the SDR and the ordered dose in the *same* units of measurement and for the same time frame: mg to mg, mcg to mcg, and hours to hours. Do not confuse the SDR and the order when performing the comparisons. When a dose has been ordered outside the SDR, contact the prescriber promptly.

RAPID PRACTICE 13-8   Intravenous Medication Calculations

ESTIMATED COMPLETION TIME: 30 minutes to 1 hour   **ANSWERS ON:** page 507

DIRECTIONS: *Examine the example shown above. Solve the IV problems using DA equations.*

1   **Ordered:** phenobarbital sodium 50 mg IV stat, for preoperative sedation of a child. SDR for children: 1–3 mg per kg per 24 hr 60–90 minutes before procedure. Patient's weight: 14 lb 8 oz. Available: phenobarbital sodium for injection 130 mg per mL.

   a. Patient's weight in kg to nearest tenth: _____

   b. SDR for this child: _____

     DA equation:

   c. Evaluation: *Safe to give* or *Hold and clarify promptly with prescriber?* (Circle one and state reason.) _____

   d. Dose to be administered if the order is safe to give:

     DA equation:

   e. Evaluation: _____

NDC 0641-0477-21

Phenobarbital
Sodium
Injection, USP   C-IV

130 mg/mL ℞ only

FOR IM OR SLOW IV USE
1 mL Vial
Do not use if discolored
or precipitated.
Manufactured by
✺ WEST-WARD

(01)00306410477211

462-351-03

Lot:

Exp.:

2 **Ordered:** furosemide, a diuretic, 25 mg IV q12h, for an infant with edema

SDR: 0.5–2 mg per kg per dose q6-12h

Patient's weight: 9 kg

FUROSEMIDE	NDC 0517-5704-25
INJECTION, USP	25 x 4 mL
40 mg/4 mL (10 mg/mL)	SINGLE DOSE VIALS

FOR INTRAVENOUS OR INTRAMUSCULAR USE   **Rx Only**
Each mL contains: Furosemide 10 mg, Water for Injection q.s. Sodium Chloride
for isotonicity, Sodium Hydroxide and, if necessary, Hydrochloric Acid to adjust pH
between 8.0 and 9.3.
WARNING: DISCARD UNUSED PORTION. USE ONLY IF SOLUTION IS CLEAR
AND COLORLESS. PROTECT FROM LIGHT.
Store at 20° to 25°C (68° to 77°F); excursions permitted to 15° to 30°C (59° to 86°F)
(See USP Controlled Room Temperature).   Directions for Use: See Package Insert.

AMERICAN REGENT, INC.
SHIRLEY, NY 11967   Rev. 11/05

Lot / Exp.

a. SDR for this infant: _____

b. Evaluation: *Safe to give* or *Hold and clarify promptly with prescriber?* (Circle one and state reason.) _____

c. Dose in mL to be administered if the order is safe to give:

DA equation:

d. Evaluation: _____

3 Use the information from problem 1. The agency has a policy that a volume-control device must be used. Agency policy states that a maximum of 2 hours' worth of volume can be placed in the device.

a. How many mL will be placed in the volume-control device? _____

b. The prescriber ordered that the dose be increased by 3 mcg per min. What will the new flow rate be?

DA equation:

c. Evaluation: _____

4 **Ordered:** KCl IV infusion 0.1 mEq per kg per hr in 100 mL D5W, ordered for a child with hypokalemia

Available from pharmacy: KCl 10 mEq per 100 mL D5W

SDR for children: up to 3 mEq per kg per 24 hr, not to exceed 40 mEq per 24 hr

Patient's weight: 8 kg

Directions in reference: Must be administered on infusion pump. Monitor electrocardiogram. Obtain order for subsequent infusion. Infuse using volume-control device with no more than 1 hour's worth of ordered fluid amount. Check potassium level every 2 hours.

a. SDR for this infant: _____

b. Amount ordered for 24 hours: _____

c. Evaluation: *Safe to give* or *Hold and clarify promptly with prescriber?* (Circle one and state reason.) _____

d. Hourly flow rate:

DA equation:

e. Evaluation: _____

5 **Ordered:** Trisenox (arsenic trioxide) IV infusion for a child with leukemia to flow at 5 mcg per min daily.

Available: Trisenox 10 mg per 250 mL NS

a. How many mcg per hr are ordered? _____
b. How many total mcg are in the available infusion? _____
c. How many mcg per mL are in the total available solution?

DA equation:

d. Evaluation: _____
e. What flow rate, to the nearest mL per hr, should be set?

DA equation:

f. Evaluation: _____

PEDS NGN

Billy Streetwater is a 8 year old with a history of asthma. He was admitted to the hospital with bacterial pneumonia. He has diminished lung sounds and some sternal retractions. Billy weighs 66 pounds. He is admitted to the pediatric ICU with the following orders:

- Admit to PICU
- Regular diet, push fluids
- IV: D5NS at 60 mL/hour
- Methylprednisolone (Solu-Medrol) 2 mg/kg/dose IV push × 1 dose now
- Sputum culture, then start Azithromycin 10 mg/kg/dose IV q 24 hours × 2 days then 5 mg/kg/dose PO q 24 hours × 3 days
- Acetaminophen 15 mg/kg/dose q 4 hours prn temp greater than 38.5 degrees Celsius.

1 How many mL of IV fluids will Billy get in 24 hours with his maintenance IV fluids?

a. 720 mL   c. 1440 mL
b. 480 mL   d. 1880 mL

2 How many milligrams of will Billy get for his first dose of IV azithromycin?

a. 500 mg   c. 200 mg
b. 300 mg   d. 100 mg

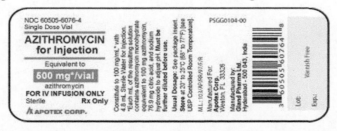

3 How many mL of Azithromycin will you need to draw out of the 500 mg vial (500 mg/5 mL) to administer the first IV dose?

a. 5 mL   c. 2 mL

b. 3 mL   d. 1 mL

4 On day 4 you need to switch Billy to the oral azithromycin. How many mL do you plan to administer?

a. 2.75 mL   c. 3.35 mL

b. 3.74 mL   d. 4 mL

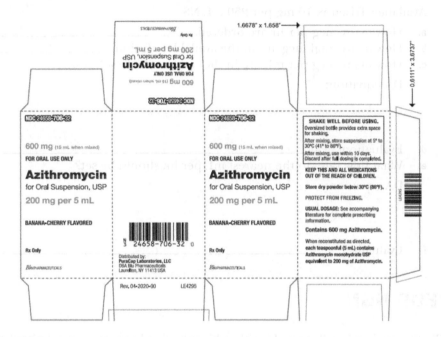

5 How many kg dose Billy weigh?

a. 32 kg   c. 32.3 kg

b. 29.9 kg   d. 28 kg

6 The pharmacy sends you a prefilled syringe of methylprednisolone 15 mg. You are prepared to give this IV push via the maintenance IV that is running. What supplies do you need? **Select all that apply**.

a. Alcohol swab

b. Betadine swab

c. Normal saline flush – 10 mL

d. Normal saline flush – 3 mL

e. Tape

f. Methylprednisone drawn up in 10 mL syringe

g. Methylprednisone drawn up in 3 mL syringe

h. Sterile gloves

i. Clean gloves

j. Hand sanitizer gel

7 How many mL of methylprednisolone (Solu-Medrol) should be in the syringe?

   a. 5.9 mL   **c.** 2 mL

   b. 0.75 mL   **d.** 59.9 mL

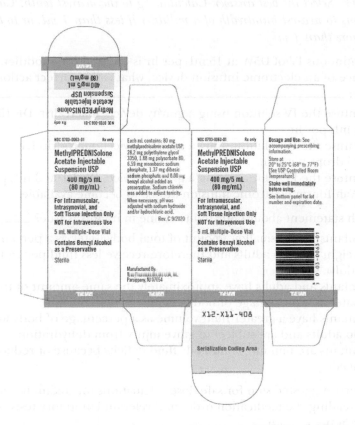

9 Acetaminophen is available in the following concentrations: 160 mg/5 mL. How many mL do you need?

   a. 10 mL   **c.** 14 mL

   b. 12 mL   **d.** 16 mL

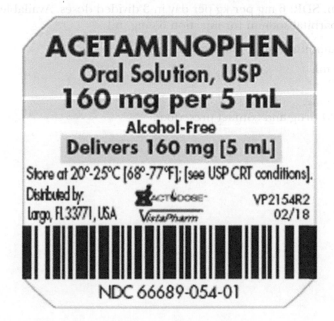

CHAPTER 13   MULTIPLE-CHOICE REVIEW

ESTIMATED COMPLETION TIME: 30 to 60 minutes   **ANSWERS ON:** page 508

DIRECTIONS: *Select the best answer. Calculate kg to the nearest tenth. Calculate medications to nearest hundredth of a milliliter if less than 1 mL or to the nearest tenth if more than 1 mL.*

1 A continuous IV of D5W at 15 mL per hr is ordered for a toddler. In the absence of an electronic infusion device, what is the correct action by the nurse? _____

   a. Infuse the IV solution using a gravity device, macrodrip DF 15, at 4 mL per hr.

   b. Infuse the IV solution using a gravity device, microdrip DF 60, at 15 drops per min.

   c. Infuse the IV solution using a gravity device, DF 10, at 3 mL per hr.

   d. Wait for an electronic infusion device to become available.

2 Which statement about body fluid volume in infants is true? _____

   a. Infants have a smaller amount of total body water as a percentage of body weight than do adults and therefore receive less fluid per kg than do adults.

   b. Infants and adults have approximately the same amount of total body water as a percentage of body weight.

   c. Infants have a greater fluid volume as a percentage of body weight than do adults and are subject to grave injury from dehydration.

   d. Infants are immune from body fluid deficits because of reduced intake needs.

3 The first suggested step for safe dose calculations for unfamiliar medications after reading the medication order and relevant laboratory tests is _____

   a. Call the prescriber.

   b. Calculate the SDR.

   c. Calculate the dose.

   d. Visit the parents and explain what you plan to do.

4 **Ordered:** phenobarbital sodium 80 mg IM for a 40-kg child who needs sedation. SDR: 6 mg per kg per day in 3 divided doses. Available: phenobarbital sodium for injection 65 mg/mL.

   Which amount would you prepare?

   a. 1.3 mL

   b. 1.23 mL

   c. 0.13 mL

   d. Hold drug and contact prescriber.

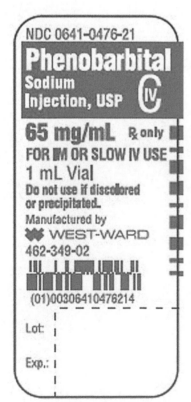

5 Two devices used in pediatric settings to help prevent drug or fluid volume overload for IV orders are _____

    a. Add-VANTAGE® systems and premixed medications

    b. Gravity infusion sets and macrodrip tubing

    c. Syringe pumps and volume-control burette chambers

    d. PCA pumps and syringe pumps

6 If an electronic pump is not available to deliver a continuous infusion to a pediatric patient, which infusion device would be the best choice? _____

    a. Gravity infusion device with microdrip tubing and a volume-control device

    b. Gravity infusion device with macrodrip tubing DF 10

    c. Direct injection with a syringe administered very slowly

    d. PCA pump

7 An IV solution of 250 mL with 250 mg of drug is to be infused at 8 mL per hr. The number of mg per hr to be delivered is _____

    a. 1   **c.** 10

    b. 8   **d.** 20

8 The nurse should avoid mixing medicines for an infant or toddler in which product: _____

    a. Applesauce   **c.** Water

    b. Sherbet   **d.** Milk

9 An IV solution of 100 mL containing 10 mg of a drug is to be infused at 20 mcg per min. The mL per hr flow rate should be set at _____

    a. 12   **c.** 100

    b. 20   **d.** 120

10 **Ordered:** 0.05 mg of a drug for a child. Available: 0.5 mg per 10 mL. How many mL will you administer? _____

    a. 15   **c.** 5

    b. 10   **d.** 1

ESTIMATED COMPLETION TIME: 1 to 2 hours   **ANSWERS ON:** page 508

DIRECTIONS: *Calculate the following medication dosages and safe dosage ranges (SDRs). Label all answers.*

1 **Ordered:** atropine sulfate 0.5 mg IV, every 4 to 6 hours as needed for a 5-year-old child with bradyarrhythmia. SDR for child with bradyarrhythmia: 0.01–0.03 mg per kg to achieve pulse rate >60 beats per minute. Maximum dose for child: 500 mcg. Patient's weight: 44 lb.

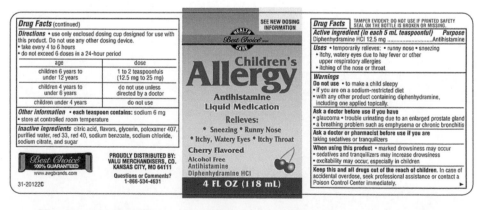

a. Weight in kg to the nearest tenth: _____
b. SDR for this child: _____

DA equation:

c. Ordered dose for this child in mcg: _____
d. Evaluation: *Safe to give* or *Hold and clarify promptly with prescriber?* (Circle one and give reason.)
e. If safe, will you give more or less than the unit dose on hand? _____
f. How many mL will you give?

DA equation:

g. Evaluation: _____

2 **Ordered:** diphenhydramine HCl (Benadryl Children's Liquid) 12.5 mg, orally now for a 10-year-old child who has developed hives from an antibiotic. He is on a regular diet.

a. How many mL will you administer? _____
b. What might you offer to follow the dose if the child does not like the taste of the medicine? _____

3 **Ordered:** Children's acetaminophen 160 mg PO every 6 hours for a 2½-year-old child. Patient's weight: 12 kg.

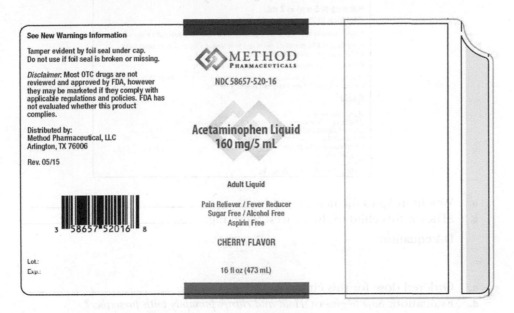

See New Warnings Information

Tamper evident by foil seal under cap.
Do not use if foil seal is broken or missing.

Disclaimer: Most OTC drugs are not reviewed and approved by FDA, however they may be marketed if they comply with applicable regulations and policies. FDA has not evaluated whether this product complies.

Distributed by:
Method Pharmaceutical, LLC
Arlington, TX 76006

Rev. 05/15

Lot.:
Exp.:

METHOD PHARMACEUTICALS

NDC 58657-520-16

Acetaminophen Liquid
160 mg/5 mL

Adult Liquid

Pain Reliever / Fever Reducer
Sugar Free / Alcohol Free
Aspirin Free

CHERRY FLAVOR

16 fl oz (473 mL)

3 58657 52016 8

a. Is the order safe? How many mL would you prepare? _____

b. What is the concentration, in mg per mL, of children's acetaminophen susp? With which device would you administer the medication?

_____

CLINICAL RELEVANCE

Parents have overdosed their children at home by giving too much of the over-the-counter product either by using household utensils or by giving it more often than the label states. Keep this in mind when teaching parents.

➤ Aspirin (acetylsalicylic acid) is not given to infants, children, and teenagers under *19 years* of age who have fever due to flu or viral symptoms. Aspirin has been associated with Reye's syndrome in those age groups.

Q & A **ASK YOURSELF** **1** Would it be safer always to clarify orders that specify only mL and do not state the total dose desired, such as 80 or 160 mg?

MY ANSWER _____

4 **Ordered:** digoxin 0.5 mg IV, now for an 18-month-old child with congestive heart failure

SDR: 7.5–12 mcg per kg divided in two q12h doses for child up to 2 years. Patient's weight 24 lb 6 oz

Directions: Administer IV over 5–10 minutes. Safe to give undiluted. If needed, dilute each mL of drug in 4 mL SW (to permit small amounts of drug to be infused over time). Use a calculator to determine SDR.

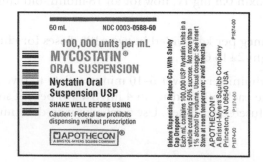

> 10 ampuls 2 mL each   NDC 24987-260-10
>
> **LANOXIN®** (digoxin) **Injection**
>
> 500 mcg (0.5 mg) in 2 mL
> (250 mcg [0.25 mg] per mL)
>
> A sterile solution for intravenous or intramuscular injection. Dilution not required.
> In a vehicle of 40% propylene glycol and 10% alcohol. Dibasic sodium phosphate
> 0.17%, citric acid anhydrous 0.08%.
>
> See prescribing information for dosage information.
>
> Store at 25°C (77°F); excursions permitted to 15° to 30°C (59° to 86°F) [see USP
> Controlled Room Temperature] and protect from light.
>
> **R only**
>
> Manufactured by
> Jubilant HollisterStier
> Kirkland, Canada H9H 4J4
> Distributed by
> Covis Pharmaceuticals, Inc.
> Cary, NC 27511
> Made in Germany
> ©2012, Covis Pharmaceuticals, Inc.

a. Weight in kg to the nearest tenth: _____

b. SDR for this child to the nearest tenth mg: _____

DA equation:

c. Ordered dose for this child: _____

d. Evaluation: *Safe to give* or *Hold and clarify promptly with prescriber?*
(Circle one and state reason.) _____

e. How many mL of digoxin will you prepare before dilution? _____

5 **Ordered:** cytarabine, an antineoplastic drug, 0.1 g per day IV to be infused in
NS over 4 hours.

SDR: 100 mg per m^2 per day

Patient's weight: 31 lb. BSA: 0.6 m^2.

a. SDR for this child for the day: _____

b. Evaluation: *Safe to give* or *Hold and clarify promptly with prescriber?*
(Circle one and state reason.) _____

c. Calculate the dose if safe.

DA equation:

d. Evaluation: _____

6 **Ordered:** Mycostatin (nystatin) oral syrup 250,000 units three times daily for a
4-month-old infant with thrush (oral candidiasis).

SDR for children and infants >3 months: 250,000-500,000 units per day

Directions: Place half the dose in either side of the mouth.

> 60 mL   NDC 0003-0588-60
>
> **100,000 units per mL**
> **MYCOSTATIN®**
> **ORAL SUSPENSION**
> **Nystatin Oral**
> **Suspension USP**
>
> SHAKE WELL BEFORE USING
> Caution: Federal law prohibits
> dispensing without prescription
>
> ☐ **APOTHECON®**
> A BRISTOL-MYERS SQUIBB COMPANY
>
> Before Dispensing Replace Cap With Safety
> Cap Dropper
> Each mL contains 100,000 USP Nystatin Units in a
> vehicle containing 50% sucrose. Not more than
> 1% alcohol by volume. Usual dosage: See insert
> Store at room temperature; avoid freezing
>
> APOTHECON®
> A Bristol-Myers Squibb Company
> Princeton, NJ 08540 USA

a. If order is safe, how many mL will you prepare? _____

DA equation:

b. Evaluation: _____

c. What device among those on p. 471 might be appropriate to administer this order to an infant of this age? _____

d. How many mL will you administer on each side of the mouth of the child? _____

7 Ordered: KCl 10 mEq per hr for 3 hrs as an intermittent infusion, for a child with hypokalemia. Check potassium levels every 4 hours and call physician. Available: 30 mEq KCl in 100 mL D5W

SDR for child with hypokalemia: 0.5 to 1 mEq per kg per dose not to exceed 40 mEq per 24 hr

Safe flow rate: maximum: 1 mEq per kg per hr. Patient's weight: 42 lb.

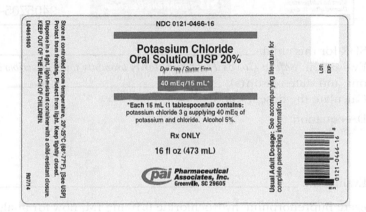

a. Weight in kg to the nearest tenth: _____

b. SDR for this child: _____

c. Ordered dose for this child: _____

d. Evaluation: *Safe to give* or *Hold and clarify promptly with prescriber?* (Circle one and state reason.) _____

e. If safe, what should the flow rate on the infusion pump be? _____

DA equation:

f. Evaluation: _____

8 Ordered: Augmentin oral suspension 1 g bid, for a 5-year-old child with tonsillitis. Patient's weight: 38 kg.

SDR: 20–40 mg per kg per day in 3–4 divided doses.

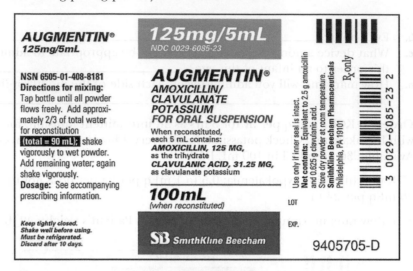

a. SDR for this child: _____

b. Evaluation: *Safe to give* or *Hold and clarify promptly with prescriber?* (Circle one and state reason(s). _____

c. Calculate the dose if safe.

DA equation:

d. Evaluation: _____

9 Ordered: buprenorphine hydrochloride 0.16 mg IM, now for analgesia.

SDR for children: 0.004 mg/kg q4-6 h

Patient's weight: 88 lb

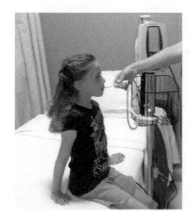

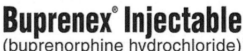

a. SDR for this child: _____

DA equation:

b. Evaluation: *Safe to give* or *Hold and clarify promptly with prescriber?* (Circle one.)

c. If safe, will you give more or less than the unit dose on hand?

DA equation:

d. What is the nearest measurable dose you will prepare for the available syringe?

DA equation:

e. Evaluation: _____

Draw a vertical line through the calibrated line on the syringe to indicate the nearest measurable dose.

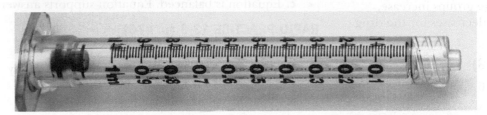

10 **Ordered:** Vancocin (vancomycin hydrochloride) 500 mg IVPB infusion q6h for a 12-year-old child with a staphylococcus infection. Directions: Dilute with 10 mL SW to withdraw from vial. Further dilute to 150 mL with D5W and infuse over 60 minutes. Patient's weight: 35 kg.

SDR IV for children. 40 mg per kg per day divided q6-12 hr not to exceed 2 g per day.

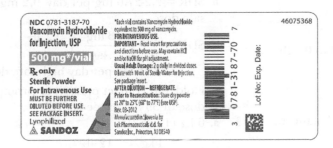

a. SDR: _____

DA equation:

b. Evaluation: _____

c. If safe, what flow rate would you set on the IV pump? _____

CHAPTER 13 ANSWER KEY

RAPID PRACTICE 13-1 (p. 466)

1 Contact prescriber.

2 Child with postoperative pain: 0.04 mg per kg per hr; child with chronic cancer pain: 2.6 mg per kg per hr

3 Child over 10 years: 12 mcg per kg; premature infant: 25 mcg per kg

Note: As the weight and age groups increase, the number of mcg per kg decreases for the drug schedule.

RAPID PRACTICE 13-2 (p. 468)

1 **a.** 12 ÷ 2 = approximately 6 kg
b. 5.5 kg

$$\text{lb} = \frac{1\,\text{lb}}{16\,\cancel{oz}} \times 3\,\cancel{oz} = \frac{3}{16}$$
$$= 0.19,\ \text{rounded to 0.2 lb}$$

0.2 lb + 12 lb = 12.2 lb

$$\text{kg} = \frac{1\,\text{kg}}{2.2\,\cancel{lb}} \times 12.2\,\cancel{lb} = 5.5\,\text{kg}$$

c. Estimate supports answer. Equation is balanced.

2 **a.** 20 ÷ 2 = approximately 10 kg
b. 9.3 kg

$$\text{lb} = \frac{1\,\text{lb}}{16\,\cancel{oz}} \times \frac{6\,\cancel{oz}}{1} = 0.375,\ \text{rounded to 0.4 lb}$$

$$\text{kg} = \frac{1\,\text{kg}}{2.2\,\cancel{lb}} \times \frac{20.4\,\cancel{lb}}{1} = 9.3\,\text{kg}$$

c. Estimate supports answer. Equation is balanced.

3 **a.** 4 ÷ 2 = approximately 2 kg
b. 2 kg

$$\text{lb} = \frac{1\,\text{lb}}{16\,\cancel{oz}} \times \frac{8\,\cancel{oz}}{1} = 0.5\,\text{lb}$$

$$\text{kg} = \frac{1\,\text{kg}}{2.2\,\cancel{lb}} \times \frac{4.5\,\cancel{lb}}{1} = 2.04,\ \text{rounded to 2 kg}$$

c. Equation is balanced. Estimate supports answer.

4 **a.** 25 ÷ 2 = approximately 12.5 kg
b. 11.6 kg

$$\text{lb} = \frac{1\,\text{lb}}{16\,\cancel{oz}} \times 9\,\cancel{oz} = \frac{9}{16}$$
$$= 0.56,\ \text{rounded to 0.6 lb}$$

$$\text{kg} = \frac{1\,\text{kg}}{2.2\,\cancel{lb}} \times 25.6\,\cancel{lb}$$
$$= 11.63,\ \text{rounded to 11.6 lb}$$

c. Equation is balanced. Estimate supports answer.

5 **a.** 18 ÷ 2 = approximately 9 kg
b. 8.5 kg

$$\text{lb} = \frac{1\,\text{lb}}{16\,\cancel{oz}} \times \frac{12\,\cancel{oz}}{1} = 0.75,\ \text{rounded to 0.8 lb}$$

$$\text{kg} = \frac{1\,\text{kg}}{2.2\,\cancel{lb}} \times \frac{18.8\,\cancel{lb}}{1} = 8.54,\ \text{rounded to 8.5 kg}$$

c. Equation is balanced. Equation supports answer.

RAPID PRACTICE 13-3 (p. 470)

1 **a.** SDR: 1–1.5 g in 4 divided doses
b. Ordered 250 mg × 4 = 1000 mg = 1 g per day
c. Safe to give. Order is within SDR.

2 **a.** 10 kg; actual weight: 9.2 kg

$$\text{lb} = \frac{1\,\text{lb}}{\underset{4}{16\,\cancel{oz}}} \times \frac{\overset{1}{4\,\cancel{oz}}}{1} = \frac{1}{4}$$
$$= 0.25,\ \text{rounded to 0.3 lb}$$

$$\text{kg} = \frac{1\,\text{kg}}{2.2\,\cancel{lb}} \times \frac{20.3\,\cancel{lb}}{1} = \frac{20.3}{2.2} = 9.2\,\text{kg}$$

b. SDR = 9.2-27.6 mg per day. 9.2 mg per day low safe dose

$$\text{SDR} = \frac{\text{mg}}{\text{day}} = \frac{3\,\text{mg}}{\cancel{kg}} \times \frac{9.2\,\cancel{lb}}{1}$$
$$= 27.6\,\text{mg per day high safe dose}$$

c. Hold and contact prescriber promptly. Ordered dose of 35 mg exceeds SDR.

3 **a.** 6 kg (12 ÷ 2);

$$\text{kg} = \frac{1\,\text{kg}}{2.2\,\cancel{lb}} \times \frac{12\,\cancel{lb}}{1}$$
$$= 5.45,\ \text{rounded to 5.5 kg actual weight}$$

Note: kg are usually calculated to the nearest tenth.

b. SDR 1100-2750 mcg per day

$$\frac{\text{mcg}}{\text{day}} = \frac{200\,\text{mcg}}{1\,\cancel{kg} \times \text{day}} \times \frac{5.5\,\cancel{kg}}{1}$$
$$= 1100\,\text{mcg per day low safe dose}$$

$$\frac{\text{mcg}}{\text{day}} = \frac{500\,\text{mcg}}{1\,\cancel{kg} \times \text{day}} \times \frac{5.5\,\cancel{kg}}{1}$$
$$= 2750\,\text{mcg per day high safe dose}$$

c. Hold and contact prescriber promptly. Overdose. Order is 15,000 mcg per day.

4 **a.** $22 \div 2 = 11$ kg; actual weight: 10 kg

$$\text{kg} = \frac{1\,\text{kg}}{2.2\,\text{lb}} \times \frac{22\,\text{lb}}{1} = 10\,\text{kg}$$

b. SDR : 5000-8000 mcg per day in 4-6 divided doses

$$\frac{\text{mcg}}{\text{day}} = \frac{500\,\text{mcg}}{1\,\text{kg} \times \text{day}} \times \frac{10\,\text{kg}}{1}$$
$$= 5000\,\text{mcg per day low safe dose}$$

$$\frac{\text{mcg}}{\text{day}} = \frac{800\,\text{mcg}}{1\,\text{kg} \times \text{day}} \times \frac{10\,\text{kg}}{1}$$
$$= 8000\,\text{mcg per day high safe dose}$$

c. Safe to give (2 mg = 2000 mcg). Order is 2 mg four times a day (or 8000 mcg per day).

5 **a.** 33 kg (66 lb ÷ 2); $\text{kg} = \dfrac{1\,\text{kg}}{2.2\,\text{lb}} \times 66\,\text{lb} = 30\,\text{kg}$

b. SDR: 300-600 mcg per hr

$$\frac{\text{mcg}}{\text{hr}} = \frac{10\,\text{mcg}}{1\,\text{kg} \times \text{hr}} \times \frac{30\,\text{kg}}{1}$$
$$= 300\,\text{mcg per hr low safe dose}$$

$$\text{mcg} = \frac{20\,\text{mcg}}{1\,\text{kg} \times \text{hr}} \times \frac{30\,\text{kg}}{1}$$
$$= 600\,\text{mcg per hr high safe dose}$$

c. Dose ordered 500 mcg per hr is within SDR. Safe to give.

RAPID PRACTICE 13-4 (p. 473)

1 **a.** BSA is not needed. The SDR is not based on m^2 of BSA.

b. 100-125 mg every 8 hr

$$\frac{\text{mg}}{\text{dose}} = \frac{2\,\text{mg}}{1\,\text{kg}} \times \frac{50\,\text{kg}}{\text{dose}}$$
$$= 100\,\text{mg low safe dose}$$

$$\frac{\text{mg}}{\text{dose}} = \frac{2.5\,\text{mg}}{1\,\text{kg}} \times \frac{50\,\text{kg}}{\text{dose}}$$
$$= 125\,\text{mg high safe dose}$$

c. Order is safe. It is within SDR.

2 **a.** $0.27\,\text{m}^2$

b. $\text{units} = \dfrac{20{,}000\,\text{units}}{1\,\text{m}^2} \times \dfrac{0.27\,\text{m}^2}{\text{dose}}$
$$= 5400\,\text{units every 24 hr}$$

c. Safe to give. The order is within in SDR (5400 ÷ 24 = 225 units per hr).

3 **a.** $1.10\,\text{m}^2$

b. $\dfrac{\text{mg}}{\text{dose}} = \dfrac{3.3\,\text{mg}}{1\,\text{m}^2} \times \dfrac{1.10\,\text{m}^2}{\text{dose}}$
$$= 3.6\,\text{mg safe daily dose}$$

c. Unsafe order. Overdose. Call prescriber promptly. Document.

4 **a.** $0.6\,\text{m}^2$

b. 0.9–1.2 mg

$$\frac{\text{mg}}{\text{week}} = \frac{1.5\,\text{mg}}{1\,\text{m}^2 \times \text{week}} \times \frac{0.6\,\text{m}^2}{1}$$
$$= 0.9\,\text{mg low safe dose once a week}$$

$$\frac{\text{mg}}{\text{week}} = \frac{2\,\text{mg}}{1\,\text{m}^2 \times \text{week}} \times \frac{0.6\,\text{m}^2}{1}$$
$$= 1.2\,\text{mg high safe dose once a week}$$

c. Safe to give. The order is within SDR.

5 **a.** BSA is not needed. The SDR is not based on m^2 of BSA.

b. 5–25 mcg per min

$$\frac{\text{mcg}}{\text{min}} = \frac{1\,\text{mcg}}{1\,\text{kg} \times \text{min}} \times \frac{5\,\text{kg}}{1}$$
$$= 5\,\text{mcg per min low safe dose}$$

$$\frac{\text{mcg}}{\text{min}} = \frac{5\,\text{mcg}}{1\,\text{kg} \times \text{min}} \times \frac{5\,\text{kg}}{1}$$
$$= 25\,\text{mcg per min high safe dose}$$

c. Safe to give. The order is within SDR.

RAPID PRACTICE 13-5 (p. 476)

1 **a.** 18.2 mg safe total daily dose
20 lb = 9.1 kg

$$\frac{\text{mg}}{\text{day}} = \frac{2\,\text{mg}}{1\,\text{kg} \times \text{day}} \times \frac{9.1\,\text{kg}}{1} = 18.2\,\text{mg per day}$$

b. Hold. Order exceeds daily safe dose.

c. N/A

2 **a.** SDR = 15 mg per kg per day
44 lb ÷ 2.2 = 20 kg

$$\frac{\text{mg}}{\text{day}} = \frac{15\,\text{mg}}{1\,\text{kg} \times \text{day}} \times \frac{20\,\text{kg}}{1}$$
$$= 300\,\text{mg per day divided}$$
$$\text{into two 150-mg doses}$$

b. Safe to give

c. Reconstitute with 55 mL of water in two portions. Shake after each addition.

d. 6 mL

$$\frac{\text{mL}}{\text{dose}} = \frac{5\,\text{mL}}{\overset{\,}{\underset{5}{125\,\text{mg}}}} \times \frac{\overset{6}{150\,\text{mg}}}{\text{dose}} = \frac{30}{5} = \frac{6\,\text{mL}}{\text{dose}}$$

3 **a.** $\text{SDR} = \dfrac{10\,\text{mg}}{1\,\cancel{\text{m}^2}} \times \dfrac{1.10\,\cancel{\text{m}^2}}{\text{dose}} = 11\,\text{mg safe dose}$

 b. Hold and clarify promptly. Ordered dose
 exceeds safe dose recommendation.

 c. N/A

 d. N/A

4 **a.** 0.06–0.12 mg per day

$\dfrac{\text{mg}}{\text{day}} = \dfrac{0.006\,\text{mg}}{1\,\cancel{\text{kg}} \times \text{day}} \times \dfrac{18\,\cancel{\text{kg}}}{1}$
$= 0.1\,\text{mg low safe dose per day}$

$\dfrac{\text{mg}}{\text{day}} = \dfrac{0.012\,\text{mg}}{1\,\cancel{\text{kg}} \times \text{day}} \times \dfrac{18\,\cancel{\text{kg}}}{1}$
$= 0.2\,\text{mg high safe dose per day}$

 b. Order of 0.1 mg bid is within safe dose range
 and frequency.

 c. 2 mL ($2 \times 0.05 = 0.1$ mg)

$\dfrac{\text{mL}}{\text{dose}} = \dfrac{1\,\text{mL}}{0.05\,\cancel{\text{mg}}} \times \dfrac{0.1\,\cancel{\text{mg}}}{\text{dose}} = \dfrac{0.1}{0.05} = \dfrac{2\,\text{mL}}{\text{dose}}$

 d. 50 mcg per mL
 Note: Microgram is abbreviated μg on the label.
 Use mcg in your written records.

5 **a.** 410–820 mg per day.

$\text{kg} = \dfrac{1\,\text{kg}}{2.2\,\cancel{\text{lb}}} \times \dfrac{36\,\cancel{\text{lb}}}{1}$
$= 16.36,\ \text{rounded to } 16.4\,\text{kg}$

$\dfrac{\text{mg}}{\text{day}} = \dfrac{25\,\text{mg}}{1\,\cancel{\text{kg}} \times \text{day}} \times \dfrac{16.4\,\cancel{\text{kg}}}{1}$
$= 410\,\text{mg low safe dose per day}$

$\dfrac{\text{mg}}{\text{day}} = \dfrac{50\,\text{mg}}{1\,\cancel{\text{kg}} \times \text{day}} \times \dfrac{16.4\,\cancel{\text{kg}}}{1}$
$= 820\,\text{mg high safe dose per day}$

 b. Safe to give. Order of 150 mg 4 × daily is within
 SDR.

 c. $\dfrac{\text{mg}}{\text{container}} = \dfrac{125\,\text{mg}}{\cancel{5\,\text{mL}}} \times \dfrac{\overset{12}{\cancel{60\,\text{mL}}}}{\text{container}}$
$= 1500\,\text{mg total in container}$

 d. Add 36 mL in two portions; shake well after
 each addition.

 e. 6 mL

$\dfrac{\text{mL}}{\text{dose}} = \dfrac{\overset{1}{\cancel{5\,\text{mL}}}}{\underset{1}{\underset{25}{\cancel{125\,\text{mg}}}}} \times \dfrac{\overset{6}{\cancel{150\,\text{mg}}}}{\text{dose}} = \dfrac{6\,\text{mL}}{\text{dose}}$

RAPID PRACTICE 13-6 (p. 481)

1 **a.** 0.3–0.9 mg per dose

$\text{kg} = \dfrac{1\,\text{kg}}{2.2\,\cancel{\text{lb}}} \times \dfrac{66\,\cancel{\text{lb}}}{1} = 30\,\text{kg}$

$30 \times 0.01 = 0.3\,\text{mg};\ 30 \times 0.03 = 0.9\,\text{mg}$

 b. Hold and clarify promptly with prescriber.
 Overdose ordered.

 c. If the drug were safe to give, Adrenalin (left
 label) 1:1000 is the correct concentration for
 this order.

 d. The 1:1000 solution is 10 times more
 concentrated than 1:10,000.

 e. N/A

 f. N/A as dose is unsafe to give.

2 **a.** 2-4 units

 b. Safe to give; within safe dose range.

 c.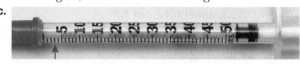

 d. Yes. Bedtime snacks needed for long-acting,
 intermediate, and evening insulin administration
 to avoid hypoglycemic events during sleep.

3 **a.** $\text{kg} = \dfrac{1\,\text{kg}}{2.2\,\cancel{\text{lb}}} \times \dfrac{44\,\cancel{\text{lb}}}{1} = 20\,\text{kg}$

$\dfrac{\text{mg}}{\text{dose}} = \dfrac{0.004\,\text{mg}}{1\,\cancel{\text{kg}} \times \text{dose}} \times \dfrac{20\,\cancel{\text{kg}}}{1} = \dfrac{0.08\,\text{mg}}{\text{dose}}$

 b. Safe to give

 c. 0.33 mL

$\dfrac{\text{mL}}{\text{dose}} = \dfrac{\text{mL}}{0.3\,\cancel{\text{mg}}} \times \dfrac{0.08\,\cancel{\text{mg}}}{\text{dose}}$
$= \dfrac{0.266\,\text{mL}}{\text{dose}}\ \text{rounds to } 0.27\,\text{mL per dose}$

 d. Equation is balanced. Only mL remain.

4 **a.** 2–5 mg once a week

 b. Safe to give. Order is within SDR.

 c. Give 0.4 mL.

$\dfrac{\text{mL}}{\text{dose}} = \dfrac{1\,\text{mL}}{\underset{5}{\cancel{10\,\text{mg}}}} \times \dfrac{\overset{2}{\cancel{4\,\text{mg}}}}{\text{dose}} = 0.4\ \text{mL per dose}$

 d. Estimate of less than 0.5 mL supports answer.
 Equation is balanced.

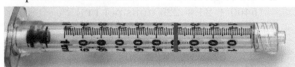

5 **a.** 0.2 mg

$\dfrac{\text{mg}}{\text{dose}} = \dfrac{0.01\,\text{mg}}{1\,\cancel{\text{kg}}} \times \dfrac{22.9\,\cancel{\text{kg}}}{\text{dose}}$
$= 0.229,\ \text{rounded to } 0.2\,\text{mg per dose}$

b. Safe to give

c. 0.5 mL

$$\frac{mL}{dose} = \frac{1\,mL}{\underset{2}{\cancel{0.4\,mg}}} \times \frac{\overset{1}{\cancel{0.2\,mg}}}{dose} = \frac{0.5\,mL}{dose}$$

d. Equation is balanced. Only mL remain.

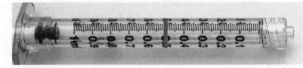

RAPID PRACTICE 13-7 (p. 489)

2 **a.** $50 - 25 = 25$ mL

  b. 25 mL

  c. 50 drops per min (drops per min = mL per hr on a microdrip set)

3 **a.** $20 - 10 = 10$ mL diluent

  b. 10 mL

  c. 40 mL per hr

$$\frac{mL}{hr} = \frac{20\,mL}{\underset{1}{\cancel{30\,min}}} \times \frac{\overset{2}{\cancel{60\,min}}}{1\,hr} = \frac{40\,mL}{hr}$$

  d. Equation is balanced. Only mL per hr remain.

4 **a.** 3 mL

  b. 30 drops per min

$$\frac{drops}{min} = \frac{\overset{2}{\cancel{60}}\,drops}{1\,\cancel{mL}} \times \frac{15\,\cancel{mL}}{\underset{1}{\cancel{30}}\,min} = \frac{30\,drops}{min}$$

  c. Only drops per min remain to be infused when the minutes are less than 1 hr; mL will not equal drops per min.

5 **a.** $30 - 15 = 15$ mL

  b. 15 mL

  c. 90 mL per hr will deliver 30 mL in 20 min. (There are three 20-minute periods in 1 hr.)

  d. Equation is balanced. Only mL per hr remains.

RAPID PRACTICE 13-8 (p. 491)

1 **a.** 6.6 kg

$$\frac{1\,kg}{2.2\,\cancel{lb}} \times \frac{14.5\,\cancel{lb}}{1} = 6.6\,kg$$

  Note: Remember to change oz (8) to lb (0.5) before solving equation.

  b. SDR: 6.6–19.8 mg $(1 \times 6.6)(3 \times 6.6)$

  c. Hold and clarify promptly with prescriber. Ordered dose of 50 mg exceeds SDR.

  d. N/A

  e. N/A

2 **a.** SDR: 4.5–18 mg per dose $(0.5 \times 9)(2 \times 9)$

  b. Hold and contact prescriber immediately. Dose ordered exceeds the SDR by 7 mg.

  c. N/A

  d. N/A

3 **a.** 16 mL (8 mL × 2 hr)

  b. 12 mL per hr

$$\frac{mL}{hr} = \frac{\overset{1}{\cancel{250}}\,mL}{\underset{1}{\cancel{10\,mg}}} \times \frac{1\,\cancel{mg}}{\underset{4}{\cancel{1000\,mcg}}} \times \frac{\overset{2}{\cancel{8\,mcg}}}{1\,\cancel{min}} \times \frac{\overset{6}{\cancel{60\,min}}}{1\,hr}$$

$$= 12\,mL\,per\,hr$$

  c. Equation is balanced. Only mL per hr remain. **Note:** It should be estimated that the flow rate would be increased from 8 mL per hr in problem 1, but not doubled.

4 **a.** SDR:

$$\frac{3\,mEq}{1\,\cancel{kg}} \times \frac{8\,\cancel{kg}}{1} = 24\,mEq\,q24h\,for\,this\,baby$$

  b. $\frac{mEq}{day} = \frac{0.1\,mEq}{1\,\cancel{kg} \times \cancel{hr}} \times \frac{8\,\cancel{kg}}{1} \times \frac{24\,\cancel{hr}}{1\,day}$

$$= 19.2\,mEq\,per\,day\,ordered$$

  c. Order is within SDR. Safe to give.

  d. 8 mL per hr

$$\frac{mL}{hr} = \frac{\overset{10}{\cancel{100}}\,mL}{\underset{1}{\cancel{10\,mEq}}} \times \frac{0.1\,\cancel{mEq}}{1\,\cancel{kg} \times hr} \times \frac{8\,\cancel{kg}}{1}$$

$$= 8\,mL\,per\,hr$$

  e. Equation is balanced. Only mL per hr remains.

5 **a.** 5 mcg × 60 min = 300 mcg per hr

  b. 10 mg = 10,000 mcg (1000 mcg = 1 mg)

  c. 40 mcg per mL

$$\frac{mcg}{mL} = \frac{10,000\,drops}{250\,mL} = \frac{40\,mcg}{mL}$$

  d. Equation is balanced. Only mcg per mL remains.

  e. 8 mL per hr

$$\frac{mL}{hr} = \frac{\overset{1}{\cancel{250}}\,mL}{\underset{1}{\cancel{10\,mg}}} \times \frac{1\,\cancel{mg}}{\underset{4}{\cancel{1000\,mcg}}} \times \frac{5\,\cancel{mcg}}{1\,\cancel{min}} \times \frac{\overset{6}{\cancel{60\,min}}}{1\,hr}$$

$$= \frac{30}{4} = \begin{array}{l}7.5,\,rounded\,to\\8\,mL\,per\,hr\end{array}$$

  f. Equation is balanced. Only mL per hr remains.

PEDS NGN (p. 493)

1 c
2 b
3 b
4 b
5 b
6 a, f, i, j
7 b
9 c

CHAPTER 13 MULTIPLE-CHOICE REVIEW (p. 496)

1 b (pediatric [microdrip] set)
2 c
3 b
4 b
5 c
6 a (Check agency policies.)
7 b
8 d (essential foods)
9 a
10 d

CHAPTER 13 FINAL PRACTICE (p. 498)

1 **a.** $kg = \dfrac{1\,kg}{2.2\,\cancel{lb}} \times \dfrac{44\,\cancel{lb}}{1} = 20\,kg$

b. SDR: 0.2–0.6 mg (200-600 mcg)
Low dose

$\dfrac{0.01\,mg}{\cancel{kg}} \times \dfrac{20\,\cancel{kg}}{dose} = 0.2\,mg\ per\ dose$

High dose

$\dfrac{0.03\,mg}{\cancel{kg}} \times \dfrac{20\,\cancel{kg}}{dose} = 0.6\,mg\ per\ dose$

c. 0.5 mg (500 mcg)
d. Safe to give; within SDR.
e. more than 1 mL
f. 1.3 mL

$\dfrac{mL}{dose} = \dfrac{mL}{\underset{4}{\cancel{4000\,mcg}}} \times \dfrac{\overset{5}{\cancel{5000\,mcg}}}{1}$

$= 1.25\,mL,\ rounded\ to\ 1.3\,mL\ per\ dose$

g. Equation is balanced. Only mL remain.

2 **a.** 5 mL (1 teaspoon)
b. Popsicle
3 **a.** Yes, it is safe. 1.6 mL
b. 32 mg per mL (160 mg per 5 mL); measuring cup
4 **a.** 11.1 kg
24 lb 6 oz = 24.4 lb
6 oz ÷ 16 = 0.38, rounded to 0.4 lb

$kg = \dfrac{1\,kg}{2.2\,\cancel{lb}} \times \dfrac{24.4\,\cancel{lb}}{1}$

$= 11.09,\ rounded\ to\ 11.1\,kg$

b. Low dose

$\dfrac{7.5\,mcg}{\cancel{kg}} \times \dfrac{11.1\,\cancel{kg}}{2\,doses} = \dfrac{83.3}{2}$

$= 41.6\,mcg\ per\ dose$

High dose

$\dfrac{12\,mcg}{\cancel{kg}} \times \dfrac{11.1\,\cancel{kg}}{2\,doses} = \dfrac{133.2}{2}$

$= 66.6\,mcg\ per\ dose$

c. 0.5 mg
d. Hold. Contact prescriber promptly. Overdose.
e. N/A
5 **a.** 60 mg per day

$\dfrac{mg}{day} = \dfrac{100\,mg}{1\,m^2 \times day} \times \dfrac{0.6\,m^2}{1} = \dfrac{60\,mg}{day}$

b. Hold and clarify promptly with prescriber. Order is greater than SDR.
c. N/A
d. N/A
6 **a.** 2.5 mL

$mL = \dfrac{1\,mL}{\underset{2}{\cancel{100,000\,units}}} \times \dfrac{\overset{5}{\cancel{250,000\,units}}}{dose}$

$= 2.5\,mL\ total\ dose$

b. Order is safe.
c. Needleless syringe or calibrated dropper
d. Place 1.25 mL on each side in the mouth of the child.
7 **a.** $kg = \dfrac{1\,kg}{2.2\,\cancel{lb}} \times \dfrac{42\,\cancel{lb}}{1} = 19.1\,kg$

b. 9.6-19.1 mEq per IV dose

$\dfrac{mEq}{dose} = \dfrac{0.5\,mEq}{\cancel{kg} \times dose} \times \dfrac{19.1\,\cancel{kg}}{1}$

$= 9.55,\ rounded\ to$
$9.6\,mEq\ low\ safe\ dose$

$\dfrac{mEq}{dose} = \dfrac{1\,mEq}{\cancel{kg} \times dose} \times \dfrac{19.1\,\cancel{kg}}{1}$

$= 19.1\,mEq\ high\ safe\ dose$

c. 30 mEq per dose
d. Overdose. Obtain new orders promptly from prescriber.
e. N/A
f. N/A
8 **a.** 760 mg to 1520 mg per day in three or four divided doses
b. Hold and clarify promptly with prescriber. A 2000 g per day order is an overdose and exceeds the required frequency.
c. N/A
d. N/A

9 **a.** 0.004 mg per kg q4-6 h

$$\frac{mg}{dose} = \frac{0.004\ mg}{1\ \cancel{kg} \times dose} \times \frac{40\ \cancel{kg}}{1}$$
$$= 0.16\ mg = safe\ dose$$

b. Safe to give; within SDR.

c. Give less than the unit dose, about 0.5 mL

d. 0.53 mL

$$\frac{mL}{dose} = \frac{1\ mL}{0.3\ \cancel{mg}} \times \frac{0.16\ \cancel{mg}}{dose}$$
$$= 0.53\ mL\ (a\ 1\text{-}mL\ syringe\ is$$
$$calibrated\ in\ hundredths)$$

e. Equation is balanced. Estimate supports answer.

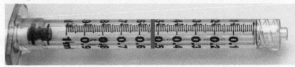

10 **a.** $SDR = \dfrac{40\ mg}{1\ \cancel{kg} \times day} \times \dfrac{35\ \cancel{kg}}{1} = 1400\ mg\ per\ day$

b. Hold medication and contact prescriber promptly. Order exceeds SDR for dose and frequency. Order of 3 g exceeds SDR for dose and frequency.

c. N/A

Suggestions for Further Reading

➤ To access many Internet references on rates and types of medication errors in pediatrics, type "children's medication errors" in your favorite search engine.

Gahart BL, Nazareno AR, Ortega: *2020 Intravenous medications: a handbook for nurses and health professionals,* ed. 37, St. Louis, 2020, Mosby.

http://www.jointcommission.org/sentinel_event_alert_issue_39_preventing_pediatric_medication_errors/

http://pediatrics.aappublications.org/content/112/2/431.full

http://www.pharmacytimes.com/publications/issue/2011/June2011/Medication-Errors-Involving-Children

http://www.fda.gov/ForConsumers/ConsumerUpdates/ucm291741.htm

https://dailymed.nlm.nih.gov/dailymed/drugInfo.cfm?setid=679af699-714d-a3a3-674b-fc9ae44a9a

https://www.drugs.com/pro/azithromycin-oral-suspension.html

https://dailymed.nlm.nih.gov/dailymed/drugInfo.cfm?setid=769cc1ae-bdf4-47e4-9a9f-c6327bd7dbf4

https://dailymed.nlm.nih.gov/dailymed/fda/fdaDrugXsl.cfm?setid=7955c2f7-38fd-4e78-87b9-a35638dea0c2&type=display

Mahmood, I, & Burckart, G. (2016) *Fundamentals of pediatric dosing.* New York; Springer.

Ⓔvolve   For additional practice problems, refer to the Pediatric Dosages section of the Elsevier's Interactive Drug Calculation Application, Version 1 on Evolve.

Comprehensive Final Practice

ESTIMATED COMPLETION TIME: 3 hours   ANSWERS ON page 528

DIRECTIONS: *Estimate and calculate doses using DA-style equations. Evaluate your answer in terms of the estimate and the equation result. If you cannot estimate the dose, estimate whether it will be more or less of the unit dose supplied. Label all answers.*

1   **Ordered:** Humulin R 6 units ⎫
     Humulin N 20 units ⎬ subcut 30 minutes ac breakfast daily
                        ⎭

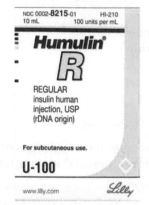
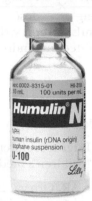

Copyright ©Eli Lilly and Company.
All rights reserved. Used with permission.

From which bottle should the insulin be withdrawn first? _____

Mark total dose on the insulin syringe provided. Place an arrow pointing to the calibration that reflects the intermediate-acting insulin dose.

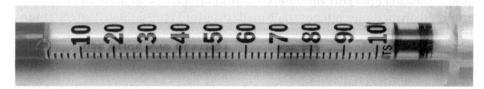

2   **Ordered:** IV D5W of 500 mL over 4 hours. Available: A gravity device. Drop factor on the tubing: 10.

a.   What flow rate will you set? _____

DA equation:

b.   Evaluation:

3 **Ordered:** insulin glargine 24 units subcut daily at bedtime.

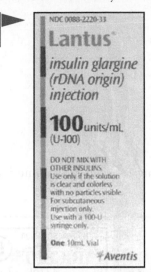

NDC 0088-2220-33

Lantus
*insulin glargine
(rDNA origin)
injection*

100 units/mL
(U-100)

DO NOT MIX WITH
OTHER INSULINS.
Use only if the solution
is clear and colorless
with no particles visible.
For subcutaneous
injection only.
Use with a 100-U
syringe only.

One 10mL Vial

Aventis

Mark the total dose on the 50-unit insulin syringe provided.*

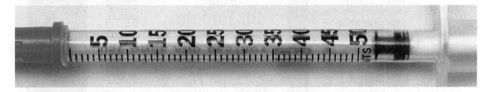

a. Is this insulin a short-, intermediate-, or long-acting insulin?

_____

b. Which is the advantage of the 50-unit 0.5 mL syringe as opposed to the
100-unit 1 mL syringe? _____

4 **Ordered:** penicillin G Procaine susp 400,000 units IM stat for a patient with a
skin infection.

Penicillin G Procaine
Injectable Suspension

600,000 UNITS per 1 mL

FOR DEEP IM INJECTION ONLY
WARNING: NOT FOR INTRAVENOUS USE

Mfg. by: King Pharmaceuticals, Inc., Bristol, TN

3000962   (01)00360793130019

Lot: Exp:

---

*Lo-Dose syringes are calibrated for U-100 insulin.

How many mL will you administer (to the nearest tenth of a mL)?

a. Estimated dose:

DA equation:

b. Evaluation:

5 **Ordered:** Aricept 10 mg PO daily at bedtime for a patient with Alzheimer's disease.

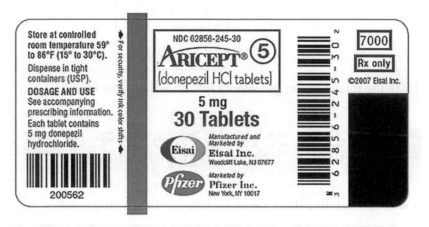

How many tablets will you administer?

a. Estimated dose:

DA equation:

b. Evaluation:

6 **Ordered:** An antibiotic 600 mg IM q6h daily for a patient with a respiratory infection. Directions for reconstitution: Add 2 mL SW for injection. Each 2.5 mL will contain 1 g of antibiotic.

How many mL will you administer (to the nearest tenth of a mL)?

a. What is the concentration of the solution in mg after reconstitution for IM injection? _____

b. Estimated dose:

DA equation:

c. Evaluation:

d. What is the amount (in mL) of water displacement by the powder?

7 **Ordered:** alprazolam 0.5 mg PO at bedtime for a patient with high anxiety.

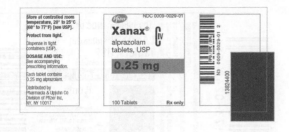

How many tablets will you administer?

a. Estimated dose:

DA equation:

b. Evaluation:

8 **Ordered:** Novolin regular insulin for a diabetic patient on a sliding scale tid 30 minutes ac and at bedtime. Current BGM is 300.

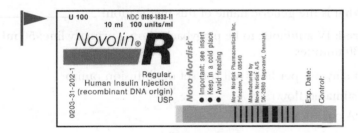

Using the sliding scale that follows, how many units of insulin will be administered? _____

Sliding Scale BG (mg/dL)	Insulin Dose (Novolin)
70–180	0 Units
181–200	2 Units
201–250	4 Units
251–300	6 Units
Over 300	Call physician

a. Mark the syringe to the nearest measurable dose:

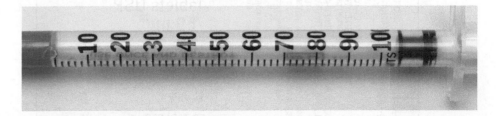

b. Is this a rapid, short, intermediate, or long-acting insulin? _____

c. Will insulin raise or lower the blood glucose level? _____

9 **Ordered:** digoxin 250 mcg PO daily for an adult with heart failure.

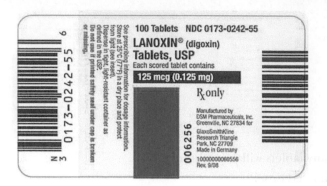

How many tablets will you administer?

a. Estimated dose:

DA equation:

b. Evaluation:

c. What is the generic name of this medication? _____

10 **Ordered:** IV antibiotic to be piggybacked on a primary line: 50 mL to infuse over 30 minutes.

How many mL per hour will you set the infusion pump?

a. Estimated flow rate:

DA equation:

b. Evaluation:

11 **Ordered:** ciprofloxacin hydrochloride 1.5 g PO for a patient with a severe infection.

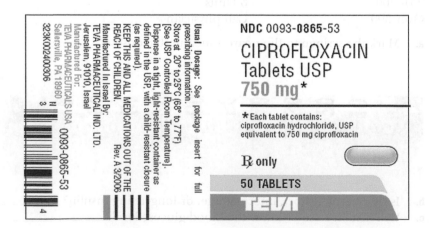

How many tablets will you administer?

a. Estimated dose:

  DA equation:

b. Evaluation:

12 Ordered: levothyroxine 0.1 mg PO daily in AM for a patient who is hypothyroid.

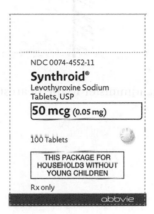

How many tablets will you administer?

a. Estimated dose:

  DA equation:

b. Evaluation:

c. What is the equivalent of the dose ordered in micrograms? _____

13 Ordered: IV antibiotic 100 mg q6h for 72 hours. Available from pharmacy: IV antibiotic solution in 30 mL of D5W to be piggybacked to a primary line. Directions: *"Infuse over 20 minutes."*

How many mL per hour will you set the infusion pump?

a. Estimated flow rate:

  DA equation:

b. Evaluation:

14 Ordered: morphine sulfate 10 mg IM stat for a patient in pain.

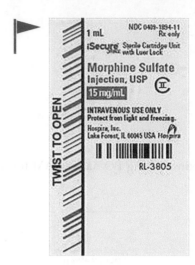

How many mL will you administer to the nearest hundredth of a mL?

a. Estimated dose:

DA equation:

b. Evaluation:

Mark the syringe to the nearest measurable amount.

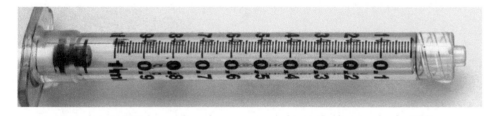

15 Ordered: IV antibiotic 250 mg q4h for 48 hrs. Available from pharmacy: IV antibiotic solution in 20 mL to be piggybacked on a primary line: Directions: *"Infuse over 60 minutes."*

a. What flow rate will you set on a gravity microdrip device? _____

b. Estimated flow rate:

DA equation:

c. Evaluation:

16 Ordered: furosemide 30 mg IM stat for a patient with urinary retention.

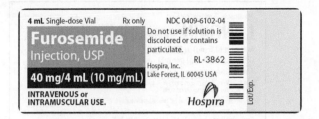

How many mL will you administer?

a. Estimated dose:

DA equation:

b. Evaluation:

Mark the syringe to the nearest measurable amount.

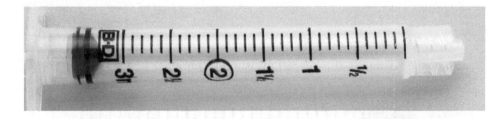

17 Ordered: IV medication for a pediatric patient of 100 mg diluted to a total volume of 20 mL in NS to be administered over 30 minutes. Agency policy requires a volume control device for all medicated IVs for pediatric patients with a maximum 1 hour's worth of fluid.

Available: medication 100 mg per 2 mL.

a. What flow rate will be set on the infusion pump for the medication administration? _____

DA equation:

b. What procedure must be followed (according to agency policy) before and after a medication is infused on a primary line? _____

18 Ordered: digoxin 0.3 mg IM on admission for a patient in heart failure.

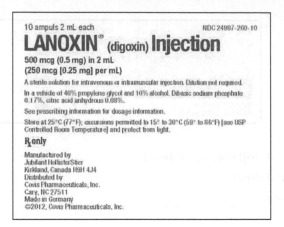

10 ampuls 2 mL each   NDC 24987-260-10

LANOXIN® (digoxin) **Injection**

500 mcg (0.5 mg) in 2 mL
(250 mcg [0.25 mg] per mL)

A sterile solution for intravenous or intramuscular injection. Dilution not required.

In a vehicle of 40% propylene glycol and 10% alcohol. Dibasic sodium phosphate 0.17%, citric acid anhydrous 0.08%.

See prescribing information for dosage information.

Store at 25°C (77°F); excursions permitted to 15° to 30°C (59° to 86°F) [see USP Controlled Room Temperature] and protect from light.

℞ only

Manufactured by
Jubilant HollisterStier
Kirkland, Canada H9H 4J4
Distributed by
Covis Pharmaceuticals, Inc.
Cary, NC 27511
Made in Germany
©2012, Covis Pharmaceuticals, Inc.

How many mL will you administer to the nearest hundredth of a mL?

a.   Estimated dose:

DA equation:

b.   Evaluation:

Mark the syringe to the nearest measurable amount.

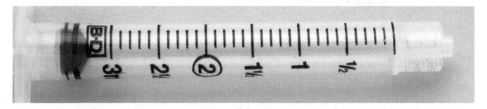

19 Ordered: hyperalimentation (TPN) continuous infusion in a central line at 60 mL per hour for a patient who has a gastrointestinal disorder. Among the contents ordered:

15% dextrose solution
4.25% amino acids

a.   How many grams of dextrose are contained in a liter of the TPN solution?*

DA equation:

b.   Evaluation:

c. How many approximate carbohydrate kilocalories will the dextrose provide per liter of PN solution?

DA equation:

d. Evaluation:

e. How many grams of amino acids are contained in a liter of the PN solution?*

DA equation:

f. Evaluation:

g. How many approximate* protein kilocalories will the amino acids provide per liter of TPN solution?

DA equation:

h. Evaluation:

20 Ordered: hydromorphone HCl 2 mg
promethazine 20 mg } IM stat for a patient in pain

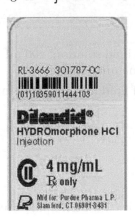

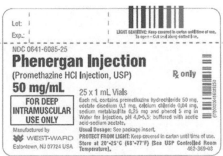

---

*A calculation of 4 calories per g of CHO, 4 calories per g of amino acids, and 9 calories per gram of fat yields an approximate amount of calories.

How many mL of hydromorphone will you prepare?

a. Estimated hydromorphone dose: _____

DA equation:

b. Evaluation:

How many mL of promethazine will you prepare?

c. Estimated promethazine dose: _____

DA equation:

d. Evaluation:

e. What is the total dose in mL to be administered?

Mark the syringe with the total dose to the nearest measurable amount.

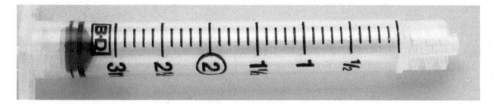

21 The prescriber orders a lipid solution: 200 mL of 20% fat emulsion to be added to the total volume once a day.

a. How many grams of lipid are contained in the 200 mL of solution?*

DA equation:

b. Evaluation:

c. How many kilocalories will each lipid solution provide?

DA equation:

d. Evaluation:

---

*A calculation of 4 calories per g of CHO, 4 calories per g of amino acids, and 9 calories per gram of fat yields an approximate amount of calories.

22 Ordered: diltiazem hydrochloride (Cartia XT) tablets 0.12 g PO daily at bedtime for a patient with hypertension.

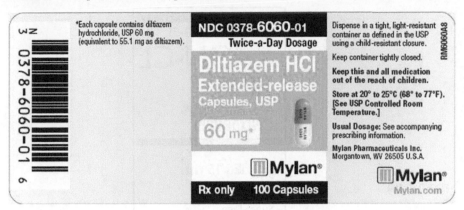

How many tablets will you administer?

a. Estimated dose:

DA equation:

b. Evaluation:

23 Ordered: dexamethasone 500 mcg PO stat for a patient with acute allergy attack.

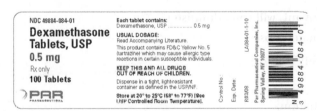

How many tablets will you administer?

a. Estimated dose:
DA equation:

b. Evaluation:

24 Ordered: 20% potassium chloride liquid 20 mEq PO daily for a patient taking a diuretic.

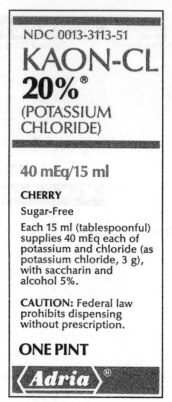

NDC 0013-3113-51

KAON-CL 20%®
(POTASSIUM CHLORIDE)

40 mEq/15 ml

CHERRY

Sugar-Free

Each 15 ml (tablespoonful) supplies 40 mEq each of potassium and chloride (as potassium chloride, 3 g), with saccharin and alcohol 5%.

CAUTION: Federal law prohibits dispensing without prescription.

ONE PINT

Adria®

How many mL will you administer?

a. Estimated dose:

DA equation:

b. Evaluation:

Shade in the medicine cup to the nearest 5 mL. Mark the syringe at the additional amount to be added.

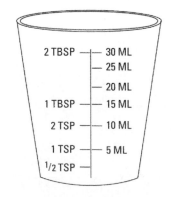

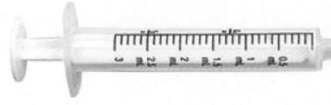

25 Ordered: phenytoin oral suspension 175 mg PO daily in the AM for a child with seizures.

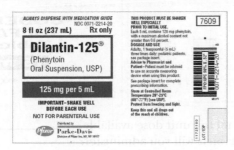

SDR child: 250 mg per m^2 per day as single dose or divided in 2 doses.

Child's BSA: 0.7 m^2

What is the safe dose for this child? _____

DA equation:

a. Evaluation:

b. If safe dose ordered, how many mL will you administer?
DA equation:

c. Evaluation:

Shade in medicine cup to nearest measurable dose. Mark the syringe at the additional amount to be added.

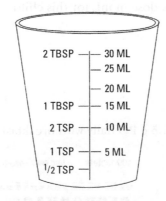

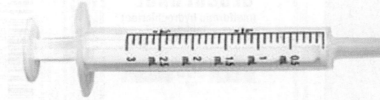

26 Ordered: codeine 45 mg PO q4-6h prn for an adult with pain.

   a. What is the metric unit dose available? _____

   b. How many tablets will you administer?

   c. Estimated dose:

       DA equation:

   d. Evaluation:

27 Ordered: epoetin alfa 5000 units IV 3 times weekly for a pediatric cancer patient. Patient's weight: 25 kg. SDR: 600 units per kg weekly.

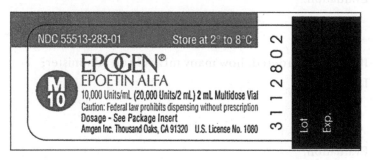

   a. What is the child's weight in kg? _____

       SDR for this child

       DA equation:

   b. Evaluation: If safe, dose in mL for this child.

       DA equation:

   c. Evaluation:

28 Ordered: metformin 1.5 g PO daily with breakfast for a diabetic patient.

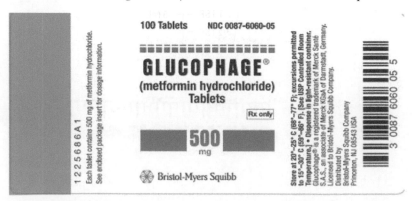

How many tablets will you administer?

a. Estimated dose:

DA equation:

b. Evaluation:

29 Ordered: heparin IV infusion 1000 units per hour. Available: heparin 20,000 units in 500 mL D5W.

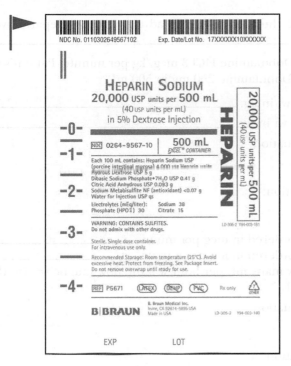

NDC No. 0110302649567102   Exp. Date/Lot No. 17XXXXXX10XXXXXX

HEPARIN SODIUM
20,000 USP units per **500 mL**
(40 USP units per mL)
in 5% Dextrose Injection

-0-
-1-

NDC 0264-9567-10 | **500 mL**
EXCEL® CONTAINER

Each 100 mL contains: Heparin Sodium USP
(porcine intestinal mucosa) 4,000 use Heparin units
Hydrous Dextrose USP 5 g
Dibasic Sodium Phosphate•7H₂O USP 0.41 g
Citric Acid Anhydrous USP 0.093 g
Sodium Metabisulfite NF (antioxidant) <0.07 g
Water for Injection USP qs

-2-

Electrolytes (mEq/liter):   Sodium 38
Phosphate (HPO₄) 30   Citrate 15

WARNING: CONTAINS SULFITES.
Do not admix with other drugs.

-3-

Sterile. Single dose container.
For intravenous use only.

Recommended Storage: Room temperature (25°C). Avoid
excessive heat. Protect from freezing. See Package Insert.
Do not remove overwrap until ready for use.

-4-

REF P5671   LATEX DEHP PVC   Rx only

B|BRAUN   B. Braun Medical Inc.
Irvine, CA 92614-5895 USA
Made in USA   LD-305-2   Y94-003-180

20,000 USP units per 500 mL
(40 USP units per mL)

HEPARIN

LD-305-2 Y94-003-181

EXP   LOT

a. How many mL per hour will you infuse?

DA equation:

b. Evaluation:

c. Which lab test must be monitored for patients receiving heparin therapy?

30 Ordered: Start Pitocin IV at 2 milliunits per minute for a patient in labor.
Available: Pitocin 5 units in 500 mL of D5W.
Conversion factors: 1000 milliunits = 1 unit; 60 minutes = 1 hour

a. At how many mL per hour will the flow rate be set?

DA equation:

b. Evaluation:

31 **Infusing:** heparin at 30 mL per hour in an IV of D5W 250 mL containing heparin 10,000 units.

    a. How many units per hour are infusing?

       DA equation:

    b. Evaluation:

    c. What is the major potential adverse effect of heparin overdose?

    _____

32 **Ordered:** Dobutamine HCl 3 mcg/kg per minute. Patient's weight: 154 lb. Available: Dobutamine 250 mg in 500 mL.

    Estimated wt in kg: _____

    a. Actual wt in kg: _____

       DA equation:

    b. Evaluation:

    c. Dose ordered in mcg per minute _____

    d. Dose ordered in mg per minute _____

    e. At how many mL per hour will the flow rate be set (to the nearest tenth of a mL)?

       DA equation:

    f. Evaluation:

33 **Infusing:** regular insulin at 7 mL per hour IV. Available: Humulin regular insulin 100 units in 100 mL of NS.

    How many units per hour are infusing?

    a. Estimated units per hour:

       DA equation:

    b. Evaluation:

    c. What is the major potential adverse effect of an insulin overdose?

    _____

34 **Ordered:** diazepam 10 mg direct IV before endoscopy procedure.

Directions: Injection undiluted at a rate of 5 mg per minute.

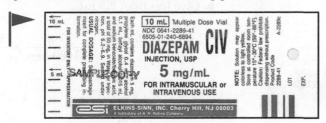

Total mL to be injected: _____

a. Estimated dose: _____

DA equation:

b. Evaluation:

c. Using a 10-mL syringe, how many mL per minute will you inject?

_____

DA equation:

d. Evaluation:

e. Over how many total minutes will you inject? _____
seconds? _____

f. How many seconds per calibration will you inject? _____

35 **Ordered:** IV KCl to infuse at 10 mEq per hour for a patient with hypokalemia.
Available: 500 mL NS with 40 mEq of KCl added premixed by pharmacy.

Directions: *"Recheck serum K levels when 40 mEq of KCl have been infused."*

a. What flow rate will you set on the infusion pump? _____
DA equation:

b. Evaluation:

c. The IV was started at 1300 hours. At what time on the 24-hr clock would
the nurse need to order and recheck a serum K level? _____

**COMPREHENSIVE FINAL PRACTICE:
CHAPTERS 1-13 (p. 510)**

1 Humulin R, the fast-acting clear insulin

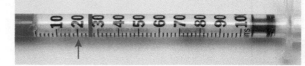

2 **a.** 21 drops per min

$$\frac{\text{drops}}{\text{min}} = \frac{\overset{1}{\cancel{10}} \text{ drops}}{1 \cancel{\text{ mL}}} \times \frac{\overset{125}{\cancel{500 \text{ mL}}}}{\underset{1}{4 \cancel{\text{ hr}}}} \times \frac{1 \cancel{\text{ hr}}}{\underset{6}{\cancel{60} \text{ min}}}$$

$$= \frac{125}{6} \times 20.83, \text{ rounded to } \frac{21 \text{ drops}}{\text{minute}}$$

b. Equation is balanced. Only drops per min remains.

3

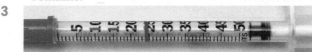

a. long acting (up to 24 hours)
b. A 50-unit syringe permits easier visualization and more accurate measurement of insulin doses of 50 units or less. It is calibrated for U-100 insulin (100 units per mL).

4 **a.** Will give slightly less than 1 mL

$$\frac{\text{mL}}{\text{dose}} = \frac{1 \text{ mL}}{\underset{6}{\cancel{600,000 \text{ units}}}} \times \frac{\overset{4}{\cancel{400,000 \text{ units}}}}{\text{dose}} = \frac{2}{3}$$

$$= \frac{0.6666}{\text{dose}} = \frac{0.67 \text{ mL}}{\text{dose}} = 0.7 \text{ mL}$$

b. Estimate supports answer.

5 **a.** 2 tabs (5 × 2 = 10 mg)

$$\frac{\text{tab}}{\text{dose}} = \frac{1}{\underset{1}{\cancel{5}}} \times \frac{\overset{2}{\cancel{10}}}{\text{dose}} = 2 \text{ tabs}$$

b. $$\frac{\text{tab}}{\text{dose}} = \frac{1 \text{ tab}}{\underset{1}{\cancel{5} \text{ mg}}} \times \frac{\overset{2}{\cancel{10}} \text{ mg}}{\text{dose}} = 2 \text{ tabs per dose}$$

6 **a.** Concentration after dilution is 1000 mg per 2.5 mL.

b. Give less than 2.5 mL.

$$\frac{\text{mL}}{\text{dose}} = \frac{\overset{0.5}{\cancel{2.5 \text{ mL}}}}{1 \cancel{\text{ g}}} \times \frac{1 \cancel{\text{ g}}}{\underset{\underset{1}{5}}{\cancel{1000 \text{ mg}}}} \times \frac{\overset{3}{\cancel{600 \text{ mg}}}}{\text{dose}}$$

$$= \frac{1.5 \text{ mL}}{\text{dose}}$$

c. Estimate supports answer.
d. 0.5 mL (2.5 mL − 2 mL SW = 0.5 mL)

7 **a.** 2 tabs (0.25 × 2 = 0.5)

$$\frac{\text{tab}}{\text{dose}} = \frac{1 \text{ tab}}{\underset{1}{\cancel{0.25 \text{ mg}}}} \times \frac{\overset{2}{\cancel{0.5 \text{ mg}}}}{\text{dose}} = 2 \text{ tabs}$$

b. Estimate supports answer.

8 6 units Novolin regular insulin*

a.

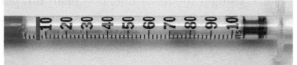

b. fast acting
c. lower

9 **a.** 2 tabs (0.125 × 2 = 0.25 mg = 250 mcg)

$$\frac{\text{tab}}{\text{dose}} = \frac{1 \text{ tab}}{\underset{1}{\cancel{125 \text{ mcg}}}} \times \frac{\overset{2}{\cancel{250 \text{ mcg}}}}{\text{dose}} = \frac{2 \text{ tabs}}{\text{dose}}$$

b. Estimate supports answer.
c. digoxin

10 **a.** 100 mL per hr (30 min × 2 = 60 min; 50 × 2 = 100 mL per hr)

$$\frac{\text{mL}}{\text{hr}} = \frac{50 \text{ mL}}{\underset{1}{\cancel{30 \text{ min}}}} \times \frac{\overset{2}{\cancel{60 \text{ min}}}}{1 \text{ hr}} = \frac{100 \text{ mL}}{\text{hr}}$$

b. Equation is balanced. Estimate supports answer.

11 **a.** 2 tabs

$$\frac{\text{tab}}{\text{dose}} = \frac{1 \text{ tab}}{\underset{3}{\cancel{750 \text{ mg}}}} \times \frac{\overset{4}{\cancel{1000 \text{ mg}}}}{1 \cancel{\text{ g}}} \times \frac{1.5 \cancel{\text{ g}}}{\text{dose}}$$

$$= \frac{6}{3} = \frac{2 \text{ tabs}}{\text{dose}}$$

b. Estimate supports answer.

---

*Note that it would be easier to visualize units on a Lo-Dose insulin syringe (see problem 30).

12 a. 100 mcg ÷ 50 mcg = 2 tabs

$$\frac{\text{tab}}{\text{dose}} = \frac{1\,\text{tab}}{\underset{1}{\cancel{50\,\text{mcg}}}} \times \frac{\overset{20}{\cancel{1000\,\text{mcg}}}}{1\,\cancel{\text{mg}}} \times \frac{0.1\,\cancel{\text{mg}}}{\text{dose}}$$

$$= 20 \times 0.1 = \frac{2\,\text{tab}}{\text{dose}}$$

b. Estimate supports answer.
c. 0.1 mg = 100 mcg

13 a. 90 mL per hr (there are three 20-minute periods in an hour)

$$\frac{\text{mL}}{\text{hr}} = \frac{30\,\text{mL}}{\underset{1}{\cancel{20\,\text{min}}}} \times \frac{\overset{3}{\cancel{60\,\text{min}}}}{1\,\text{hr}} = \frac{90\,\text{mL}}{\text{hr}}$$

b. Estimate supports answer.

14 a. Give less than 1 mL.

$$\frac{\text{mL}}{\text{dose}} = \frac{1\,\text{mL}}{\underset{3}{\cancel{15\,\text{mg}}}} \times \frac{\overset{2}{\cancel{10\,\text{mg}}}}{\text{dose}} = \frac{0.67\,\text{mL}}{\text{dose}}$$

b. Estimate supports answer.

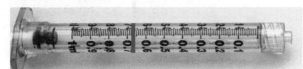

15 a. 20 drops per min with a DF60 set = 20 mL per hr
b. 20 drops per min

$$\frac{\text{drops}}{\text{min}} = \frac{\overset{1}{\cancel{60}}\,\text{drops}}{1\,\cancel{\text{mL}}} \times \frac{20\,\cancel{\text{mL}}}{\underset{1}{\cancel{60}}\,\text{min}} = \frac{20\,\text{drops}}{\text{minute}}$$

c. Estimate supports answer.

16 a. Give less than 4 mL, about one quarter less.

$$\frac{\text{mL}}{\text{dose}} = \frac{4\,\text{mL}}{\underset{4}{\cancel{40\,\text{mg}}}} \times \frac{\overset{3}{\cancel{30\,\text{mg}}}}{\text{dose}} = \frac{12}{4} = \frac{3\,\text{mL}}{\text{dose}}$$

b. Estimate supports answer.

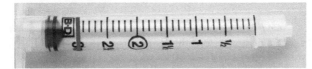

17 a. 40 mL per hr using 2 mL of medication and 18 mL of diluent

$$\frac{\text{mL}}{\text{hr}} = \frac{20\,\text{mL}}{\underset{1}{\cancel{30\,\text{min}}}} \times \frac{\overset{2}{\cancel{60\,\text{min}}}}{1\,\text{hr}} = \frac{40\,\text{mL}}{\text{hr}}$$

b. The volume control device must be flushed with a compatible solution according to agency policies and manufacturer's recommendations.

18 a. Give less than 2 mL.

$$\frac{\text{mL}}{\text{dose}} = \frac{2\,\text{mL}}{0.5\,\cancel{\text{mg}}} \times \frac{0.3\,\cancel{\text{mg}}}{\text{dose}} = \frac{0.6}{0.5} = \frac{1.2\,\text{mL}}{\text{dose}}$$

b. Estimate supports answer.

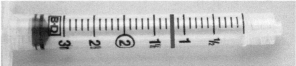

19 a. 150 g Dextrose

$$\text{g Dextrose} = \frac{15\,\text{g}}{\underset{1}{\cancel{100\,\text{mL}}}} \times \overset{10}{\cancel{1000}}\,\text{mL}$$

$$= 150\,\text{g of Dextrose}$$

b. Equation is balanced. Only g remain.
c. 600 kcal CHO

$$\text{kcal} = \frac{4\,\text{kcal}}{1\,\cancel{\text{g}}} \times \frac{150\,\cancel{\text{g}}}{1} = 600\,\text{kcal CHO}$$

d. Equation is balanced. Only kcal remain.
e. 42.5 g amino acids

$$\text{g amino acids} = \frac{4.25\,\text{g}}{\underset{1}{\cancel{100\,\text{mL}}}} \times \frac{\overset{10}{\cancel{1000\,\text{mL}}}}{1}$$

$$= 42.5\,\text{g of amino acids}$$

f. Equation is balanced. Only amino acids remain.

g. kcal amino acids $= \dfrac{4\,\text{kcal}}{1\,\cancel{\text{g}}} \times \dfrac{42.5\,\cancel{\text{g}}}{1}$
$= 170$ kcal amino acids

h. Equation is balanced. Only kcal remain.

20 a. about 0.5 mL

$$\frac{\text{mL}}{\text{dose}} = \frac{1\,\text{mL}}{\underset{2}{\cancel{4\,\text{mg}}}} \times \frac{\overset{1}{\cancel{2\,\text{mg}}}}{\text{dose}} = \frac{1}{2}$$

$$= \frac{0.5\,\text{mL}}{\text{dose}}\ \text{Hydromorphone}$$

b. Estimate supports answer.

c. less than $\dfrac{1}{2}$ mL

$$\frac{\text{mL}}{\text{dose}} = \frac{\text{mL}}{\underset{5}{\cancel{50\,\text{mg}}}} \times \frac{\overset{2}{\cancel{20\,\text{mg}}}}{\text{dose}}$$

$$= \frac{0.4\,\text{mL}}{\text{dose}}\ \text{Promethazine}$$

d. Estimate supports answer.

e. $0.5 + 0.4 = 0.9$ mL

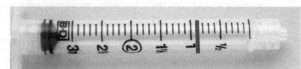

21 a. 40 g lipids

$$\text{g Lipid} = \frac{20 \text{ g}}{\cancel{100 \text{ mL}}_{1}} \times \frac{\cancel{200 \text{ mL}}^{2}}{1} = 40 \text{ g lipids}$$

b. Equation is balanced. Only g remain.

c. 360 kcal lipids

$$\text{kcal lipids} = \frac{9 \text{ kcal}}{1 \cancel{\text{ g}}} \times 40 \cancel{\text{ g}} = 360 \text{ kcal lipids}$$

d. Equation is balanced. Only kcal remain.

22 a. 2 tabs

$$\frac{\text{tab}}{\text{dose}} = \frac{1 \text{ tab}}{60 \cancel{\text{ mg}}} \times \frac{1000 \cancel{\text{ mg}}}{1 \cancel{\text{ g}}} \times \frac{0.12 \cancel{\text{ g}}}{\text{dose}}$$

$$= \frac{120}{60} = \frac{2 \text{ tabs}}{\text{dose}}$$

b. Equation is balanced. Answer equals estimate.

23 a. 1 tab

$$\frac{\text{tab}}{\text{dose}} = \frac{1 \text{ tab}}{0.5 \cancel{\text{ mg}}} \times \frac{1 \cancel{\text{ mg}}}{\cancel{1000 \text{ mcg}}_{2}} \times \frac{\cancel{500 \text{ mcg}}^{1}}{\text{dose}}$$

$$= \frac{1 \text{ tab}}{\text{dose}}$$

b. Estimate supports answer.

24 a. $\frac{1}{2}$ of $40 = 20$; $\frac{1}{2}$ of $15 \text{ mL} = 7.5 \text{ mL}$

$$\frac{\text{mL}}{\text{dose}} = \frac{15 \text{ mL}}{\cancel{40 \text{ mEq}}_{2}} \times \frac{\cancel{20 \text{ mEq}}^{1}}{\text{dose}} = \frac{15}{2}$$

$$= \frac{7.5 \text{ mL}}{\text{dose}} \quad \begin{array}{l}(5 \text{ mL in cup, } 2.5 \text{ mL} \\ \text{in syringe})\end{array}$$

b. Estimate supports answer.

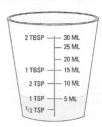

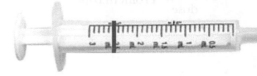

25 175 mg per day

$$\frac{\text{mg}}{\text{day}} = \frac{250 \text{ mg}}{\text{mg} \times \text{day}} \times \frac{0.7 \cancel{\text{ m}^2}}{\text{dose}}$$
$$= 175 \text{ mg per day safe dose}$$

a. Equation is balanced. Only mg remain.

b. 7 mL

$$\frac{\text{mL}}{\text{dose}} = \frac{5 \text{ mL}}{\cancel{125 \text{ mg}}_{5}} \times \frac{\cancel{175 \text{ mg}}^{7}}{1} = \frac{35}{5} = \frac{7 \text{ mL}}{\text{dose}}$$

c. Equation is balanced. Only mL remain.

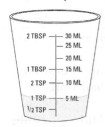

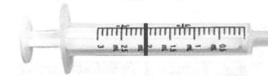

26 a. 15 mg per tab*

b. $45 \div 15 = 3$ tabs

c. $\dfrac{\text{tab}}{\text{dose}} = \dfrac{1 \text{ tab}}{\cancel{15 \text{ mg}}_{1}} \times \dfrac{\cancel{45 \text{ mg}}^{3}}{\text{dose}} = \dfrac{3 \text{ tabs}}{\text{dose}}$

d. Estimate supports answer. Recheck orders for more than 1-2 tablets.

*Use the metric dose.

27 a. 25 kg
SDR:

$$\frac{\text{units}}{\text{week}} = \frac{600 \text{ units}}{1 \cancel{\text{ kg}} \times \text{week}} \times \frac{25 \cancel{\text{ kg}}}{1}$$
$$= 15,000 \text{ units per week}$$

b. Safe order

$$\frac{\text{mL}}{\text{dose}} = \frac{\cancel{2}^{1} \text{ mL}}{\cancel{20,000 \text{ units}}_{10}} \times \frac{\cancel{5000 \text{ units}}^{5}}{\text{dose}}$$
$$= 0.5 \text{ mL per dose}$$

28 a. $1.5 \text{ g} = 1500 \text{ mg} \div 500 \text{ mg} = 3$ tabs*

$$\frac{\text{tab}}{\text{dose}} = \frac{1 \text{ tab}}{\cancel{500 \text{ mg}}_{1}} \times \frac{\cancel{1000 \text{ mg}}^{2}}{1 \cancel{\text{ g}}} \times \frac{1.5 \cancel{\text{ g}}}{\text{dose}} = \frac{3 \text{ tabs}}{\text{dose}}$$

b. Estimate supports answer.

*Recheck dose order and amount when it exceeds two times the unit dose.

29 a. 25 mL per hr

$$\frac{mL}{hr} = \frac{500\ mL}{\underset{20}{20,000\ \text{units}}} \times \frac{\overset{1}{1000\ \text{units}}}{1\ hr}$$

$$= \frac{50\cancel{0}}{2\cancel{0}} = \frac{25\ mL}{hr}$$

b. Equation is balanced. Only mL per hr remains.
c. The aPTT must be monitored.

30 a. 12 mL per hr

$$\frac{mL}{hr} = \frac{\overset{1}{500}\ mL}{5\ \text{units}} \times \frac{1\ \text{unit}}{\underset{\underset{1}{2}}{1000\ \text{milliunits}}} \times \frac{\overset{1}{2\ \text{milliunits}}}{1\ \text{min}}$$

$$\times \frac{60\ \text{min}}{1\ hr} = \frac{12\ mL}{hr}$$

b. Equation is balanced. Only mL per hr remains.

Note: "milli" means $\frac{1}{1000}$.

31 a. 1200 units per hr

$$\frac{units}{hr} = \frac{\overset{40}{10,000}\ units}{\underset{1}{250\ mL}} \times \frac{30\ \text{mL}}{1\ hr} = \frac{1200\ units}{hr}$$

b. Equation is balanced. Only units per hr remains.
c. hemorrhage

32 77 kg (154 lb ÷ 2)
a. 70 kg

$$\frac{1\ kg}{2.2\ \text{lb}} \times \frac{154\ \text{lb}}{1} = 70\ kg$$

b. Estimate supports answer. Only kg remain.

c. $\dfrac{mcg}{min} = \dfrac{3\ mcg}{1\ \text{kg}} \times \dfrac{70\ \text{kg}}{1} = \dfrac{210\ mcg}{minute}$

d. $\dfrac{mg}{min} = 0.21$ mg per min (210 ÷ 1000)

e.

$$\frac{mL}{hr} = \frac{\overset{2}{500}\ mL}{\underset{1}{250\ mg}} \times \frac{1\ \text{mg}}{1000\ \text{mcg}} \times \frac{210\ \text{mcg}}{1\ \text{min}} \times \frac{60\ \text{min}}{1\ hr}$$

$$= \frac{25,200}{1000} = \frac{25.2\ mL}{hour}$$

f. Equation is balanced. Only mL per hr remains.

33 a. 7 units per hr (100 units per 100 mL is a 1:1 solution)

$$\frac{units}{hr} = \frac{\overset{1}{100}\ units}{\underset{1}{100\ mL}} \times \frac{7\ \text{mL}}{hr} = \frac{7\ units}{hr}$$

b. Equation is balanced. Only mL per hr remains.
c. hypoglycemia

34 a. 2 mL (5 mg × 2 = 10 mg)

$$\frac{mL}{dose} = \frac{1\ mL}{5\ \text{mg}} \times \frac{\overset{2}{10\ \text{mg}}}{dose} = \frac{2\ mL}{dose}$$

b. Equation is balanced. Only mL remain.

c. $\dfrac{mL}{min} = \dfrac{\frac{1}{2}\ mL}{\underset{\underset{1}{2}}{10\ \text{mg}}} \times \dfrac{\overset{1}{5\ \text{mg}}}{1\ min} = \dfrac{1\ mL}{minute}$

d. Equation is balanced. Only mL per minute remain.

e. Total minutes $= 2\left(\dfrac{1\ min}{\underset{1}{5\ \text{mg}}} \times \dfrac{\overset{2}{10\ \text{mg}}}{1} = 2\ min \right)$

Total seconds $= 120\left(\dfrac{60\ sec}{1\ \text{min}} \times \dfrac{2\ \text{min}}{1} = 120\ sec \right)$

f. $\dfrac{seconds}{calibration} = \dfrac{120\ sec}{10\ calibration} = \dfrac{12\ sec}{calibration}$

35 a. 125 mL per hr

$$\frac{mL}{hr} = \frac{\overset{125}{500}\ mL}{\underset{\underset{1}{4}}{40\ mEq}}\ KCl \times \frac{\overset{1}{10\ mEq}}{1\ hr} = \frac{125\ mL}{hr}$$

b. Equation is balanced. Only mL per hr remains.
c. 1300 + 4 hr = 1700 hr. At 1700 the nurse needs to recheck serum K level.

$$hr = \frac{1\ hr}{10\ \text{mEq}} \times 40\ \text{mEq} = 4\ hr$$

The Joint Commission "Do Not Use" List

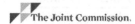 The Joint Commission.

Official "Do Not Use" List

- This list is part of the Information Management standards
- Does not apply to preprogrammed health information technology systems (i.e. electronic medical records or CPOE systems), but remains under consideration for the future

Organizations contemplating introduction or upgrade of such systems should strive to eliminate the use of dangerous abbreviations, acronyms, symbols and dose designations from the software.

Official "Do Not Use" List[1]

Do Not Use	Potential Problem	Use Instead
U, u (unit)	Mistaken for "0" (zero), the number "4" (four) or "cc"	Write "unit"
IU (International Unit)	Mistaken for IV (intravenous) or the number 10 (ten)	Write "Inaternational Unit"
Q.D., QD, q.d., qd (daily)	Mistaken for each other	Write "daily"
Q.O.D., QOD, q.o.d, qod (every other day)	Period after the Q mistaken for "I" and the "O" mistaken for "I	Write "every other day"
Trailing zero (X.0 mg)* Lack of leading zero (.X mg)	Decimal point is missed	Write X mg Write 0.X mg
MS	Can mean morphine sulfate or magnesium sulfate	Write "morphine sulfate" Write "magnesium sulfate"
MSO_4 and $MgSO_4$	Confused for one another	

[1]Applies to all orders and all medication-related documentation that is handwritten (including free-text computer entry) or on pre-printed forms.

*Exception: A "trailing zero" may be used only where required to demonstrate the level of precision of the value being reported, such as for laboratory results, imaging studies that report size of lesions, or catheter/tube sizes. It may not be used in medication orders or other medication-related documentation.

Development of the "Do Not Use" List

In 2001, The Joint Commission issued a *Sentinel Event Alert* on the subject of medical abbreviations. A year later, its Board of Commissioners approved a National Patient Safety Goal requiring accredited organizations to develop and implement a list of abbreviations not to use. In 2004, The Joint Commission created its "Do Not Use" List to meet that goal. In 2010, NPSG.02.02.01 was integrated into the Information Management standards as elements of performance 2 and 3 under IM.02.02.01.

8/20

The Joint Commission

FACT SHEET

For more information

- Complete the Standards Online Question Submission Form.
- Contact the Standards Interpretation Group at 630-792-5900.

Appendix B

Institute for Safe Medication Practice's List of High-Alert Medications

ISMP List of High-Alert Medications
in Acute Care Settings

High-alert medications are drugs that bear a heightened risk of causing significant patient harm when they are used in error. Although mistakes may or may not be more common with these drugs, the consequences of an error are clearly more devastating to patients. We hope you will use this list to determine which medications require special safeguards to reduce the risk of errors. This may include strategies such as standardizing the ordering, storage, preparation, and administration of these products; improving access to information about these drugs; limiting access to high-alert medications; using auxiliary labels; employing clinical decision support and automated alerts; and using redundancies such as automated or independent double checks when necessary. (Note: manual independent double checks are not always the optimal error-reduction strategy and may not be practical for all of the medications on the list.)

Classes/Categories of Medications

adrenergic agonists, IV (e.g., **EPINEPH**rine, phenylephrine, norepinephrine)

adrenergic antagonists, IV (e.g., propranolol, metoprolol, labetalol)

anesthetic agents, general, inhaled and IV (e.g., propofol, ketamine)

antiarrhythmics, IV (e.g., lidocaine, amiodarone)

antithrombotic agents, including:
- anticoagulants (e.g., warfarin, low molecular weight heparin, unfractionated heparin)
- direct oral anticoagulants and factor Xa inhibitors (e.g., dabigatran, rivaroxaban, apixaban, edoxaban, betrixaban, fondaparinux)
- direct thrombin inhibitors (e.g., argatroban, bivalirudin, dabigatran)
- glycoprotein IIb/IIIa inhibitors (e.g., eptifibatide)
- thrombolytics (e.g., alteplase, reteplase, tenecteplase)

cardioplegic solutions

chemotherapeutic agents, parenteral and oral

dextrose, hypertonic, 20% or greater

dialysis solutions, peritoneal and hemodialysis

epidural and intrathecal medications

inotropic medications, IV (e.g., digoxin, milrinone)

insulin, subcutaneous and IV

liposomal forms of drugs (e.g., liposomal amphotericin B) and conventional counterparts (e.g., amphotericin B desoxycholate)

moderate sedation agents, IV (e.g., dexmedetomidine, midazolam, **LOR**azepam)

moderate and minimal sedation agents, oral, for children (e.g., chloral hydrate, midazolam, ketamine [using the parenteral form])

opioids, including:
- IV
- oral (including liquid concentrates, immediate- and sustained-release formulations)
- transdermal

neuromuscular blocking agents (e.g., succinylcholine, rocuronium, vecuronium)

parenteral nutrition preparations

sodium chloride for injection, hypertonic, greater than 0.9% concentration

sterile water for injection, inhalation and irrigation (excluding pour bottles) in containers of 100 mL or more

sulfonylurea hypoglycemics, oral (e.g., chlorpro**PAMIDE**, glimepiride, gly**BURIDE**, glipi**ZIDE**, **TOLBUT**amide)

Specific Medications

EPINEPHrine, subcutaneous

epoprostenol (e.g., Flolan), IV

insulin U-500 (special emphasis*)

magnesium sulfate injection

methotrexate, oral, nononcologic use

nitroprusside sodium for injection

opium tincture

oxytocin, IV

potassium chloride for injection concentrate

potassium phosphates injection

promethazine injection

vasopressin, IV and intraosseous

All forms of insulin, subcutaneous and IV, are considered a class of high-alert medications. Insulin U-500 has been singled out for special emphasis to bring attention to the need for distinct strategies to prevent the types of errors that occur with this concentrated form of insulin.

Background

Based on error reports submitted to the ISMP National Medication Errors Reporting Program (ISMP MERP), reports of harmful errors in the literature, studies that identify the drugs most often involved in harmful errors, and input from practitioners and safety experts, ISMP created and periodically updates a list of potential high-alert medications. During June and July 2018, practitioners responded to an ISMP survey designed to identify which medications were most frequently considered high-alert medications. Further, to assure relevance and completeness, the clinical staff at ISMP and members of the ISMP advisory board were asked to review the potential list. This list of medications and medication categories reflects the collective thinking of all who provided input.

Appendix C
5-Minute Sample Verbal Communication Hand-off Report

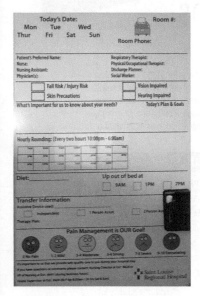

A whiteboard in the patient's room can be updated as needed and assist with communication between nurses giving hand-off report when "walking rounds" is done simultaneously.

A hand-off report is the transfer and acceptance of patient care responsibilities through effective communication between caregivers at shift change or for transfer between units, agencies, or to home, in order to ensure patient safety. Many errors, *including medication errors,* have been attributed to inadequate hand-off communication. The highlighted areas in the sample report presented here pertain to key medication-related information. Additional information would be given for discharge communication to home, including accompanying written materials about all medications and treatments and when to make appointments for checkups. Whereas only major medication issues are verbally reported for a shift change, complete medication information must be provided in writing for all physical patient transfers. Check agency procedures and forms for hand-off communication and medication information for transfer.

Situation: Nurse giving report to next caregiver at shift change on a medical-surgical unit

(Sex, Age, Mental/Emotional Status, Main Diagnoses, Dates of Admission and Transfers, Additional Diagnoses, Allergies)

Mr. G is a 73-year-old, moderately hard-of-hearing, alert, oriented (to person, time, and place), cooperative English-speaking male in no acute distress, admitted to ICU with uncontrolled hypertension and acute bronchitis on the 3rd of October and transferred to our unit on the 6th. He also has chronic prostatitis, mild anemia, an artificial hip replacement as of a year ago that requires use of a cane for stability, and occasional asthmatic episodes controlled with an inhaler. He is allergic to penicillin and aspirin, reacting with hives and wheezing as well as diarrhea from penicillin, and is a fairly reliable historian. He lives with his daughter, so it's best to include her in all teaching, particularly because of the hearing loss.

(Vital Signs)

His vital signs are all stable today.

(Meds: Med Changes, Meds Due, Related Orders)

He had a central line removed before transfer here. His main medications are an intravenous antibiotic piggyback (IVPB) every 6 hr for 24 more hr for his bronchitis. His next one is due soon at 1700 hr. He is on digoxin every morning and two new blood pressure meds, one a diuretic in the morning and the other an ACE inhibitor in the evening. His blood pressure needs to be recorded each shift and after any complaint of weakness or extreme fatigue. Notify the attending physician if the systolic pressure exceeds 170. Make sure his inhaler is within reach and record his use.

(Labs)

His white blood count is still elevated at 13,000 but has been improving steadily. He is NPO after midnight for fasting blood work and also has a lung function test scheduled in the morning. His other labs are within normal limits. Hold the diuretic in the morning until the labs are completed.

(Treatments)

The discontinued central line site needs to be assessed once a day. He is receiving respiratory therapy every morning between 0800 and 0900 and wants to bathe before the treatments come.

(Nutrition/Intake and Output)

He is now tolerating a regular diet well but needs encouragement to drink more fluids. Since he started on the diuretic, he self-limits fluids to try to reduce urination. The fluid intake and urinary output is to be recorded until discharge. Notify the attending physician if the intake or output drops below 1000 mL per day.

(Activity Level: Mobility)

He does need assistance and encouragement getting in and out of bed but does not need assistance walking as long as he has the cane. The doctor wants him to be out of bed most of the day if possible. Bedrails are up at bedtime and a urinal within reach at all times because of the diuretic and urinary frequency.

(Other Needs/Discharge Planning)

His discharge is tentatively planned for next Monday, so special emphasis needs to be given to teaching Mr. G about the new medication regime and need for fluids and activity. He lives with his daughter, who visits after work daily. Be sure to include her in all teaching and discharge because the day shift doesn't see her often. A main issue is that he is unhappy about having to take "new pills," so we've already started reinforcing the importance of compliance with him and the daughter. Be sure to get feedback because he does not always mention that he did not hear everything.

Note: Although this seems like a lot of information, the nurse who cares for the patient for a full shift and who has established a sequential format for the reporting information can communicate this information verbally on each assigned patient with ease. It helps to keep a checklist on hand with abbreviated cues (see the sample boldfaced subheadings) to ensure the verbal hand-off report covers all the major areas. The receiving nurse refers to the written record for further details. There are many potential variations for reporting; for example, fasting could be included under Nutrition/Intake and Output instead of Labs.

Appendix D

Sample Medication Administration Errors and Potential Clinical Outcomes

Medication errors may be made in each step of the process, including a prescription order error, pharmacy misinterpretation, pharmacy preparation, labeling and dispensing, and finally, nurse interpretation, calculation, and administration. The nurse who administers the medication is the last protector. The nurse must review the order, patient allergies, and idiosyncrasies, followed by a check for drug interactions, before preparing and administering the medication. Each of the foregoing processes, including checking safe dose range, is necessary to protect the patient from an adverse drug event (ADE). Failure to do so not only may harm the patient, but may result in disciplinary actions by the agency and/or the State Board of Nursing. There may be additional legal implications should an injury occur.

Sample Order	Error	Type of Error and Comments	Potential Outcomes
Morphine SO$_4$ 10 to 20 mg q4h IM prn severe pain	Morphine SO$_4$ (10 mg per mL supplied in CarboJet) 20 mg given for initial dose	Lack of knowledge: initial dose should be lowest of the range Failure to monitor patient for side effects	Respiratory depression Coma Death
Blood administration	Administered with dextrose solution instead of normal saline Dextrose solution also administered through same line after transfusion	Lack of knowledge Failure to check the solutions for compatibility Failure to change line after transfusion	Hemolytic reaction (jaundice) and coagulation of blood in infusion line because of dextrose
Ordered: Furosemide, a diuretic, 0.05 mg per kg per hr initial rate for a continuous IV for a 25-kg child	Programmed: Furosemide, 0.5 mg per kg per hr The nurse overrode the dose limit alarm on the smart pump, which resulted in a tenfold dosage error.	Lack of knowledge of initial safe dose range and failure to focus Failure to double-check the order and safe dose range for this weight of child when the alarm sounded	Diuresis Dehydration Electrolyte imbalances Nephrocalcinosis Death
IV potassium chloride solution (KCl)	Administered undiluted or improperly diluted by nurse who obtained concentrated KCL 20 mEq per mL from pharmacy cabinet after hrs per agency policy	Lack of knowledge related to potassium dilution and administration procedures when adding to IV solutions to ensure dilution is achieved	Burning pain Damage to the lining of the vein Arrhythmias Cardiac arrest
Gabapentin (Neurontin) for seizures	Two doses omitted because patient nauseated Recorded on MAR Discovered by pharmacy when medication cart returned and checked	Lack of knowledge of actions and dangers of omitted drugs Failure to report promptly to prescriber	Seizures Status epilepticus (continuous seizures) Prolonged hospitalization
Risperidone (Risperdal) 4 mg bid po, an antipsychotic to treat a patient with schizophrenia Supplied: Requip (ropinirole) 2 mg tid po	Given: Requip (ropinirole) two 2-mg tablets (a sound-alike/look-alike drug) An anti-Parkinson's disease drug also used for restless legs syndrome	Lack of knowledge re: patient illness and drug: inappropriate medication Failure to check medication with prescriber order	Some side effects of Requip: Nausea Vomiting Low blood pressure Dizziness Relapse of psychotic behavior because of missed dose of risperdal

Consequences depend upon the history of errors, type of error, severity of error, whether corrective measures were sought and/or instituted promptly and by whom, patient outcome, and perceptions of those evaluating the incident, including the patient and family.

Action may be taken by the employing agency, the State Board of Nursing, and legal representatives of the patient. The actions can range from a discussion, a letter of reprimand, required course(s) of study, probation with or without clinical supervision followed by reinstatement if probation period reflects competence, loss of employment, suspension of license, revocation of license, and lack of renewal of malpractice insurance. A civil and/or criminal lawsuit by the client may be brought against the employee and the employer regardless of the foregoing actions.

Nurses should carry their own private malpractice insurance for personal representation, even if the employer "covers malpractice insurance." There may be occasional conflicts of interest when the nurse depends upon the employer's insurance.

Appendix E

Apothecary System and Household Measurements

The change to the metric system has been recommended by all the major national agencies dealing with patient safety and medication errors. Metric measurements appear in physician orders, patient records, and medication labels in order to reduce medication errors. Only a few countries in the world have not completely "metrified." Celsius temperatures, liters of gas and milk, milligrams and grams of medication, and kilograms of weight are the norm in most countries of the world. The metric measurements are the most precise.

Other measurements such as those seen with household equipment and the outdated apothecary system do not provide accurate doses and cannot be converted to or from the metric system.

Two important safety measures to keep in mind:
- Consult the pharmacy or the prescriber when unfamiliar medication-related abbreviations, measurements, doses, or terms are encountered.
- Instruct the patient on discharge to only use the metric-calibrated equipment that is supplied with liquid medicines.

Use metric, but be able to recognize apothecary and household measurements!

Metric, Household, and Apothecary Liquid Equivalents*

Metric	Household	Apothecary
1 mL		15–16 minims*
5 mL	1 teaspoon (tsp)	1 dram*
15 mL	1 tablespoon (tbs)	4 drams* (oz ss) (½ ounce) (oz)
30 mL	2 tablespoons (1 oz)	8 drams (oz i)
240 mL	1 measuring cup (8 oz)	8 oz (oz viii)
500 mL	1 pint (pt) (16 oz)	1 pint (16 oz)
1000 mL (1 liter)	1 quart (qt) (32 oz)	1 quart (32 oz)
4 liters	1 gallon (gal) (4 quarts)	1 gallon (4 quarts)

Note: These equivalents are approximate.

*Minims and drams are no longer used in medication orders in the United States.

Comparison of Metric and Apothecary Weights

Metric	Apothecary
1000 g = 1 kg	2.2 lb
1000 mg = 1 g	15 grains (gr xv)
60 mg	1 gr
30 mg	$gr_{1/2}$ or ss
0.6 mg	$gr_{1/100}$
0.4 mg	$gr_{1/150}$
0.3 mg	$gr_{1/200}$

➤ Please refer to the TJC and ISMP lists on pp. 526–527

➤ Consult a pharmacist or the prescriber for when all unfamiliar medication-related abbreviations, measurements, doses or terms are encountered.

Index

Note: Page numbers followed by f, t, or b indicate figures, tables, or boxes, respectively.